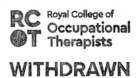

Manual
of
Physical Therapy

Manual
of
Physical Therapy

Edited by

Otto D. Payton, Ph.D., P.T.

Professor, Department of Physical Therapy,
Virginia Commonwealth University Medical College of Virginia,
Richmond, Virginia

Associate Editors

Richard P. Di Fabio, Ph.D., P.T.

Director, Department of Physical Therapy,
University of Wisconsin Hospital and Clinics;
Research Scientist and Clinical Assistant
Professor, Department of Rehabilitation
Medicine, University of Wisconsin Medical
School, Madison, Wisconsin

Stanley V. Paris, Ph.D., P.T., M.C.S.P., N.Z.S.P.

President, Institute of Graduate Health Sciences,
Atlanta, Georgia; Clinical Professor, Institute
of Graduate Health Sciences, St. Augustine,
Florida

Elizabeth J. Protas, Ph.D., P.T.

Professor and Coordinator, School of Physical
Therapy, Texas Woman's University,
Houston, Texas

Ann F. VanSant, Ph.D., P.T.

Associate Professor, Department of Physical
Therapy, Virginia Commonwealth University
Medical College of Virginia, Richmond,
Virginia

With a contribution from Osa Littrup Jackson, Ph.D., P.T.
Illustrated by Susan Seif, A.M.I.

Churchill Livingstone
New York, Edinburgh, London, Melbourne   1989

Library of Congress Cataloging-in-Publication Data

Manual of physical therapy / edited by Otto D. Payton . . . [et al.];
  with a contribution from Osa Jackson; illustrated by Susan Seif.
      p.   cm.
    Includes bibliographies and index.
    ISBN 0-443-08499-8
    1. Physical therapy—Handbooks, manuals etc.   I. Payton, Otto D.
  II. Jackson, Osa.
    [DNLM: 1. Physical Therapy—methods.   WB 460 M2935]
  RM700.M37 1989
  615.8′2—dc19
  DNLM/DLC
  for Library of Congress   88-8311
                                                                  CIP

© **Churchill Livingstone Inc.   1989**

Distributed in the United Kingdom by Churchill Livingstone, Robert Stevenson
House, 1–3 Baxter's Place, Leith Walk, Edinburgh EH1 3AF, and by associated
companies, branches, and representatives throughout the world.

Accurate indications, adverse reactions, and dosage schedules for drugs are provided
in this book, but it is possible that they may change. The reader is urged to review the
package information data of the manufacturers of the medications mentioned.

The Publishers have made every effort to trace the copyright holders for borrowed
material. If they have inadvertently overlooked any, they will be pleased to make the
necessary arrangements at the first opportunity.

Acquisitions Editor: *Kim Loretucci*
Copy Editor: *Kimberly Quinlan*
Production Designer: *Charlie Lebeda*
Production Supervisor: *Sharon Tuder*

Printed in the United States of America

First published in 1989

Contributors

Gary E. Adams, Ph.D., F.A.C.S.M.
Associate Professor, Department of Medicine, University of Nevada School of Medicine, Reno, Nevada; Director, Department of Cardiac Rehabilitation, University Medical Center of Southern Nevada, Las Vegas, Nevada

Kent Allsop, Ph.D., P.T.
Associate Professor, Department of Physical Therapy, College of Health, University of Utah; Physical Therapist, Muscle Disease Clinic, University of Utah Medical Center, Salt Lake City, Utah

Mary Beth Badke, M.S., P.T.
Associate Director, Department of Physical Therapy, University of Wisconsin Hospital and Clinics; Clinical Assistant Professor, Department of Physical Therapy, University of Wisconsin School of Allied Health Professions, Madison, Wisconsin

Richard Balliet, Ph.D.
Associate Professor, Department of Rehabilitation Medicine, University of Wisconsin Medical School; Clinical Director, NeuroMuscular Retraining Clinic, Madison, Wisconsin

Sandra C. Brooks, M.S., P.T.
Associate Professor, Department of Physical Therapy, Maryville College; President, Pediatric Physical Therapy, Inc., St. Louis, Missouri

Anita C. Bundy, Sc.D., O.T.R.
Assistant Professor, Department of Occupational Therapy, College of Associated Health Professions, University of Illinois at Chicago, Chicago, Illinois

Richard P. Di Fabio, Ph.D., P.T.
Director, Department of Physical Therapy, University of Wisconsin Hospital and Clinics; Research Scientist and Clinical Assistant Professor, Department of Rehabilitation Medicine, University of Wisconsin Medical School, Madison, Wisconsin

Pamela W. Duncan, M.S., P.T.
Assistant Professor, Graduate Program in Physical Therapy, Duke University, Durham, North Carolina

Ann Winkel Fick, M.S., P.T.
Senior Therapist, Department of Rehabilitation, St. Luke's Episcopal Hospital, Houston, Texas

Anne G. Fisher, Sc.D., O.T.R.
Assistant Professor, Department of Occupational Therapy, College of Associated Health Professions, University of Illinois at Chicago, Chicago, Illinois

Robert Friberg, Ph.D., P.T.
Associate Professor and Director, Department of Physical Therapy, College of Biological Sciences, University of Osteopathic Medicine and Health Sciences, Des Moines, Iowa

Mary Lou Galantino, P.T.
Director, Department of Physical Therapy, Institute for Immunologic Disorders, Houston, Texas

Manuela J. Giannini, M.S., P.T.
Doctoral Fellow, School of Physical Therapy, Texas Woman's University, Houston, Texas

Mary Jo Given, M.S., P.T.
Supervisor of Neurological Disorders, Department of Physical Therapy, Northwestern Memorial Hospital, Chicago, Illinois

Peggy Blake Gleeson, Ph.D., P.T.
Director, Physical Therapy Services, Westside Orthopaedic and Sports Medicine Associates, Houston, Texas

Viola Holloway, P.T.
Supervisor, Department of Rehabilitation, St. Luke's Episcopal Hospital, Houston, Texas

Osa Littrup Jackson, Ph.D., P.T.

Director and Associate Professor, Department of Physical Therapy, and Chairman, Department of Kinesiological Science, School of Health Sciences, Oakland University, Rochester, Michigan

Robert Kellogg, P.T.

Associate, Department of Physical Therapy, University of Kentucky, Lexington, Kentucky

Betti J. Krapfl, P.T.

Assistant Director, Department of Physical Therapy, Craig Hospital, Englewood, Colorado

Steven L. Kraus, P.T.

Clinical Assistant Professor, Orthodontic Residency Program, Part-time Faculty, TMJ/Facial Pain Clinic, Emory University School of Dentistry; Adjunct Faculty and Clinical Educator, Orthopedic Physical Therapy Master's Program, Emory University; Co-director, Physical Therapy Associates of Metro Atlanta, Atlanta, Georgia

Pamela May, P.T.

Co-director, Atlanta Back Clinic Orthopedic Physical Therapy and Training Center; Instructor, Institute of Graduate Health Sciences, Atlanta, Georgia

Grace Moffat Minerbo, M.D., Ph.D.

Visiting Associate Professor, School of Physical Therapy, Texas Woman's University, Houston, Texas

Richard Nyberg, M.M.Sc., P.T.

Co-director and Clinician, Atlanta Back Clinic Orthopedic Physical Therapy, and Training Center; Instructor, Division of Physical Therapy, Emory University; Instructor, Institute of Graduate Health Sciences, Atlanta, Georgia

Bill O'Daniel, P.T.

Director, Department of Physical Therapy, Craig Hospital, Englewood, Colorado

Carolyn M. Oddo, P.T.

Coordinating Physical Therapist, Meyer Center for Developmental Pediatrics, Baylor College of Medicine, Houston, Texas

Barbara S. Oremland, M.Ed., P.T.

Adjunct Assistant Professor of Physical Therapy, Department of Health Sciences, Cleveland State University; Director, Parkinson's Physical Therapy Program, Mitchell-Zoltowicz-Holtz Physical Therapy (a division of InSpeech, Inc., Valley Forge, Pennsylvania) Cleveland, Ohio

Stanley V. Paris, Ph.D., P.T., M.C.S.P., N.Z.S.P.

President, Institute of Graduate Health Sciences, Atlanta, Georgia; Clinical Professor, Institute of Graduate Health Sciences, St. Augustine, Florida

Catherine E. Patla, P.T.

Clinical Instructor, Institute of Graduate Health Sciences, Atlanta, Georgia; Partner, Paris, Irwin, and Associates, Orthopaedic Physical Therapy, St. Augustine, Florida

Otto D. Payton, Ph.D., P.T.

Professor, Department of Physical Therapy, Virginia Commonwealth University Medical College of Virginia, Richmond, Virginia

Elizabeth J. Protas, Ph.D., P.T.

Professor and Coordinator, School of Physical Therapy, Texas Woman's University, Houston, Texas

L. Gail Robinson, P.T.

Instructor, Department of Rehabilitation Sciences, College of Allied Health Sciences, University of Tennessee, Memphis, Tennessee

Ann F. VanSant, Ph.D., P.T.

Associate Professor, Department of Physical Therapy, Virginia Commonwealth University Medical College of Virginia, Richmond, Virginia

Preface

The editors of this text have worked together to develop a comprehensive reference of assessment and treatment strategies in the three major specialty areas of physical therapy practice—neurology, orthopaedics, and cardiopulmonary practice. The purpose of this book is to provide, in one readily accessible source, a foundation of knowledge for the management of most types of patients that physical therapists are likely to see in the course of their practice.

The approach and methods in this book are those suggested by five nationally recognized physical therapists (the editors) and their colleagues. In making their recommendations, the editors and contributors have faced the same dilemma that confronts all practitioners: They have had to make judgments based both on available research and on their own clinical experience. The process and methods recommended in this book can be considered state-of-the-art within each specialty. Clinicians can, therefore, use this volume as a means for updating their own strategies for problem solving or for providing care to patients who are not typical in terms of the usual caseload.

In most instances, the book outlines evaluation and treatment procedures, as well as provides reference sources for further reading. Because of the diversity and breadth of the topics, however, the style of presentation cannot be totally uniform from subject to subject. Content won out over format, to the advantage of the readers. The section on orthopaedic dysfunction is presented as a concise overview of the practice of orthopaedic physical therapy for dysfunction of the spine and extremities. No one book could possibly contain all that is necessary to know in orthopaedics, let alone the other disciplines covered in this text. But the section editors and contributors do feel that what has been achieved here is a complete guide to one possible approach.

The section on neurologic dysfunction is a comprehensive guide to assessment and treatment of a wide range of neuromuscular and sensorimotor pathologies. The organization of content parallels an anatomical model, addressing management of peripheral nervous system lesions, spinal cord injury, and supraspinal pathology. While only selected general diagnostic categories have been included, the information in the neurologic section provides a basis for treating patients with differing mixes of signs, symptoms, and functional levels.

The final section is a comprehensive presentation of both cardiac and pulmonary rehabilitation. Areas that are traditionally associated with cardiopulmonary rehabilitation, such as postoperative and community-based cardiac programs, as well as less traditional concerns, such as health risk appraisal and the patient with acquired immune deficiency syndrome, have been included. The addition of chapters on the medical management of cardiac and pulmonary pathology should make this a useful reference for all physical therapists.

The size and scope of this volume reflect the diversity of physical therapy practice— and still we acknowledge that we have not included everything that we might have included. We feel that this manual can be used as a clinical reference and as a vital supplement to the knowledge base of the working therapist. However, the editors wish to emphasize most strongly that this manual is not meant to cover all aspects of clinical practice—scientific rationale, signs and symptoms, techniques of assessment, or treatment. It is meant to be a guiding reference, and as such to assist clinicians in their daily practice of physical therapy.

Otto D. Payton, Ph.D., P.T.
Richard P. Di Fabio, Ph.D., P.T.
Stanley V. Paris, Ph.D., P.T., M.C.S.P., N.Z.S.P.
Elizabeth J. Protas, Ph.D., P.T.
Ann F. VanSant, Ph.D., P.T.

Contents

Section II.   Orthopaedic Dysfunction
               Stanley V. Paris

Pediatric Orthopaedic Dysfunction

Section I

Neurologic Dysfunction

Edited by
Richard P. Di Fabio

1 Mobility Impairment: The Juncture of Neural Lesion and Biomechanics

Richard P. Di Fabio

Models predicting mobility dysfunction are important to physical therapists because they help the practitioner identify the underlying characteristics of motor impairment. Complex neurological problems require a combination of models to explain the type, extent, and duration of signs and symptoms, as well as the prognosis for successful therapeutic intervention. The neuroanatomical model for understanding pathology is helpful as a first layer of organization. For example, certain pathologies are often associated with specific anatomical systems:

1. Peripheral nerves—Neuropathy
2. Spinal cord—Paralysis and sclerosis
3. Brain stem—Coma
4. Vestibular apparatus—Equilibrium dysfunction
5. Basal ganglia—Parkinson's disease
6. Cerebral cortex—Stroke

The neuroanatomical model is supplemented by a behavioral approach to explain disorders of complex integrated movement such as balance and coordinated motor patterns. The behavioral perspective, which is found in every chapter of this volume, is necessary because

1. Lesion of a neural structure does not always correlate directly with loss of a specific function.[1]
2. Patients with neurological deficits rarely present with lesions localized to a specific neural system.

3. Disorders of complex integrated behaviors can not be attributed to isolated neuroanatomical structures.

Mobility requires the interaction of muscle contraction with the physical realities of biomechanics. The torque produced on limb segments and the velocity, amplitude, and duration of joint movement are not only created by neural impulse but also influence the response of the nervous system.[2] This chapter will focus on selected biomechanic and neuromuscular factors underlying mobility impairment.

COMPONENT PARTS OF MOBILITY

Joints can be thought of as the smallest common denominator for limb or trunk mobility. The causes of joint dysfunction can be numerous and include

1. Contracture
2. Swelling
3. Ligamentous laxity
4. Hypomobility of supporting structures
5. Muscle weakness

Neurological and orthopaedic principles are combined in Chapter 6 to describe the assessment and treatment of joint pathology. Joint dysfunction can cause mobility impairment independent of a neurological lesion or may only indirectly be influenced by neurological function. Consider a cycle

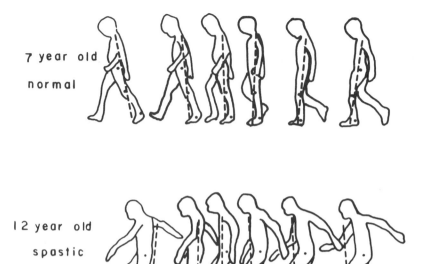

Fig. 1-1 Progressive deterioration of limb segment alignment during gait in normal and spastic diplegic conditions. Vertical dotted line represents location of the composite floor reaction force with respect to the approximate centers of the hip, knee, and ankle joint axes. As the composite line of force moves away from the joint axis, greater joint torque requires additional compensatory muscle activity. The diplegic requires excessive activity of the gluteus and quadriceps muscles at the beginning and end of stance respectively. (From Sutherland et al.,[3] with permission.)

of biomechanical events triggered by a neuromuscular deficit that caused weakness in the lower extremity during stance (Fig. 1-1).

1. Weight is applied to the lower limb in standing.
2. The ankle-knee-hip alignment is distorted and requires co-contraction of stabilizing muscles.
3. The muscles are weak and only partially stabilize the stance limb.
4. Distortion of the ankle-knee-hip alignment increases.
5. More co-contraction of antagonists is required to stabilize the limb.
6. Mobility is compromised by excessive stability.

The deterioration of limb segment alignment during gait has been observed with spastic diplegics.[3] The biomechanical effects of poor segmental alignment create the superficial impression that the neurological deficit extends beyond muscle weakness (i.e., involves poor sequencing of lower extremity synergists). Intervention to improve limb segment alignment would reduce the abnormal requirements for antagonistic muscle co-contraction.

KINEMATIC CHAINS

A kinematic chain is a series of joints coupled together to perform a given function. The two types of kinematic chains are

1. Open—The distal most joint is free to move in space and provides maximum mobility. *Example*: the swing leg during gait.
2. Closed—The distal most joint is fixed and provides maximum stability. *Example*: the stance leg during gait.

During normal motion a finely graded trade-off between mobility and stability makes movement highly efficient. However, in many cases of neurological disease or trauma the following are common:

1. Stability is excessive, limiting mobility as in Parkinson's disease (see Ch. 8).

2. Mobility is excessive due to a lack of proximal stability as in some cases of hemiplegia (see Ch. 9).
3. Mobility is initially excessive due to peripheral nerve lesion but then becomes limited due to joint contracture (see Ch. 2).
4. Stability is excessive due to inappropriate orthotic devices or ambulation aids.

In each of these cases, the trade-off between mobility and stability is exaggerated. Coordinated movement requires a dynamic balance between mobilizing and stabilizing forces.

DEGREES OF FREEDOM

The number of independent axes in each joint equals the number of degrees of freedom. The glenohumeral joint, for example, has three degrees of freedom (DF):

1. Flexion-extension
2. Abduction-adduction
3. Medial-lateral rotation

All other movements of the glenohumeral joint can be defined by a combination of two or more of these primary movements. Degrees of freedom provide an index of unique movement patterns and are cumulative when measured from proximal

to distal. The lower extremity has an accumulation of at least 27 primary movements.

1. Hip—3 df
2. Knee—2 df
3. Ankle/foot—3 df
4. Toes—19 df
5. Total = 3 + 2 + 3 + 19 = 27 df

Pathology involving the nervous system will often result in a limitation of degrees of freedom by

1. Preventing the timely onset of joint motion
2. Preventing joint motion in a functional range
3. Forcing a joint to move out of sequence (rendering joint motion ineffective)

When a mobility task requires multiple degrees of freedom, the patient with limited df is at a disadvantage because

1. During gait, many df are required to accommodate changing support surface conditions. Limited df decrease the margin of error and increase the risk of falling.
2. During stance, many df are used so that joint position may change within the kinematic chain without altering the projection of the center of gravity within the base of support (Fig. 1-2). Limited df again decrease the margin of error and increase the risk of falling.

BASE OF SUPPORT

The base of support (BOS) is an area that defines the limits of stability. A small BOS is associated with instability.

For symmetrically standing patients, the BOS is roughly equivalent to an outline of the outer borders of the feet (Fig. 1-3). Toe walkers (seen with spastic diplegics) have a BOS limited to the area under the balls of the feet, whereas hemiplegics use primarily one limb for their BOS. A biomechanical component to postural instability may exist because normal subjects who stand with their weight biased to one side show electromyographic patterns similar to hemiplegic patients (Fig. 1-4).

During some functional activities, the center of gravity (COG) normally moves outside the BOS.

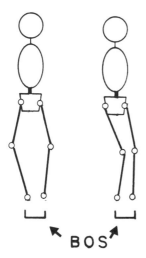

Fig. 1-2 Center of gravity remains within the base of support (BOS) regardless of the variation in lower limb position.

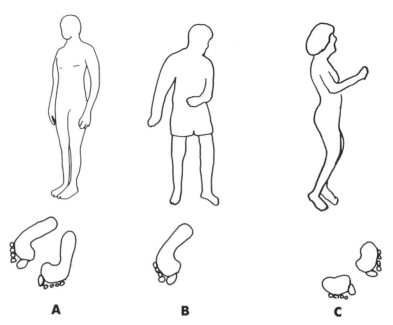

Fig. 1-3 Resting posture (top) and the outline of the base of support (bottom) for a normal (**A**), hemiplegic (**B**), and spastic diplegic (**C**).

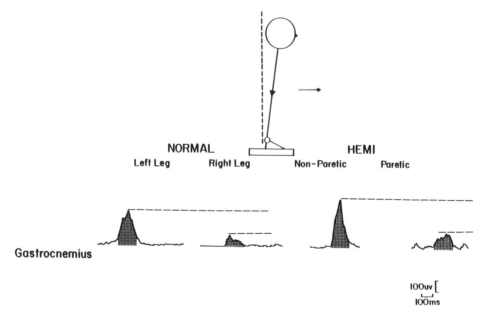

Fig. 1-4 Bilateral integrated electromyographs of gastrocnemius muscle activity during induced forward body sway. Normal subject was standing with body weight biased to the left side to mimic hemiplegic stance. Gastrocnemius shows an increase in burst amplitude on the normal loaded limb, which is similar to the hemiplegic pattern. Electrode placement, interelectrode resistance, and gain settings were standardized in both subjects.

Gait may be referred to as a process of controlled falling because the COG falls outside the BOS during a significant portion of the gait cycle. Selected activities that do not require excursions of the COG beyond the limits of stability are compared with gait.

Control of the COG within the base of support may be an appropriate activity for mobility training in the early stages of therapy or for simple movements requiring relatively few degrees of freedom. Sitting balance does not require lower extremity weight-bearing and effectively limits the df to trunk and upper extremity. Knowledge of the limits of stability is necessary for effective balance. Kneel-standing incorporates hip and some knee df but eliminates ankle-foot components. Bilateral stance requires use of df from both lower extremities. However, excursions of the COG beyond the limits of stability are not a component of symmetrical standing.

Ambulation requires an excursion of the center of gravity beyond the base of support. Upon initial contact of the foot to the floor, the floor provides an equal and opposite force to stabilize the foot. This three-dimensional force is the floor reaction force. Dynamic control of joint movement is influenced less by gravity and more by external forces (i.e., the composite floor reaction force). In contrast, during "static" activities such as sitting and standing balance, gravitational influences on joint equilibrium become more critical. Location of the line of force with respect to each joint axis in the kinematic chain will determine the direction of torque on the joint. The farther away the composite line of force from the joint axis, the more muscle action required to stabilize the joint (Fig. 1-1).

The sequence of mobility patterns from sitting to standing has been traditionally referred to as a *developmental sequence* because during the developmental process, the subordination of primitive reflex patterns paves the way for more advanced activity. Significant biomechanical considerations are not necessarily emphasized by the term "developmental sequence." Also, in many cases, the existence of primitive reflex patterns in the adult neurological patient may have little to do with functional outcomes.[4,5] In contrast, the df required for the task, limb segment alignment, and relative movement within the kinematic chain may play a major role in the quality of movement observed. Therefore, mobility patterns used in therapy are related in terms of a *"functional sequence."*

PATHOMECHANICS OF STANCE

Stance is a part of the gait cycle, as well as a fundamental activity that provides the foundation for goal-directed limb movements. The nature of compensatory activity when components of the kinematic chain malfunction or when spasticity dominates the lower extremities provides insight into the assessment of mobility impairment because the foundation for movement is affected. A detailed summary of the following selected compensatory postures appears elsewhere.[6]

Gait: Initial Foot Contact (Fig. 1-5)

1. Normal—Dorsiflexed ankle creates a composite reaction force that encourages plantar flexion. Knee absorbs limb loading force with slight flexion.
2. Pathological—Initial contact is made with the foot flat. The most common assumption for this compensatory strategy is weak pretibial

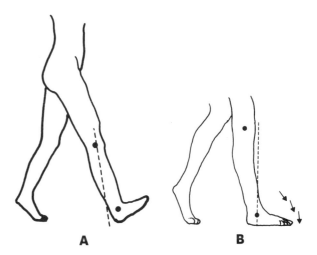

Fig. 1-5 Normal heel strike during gait (**A**) and pathological flat foot position (**B**). Vertical dotted line represents the location of the composite floor reaction force with respect to the knee and ankle joint axes. See text for discussion.

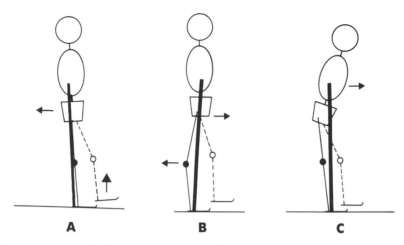

Fig. 1-6 Uncompensated (**A**) and compensated (**B** and **C**) postures when the ankle assumes a plantar flexed position during initiation of contralateral lower limb movement. The thick solid line represents the composite floor reaction force. Arrows indicate direction of limb segment or body displacement. (From Cerny,[6] with permission.)

muscles. However, apparent foot drop could also be caused by weak quadriceps[6] or hypermobility at the talocrural junction. Therefore, a biomechanical component for the compensatory strategy should be considered. Mobility testing of the talocrural joint will assist a definitive assessment.

Initiation of Movement from Bilateral Stance

1. Normal—One lower limb is advanced, the pelvis moves forward, and the stance limb shifts the line of the composite floor reaction force in front of the tibia. Forward motion is facilitated.
2. Pathological (Fig. 1-6)—An attempt is made to advance one lower limb, but as the foot rises off the floor, the body begins to fall backward. If the distal component of the kinematic chain (the ankle) is at fault, at least two compensatory strategies may be used to shift the composite reaction force anterior to the ankle joint: forward bend at the trunk and hyperextension at the knee.

Compensatory joint movements are largely subconscious and normally accompany other goal directed movements of the limbs. Rapid arm movements are normally preceded by activation of the hamstrings to offset an impending forward displacement of the COG.[7] Certain hemiplegics lack preparatory muscle responses.[8]

Rapid rise on the toes (caused by gastrocsoleus activation) is normally preceded by activation of the tibialis anterior to offset an impending backward displacement of the COG. Parkinson's patients lack this preparatory muscle response.[9] Patients with spinocerebellar degeneration have a normal pattern of preparatory muscle activation.[9]

REACTIVE POSTURAL ADJUSTMENTS

Patients need to develop not only postural responses that accompany self-initiated movement, but also a functional response to unexpected support surface displacements. The latter, termed reactive postural adjustments, have three components: activation, sequencing, and adaptation.

Activation of Postural Synergists

Normal control of postural sway occurs in a distal-to-proximal sequence, with the distal muscle activating 100 ms after a postural disturbance.[10] For example, during an induced forward sway, postural muscles are activated in the following order: (1) gastrocnemius, (2) hamstring, and (3) paraspinal.

Adult hemiplegics tend to co-contract postural synergists. Activation of distal and proximal lower extremity muscles occurs closer in time than normal. When muscles are not simultaneously activated the latency of activation occurs in a diagonal pattern.[11]

1. Response of paretic distal muscles is delayed.
2. Response of nonparetic proximal muscles is accelerated.
3. Latency of nonparetic distal and paretic proximal muscles is normal.

Children with cerebral palsy have delayed activation patterns.[12]

1. Hemiplegics have some delay in the nonparetic lower extremity and even greater delays in the paretic lower limb.
2. Ataxics have the longest delays in postural muscle activation of the children studied. This means they have the greatest risk of falling.

Sequencing

Normal distal-to-proximal sequencing of postural synergists is disrupted when spastic patients attempt to regain their balance. The spastic pattern of activation uses a proximal-to-distal strategy when co-contraction is not predominate. If proximal muscles contract first, the line of force applied to the knee joint is displaced and flexion/extension torques are no longer balanced. Altering knee joint equilibrium by activating the proximal synergists out of sequence will cause the knee to collapse during forward sway (or cause a peg leg stance with backward sway).[12] In this example, there is not a smooth gradation between mobility and stability of the knee joint. This gradation is necessary for normal corrective posture.

Adaptation

Given the same adequate stimulus (muscle stretch) under different conditions, the extent of patient adaptation can be evaluated. Consider two situations that result in identical stretch on the tibialis anterior. The first case involves a subject slipping on the floor and nearly falling backwards. In this example, facilitation of tibialis anterior is appropriate because activation will right body posture

to the vertical position. The second case involves a subject catching a heel on descending a stair, forcing the ankle into plantar flexion. A stretch is still applied to the tibialis anterior, but this time muscle activation will destabilize balance and cause a fall forward.[13]

Normal subjects are able to facilitate muscle activity when appropriate and attenuate muscle activation when it is potentially destabilizing. Therefore, a stretch stimulus may not necessarily result in a vigorous contraction. This context-dependent alteration in muscle burst amplitude allows the intact nervous system to adapt to changing environmental conditions independent of the segmental stretch reflex.[13]

Patients with spinocerebellar degeneration[13] and children below the age of 9 years[14] lack the ability to make context-dependent alterations in muscle activity. They will respond identically given a variety of environmental conditions and, therefore, lack an adaptable equilibrium response.

Adult hemiplegics in an advanced stage of recovery have normal patterns of postural adaptation.[11] However, it is not clear at this time whether stroke patients retain or relearn context-dependent responses to balance perturbations.

REFLEX SUBORDINATION AND POSTURAL CONTROL

The developmental approach to therapy has been traditionally reinforced by the clinical necessity of dealing with primitive reflex patterns associated with central nervous system (CNS) damage. Unfortunately, there is little correlation between the mere presence of abnormal muscle tone and the patient's function (see Ch. 9). For CNS lesions above the level of the brain stem, the presence or absence of primitive reflex patterns influencing equilibrium will be considered with reference to balance behavior in young children.

Normal children below the age of 9 years demonstrate

1. Visual dependence for balance
2. Delay of muscle activation (prolonged latency)
3. Poor adaptation (undeveloped context dependent balance behaviors)[14]

Primary vestibular deficits (patients presenting with a positive Rhomberg sign and measurable vestibular ocular deficits) show

1. Visual dependence for balance
2. Normal latency of muscle activation to regain balance
3. Poor postural adaptation.[15] Severely affected patients do not attenuate inappropriate muscle activity (see Ch. 7 for treatment strategies).

Elderly patients with diffuse cortical degeneration demonstrate a somatosensory dependence for balance control.[16] When visual cues are disrupted, this group of patients will continue to demonstrate effective balance strategies. Somatosensory dependence on equilibrium function in the elderly is in contrast to the visual dependence seen in normal children and in patients with vestibular deficits. However, the elderly, normal children, and vestibular patients all share a loss (or lack of development) of the redundant functions normally available when integrating visual, somatosensory, and vestibular inputs. Dependence on one source of sensory input will limit the range of balance behaviors and will ultimately constrain patient mobility.

Adult hemiplegics require a longer period of time to correct body alignment in the paretic limb than in the nonparetic lower extremity. These patients experience normal context-dependent modifications of muscle activity to remain upright.[16]

Cerebral palsy patients experience delays in the postural response similar to those experienced by adult hemiplegics, whereas ataxics demonstrate longer delays.[12] When vision and somatosensory inputs are stabilized (presented in a way to nullify their meaning), both hemiplegics and ataxics became increasingly unstable.

In Parkinson's disease, the latency of postural activation is normal,[17,18] but the amplitude of the response is diminished.[9,17] Parkinson's disease creates fixed postural responses regardless of the environmental conditions. Adaptation is poor.[18]

In spinocerebellar degeneration, sway compensations occur at normal latencies, but there is a marked loss of context-dependent alterations in postural activity.[13,19]

It is clear that a loss of reflex subordination is *not* a primary factor in reactive postural stabilization with lesions above the brain stem. Rather, disorders in the sequence, amplitude, and timing of preprogrammed muscle patterns alter normal balance function.

ROLE OF PROPRIOCEPTION IN BALANCE

The literature concerning proprioception and motor control is massive. Only one small aspect has been selected to refine accepted therapeutic approaches. For the purpose of discussion, proprioception will be divided into two categories:

1. Category I—Cutaneous, joint, and pressure inputs
2. Category II—Muscle afferents

Many therapeutic procedures use proprioceptive inputs to improve motor behavior. Some examples include (1) joint approximation,[20] (2) stroking,[21] and (3) quick stretching.[21] Preliminary evidence indicates that Category I proprioceptors contribute to coordinated balance reactions only when velocity of movement is relatively low.[22] At rapid velocities, elimination of Category I proprioceptors by ischemic block has no effect on the control of body sway. It is generally accepted that Category II proprioceptors act as a trigger for preprogrammed postural responses during rapid equilibrium reactions. Therefore, velocity sensitivity may be a factor to consider during the rehabilitation process.

TREATMENT IMPLICATIONS

Interdependence of Joint Motion

The position of one joint in the kinematic chain will affect the movement of other joints within the kinematic chain.

1. *Example*—A low level paraplegic with hip flexion contractures will be unable to achieve the appropriate degree of lumbar lordosis to effectively balance in a knee-ankle-foot orthosis. In this case, the interdependence between lumbar mobility and hip position is critical to balance (see Ch. 4).

2. *Example*—Hypermobility of the tibia gliding posteriorly on the talus at heel strike during gait will cause knee hyperextension.
3. *Example*—Hypomobility of the lumbar spine will accelerate pelvic movement and limit sequential rolling during bed mobility.

Variability of Response

The large number of degrees of freedom in the human body create a large repertoire of potential motor patterns. Variability of response will prepare a patient for responding in a unique way to unexpected environmental demands.

1. *Example*—Patients with facial paralysis (see Ch. 5) often attempt mass movements for expression and are unable, at first, to differentiate specific muscle responses. Rehabilitation involves recognition and practice of slow constant velocity, rapid-hold, and rapid-release motor patterns. Each type of contraction contributes to a variety of expressions necessary for normal facial function.
2. *Example*—A low level paraplegic relearning ambulation skills will find that different inclines will require a different style of gait (i.e., swing-to versus swing-through). These patients should practice different gait styles on different surfaces, with different inclines, and different step sizes (see Ch. 4).

Balance Versus Controlled Falling

Balance is not the same as controlled falling. The task requirements of balance focus on maintaining the center of gravity within the base of support. In contrast, controlled falling is a goal-directed behavior that requires excursions of the center of gravity outside the base of support.

1. *Example*—Sitting balance is an activity that requires the center of gravity to remain within the limits of stability defined by the pelvic base. Patients are taught to approach but not exceed the limits of stability before attempting more complex activities that require additional degrees of freedom.
2. *Example*—During the gait cycle, the center of gravity moves outside the base of support.[6]

Activities that prepare a patient for gait should focus on graded control of falling as the patient exceeds the limits of stability (see Chs. 7–9).

Self-Initiated Versus Reactive Postural Adjustment

The excursion of the center of gravity is much smaller during self-initiated movements when compared to reactive postural adjustments.[23] Therefore, the magnitude of postural sway and the ability to anticipate postural disturbances are variables that change with intentional movement. During normal mobility, constant alternations between self-initiated and reactive motor patterns occur. To insure appropriate adaptation to changing environmental demands, both reactive and self-initiated motor tasks should be practiced in therapy.

Altering the Base of Support

In some patients, the base of support is too wide (i.e., Parkinson's disease), and mobility is compromised for excessive stability. In other patients (i.e., hemiplegics), the base of support is too narrow and stability is compromised due to excessive mobility. During initiation of movement, the base of support will also influence kinematic chain function. For example, when standing from a sitting position, if the feet are too close together, the range and timing of hip and knee components will be altered and standing is inhibited.[24] Therefore, activities that alter the base of support or afford more control over its size should be considered during therapy (see Ch. 8).

Treating in and out of Context

Currently, there is a good deal of emphasis for designing treatment programs for patients that incorporate joint movement together with some meaningful context.[25] For example, isolated knee motion performed on a mat with a spastic hemiplegic may not meet the requirements of functional knee joint motion when standing or walking. However, if the knee joint cannot function in isolation, we would not expect normal integration of knee joint function when it is required to move with other joints in a kinematic chain. Therefore, a sound treatment approach should consider the part (isolated joint) as well as the whole (the entire kinematic chain). Rehabilitation of isolated joint function may be out of context from functional activity, but it is necessary as a prerequisite to normal body mobility (see Ch. 6).

Proprioception

The type of proprioceptive input to the CNS may be dependent on the velocity of movement.[22] During the rehabilitation process, velocity of movement can be altered to enhance proprioceptive functions. Generally, during slow movements the CNS may use optimally cutaneous, joint, and pressure receptors. In contrast, rapid movement may require a "fixed" preprogrammed response triggered by muscle afferents.

Influencing Abnormal Tone

Stretch reflex sensitivity has little to do with functional movement.[4] Given the poor correlations between abnormal synergies and functional capability, it does not make sense to focus on treatment techniques designed to decrease abnormal muscle tone unless the goal is isolated joint rehabilitation. The components of joint movement as segments of a kinematic chain are discussed in Chapter 6. Alternative and supplemental treatment strategies are provided in Chapter 9.

SUMMARY

A biochemical perspective can add another dimension to understanding mobility dysfunction in the neurologically impaired patient. The syndromes directly caused by neural lesion all have a biomechanical component if the symptoms influence movement. Clinicians must identify the interaction between biomechanics and primary lesion characteristics in order to optimize therapeutic intervention.

REFERENCES

1. Hertanu JS, Demopoulos JT, Yang WC, Calhoun WF, Fenigstein HA: Stroke rehabilitation: correlation and prognostic value of computerized tomography and sequential functional assessments. Arch Phys Med Rehabil 65:505, 1984
2. Wyke B: The neurology of joints. Ann R Coll Surg Engl 41:25, 1967
3. Sutherland DH, Cooper L: The pathomechanics of progressive crouch gait in spastic dysplegia. Orthop Clin North Amer 9:143, 1978
4. Sahrmann SA, Norton JB: The relationship of voluntary movement to spasticity in the upper motor neuron syndrome. Ann Neurol 2:460, 1977
5. Van Sant A: Designing a definitive clinical study of spasticity. Neurology Report 9:17, 1985
6. Cerny K: Pathomechanics of stance: clinical concepts for analysis. Phys Ther 64:1851, 1984
7. Belenkii VY, Gurfinkel VS, Pal'tsev YI: Elements of control of voluntary movements. Biophysics 12:135, 1967
8. Pal'tsev YI, El'Ner AM: Preparatory and compensating period during voluntary movement in patients with involvement of the brain in different localization. Biophysics 12:142, 1967
9. Dichgans J, Mauritz KH: Patterns and mechanisms of postural instability in patients with cerebellar lesions. pp. 633. In JE Desmedt (ed): Motor Control Mechanisms in Health and Disease. Raven Press, New York, 1983
10. Nashner LM: Fixed patterns of rapid postural responses among leg muscles during stance. Exp Brain Res 30:13, 1977
11. DiFabio RP, Badke MB, Duncan PW: Adapting human postural reflexes following localized cerebrovascular lesion: analysis of bilateral long latency responses. Brain Research 363:257, 1986
12. Nashner LM, Shumway-Cook A, Marin O: Stance postural control in select groups of children with cerebral palsy: deficits in sensory organization and muscular co-ordination. Exp Brain Res 49:393, 1983
13. Nashner LM: Adapting reflexes controlling human posture. Exp Brain Res 26:59, 1976
14. Forssberg H, Nashner LM: Ontogenetic development of postural control in man: adaptation to altered support and visual conditions during stance. J Neurosci 2:545, 1982
15. Nashner LM, Black FO, Wall C: Adaptation to altered support and visual conditions during stance: patients with vestibular deficits. J Neurosci 2:536, 1982
16. Wollacott MH, Shumway-Cook A, Nashner LM: Postural reflexes and aging. p. 98 Mortimer JA, Pirozzolo FJ, Maletta JG (eds): The Aging Motor System, Praeger, New York, 1983
17. Traub MM, Rothwell JC, Marsden CD: Anticipatory postural reflexes in Parkinson's disease and other akinetic-rigid syndromes and in cerebellar ataxia. Brain 103:393, 1980
18. Horak FB, Nashner LM, Nutt JG: Postural instability in Parkinson's disease: motor coordination and sensory organization. Soc Neurosci Abst, 1984
19. Nashner LM, Grimm RJ: Analysis of multiloop dyscontrols in standing cerebellar patients. pp. 300–319. In JE Desmedt (ed): Cerebral Motor Control in Man: Long Loop Mechanisms. Raven Press, New York, 1978

In JE Desmedt (ed): Cerebral Motor Control in Man: Long Loop Mechanisms. Raven Press, New York, 1978

20. Knott M, Voss DE: Proprioceptive neuromuscular facilitation. Harper & Row Publishers, New York, 1968

21. Goff B: Appropriate afferent stimulation. Physiotherapy 55:9, 1969

22. Diener HC, Dichgans J, Guschlbauer B, Mau H: The significance of proprioception on postural stabilization as assessed by ischemia. Brain Research 196:103, 1984

23. Badke MB, Di Fabio RP: Effects of postural bias during support surface displacements and rapid arm movements. Phys Ther 65:1490, 1985

24. Carr JH, Sheperd RB: A Motor Relearning Program for Stroke. Aspen Systems Corporation, London, 1983

25. Craik RL: Biomechanics: a neural control perspective. Phys Ther 64:1810, 1984

SUGGESTED READING

Soderberg GL: Kinesiology: Application to Pathological Motion. Williams & Wilkins, Baltimore, 1986

2 Peripheral Neuropathies and Entrapment Syndromes

Robert Kellogg

PERIPHERAL POLYNEUROPATHIES

Peripheral polyneuropathy is a general term used to describe a symmetrical motor and sensory neuropathy involving many nerves. The general etiological causes include genetic predisposition, metabolic abnormalities, exposure to various toxins, immunological reactions, nutritional deficiency states, infectious states, and a remote effect in some cases of malignancy; in a certain percentage of cases the etiology remains undetermined.[1-3]

Classification of Peripheral Polyneuropathies Based on Anatomical Site of Pathology

A neuron in the peripheral nervous system (PNS) can be divided into four component parts: (1) the neuron cell body, (2) the axon, (3) the Schwann cells/myelin sheath, and (4) motor nerve end plates and sensory nerve end organs. When discussing the site of primary pathological change in relation to peripheral neuropathies, we are most often speaking of changes in the nerve cell bodies, axons, and myelin sheaths. The classification for these conditions is as follows:

Neuronopathy—A condition in which the lesion primarily affects the nerve cell body
Axonopathy—A condition in which the lesion primarily affects the nerve cell axon
Myelinopathy—A condition in which the lesion primarily affects myelin or the Schwann cell[4]

This chapter will be limited to a discussion of axonopathies and myelinopathies. For a discussion of neuronopathies and diseases of the neuromuscular junction please see the appropriate chapters of this text.

Axonopathies

Pathology

Axonal degeneration is thought to be the most common reaction of the PNS to pathological states. Other terms often used for this phenomenon include distal axonopathy, central-peripheral distal axonopathy, and dying-back neuropathy. When dealing with axonopathies two factors are of significance: increased diameter of the axon fiber and increase in distance between the motor end plate or sensory receptor and the nerve cell body. Essentially, this breaks down into metabolic demand. The larger the fiber and the farther it is from the cell body, the more susceptible it is to alterations in normal metabolism.

Peripheral neuropathies that are primarily axonal in nature include

1. Diabetic
2. Uremic
3. Endocrine related
4. Charcot-Marie-Tooth disease (hereditary motor/sensory neuropathy HMSN type II)
5. Alcoholic
6. Most nutritional deficiencies
7. Most toxins
8. Certain malignancies (e.g., oat cell carcinoma)

Clinical Presentation of Axonopathies

In the typical picture, the hallmarks of an axonopathy include

1. Symmetrical complaints of altered sensations. These may be described as numbness, heaviness, burning, crawling, or itching. These symptoms usually involve the distal lower extremities; however, these symptoms may be restricted to the upper extremities.
2. Gradual onset of symptoms that have steadily progressed
3. Complaints of weakness involving primarily the foot and ankle musculature and possibly the hand intrinsics
4. Complaints of altered sense of balance with falls occurring at night. This is a good illustration of selective large fiber involvement causing either weakness (unrecognized foot drop) or altered proprioception (loss of balance) (Table 2-1).

Clinical Examination and Findings

To identify correctly the presence of a peripheral neuropathy and its cause the patient should undergo a thorough physical examination, various laboratory studies, and electrophysiological testing.[5]

The physical findings indicative of peripheral neuropathy are

1. Stocking-glove sensory loss. Joint position and vibratory sensation abnormalities may be the early findings (Fig. 2-1).
2. Stocking-glove motor weakness. Patients often will have detectable weakness or visible atrophy in the hand and foot intrinsics.
3. Symmetrical loss of ankle jerks
4. Possible gait ataxia[6,7]
5. Possible trophic changes of the feet

Laboratory findings are quite variable depending on the suspected etiology. Examples include

1. Diabetics—Increased blood glucose levels
2. Kidney disease—Elevated serum creatinine or BUN
3. Toxins—Elevated levels of the toxin detected during laboratory testing.

Electrophysiological testing should include both electromyography and nerve conduction velocity testing.

Electromyography (EMG)

As this is a pathology involving primarily the nerve axons, the following abnormalities are typically found during the EMG examination:

1. Fibrillation potentials and positive sharp waves
2. Diminished interference patterns with motor units possibly being polyphasic and of increased amplitude and duration
3. Abnormalities limited to the distal musculature of the legs and arms
4. Distribution pattern of multiple peripheral nerves in different myotomal distributions.[8]

Nerve Conduction Velocity Testing (NCV)

In diseases that are primarily axonopathies, actual nerve conduction velocity changes are minor and thought to be secondary to axonal shrinkage and

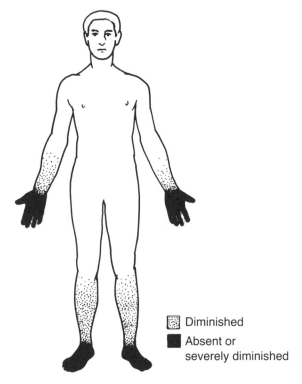

Diminished

Absent or severely diminished

Fig. 2-1 Diagram of the sensory losses seen in distal axonopathies.

Table 2-1 Comparison of Nerve Fiber Type by Size, Conduction Velocity, and Function

Fiber Type	Size	Velocity	Function
Class A Sensory Group Ia/Ib	20 μm	100 m/sec	Sensory from muscle Spindle and golgi tendon organ
Group II	5–15 μm	20–90 m/sec	Vibration and position sense
Group III	1–7 μm	12–30 m/sec	Certain pain impulses
Motor Alpha	17 μm	50–100 m/sec	Extrafusal muscle
Gamma	2–10 μm	10–45 m/sec	Intrafusal muscle
Class B B Fibers	<3 μm	3–15 m/sec	Preganglionic autonomic
Class C C Fibers	.2–1.5 μm	.3–1.6 m/sec	Postganglionic autonomic efferents Many pain fibers

subsequent myelin changes rather than primary myelin disease.[9] Changes that can be noticed during NCV testing are

1. Mild slowing of the motor nerve conduction velocities
2. Mild slowing of sensory nerve conduction velocities
3. Decreased amplitudes of the motor and sensory nerve evoked responses
4. A pattern of multiple peripheral nerves in at least three extremities

Rehabilitation

The prognosis for any given axonopathy is greatly dependent on many factors, all of which must be considered when developing a treatment program. In the best of situations axons regenerate at 1 to 4 mm per day.[10] Accordingly, the patient should be prepared from the beginning for a potentially lengthy duration of rehabilitation. Factors influencing prognosis are

1. Etiology
2. Patient's age
3. Patient's overall state of health
4. Severity of the polyneuropathy
5. Control of metabolic factors, nutrition deficits, and toxin exposure
6. Patient's compliance with treatment program
7. Patient's support systems

Role of the Physical Therapist

The roles of the physical therapist in the treatment of patients with peripheral neuropathies include:

1. Assisting in pain management
2. Maintaining or increasing range of motion
3. Maintaining or increasing strength
4. Gait training
5. Instructing activities of daily living and energy saving tips
6. Counseling

Modalities

Physical therapists have at their disposal a wide variety of therapeutic modalities and techniques for each of the preceding categories. What follows is only a partial discussion of available interventions for specific complaints and physical findings.

Pain Management—Use of Heat or Cold. The use of heat or cold can be of benefit to some in the temporary relief of pain.[11]

1. Usefulness is best evaluated by clinical trial as indicated for the particular patient.
2. Approach with caution secondary to the patient's diminished sensory capabilities and the possibility of altered vascular responses.
3. Safest applications maintain skin visibility during the treatment[12] (e.g., hydrotherapy, infrared lamps, etc.).
4. Generally the treatment intensity will be lessened and the duration shortened.

Pain Management—Transcutaneous Electrical Nerve Stimulators (TENS). TENS has been of some value in the treatment of pain complaints in patients with peripheral polyneuropathy.

1. Methods include both high and low frequency techniques.
2. Successful use will often require multiple trials with variable electrode placements.
3. Caution must be exercised because of the patient's sensory deficit. Patients suffering from polyneuropathies (particularly diabetics) can ill afford any type of skin disruption that may result from the electrical current or electrode adhesives.[13]

Pain Management—Massage. Therapeutic massage can be a useful technique in pain relief. Pain relief can occur based both on the counter-irritation theory and by assisting vascular return in patients with edema in the distal extremities.

Before considering any of the preceding techniques for pain control, the patient's response to cutaneous stimulation must be considered. Quite often patients with peripheral polyneuropathies find cutaneous stimulation disagreeable. If this is the case, pain relief by modalities that depend on cutaneous stimulation may prove ineffective.

Range of Motion (ROM)

Maintenance or improvement in a patient's ROM can be of vital importance in patients with polyneuropathies. The various techniques used will depend in great part on the patient's level of disability.

1. Active ROM exercises would be the ideal in patients able to perform them. The active ROM exercise program should be structured so that the patient does not become fatigued.
2. Active assisted ROM may be required for those patients with moderate to severe disability. Caution should be exercised because of the patient's altered sensibility.
3. Passive ROM exercises will be needed for those individuals with complete motor function loss or those with already limited ROM. Because these patients most likely have severe disease, they are more prone to those afflictions that plague the bedridden or wheelchair-bound patient, such as multiple

joint contractures (hips, knees, and ankles), decubitus ulcers, postural hypotension, and osteoporosis. These possibilities in conjunction with the patient's altered sensibility require that therapeutic exercises be closely monitored.

Strengthening Exercises

The degree of success of muscle strengthening exercises will depend on the state of control of the patient's disease process. Many different techniques are advocated to strengthen muscles. The techniques you choose will depend on the patient's level of disability, available equipment, and your personal preference.

1. Isometrics are easily accomplished by bedridden or wheelchair-bound patients and are frequently used as an initial starting exercise in a progressive strengthening program. When using isometrics, as with all active exercises in patients with polyneuropathies, patient fatigue should be avoided.
2. Isotonic strengthening exercises may be developed readily for patients using manual resistance, weights, rubber tubing, or dental dam.
3. Isokinetic strengthening can be used effectively in those patients with mild axonopathies or in certain instances with those patients demonstrating ambulation difficulties. For these patients, the strengthening program will be more aggressive with the additional emphasis on endurance training.
4. Electrical stimulation as a method of strengthening continues to be a subject of considerable controversy.[14,15] In particular its usefulness in patients with axonopathies may be limited. Because of the widespread changes in peripheral neuropathies and the often hypersensitive response to noxious stimuli, electrical muscle stimulation is not generally used. A possible exception to this would be the use of electrical muscle stimulation for re-education purposes as opposed to actual strengthening. In these cases one would be working with at least partially innervated musculature using stimulation parameters that are generally more comfortable than those necessary for completely denervated muscles.

Gait Training

Ambulation aids may be required for patients with moderate to severe axonopathies. Most often the only form of assistive device needed is a cane. This is particularly effective in assisting the patient who has diminished proprioception. The use of crutches or walkers may be needed for patients with more involved disease.

The use of braces will depend on the amount and distribution of the patient's weakness. Most often all that is required is an ankle foot orthosis or perhaps a more supportive double upright-type brace. The brace should be lightweight and well fitted because of the patient's weakness, sensation deficits, and their often fragile skin integrity status.

Activities of Daily Living

1. Instruction in energy saving techniques should include work simplification and task organization education.
2. Home and work place structuring is best accomplished by a home visit if possible.
3. Techniques of wheelchair living (if appropriate)

Counseling

1. Compliance with treatment regimen
2. Education concerning the need for meticulous foot care
3. Sexual counseling

Unfortunately patients with polyneuropathic diseases suffer in most cases from pain, altered body image, loss of function, changes in life style etc. With this in mind the need for additional supportive measures, such as psychological, occupational, social, and financial counseling, becomes evident, necessitating the appropriate referrals.

Myelinopathies

Pathology

Diseases that primarily affect myelin or the Schwann cell are much less frequently encountered than those that affect the axon. One would be most likely to encounter myelinopathies of a toxic, immunological, inflammatory, or genetic etiology. The overall neuropathological process is illustrated in Figure 2-2.

A list of polyneuropathies characterized as myelinopathies includes

1. Acute idiopathic inflammatory polyneuropathy (Guillain-Barré)
2. Chronic inflammatory polyneuropathy
3. Diphtheric
4. Certain types of diabetic neuropathies (both mononeuropathies and polyneuropathies)
5. Possibly HMSN type I

Clinical Presentation of Myelinopathies

Because acute idiopathic inflammatory polyneuropathy (Guillain-Barré) is the most frequently encountered myelinopathy, it will serve as our clinical picture.[16] Symptoms include generalized weakness with often only mild sensory loss that may develop quite rapidly over hours to days. Symptoms usually start in the lower extremities but not necessarily in the distal musculature.

Clinical Examination and Findings

Physical findings include

1. Diffuse weakness in all four extremities, not related to isolated peripheral nerves or a myotomal distribution
2. Variable sensory loss, which may be quite mild or not involved. Often sensory findings may be in a distal distribution, involving only fingers and feet.
3. Loss of deep tendon reflexes in all extremities, which reflects nerve fiber specificity with highly myelinated sensory Ia and motor fibers being primarily affected
4. No signs of central nervous system disease such as clonus or positive Babinski response

Laboratory findings indicative of Guillain-Barré syndrome are

1. Increased levels of serum immunoglobulins
2. Increased percentages of leukocytes and lymphocytes
3. Elevated cerebrospinal fluid protein

Electrophysiological testing includes both EMG and NCV.

Electrophysiological findings most indicative of a good recovery include normal amplitude of muscle action potentials during NCV studies and

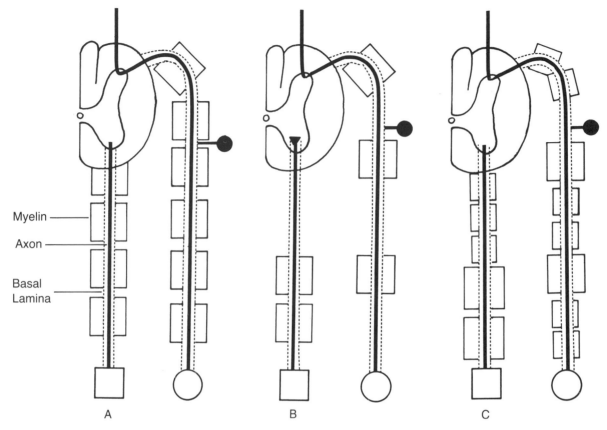

Myelin

Axon

Basal
Lamina

A   B   C

Fig. 2-2 Diagram of the pathological changes associated with a myelinopathy. **(A)** Normal motor
and sensory peripheral nerves. **(B)** Segmental sites of demyelination. **(C)** Myelin regeneration
illustrating the formation of more numerous smaller internodes of myelin.

lack of fibrillation potentials and positive sharp
waves during the EMG examination. Both of these
findings illustrate relative lack of axonal involvement.

EMG
1. EMG changes in early disease are generally
   limited to showing decreased or absent motor
   unit interference patterns.
2. If the inflammatory response is severe enough,
   axonal damage can occur leading to the
   development of fibrillation potentials and
   positive sharp waves.
3. The presence of profuse fibrillation potentials
   and positive sharp waves is a poor prognostic
   sign.[8,17]

NCV
NCV changes are the hallmark of myelinopathies. The changes that occur are quite striking.
For patients with Guillain-Barré syndrome these
changes include

1. Motor nerve conduction velocity reduced by
   30 to 40 percent
2. Muscle action potential may be polyphasic with
   increased temporal dispersion.
3. In early disease, conduction abnormalities may
   only be noticeable in "F" wave studies. This
   reflects the more proximal nature of the
   segmental demyelination.[18]
4. Sensory nerve conduction studies may be
   normal.

Rehabilitation

The rehabilitation of the patient with Guillain-Barré syndrome initially consists of intensive supportive care during the initial stages of the acute paralysis. Depending on the severity of the disease, patients may need mechanical ventilation, nasogastric tube feeding, urinary catheterization, etc. The overall status of the patient can change rapidly during the first 4 weeks of the acute stage. Ideally, the patient's involvement with the rehabilitation program begins at this time.

The rehabilitation of patients with Guillain-Barré syndrome can be a most rewarding experience. Prognosis is very good with recovery starting within 2 to 4 weeks from the period of maximal deficit. This rapid recovery is related to the type of pathology (myelinopathy). Myelin regeneration is much quicker than axonal regeneration. The rehabilitation process is organized into three stages: acute, intermediate, and chronic.

Acute Stage

During this stage, the patient demonstrates a complete loss of muscular strength or a steady decline in muscular strength. The physical therapist's primary goals are the preservation of ROM, maintenance of skin integrity, and psychological support.

ROM exercises may be passive to active assisted in nature. The following points should be followed when using ROM exercises:

1. Avoid fatigue.
2. Exercises should be done gently to avoid over stretch type injuries.
3. Resting/positional splints may be needed, particularly for the feet and hands (Figs. 2-3 and 2-4).

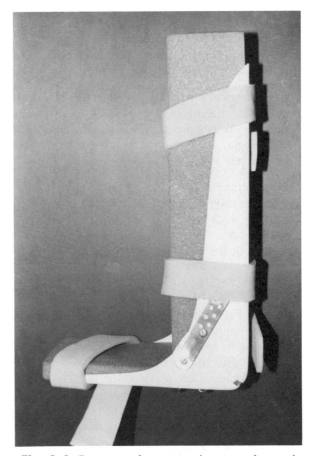

Fig. 2-3 Illustration of a positional resting splint used for the foot and ankle.

Skin integrity is threatened by the patient's inability to move independently. The following points should be kept in mind.

1. Patients require frequent position changes, at least every 2 hours.

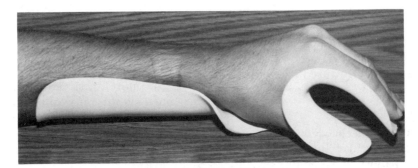

Fig. 2-4 Illustration of a positional resting splint used for the hand and wrist.

2. Use of bedding to lessen friction/pressure (i.e., sheepskin or Roho cushion).
3. Regular skin inspection to observe for areas of potential breakdown.

Psychological support for these patients is mandatory. Because of the acute onset of what may become a severe (although it is hoped temporary) quadriplegia, these patients undergo great feelings of stress and loss.

1. Devise methods by which patients can communicate with you.
2. Explain what you are doing and why you are doing it.
3. Talk with the patient.

Intermediate Stage

At times, this stage is a period of remarkable recovery. During this phase the physical therapist's goals are maintaining or increasing ROM, increasing strength, re-educating weak muscles, gait retraining, and return to independence in activities of daily living. This period usually starts 1 to 2 months after the onset of the original symptoms and can last a variable amount of time depending on the severity of demyelination and the degree of axonal damage.

The following points should be kept in mind when instituting ROM exercises:

1. Progress exercises according to the level of strength returning.
2. Direct attention toward maintaining proper mobility of the heelcords, hamstrings, hip adductors, and shoulder structures.

Strengthening exercises should

1. Be instituted as patients start to demonstrate voluntary motor activity
2. Incorporate isometric, isotonic, and isokinetic forms of exercise
3. Be well supervised and structured to avoid fatigue and injuries from overuse or overstretching

Muscular re-education is needed in the early stages of returning muscular function. Various techniques include patterning, tapping, stroking,

positioning, EMG biofeedback, and the use of electrical stimulation. It is important to avoid patient fatigue.

The therapist should keep the following points in mind when instituting gait training:

1. Ambulation should not be attempted until the hip and thigh musculature is at least fair to good in strength to avoid injury by overstretching and the development of abnormal gait patterns.[14]
2. Early gait training activities may include the use of a therapeutic pool, stationary bicycle, and/or other therapeutic equipment designed to strengthen the lower extremities.
3. Early therapeutic exercises should emphasize pelvic stability and trunk balance.
4. Early ambulation may require the use of a walker or crutches.
5. The patient should progress to the use of a cane or unassisted ambulation when appropriate.
6. Use of ankle foot orthoses, short leg braces, or full leg braces may be needed by those with moderate to severe unresolving weakness.

During the intermediate stage, patients may regain independence in the activities of daily living.

1. Training should start as soon as the patient is able to generate voluntary activity.
2. The amount of assistance needed will depend on the level of disability.
3. Early emphasis should be placed on self-care activities to re-establish the patient's sense of independence.
4. The fabrication of hand and wrist splints may be needed to accomplish self-care. (See section on peripheral nerve injuries of the upper extremities in this chapter.)

Chronic Stage

If patients continue to demonstrate severe weakness for more than 6 months, they may have sustained significant axonal damage. If this is the case, an ongoing rehabilitation program is very important.[19] This type of program would be the same as that described earlier for patients with axonopathies.

Table 2-2 Comparison of Various Classification Terminologies Concerning Peripheral Nerve Injuries

Sheddon	Sunderland	Schaumburg Spencer Thomas	Anatomic Lesion
Neuropraxia	First Degree	Class 1	Conduction block Ischemic or demyelinating
Axonotmesis	Second Degree	Class 2	Axonal interruption

Neurotmeses
Partial
Complete
	Third Degree
	Fourth Degree
	Fifth Degree
		Class 3	Nerve fiber interruption
			    with connective tissue damage
			    with nerve severance

NERVE ENTRAPMENT SYNDROMES

The classification of isolated peripheral nerve lesions can also be based on the anatomical site of pathology.[4] A comparison of various classification systems for isolated peripheral nerve injuries is given in Table 2-2. The most common description of nerve injuries relates to the terms neuropraxia, axonotmesis, and neurotmesis.

Neuropraxia

Pathology

Neuropraxia is a temporary interruption of conduction without loss of axonal continuity (Fig. 2-5). Neuropraxia is present when

1. The lesion is localized to isolated nerve segment
2. There is no loss of axonal continuity
3. There is no Wallerian degeneration
4. Nerve conduction deficit is completely reversible with removal of the cause

Clinical Examination and Findings
1. Muscle strength distal to the lesion is absent or decreased in a specific distribution.
2. Sensation distal to the lesion is absent or decreased in a specific distribution.
3. Nerve conduction across the site of injury is slowed or absent.
4. Nerve conduction in the segments above and below the lesion is normal.
5. EMG shows absent or decreased motor unit

interference patterns without the presence of positive sharp waves or fibrillation potentials.

Rehabilitation
1. Maintain ROM for those joints affected.
2. Strengthen affected muscles if voluntary function is present.
3. Use electrical stimulation to limit disuse atrophy.
4. Use splinting or orthotics as needed to preserve function.

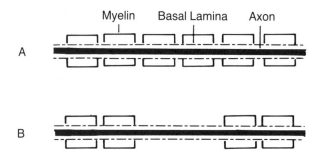
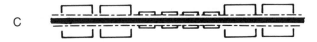

Fig. 2-5 Diagram of the pathological changes associated with a neuropraxic lesion. **(A)** Normal peripheral nerve fiber. **(B)** Segmental demyelination with an intact axon and basal lamina. **(C)** Remyelination of the lesion site with myelin internodes of decreased size and increased number.

5. Counseling and protection should be employed to avoid injury to desensate body parts.
6. Reassure the patient that the loss of function/ sensation returns, generally within a few weeks to a few months.

Axonotmesis

Pathology

Axonotmesis is a disruption of the nerve cell axon, with Wallerian degeneration occurring below and slightly proximal to the site of injury. The Schwann cell basal lamina and endoneurial connective tissue remain intact.[4] Axonotmesis is characterized by

1. Complete axonal failure at the site of injury
2. Wallerian degeneration of the axon distal and one node of Ranvier proximal to the site of injury.
3. Loss of nerve conduction distal to the site of injury 3 to 4 days postinjury.
4. Good prognosis for recovery as the basal lamina forms channels facilitating appropriate regeneration.

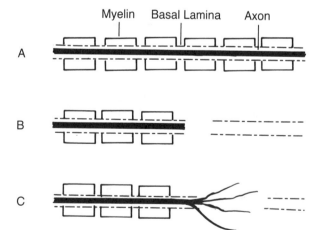

Fig. 2-6 Diagram of the pathological changes associated with a neurotmetic lesion. **(A)** Normal peripheral nerve fiber. **(B)** Axonal and myelin degeneration distal and one node of Ranvier proximal to the site of the lesion. **(C)** Poor chance of regeneration because of the complete separation of the basal lamina.

Clinical Examination and Findings

1. Muscle strength distal to the lesion is absent or decreased in a specific distribution.
2. Sensation distal to the lesion is absent or decreased in a specific distribution.
3. NCV study shows an absence of distal motor and sensory responses. In cases of partial injury, the motor and sensory responses will be of decreased amplitude. Motor conduction studies may show segmental slowing at the site of injury.
4. EMG shows fibrillation potentials and positive sharp waves in associated muscle fibers 14 to 21 days postinjury. Motor unit recruitment is decreased or absent, depending on the severity of nerve injury.

Rehabilitation

1. Maintain ROM for those joints affected.
2. Strengthen affected muscles if voluntary function is present.
3. Use electrical stimulation to attempt to delay the effects of denervation atrophy.
4. Use splinting or orthotics as needed to preserve function.
5. Counseling and protection should be instituted to avoid injury to desensate body parts.
6. Reassure patients that their prognosis is good in most cases. Rate of recovery depends on the distance from the site of injury, with axonal regeneration occurring at 1 to 4 mm/day.[10]

Neurotmesis

Pathology

Neurotmesis is a total severance or disruption of the entire nerve fiber (Fig. 2-6). It is characterized by

1. Wallerian degeneration of the axon distal and one node of Ranvier proximal to the site of injury
2. Disruption of the Schwann cell basal lamina and endoneurial connective tissue
3. Loss of nerve conduction distal to the site of injury 3 to 4 days postinjury
4. Poor prognosis because of total fiber disruption. Generally, this condition requires surgical repair

Clinical Examination and Findings

Examination and findings are the same as for axonotmetic lesions.

Rehabilitation

Rehabilitation goals and techniques are the same as for axonotmetic lesions. Overall, rehabilitation may be significantly prolonged with the final results being quite variable depending on the location and severity of the lesion.

UPPER EXTREMITY PERIPHERAL NERVE LESIONS

Generally, all patients presenting with complaints of neck and/or arm pain require a thorough physical examination of the neck and upper extremities as a minimum. Even though the greatest percentage of pathologies can be localized by patient history, it is not unusual for a first impression to be wrong. A typical screening examination for the cervical spine and upper extremities would include

1. Active and passive cervical spine ROM with compression, distraction, and overpressure testing
2. Active upper extremity ROM including shoulder, elbow, wrist, and fingers
3. Manual muscle testing of the cervical and upper extremity musculature in a gross motion pattern
4. Deep tendon reflexes of the biceps, brachioradialis, and triceps.
5. Sensory testing to light touch.

Based on the findings of your screening examination you are now ready to focus on areas of established or suspected pathology. Further examination would include

1. Palpation of specific cervical or upper extremity structures
2. Specific isolated manual muscle testing. This testing should follow specific peripheral nerve or myotomal distributions.
3. Specific sensory testing to multiple modalities (sharp/dull, hot/cold, two point discrimination etc.). This testing should follow specific peripheral nerve or dermatomal distributions (see Fig. 4-2 in Ch. 4).

4. Specialty tests for suspected pathologies (Phalen's, Tinel's, and Adson's etc.)[20]

During the examination process, it is important to be aware of the possibility of more than one site of pathology. In this double crush syndrome, a proximal nerve lesion makes the distal portion of that nerve more susceptible to compression/entrapment injuries.[10] The other point to keep in mind is that partial lesions are going to be more difficult to isolate than complete lesions. To compound this, partial lesions are more often the rule than the exception.

CERVICAL RADICULOPATHIES

Pathology

Injuries to the cervical nerve roots can be caused by many different forms of pathology. Those most commonly encountered by the physical therapist include cervical spondylosis, herniated cervical disc, and traumatic cervical root avulsions. Typically, injuries to cervical nerve roots will demonstrate sensory and motor deficits in well-delineated dermatomal and myotomal distributions.

Clinical Examination and Findings

Primary physical findings for specific cervical nerve root lesions are summarized in the following sections.

C5 Root Lesions
1. Motor deficits are most noticeable in the rhomboids, supraspinatus/infraspinatus, deltoids, and biceps.
2. Sensory loss can be slight. When present it extends over the lateral shoulder and lateral upper arm.
3. There is a loss or decrease in the biceps deep tendon reflex.
4. Pain is frequently described as radiating into medial scapula and/or shoulder.
5. Symptoms may be reproduced with cervical rotation and extension to the involved side.

C6 Root Lesions
1. Motor deficits are most noticeable in the deltoids, biceps, brachioradialis, and the radial wrist extensors.

2. Sensory loss occurs along the radial forearm and radial dorsal hand.
3. There is a loss or decrease in the biceps and/or brachioradialis deep tendon reflexes.
4. Pain is frequently described as radiating into the scapula and dorsal radial forearm.
5. Symptoms may be reproduced with cervical spine rotation and extension to the involved side.

C7 Root Lesions

1. Motor deficits are most noticeable in the triceps, finger extensors, and pronator teres.
2. Sensory loss occurs over the dorsal medial and ulnar hand.
3. There is a loss or decrease in the triceps deep tendon reflex.
4. Pain is described as radiating into dorsal forearm and dorsal hand.
5. Symptoms may be reproduced by cervical rotation and extension to the involved side.

C8 Root Lesions

1. Motor deficits are most noticeable in the long thumb flexor, hand intrinsics, and ulnar wrist flexor/extensor.
2. Sensory loss occurs over the fourth and fifth fingers and along the ulnar forearm.
3. Pain is frequently described as radiating into the ulnar hand.
4. Symptoms may be reproduced by cervical rotation and extension to the involved side.

T1 Root Lesion

1. Motor deficits are most often restricted to the hand intrinsics.
2. Sensory loss occurs along the medial upper arm.
3. Pain is frequently described as radiating into the axilla and medial upper arm.
4. Horner's syndrome may be present with constricted pupil, ptosis, and enophthalmos.
5. Symptoms may be reproduced by cervical rotation and extension to the involved side.

Special Evaluation Procedures

1. X-rays, CT scan, and myelography. Used to demonstrate and localize the presence of structural abnormality, pathology, or impingement

2. Bone scan. Used to evaluate the possibility of pathologies that involve primarily bone
3. Electrophysiological testing. Useful in localizing the level of the neurological lesion but does not provide information as to the cause of the lesion.

EMG Studies

EMG studies typically show reduced voluntary motor unit interference patterns in early disease, restricted to a myotomal distribution. With symptoms of greater than 3 weeks' duration fibrillation potentials and positive sharp waves may be found in a myotomal distribution including the paraspinal musculature.

NCV Studies

NCV studies show normal nerve conduction velocity. Motor response amplitude may be decreased in clinically weak muscles. Sensory responses are normal. This is an important differentiating point between root lesions and lesions distal to the dorsal root ganglia.

Rehabilitation

Many techniques are available to the physical therapist in treating patients with cervical radiculopathies. Goals for treatments include pain relief, postural correction, and strengthening of weak musculature.

Pain Relief

1. Cryotherapy is very effective in the acute stages or in those injuries cause by trauma.
2. Heating modalities such as infrared radiation, short wave diathermy and ultrasound all have been demonstrated to be beneficial in the treatment of pain.
3. TENS of varying types and frequencies may be helpful.
4. Certain mobilization and muscle energy techniques may help relieve pain.[21] (For specifics refer to the orthopaedic section of this text.)
5. Cervical traction may be used with either constant or intermittent pull in the sitting or supine position.
6. Cervical collars may be used to improve patient comfort and maintain proper posture if appropriate.

Postural Correction

1. Mobilization or muscle energy techniques assist in postural correction.
2. Specific exercises to relax, stretch and/or strengthen cervical and shoulder girdle musculature should be instituted.
3. EMG biofeedback
4. Counseling concerning activities of daily living, sitting, standing, and resting positions

Strengthening Exercises

1. Specific strengthening of weak extremity musculature may have to wait until the acute pain has resolved. Strengthening exercises should be structured to initially stress the involved muscles.
2. As the patient improves, the exercise program should be progressed to include endurance-type exercises, the ultimate goal being to return to unrestricted activity.

Brachial Plexus Lesions

Pathology

Lesions of the brachial plexus can present in a multitude of ways. Quite often it is very difficult to locate the precise level of the lesion in partial injuries. Causes of brachial plexus injuries include trauma, compression in the thoracic outlet, familial tendency, radiation (secondary to the treatment of cancer), and idiopathic.[22–25]

Clinical Examination and Findings

The patient presenting with an acute injury to the brachial plexus can be difficult to evaluate and treat depending on the severity of injury.

1. Localize the majority of clinical findings to a root, trunk, division, or cord level. (Motor loss is somewhat more helpful than sensory changes.) In many cases, this localization may not be clear cut.
2. Pain is reproduced with lateral side bending and rotation of the neck away from the side of complaints.
3. EMG studies provide the needed information in localizing and defining the extent of the lesion based on the anatomical distribution of electrical findings.

4. NCV studies are beneficial in localizing the level of the lesion. Sensory studies are particularly important to differentiate between lesions of the plexus and the cervical roots.

Rehabilitation

The overall treatment goals of patients with brachial plexus lesions follows the same guidelines as those outlined for cervical radiculopathies.

Pain Management

1. Pain is often difficult to manage.
2. TENS of either high and/or low frequency techniques to appropriate sensory intact areas should be performed.
3. The use of heat or cold should be approached cautiously secondary to sensory impairment.

ROM Exercises

1. Passive to active ROM should be undertaken to the shoulder, elbow, wrist and fingers.
2. Positional splinting may be needed for wrist and hand.
3. Shoulder sling may be needed if shoulder musculature is involved.

Strengthening Exercises

1. Progressive strengthening of weakened muscles is indicated as soon as voluntary activity is demonstrated.
2. Electrical stimulation may help in some cases.

Edema Control

1. The involved extremity should be elevated whenever possible.
2. A pressure gradient glove and sleeve should be used.
3. Massage is appropriate if needed.

Counseling

1. The patient may require extensive life style changes such as hand dominance and occupation.
2. The patient should be counseled in stress management to assist in chronic pain control.

Thoracic Outlet Syndrome

Pathology

Thoracic outlet syndrome diagnosis and management has been and continues to be a subject of considerable controversy. Potential etiologies for thoracic outlet include a cervical rib, postural changes, entrapment by the first rib/clavical, scalene muscles, or a fibrous band. The portion of the plexus most often involved is the lower trunk and/or the medial cord.

Clinical Examination and Findings

1. The patient will present with complaints of pain or aching throughout the arm or restricted to the medial aspect of the hand and arm.
2. The patient may note that symptoms are worse when working or sleeping with arm held above the head.
3. The patient may complain of intermittent paresthesias into the involved hand, in an ill-defined distribution.
4. In later stages, the patient may note diffuse hand weakness or clumsiness, which worsens with repetitive use of the hand.
5. The patient may have poor posture with forward head or depressed or protracted shoulders. (Large breasts may contribute to this syndrome in women.)
6. Except in severe cases, muscular strength is normal. When weakness is present, it is usually isolated to the hand intrinsics and the ulnar wrist and finger flexors.
7. Sensory loss may occur in a C8-T1 distribution.
8. Special tests include the stress abduction test, Adson's test, costoclavicular, and hyperabduction maneuvers.[20,26] These tests should be interpreted on their ability to reproduce the patient's symptoms and not by the change in the radial pulse, as many normal patients will have some pulse changes (Fig. 2-7).
9. Tinel's sign may be present in the supraclavicular fossa.
10. EMG examination may show changes consistent with a chronic compression syndrome, such as (1) reduction in the number of voluntary motor units, (2) motor units may be of increased duration and amplitude, possibly showing an increased percentage of polyphasic potentials, and (3) findings usually limited to those muscles

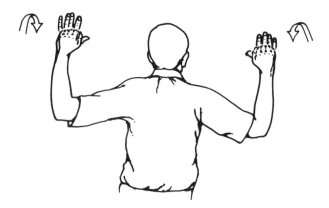

Fig. 2-7 Stress abduction test: With shoulders abducted to 90° and elbows flexed to 90° the patient is asked to open and close his hands as rapidly as possible for 2 minutes. A positive test will show early fatigue or coordination loss on the involved side along with coloration changes of the involved hand.

innervated by the lower trunk or medial cord of the brachial plexus.
11. NCV studies may show the following: (1) normal median and ulnar motor conduction velocities from the axilla down, (2) decreased amplitude of the ulnar and medial forearm cutaneous sensory nerve responses, and (3) prolonged latencies across the brachial plexus when "F" wave and root stimulation techniques are employed.

Rehabilitation

The goals of the physical therapist include postural correction, restoration of normal mobility, and strengthening of weak musculature.[27]

Posture correction is the main area of emphasis. The areas of greatest concern are (1) forward head, (2) protracted shoulders, and (3) depressed shoulders. Patients should be educated regarding the importance of maintaining a balanced neutral posture.

ROM exercises include stretching exercises, which may be needed for the scalenes, pectorals, and other shoulder girdle musculature. Mobilization techniques may be needed to restore normal shoulder accessory joint motions.

Strengthening exercises are usually needed for the shoulder girdle muscles, including the shoulder elevators and retractors. In addition, exercises should be geared toward gentle strengthening of the cervical and thoracic extensors. The patient should advance to a progressive generalized conditioning program as symptoms improve.

During activities of daily living, patients should avoid working with arms above the head and should maintain proper standing, sitting, and resting postures. Supportive bras are recommended for women with large breasts.

Suprascapular Nerve

Pathology

Isolated injuries of the suprascapular nerve occur infrequently. Generally, injuries are traumatic and can be closely associated with lesions of the upper trunk of the brachial plexus.[28]

Clinical Examination and Findings
1. Pain may be described as a deep ache into the shoulder.
2. Patients will demonstrate weakness limited to the shoulder external rotation and abduction/ flexion. Specific testing will isolate weakness to the supraspinatus and infraspinatus muscles.
3. Patients may have visible atrophy of the supraspinatus and infraspinatus muscle masses.
4. There are no sensory changes.
5. There is no loss of deep tendon reflexes.
6. EMG examination may show (1) fibrillation potentials and positive sharp waves in the supraspinatus and infraspinatus, (2) decreased or absent interference patterns of voluntary motor units in the infraspinatus and/or supraspinatus muscles.
7. NCV studies may demonstrate delayed or absent conduction to the supraspinatus and/or infraspinatus muscles.

Rehabilitation

The treatment goals for isolated injuries to peripheral nerves are to decrease pain, maintain joint mobility, increase strength, protect the limb, maintain muscle mobility, and maximize functional ability.

Pain Management
1. Use of a sling may be helpful during the acute stages.

2. Therapeutic modalities such as heat, cold, and TENS may be used if needed for pain control.

ROM Exercises
1. Passive to active ROM exercises should be started to preserve normal joint function.
2. Specific emphasis should be placed on maintaining shoulder external rotation and abduction.

Strengthening Exercises
1. Exercises should begin as soon as voluntary contraction of the affected muscles becomes evident.
2. Exercises should be slowly progressive to avoid overstress injuries.
3. Electrical stimulation may be considered as a modality to help with early strengthening.
4. Functional motions to be stressed are shoulder external rotation and abduction.

Limb Protection

The patient should be counseled to avoid heavy lifting or high velocity movements with the involved shoulder.

Maintaining Muscle Mobility

The use of electrical stimulation, though controversial, takes on more clinical significance when dealing with isolated peripheral nerve injuries. For both neuropraxic and axonotmetic/neurotmetic lesions, an early and long-term goal is to maintain the contractile functioning of the muscle fiber.[15]

1. For neuropraxic lesions the use of faradic or alternating current generators will suffice, as the muscle fiber has an intact nerve supply.
2. Axonotmetic/neurotmetic lesions require the use of interrupted galvanic/direct currents or alternating currents of less than 10 Hz, as the muscle fibers do not have an intact nerve supply.

Musculocutaneous Nerve

Pathology

Isolated lesions of the musculocutaneous nerve are uncommon. Injury to this nerve can occur with humeral fractures, trauma to the upper arm, and as surgical complications during shoulder procedures.

Clinical Examination and Findings

1. Patients may complain of pain in the shoulder, axilla, or elbow.
2. Patients experience loss of function or weakness of the biceps, brachialis, and possibly the coracobrachialis. Weakness may be noted in elbow flexion and forearm supination.
3. There is loss of the biceps deep tendon reflex.
4. There is sensory loss or decrease over the lateral forearm.
5. Visible atrophy of the biceps and brachialis may occur.
6. EMG may show (1) fibrillation potentials and positive sharp waves in the biceps and brachialis and (2) decreased motor unit unit interference patterns limited to those muscles innervated by the musculocutaneous nerve distal to the lesion.
7. NCV studies may show (1) absent or prolonged distal motor latencies to the biceps and (2) absent or diminished lateral forearm cutaneous nerve sensory response.[29,30]

Rehabilitation

ROM Exercises

Passive to active ROM should be done for the shoulder, elbow, and wrist (pronation/supination).

Strengthening Exercises

1. Primary strengthening emphasis is directed to the brachialis as an elbow flexor and the biceps as an elbow flexor and forearm supinator.
2. Early strengthening may be facilitated by the use of electrical stimulation.

Maintaining Muscle Contractility

Electrical stimulation can be performed. The technique used will vary depending on whether the musculature is innervated or denervated.

Limb Protection

1. A sling may prove helpful in the acute phase.
2. Counsel the patient to avoid heavy lifting or high velocity elbow extension with the involved arm.

Long Thoracic Nerve

Pathology

Lesions of the long thoracic nerve can occur as a result of trauma, heavily loaded shoulder straps, surgical complication, and idiopathic causes.[31]

Clinical Examination and Findings

1. Patients may notice shoulder blade winging or catching on chair backs.
2. Weakness of the serratus anterior may be present, causing altered scapular mechanics. This would produce a winging of the inferior angle of the scapula.
3. There may be weakness of functional shoulder flexion and abduction secondary to altered scapular mechanics.
4. There is no sensory loss.
5. There are no changes in deep tendon reflexes.
6. EMG exam may show (1) fibrillation potentials and positive sharp waves in the serratus anterior and (2) decreased motor unit interference patterns isolated to the serratus anterior.

Rehabilitation

ROM Exercises

1. Passive to active ROM exercises should be initiated to maintain shoulder motion.
2. The patient may benefit from mobilization of clavicle and scapula to maintain shoulder accessory motions.
3. Exercises should avoid creating a shoulder impingement syndrome secondary to the altered scapular mechanics.

Strengthening Exercises

1. Exercises may begin as soon as there is evidence of voluntary activity.
2. Functional strengthening of the serratus anterior occurs by exercising it as a shoulder protractor and as a scapular stabilizer.
3. Electrical stimulation is not useful for this muscle.

Limb Protection

1. Advise the patient to avoid heavy or prolonged lifting with the involved shoulder.
2. If the injury is thought to be caused by compressive external forces (backpack straps), those stresses should be avoided.

Axillary Nerve

Pathology

Axillary nerve injuries can occur because of trauma, shoulder dislocations, humeral fractures, pressure from axillary crutches, and from hyperextension shoulder motions.[32,33]

Clinical Examination and Findings

1. Patients will have complaints of weakness involving shoulder flexion, abduction, and possibly external rotation.
2. Patients may complain of shoulder pain.
3. Patients will demonstrate weakness or no function of the deltoids and teres minor.
4. Sensory loss may occur over the lateral shoulder, though this finding is not always present.
5. Deep tendon reflexes of biceps, brachioradialis, and triceps are intact.
6. There is visible atrophy of the deltoids.
7. EMG exam may show (1) fibrillation potentials and positive sharp waves in the deltoids and/or the teres minor and (2) decreased motor unit interference patterns in the deltoids and possibly the teres minor.
8. NCV study may show delayed or absent distal motor latency to the deltoids.

Rehabilitation

ROM Exercises

1. Passive to active ROM exercises should be instituted in all planes of shoulder motion.
2. Clavicular and scapular mobilization may be indicated to prevent the loss of shoulder accessory joint motions.

Strengthening Exercises

1. Strengthening of the deltoids and teres minor should begin as soon as there is evidence of voluntary activity.
2. Electrical stimulation may be helpful as an early form of strengthening.
3. Early exercises should avoid positions that may create an impingement syndrome.

Pain Management

1. The use of a sling may be beneficial during the early stages.
2. Therapeutic modalities such as heat, cold, and TENS can be used.

Maintaining Muscle Contractility

1. Electrical stimulation can be used to maintain muscle fiber contractility and delay disuse or denervation atrophy.
2. Stimulating parameters will vary according to the electrical evidence for muscle innervation or denervation.

Limb Protection

1. Counsel patients to avoid heavy or repeated overhead lifting.
2. Patients should avoid sitting and sleeping positions that create impingement stresses.

Radial Nerve

The radial nerve is subject to many forms of injury along its course. The most common sites of compression will be discussed in the following sections.

Injury at the Level of the Axilla

Pathology

Injuries can occur from shoulder dislocation, trauma, and compression from axillary crutches.

Clinical Examination and Findings

1. Weakness or loss of function of all radial nerve innervated musculature, including the triceps
2. Sensory loss over dorsal radial hand
3. Loss of brachioradialis and triceps deep tendon reflexes
4. Loss of functional finger, wrist, and elbow extension, with subsequent varying wrist flexion posture.
5. Don't be fooled by the ability of the lumbricals to extend the proximal interphalangeal and distal interphalangeal joints, giving the appearance of a partially intact extensor digitorum.
6. Don't be fooled by the tenodesis effect of wrist flexion on the extensor digitorum appearing actively to partially extend the fingers.
7. May have a Tinel's sign in the axilla
8. EMG exam may show (1) fibrillation potentials and positive sharp waves in all muscles innervated by the radial nerve and (2) decreased motor unit interference patterns in all muscles innervated by the radial nerve.
9. NCV study may show (1) decreased amplitude or no response from radial nerve innervated muscles, (2) segmental delay or complete block of motor nerve conduction velocities at the site of the lesion if the motor response is intact, and (3) absent or decreased amplitude of the sensory radial nerve response.

Injury at the Level of the Humeral Spiral Groove

Pathology

Injuries of the radial nerve at this level can be secondary to humeral fractures, trauma, and pressure palsies from rifle slings and sleeping against a hard surface.

Clinical Examination and Findings

1. Weakness or loss of function of the radial nerve innervated musculature distal to and including the brachioradialis
2. Sparing of triceps function
3. Functional loss of wrist extension and finger extension
4. Sensory loss over dorsal radial hand
5. Loss of brachioradialis deep tendon reflex; triceps reflex intact
6. Possible Tinel's sign at the spiral groove
7. EMG exam may show (1) fibrillation potentials and positive sharp waves in radial nerve innervated muscles distal to the triceps and (2) decreased motor unit interference patterns in all muscles innervated by the radial nerve distal to the triceps.
8. NCV study may show (1) decreased amplitude or no response from radial nerve innervated muscles distal to the triceps, (2) segmental delay or complete block of motor nerve conduction velocities at the spiral groove if the motor response is intact, and (3) absent or decreased amplitude of the radial sensory nerve response.

Injury of the Radial Nerve in the Proximal Forearm

Pathology

The radial nerve has many potential sites of injury in the forearm. Fractures and dislocations of the radial head, trauma, entrapment in the arcade of Frohse, elbow joint pathology, and tumors have all been sources of radial nerve injury.

Clinical Examination and Findings

1. Weakness or loss of function of muscles distal to the extensor carpi radialis and supinator
2. No sensory loss
3. Deep tendon reflexes of triceps and brachioradialis intact

4. Functional loss of finger extension and ulnar wrist extension
5. Possible Tinel's sign over radial nerve in the forearm at the radial head
6. Hand resting attitude may resemble an "ulnar claw" in partial injuries (see Fig. 2-12).
7. Pain complaints may mimic those of tennis elbow
8. EMG exam may show (1) fibrillation potentials and positive sharp waves in all muscle innervated by the posterior interosseous branch of the radial nerve distal to the supinator and (2) decreased motor unit interference patterns in all muscles innervated by the posterior interosseous branch of the radial nerve distal to the supinator.
9. NCV study may show (1) decreased amplitude or no response from radial nerve innervated muscles distal to the supinator, (2) segmental delay or complete block of motor nerve conduction velocites at the level of the radial head if the motor response is intact, and (3) intact radial sensory nerve response.[34]

Lesions of the Superficial Sensory Branch of the Radial Nerve

Pathology

Isolated lesions of the superficial radial sensory nerve can occur with compression or trauma to the dorsal radial forearm.

Clinical Examination and Findings

1. Sensory loss of the dorsal radial hand
2. No motor loss
3. No loss of deep tendon reflexes
4. Possible Tinel's sign over the radial sensory nerve
5. Normal EMG
6. NCV studies may show (1) delay or absence of radial sensory distal latency and (2) decreased amplitude of the sensory response if it is intact.[35]

Rehabilitation
Pain Management
1. The use of therapeutic modalities such as heat, cold and TENS can be helpful.
2. Caution must be exercised if using such modalities over desensate areas.

3. Soft tissue mobilization of scar tissue should be performed if present.

ROM Exercises. Passive to active ROM exercises should be started to maintain the mobility of the elbow, wrist and fingers. Specific attention should be placed on wrist and finger motions using both gross and component motion techniques. Be aware that exercise progression may be limited secondary to surgical repair of injured nerve and/or bones and tendons.

Strengthening Exercises
1. Strengthening exercises should begin as soon as voluntary contraction becomes possible.
2. Exercises should be directed at those muscles demonstrating clinical weakness. The pattern of weakness will vary depending on the level of the radial nerve injury.
3. Early strengthening may be facilitated by the use of electrical stimulation.
4. Functional motions to be stressed are elbow extension, wrist extension, and finger/thumb extension.
5. Care should be taken to avoid fatigue.

Maintaining Muscle Contractility. Electrical stimulation may be employed to maintain muscle contractility and to delay disuse or denervation atrophy. The stimulation parameters will depend on the electrical evidence concerning the innervation or denervation of the muscle.

Limb Protection
1. Fit with wrist/finger extension splint. Splint can be static or dynamic, holding the wrist and fingers in mild extension (Fig. 2-8).

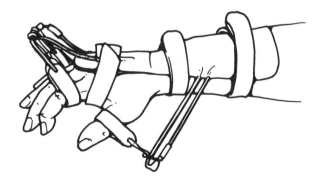

Fig. 2-8 Example of a dynamic wrist splint used for radial nerve palsies.

2. Counsel the patient to avoid heavy lifting with the involved extremity.
3. High velocity elbow flexion motions should be avoided with high level radial nerve injuries.
4. Educate the patient concerning their vulnerability to injury secondary to hand sensory deficit.
5. Activities that reproduce symptoms (resisted wrist extension or forearm supination) should be avoided.

Median Nerve Lesions

The median nerve is subject to many forms of injury/compression along its course. The most common sites of injury are in the upper arm, at the elbow, in the forearm, and at the wrist.

Upper Arm Lesions of the Median Nerve
Pathology
The median nerve can be injured in the upper arm by shoulder dislocations, humeral fractures, trauma, and compression-type injuries (tight rifle slings and improper axillary crutch use.

Clinical Examination and Findings
1. Weakness or loss of function of all median nerve innervated musculature including the pronator teres
2. Sensory loss in median nerve distribution including the thenar eminence
3. Atrophy of median nerve innervated forearm and thenar musculature
4. Functional loss of thumb oppositon, index finger flexion, distal thumb flexion, radial wrist flexion, and forearm pronation
5. Possible Tinel's sign along median nerve in upper arm
6. Deep tendon reflexes of triceps, brachioradialis, and biceps intact
7. Hand posture may demonstrate slight hyperextension of the MCP joints of the index and long fingers. The thumb will be held beside the index finger
8. EMG examination may show (1) positive sharp waves and fibrillation potentials in all median nerve innervated muscles and (2) decreased or absent interference patterns of voluntary

motor units in all median innervated muscles distal to and including the pronator teres.

9. NCV study may show (1) decreased or absent median nerve innervated muscle responses, (2) decreased or absent median nerve sensory response, and (3) segmentally delayed or complete block of motor nerve conduction velocity at the site of the arm lesion if motor response is present.

Lesions of the Median Nerve at or about the Elbow

Pathology

The most common cause of a median nerve entrapment syndrome at the elbow is the pronator teres syndrome. An additional entrapment syndrome is caused by the ligament of Struthers. Other causes of median nerve lesions at the elbow include distal humeral fractures, proximal radius or ulna fractures, and soft tissue trauma.

Clinical Examination and Findings of the Pronator Teres Syndrome

1. Weakness or loss of function of median nerve innervated musculature distal to the pronator teres. (Entrapment by the ligament of Struthers would cause weakness in the pronator teres.)
2. Sensory loss in the median nerve distribution including the thenar eminence
3. Functional loss or deficit of thumb opposition, radial wrist flexion, distal thumb flexion, and index finger flexion. Forearm pronation is functionally intact, although it may be weak (no pronator quadratus)
4. Symptoms worse with resisted forearm pronation[36]
5. Tenderness over the pronator teres
6. Atrophy of thenar eminence and median innervated forearm muscles distal to the pronator teres
7. Deep tendon reflexes of biceps, triceps, and brachioradialis intact
8. Posturing of the hand the same as with high median nerve lesions
9. Possible Tinel's sign over the pronator teres
10. EMG examination may show (1) positive sharp waves and fibrillation potentials in all

median nerve innervated muscles distal to the pronator teres and (2) decreased or absent interference patterns of voluntary motor units in all median innervated muscles distal to the pronator teres

11. NCV study may show (1) decreased or absent median nerve innervated muscle responses distal to the pronator teres, (2) decreased or absent median nerve sensory response, and (3) segmentally delayed or complete block of motor nerve conduction velocity at the site of the lesion if motor response present.[37]

Lesions of the Anterior Interosseous Nerve

Pathology

The anterior interosseous nerve is subject to compression from many sources including the deep head of the pronator teres, multiple accessory or variant muscles, enlarged bursa, and unusual vasculature. Of course injury can occur from trauma, and occasionally brachial plexus lesions can manifest as anterior interosseous lesions.[38,39]

Clinical Examination and Findings

1. Weakness or loss of function of flexor pollicis longus, flexor digitorum profundus to the index and long fingers, and the pronator quadratus
2. No sensory loss
3. May have visible atrophy with hollowing of distal radial volar forearm
4. Inability to make a zero with thumb and index finger (Fig. 2-9)
5. Patient may give history of proximal forearm pain of recent onset and short duration
6. Deep tendon reflexes for biceps, brachioradialis, and triceps intact.
7. EMG examination may show (1) positive sharp waves and fibrillation potentials in the anterior interosseous nerve innervated musculature, and (2) decreased or absent interference patterns of voluntary motor units in the anterior interosseous nerve innervated musculature.
8. NCV study may show (1) decreased or absent motor responses of the anterior interosseous innervated musculature, (2) anterior interosseous motor nerve distal latency may be

Fig. 2-9 Finger position assumed by patients with anterior interosseous nerve palsies when trying to make a zero with thumb and index finger.

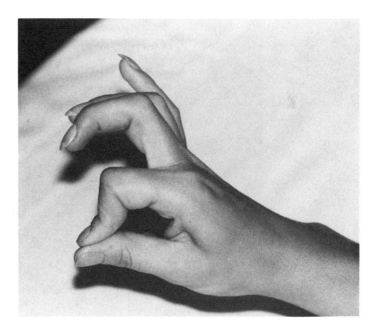

delayed or absent, (3) normal median nerve sensory response, and (4) normal median motor nerve conduction velocity to the thenar muscles.

Lesions of the Median Nerve at the Wrist

Median nerve lesions at the wrist can occur as a result of distal radius or ulna fractures and trauma. The most common cause is carpal tunnel syndrome (CTS), which will be used as the example of the median nerve lesion.

Pathology
CTS is an entrapment of the median nerve as it passes through the carpal tunnel, being accompanied by the nine finger flexor tendons. This crowded arrangement can be complicated by any tissue inflammatory condition, wrist joint abnormality, or space-occupying lesion leading to median nerve compression.

Clinical Examination and Findings
1. Complaints of paresthesias, numbness, pain and/or weakness in the first three fingers of the hand
2. Patient may describe pain as radiating up the arm to the elbow and occasionally the shoulder
3. Symptoms worse when sleeping, driving, or when using hand while typing, etc.
4. Symptoms relieved by shaking hand or dangling hand and working the fingers
5. Weakness or loss of function of thumb opposition and to a lesser degree thumb abduction
6. Sensory loss to the fingers in a median nerve distribution. Intact sensation over the thenar eminence
7. Positive Phalen's test (Fig. 2-10)
8. Possible Tinel's sign over the carpal tunnel
9. Atrophy of the thenar eminence
10. Deep tendon reflexes of the biceps, brachioradialis, and triceps intact
11. EMG testing may demonstrate (1) fibrillation potentials and positive sharp waves in the median nerve innervated thenar muscles and (2) decreased or absent interference patterns of voluntary motor units in the median innervated hand intrinsics[40]
12. NCV studies may demonstrate (1) decreased amplitude of the thenar muscle response, (2)

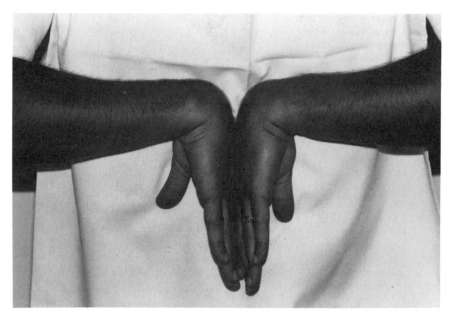

Fig. 2-10 Phalen's test. Wrists held in maximal flexion attempting to reproduce symptoms of median nerve compression at the wrist.

prolonged distal motor latencies when stimulating the median nerve at the wrist, (3) decreased amplitude of median nerve sensory responses to the fingers, (4) prolonged sensory distal latencies when stimulating the median nerve at the wrist, and (5) normal motor conduction velocities of the median nerve above the wrist.

Rehabilitation
Pain management
1. Use of heat, cold, and/or TENS may assist in pain relief.
2. For patients with CTS, contrast baths can be helpful.
3. A wrist resting splint will assist the patient with CTS by maintaining the wrist in the neutral position. The splint should be worn when doing activities that cause symptoms or when sleeping at night.
4. Soft tissue mobilization is appropriate for post-traumatic or surgical scars.

ROM Exercises
1. Passive to active exercises should be prescribed for the elbow, wrist, and fingers.

2. For complete nerve lesions graded articulations of the wrist and first three digits may prove helpful.
3. In conditions caused by entrapment, the ROM exercises should be structured to avoid reproducing symptoms. For CTS, avoid extremes of wrist flexion and extension. For the pronator teres syndrome avoide extremes of forearm supination with elbow extension.

Strengthening Exercises
1. Begin strengthening exercises as soon as there is evidence of voluntary muscle activity.
2. The motions to be stressed functionally are forearm pronation, radial wrist flexion, finger flexion (digits I-III), plus thumb abduction and opposition. The actual distribution of clinical weakness will dictate the motions to be strengthened.
3. For early strengthening, electrical stimulation may be helpful.
4. Avoid fatigue and overstretching of the weak musculature.

Maintaining Muscle Contractility. Electrical stimulation can be used to help maintain muscle fiber contractility and delay disuse of denervation

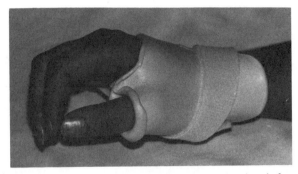

Fig. 2-11 Thenar splint to help stabilize the thumb for patients with median nerve injuries.

atrophy. The electrical parameters will vary according to the electrical evidence concerning the muscle's degree of denervation.

Limb Protection

1. The CTS patient should use wrist splints during activity and at night.
2. Counseling patients to avoid traumatic injuries to the first three digits secondary to diminished sensation.
3. Fit patient with functional splint to hold the thumb in abduction. This compensates for the unopposed action of the extensor pollicis longus and adductor pollicis (Fig. 2-11).

Ulnar Nerve Lesions

The ulnar nerve can be subjected to many forms of trauma, injury, and compression along its entire course. The most common sites of nerve injury are in the upper arm, at the elbow, and as it crosses the wrist.

Injuries of the Ulnar Nerve in the Upper Arm

Pathology

The ulnar nerve can be injured in the upper arm by humeral fractures, trauma and compression forces.

Clinical Examination and Findings

1. Patient will demonstrate weakness or loss of function of all ulnar nerve innervated musculature

2. Functional loss of finger abduction and adduction in digits II-V, loss of DIP flexion in digits IV-V, and loss of ulnar wrist flexion
3. Sensory loss in the entire ulnar nerve distribution
4. Mild claw attitude of the hand (Fig. 2-12)
5. Atrophy of ulnar innervated hand intrinsics and ulnar forearm musculature
6. Deep tendon reflexes of biceps, brachioradialis, and triceps intact
7. Positive Froment's sign. Inability to pinch using the adductor pollicis and first dorsal interossei. Patient will substitute and use the flexor pollicis longus (Fig. 2-13).
8. Possible Tinel's sign over ulnar nerve along the upper arm
9. EMG examination may show (1) fibrillation potentials and positive sharp waves in all ulnar nerve innervated musculature, and (2) decreased or absent voluntary motor unit interference patterns in all muscles innervated by the ulnar nerve.
10. NCV studies may show (1) decreased amplitudes or no responses from ulnar nerve innervated musculature, (2) diminished or

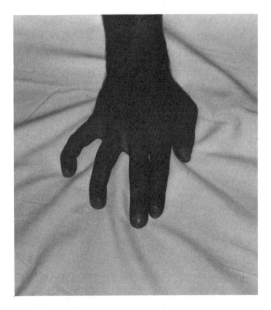

Fig. 2-12 Ulnar claw. Resting posture of the hand for patients with ulnar nerve lesions. This posture is most severe in patients with lesions of the ulnar nerve at the wrist.

Fig. 2-13 Froment's sign. **(A)** Normal lateral pinch between the thumb and index finger. **(B)** Patient with an ulnar nerve lesion will substitute the long thumb flexor for the weak thumb adductor and the first dorsal interosseous.

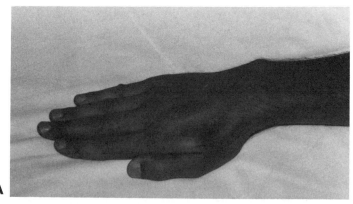

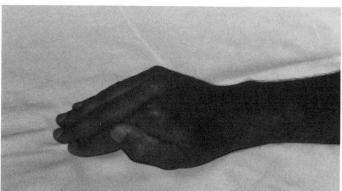

absent ulnar nerve sensory responses, and (3) segmental delay or complete blocking of motor nerve conduction velocity at the site of the arm lesion if motor response intact.

Lesions of the Ulnar Nerve at or about the Elbow

The ulnar nerve is subject to many forms of injury at the elbow level including distal humerus fractures, proximal ulna fractures, and soft tissue trauma. Many forms of entrapment within the cubital tunnel also cause these lesions[36] and will be described in this section.

Pathology

Entrapment of the ulnar nerve in the cubital tunnel as it passes under the aponeurosis connecting the two heads of the flexor carpi ulnaris may be the most common cause of compression. The compressive forces may be of an acute or chronic nature, frequently associated with an occupational cause.

Clinical Examination and Findings

1. Complaints of constant or intermittent sensory loss or paresthesias in the entire ulnar nerve distribution
2. Weakness or loss of function of the flexor digitorum profundis to digits IV and V, the anterior and dorsal interossei, the hypothenar muscles, and the lumbricals of digits IV and V
3. Functional loss of finger abduction, finger adduction, and DIP flexion of digits IV and V
4. Sparing of the flexor carpi ulnaris
5. Sensory loss in entire ulnar nerve distribution
6. Intact deep tendon reflexes of the biceps, brachioradialis, and triceps
7. Positive Froment's sign
8. Possible Tinel's sign at the elbow
9. Hand may demonstrate a mild claw position
10. EMG examination may show (1) fibrillation potentials and positive sharp waves in all muscles innervated by the ulnar nerve distal

to the flexor carpi ulnaris and (2) decreased or absent voluntary motor unit interference patterns in all muscles innervated by the ulnar nerve distal to the flexor carpi ulnaris.

11. NCV studies may show (1) decreased amplitudes or no responses from ulnar nerve innervated musculature distal to the flexor carpi ulnaris, (2) diminished or absent ulnar nerve sensory responses, and (3) segmental delay or complete blocking of motor nerve conduction velocity at the site of elbow compression if motor response intact.

Ulnar Nerve Lesions at the Wrist

Pathology

Compression of the ulnar nerve in Guyon's canal (depression between the pisiform and the hook of the hamate) may present with either mixed motor and sensory symptoms or with isolated motor or sensory deficits. Injury to the ulnar nerve can be secondary to fractures of the hamate or pisiform, soft tissue trauma, and acute or chronic occupational compressive forces.[41]

Clinical Examination and Findings

1. Sensory loss if present, will be restricted to the ulnar palm, volar surface of the V digit and ulnar half of the digit IV. Dorsal hand and dorsal finger V sensation will be spared.
2. Motor loss is restricted to the ulnar nerve innervated hand intrinsic musculature and may present as affecting only the deep branch and/or the hypothenar muscles.
3. Marked hand posturing or ulnar claw
4. Tinel's sign at wrist
5. Positive Froment's sign
6. Functional loss of thumb adduction, finger abduction, and finger adduction
7. Visible atrophy of ulnar innervated hand intrinsics
8. Intact function of ulnar innervated flexor digitorum profundis and flexor carpi ulnaris
9. EMG examination may show (1) fibrillation potentials and positive sharp waves in the ulnar nerve innervated hand intrinsics and (2) decreased or absent voluntary motor unit interference patterns in the ulnar nerve innervated hand intrinsic muscles.
10. NCV studies may show (1) decreased amplitudes or no responses from ulnar nerve innervated hand intrinsic musculature, (2) diminished or absent ulnar nerve sensory finger responses, (3) spared dorsal ulnar cutaneous sensory response, and (4) delayed distal motor latency if motor response intact.

Rehabilitation

Pain Management

1. Use of heat, cold, and/or TENS can be beneficial.
2. For lesions at the wrist, contrast baths may be beneficial.
3. Wrist splints are indicated for lesions at the wrist.
4. For ulnar nerve lesions at the elbow, elbow pads may prove helpful.
5. Soft tissue mobilization to traumatic or surgical scars is indicated.

ROM Exercises

1. Begin immediately to preserve elbow, wrist, and finger mobility.
2. Traditional exercises may be passive to active in nature.
3. In complete lesions, isolated articulations of the wrist and fingers may be beneficial.
4. Progression of exercises may depend on the presence of other pathologies, such as bone or tendon injuries.

Strengthening Exercises

1. Exercise should begin as soon as there is voluntary muscular activity.
2. Functional motions to be stressed are ulnar wrist flexion, finger abduction, finger adduction, and finger flexion of digits IV and V. The actual muscles to be strengthened will depend upon the level of the lesion and the presentation of clinical weakness.
3. Electrical stimulation may be helpful in early strengthening.
4. Avoid overstress-type injuries and muscle fatigue.
5. Program progression may be limited secondary to additional trauma, such as fractures and tendon repairs.

Maintaining Muscle Contractility. The use of electrical stimulation may maintain muscle fiber

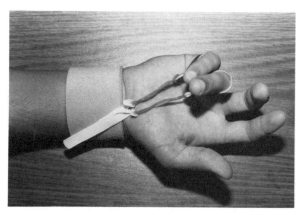

Fig. 2-14 Example of a splint designed to help minimize the hyperextension of the MCP joints of patients with ulnar nerve lesions.

contractility and help delay disuse or denervation atrophy. The electrical parameters needed will depend on the muscle's state of innervation or denervation.

Limb Protection

1. Counseling to avoid injury to desensate areas
2. Use of elbow pads for ulnar nerve lesions at the elbow
3. Wrist splint for ulnar nerve injuries at the wrist
4. Use of a hand splint to compensate for the unopposed pull of the extensor digitorum. Because of the loss of lumbrical function, the MCP joints of digits IV and V are pulled into varying degrees of hyperextension (Fig. 2-14).
5. Counseling the patient on the possible occupational/postural conditions that may aggravate ulnar nerve compressions at the wrist or elbow.

LOWER EXTREMITY PERIPHERAL NERVE LESIONS

Localizing neurological lesions in the lower extremities is not quite as difficult as localizing lesions in the upper extremities primarily because of fewer common entrapment sites and a less complex sensory distribution.

Generalized Screening Examination

A general screening examination is recommended for all patients presenting with complaints of pain,

numbness, paresthesias, or motor loss that involves the back and or lower extremities. After a detailed patient history is obtained, the initial screening examination should include

1. Gait analysis
2. Postural observation
3. Active ROM of the lower extremities
4. ROM of the trunk
5. Manual muscle testing of the lower extremities. This can test major functions rather than isolated muscles.
6. Sensory examination with light touch
7. Deep tendon reflexes of the quadriceps, gastrocsoleus, and possibly the posterior tibialis

Specialized Screening Examination

Based on the patient's history and the results of the screening examination, a more detailed examination with special tests can be started.

1. Specific manual muscle testing should follow a peripheral nerve and/or a myotomal pattern.
2. Specific sensory examination using different modalities could include sharp, dull, vibration, and proprioception testing. The sensory testing should follow a peripheral nerve and/or a dermatomal distribution (see Fig. 4-2 of Ch. 4).
3. Specific palpation of appropriate joints, vertebral segments, and soft tissue structures.
4. Other special tests include flexion abduction and external rotation (FABER), straight leg raising (SLR), and sacroiliac (SI) joint compression.[20]

Lumbosacral Radiculopathies

Pathology

Injuries to the lumbar and sacral nerve roots can occur with a wide variety of pathologies. Vertebral fractures, herniated intervertebral discs, degenerative joint disease, metastatic disease, pelvic or sacral fractures, and diabetic neuropathies have all been implicated in injury to the lumbosacral roots. Typically injury to the nerve root will cause well-delineated sensory and motor deficits in a dermatomal and myotomal distribution. When dealing with root level pathology, the sensory pattern may better localize the lesion because the lower extremity muscles frequently have heavy segmental supplies from multiple root levels.[42,43]

Clinical Examination and Findings

The clinical findings for the most common lower extremity radiculopathies are summarized in the following sections.

L4 Root Lesion

1. Motor deficit most noticeable in the quadriceps and anterior tibialis
2. Sensory deficit along medial lower leg to the medial great toe
3. Pain radiating to the great toe
4. Loss or decrease of quadriceps deep tendon reflex
5. Possible positive femoral nerve stretch test
6. Gait may demonstrate foot drop on the involved side or knee hyperextension during stance phase
7. Posture may show lateral shift

L5 Root Lesion

1. Motor deficit most noticeable in the extensor hallucis longus, posterior tibialis, anterior tibialis, and gluteus medius
2. Sensory loss over the dorsum of the foot
3. Pain radiating down lateral leg and onto the dorsal foot
4. May have loss of posterior tibialis deep tendon reflex
5. May have positive sitting and supine straight leg raise test
6. Gait may demonstrate gluteus medius limp or foot drop
7. Posture may show a lateral shift

S1 Root Lesion

1. Motor deficit most noticeable in the gastrocsoleus, flexor hallucis longus, and gluteus maximus
2. Sensory loss along the lateral foot to small toe
3. Pain radiating down posterior leg to little toe
4. Loss or decrease in the gastrocsoleus deep tendon reflex
5. May have positive sitting or supine straight leg raise test
6. Gait may demonstrate decreased toe off on the involved side
7. Posture may show lateral shift

8. EMG is useful in localizing the level and extent of the neurological lesion but does not provide information about the cause of the lesion. Studies will typically show reduced voluntary motor unit interference patterns in early disease restricted to a myotomal distribution. With symptoms of greater than 3 weeks' duration fibrillation potentials, positive sharp waves, and polyphasic motor units of increased or normal amplitude may be found in a myotomal distribution including the paraspinal musculature.
9. NCV studies generally show (1) normal motor nerve conductions, (2) decreased motor response amplitude in clinically weak muscles, and (3) normal sensory responses, an important differentiating point between root lesions and lesions distal to the dorsal root ganglia. Evaluation of "H" reflex latencies may be of value in S1 radiculopathies.

Rehabilitation

Many techniques are available to the physical therapist for treating patients with lumbar radiculopathies. Goals for treatments include pain relief, postural correction, strengthening of weak musculature, and back care education.

Pain Relief

1. Cryotherapy is often very effective in the acute stages or in those injuries cause by trauma.
2. Heating modalities, such as infrared radiation, short wave diathermy, and ultrasound, have been demonstrated to be beneficial in the treatment of pain.
3. Varying types and frequencies of TENS can be used.
4. Certain mobilization and muscle energy techniques are appropriate.
5. Pelvic traction can be used with either constant or intermittent pull in the prone or supine position.
6. The importance of proper bed rest during the acute stage should be stressed.

Postural Correction

1. Mobilization or muscle energy techniques (see orthopaedic section of this text)

2. Specific exercises to relax, stretch and/or strengthen the trunk, pelvic, and lower extremity musculature
3. EMG biofeedback
4. Counseling concerning activities of daily living, sitting, standing, and resting positions

Strengthening Exercises

Specific strengthening of weak extremity musculature may have to wait until the acute pain has resolved. Strengthening exercises should be structured initially to stress the involved muscles. As the patient improves, the exercise program should be progressed to include endurance-type exercises, the ultimate goal being to return to unrestricted activity.

Femoral Nerve Lesions

Pathology

The femoral nerve is subject to injury from penetrating wounds, soft tissue trauma, severe pelvic trauma, retroperitoneal hematomas, femur fractures, and diabetic neuropathy.[44] When dealing with a suspected femoral nerve lesion, be aware that the lesion may be more proximal in the lumbar plexus. The following sections outline the examination and rehabilitation for femoral nerve compression at or about the inguinal ligament.

Clinical Examination and Findings

1. Tendency to hyperextend knee to increase stance stability
2. Sensory loss over the anteromedial aspect of thigh, leg, and foot
3. Weak hip flexor strength and absent or weak quadriceps strength
4. Absent or diminished quadriceps deep tendon reflex
5. Functional loss of knee extension. If hip flexion is extremely weakened, be suspicious of a lesion in the lumbar plexus.
6. Atrophy of quadriceps
7. EMG examination may show (1) fibrillation potentials and positive sharp waves in the quadriceps muscles and (2) diminished or absent interference patterns of voluntary motor units in the quadriceps.

8. NCV studies may show (1) motor responses to be reduced in amplitude or absent in the femoral nerve innervated muscles, (2) delay or complete block of the motor conduction velocity across the inguinal ligament, and (3) saphenous sensory response decreased in amplitude or absent.

Rehabilitation

Pain Management

1. Heat, cold, massage and/or TENS can be helpful in controlling pain.
2. A cane or crutches can be used if pain occurs with ambulation.

ROM Exercises

Passive to active ROM exercises should be started immediately. Emphasis should be placed on hip and knee motions.

Strengthening Exercises

1. Begin exercises as soon as the patient demonstrates voluntary muscle activity.
2. Functional motions to be stressed include hip flexion, knee extension, and hip external rotation.
3. Electrical stimulation may be beneficial in the early stages.
4. The use of bicycling with toe clips can strengthen both the hip flexors and the knee extensors.

Maintaining Muscle Contractility

Electrical stimulation can maintain muscle contractility and delay the effects of disuse or denervation atrophy. The electrical parameters will vary depending on the state of muscle innervation or denervation.

Limb Protection

1. Cane or crutches as needed
2. Caution patient to be aware of knee stability while weight bearing on the involved side.
3. Caution patient concerning their loss of sensation.

Sciatic Nerve Lesions

Pathology

The sciatic nerve can be injured by pelvic fractures, hip fractures, femoral shaft fractures, pelvic neoplastic disease, hip surgery, and compression syndromes such as the pyriformis syndrome. The following sections outline the examination and rehabilitation for sciatic nerve lesions of the proximal thigh.

Clinical Examination and Findings

1. Weakness or loss of function of hamstrings and distal tibial and/or peroneal nerve innervated musculature
2. Loss of sensation over dorsal, lateral, and plantar foot
3. Diminished or absent gastrocsoleus and posterior tibial deep tendon reflexes.
4. Functional loss of knee flexion, ankle dorsi/plantar flexion, ankle inversion/eversion, and toe flexion/extension.
5. Gait deficits may include a drop foot with a high steppage gait and decreased toe off.
6. EMG examination may show (1) fibrillation potentials and positive sharp waves in the hamstrings and all muscles in the tibial and peroneal nerve distributions and (2) diminished or absent interference patterns of voluntary motor units in the hamstrings and in all muscles in the tibial and peroneal nerve distributions.
7. NCV studies may show (1) motor responses reduced in amplitude or absent in the tibial and/or peroneal nerve innervated muscles, (2) delay or complete block of the motor conduction velocity across the site of the lesion, and (3) tibial and peroneal sensory responses absent or decreased in amplitude.

Rehabilitation

Pain Management

1. Use of heat, cold, massage, and/or TENS. Caution should be exercised when using the above modalities over desensate areas.
2. Leg elevation and the use of support hose to assist in venous return.
3. Use of cane or crutches if ambulation is painful.

ROM Exercises

1. Begin immediately to maintain hip, knee, ankle, and toe mobility.

2. May need to provide patient with prolonged gentle stretches for the hamstrings and heelcords.
3. Resting ankle splints may help with bed positioning.

Strengthening Exercises

1. Begin as soon as there is evidence of voluntary muscle activity.
2. Functional motions to be stressed are knee flexion, ankle dorsi/plantar flexion, ankle inversion/eversion, and toe flexion/extension. The actual muscles that need strengthening will depend on the pattern of clinical weakness.
3. Electrical stimulation may be used as an early form of strengthening.
4. Be careful to avoid overstress injuries.

Maintaining Muscle Contractility

1. The use of electrical stimulation may maintain muscle fiber contractility and help delay disuse or denervation atrophy.
2. Electrical parameters needed will vary depending on the status of muscle innervation or denervation.
3. Electrical stimulation may not be practical, depending on the severity and level of the sciatic nerve lesion.

Limb Protection

1. Use of an ankle foot orthosis or double upright lower leg brace
2. Use of a cane or crutches if needed
3. Counsel patient to exercise caution when ambulating
4. Instruct patient in proper care of involved foot secondary to sensory impairment

Peroneal Nerve Lesions

Pathology

The peroneal nerve is commonly injured at the fibular head because of traumatic or compressive lesions. In sciatic nerve injuries, the peroneal portion of this nerve is often selectively involved with trauma secondary to hip fractures or dislocations. The clinical differential between sciatic nerve lesions and common peroneal nerve lesions is the involvement of the short head of the biceps femoris and possible findings of weakness in tibial nerve innervated musculature. The following sections outline the examination and rehabilitation recommendations for compression of the peroneal nerve at the fibular head.

Clinical Examination and Findings
1. Ambulation with a high steppage gait secondary to foot drop.
2. Weakness or absent function of ankle dorsiflexors, ankle everters, and toe extensors. It should be noted that patients can have lesions isolated to the deep peroneal or superficial peroneal nerves.
3. Sensory loss over the dorsal foot and/or great toe web space
4. Loss of funcitonal toe extension, ankle dorsiflexion, and ankle eversion
5. Possible Tinel's sign over the fibular head
6. EMG examination may show (1) fibrillation potentials and positive sharp waves in the muscles innervated by the deep and superficial peroneal nerves and (2) diminished or absent interference patterns of voluntary motor units in the muscles innervated by the deep and superficial peroneal nerves.
7. NCV studies may show (1) motor responses reduced in amplitude or absent in the peroneal nerve innervated muscles, (2) delay or complete block of the motor nerve conduction velocity around the fibular head, and (3) peroneal nerve sensory responses decreased in amplitude or absent.[45]

Rehabilitation

Pain Management
1. Heat, cold, massage and TENS
2. Supportive hose
3. Bracing with an ankle-foot orthosis (AFO) or more supportive brace if ankle lateral stability is a problem.

ROM Exercises
Passive to active exercises should begin as soon as possible to maintain ankle and toe mobility. An ankle resting splint may be worn at night.

Strengthening Exercises
1. Begin as soon as there is evidence of voluntary muscle activity.

2. Functional motions to be stressed include ankle dorsiflexion, ankle eversion, and toe extension.
3. Electrical stimulation may be used as an early form of strengthening exercise.
4. Avoid overstress injuries.

Maintaining Muscle Contractility
Use of electrical stimulation can maintain muscle fiber contractility and delay disuse or denervation atrophy. Electrical stimulation parameters will vary depending on the status of muscle innervation or denervation.

Limb Protection
1. Fit with a brace. An AFO is usually all that is needed to prevent foot drop while ambulating. In cases with severe lateral ankle instability, a more supportive brace should be considered.
2. Counsel patient to avoiding positions that may compress the nerve as it crosses the fibular head. These can include sitting cross-legged, sleeping with the legs externally rotated, and leaning the leg against the car door while driving.
3. Instruct the patient in proper foot care.

Posterior Tibial Nerve Injuries

Pathology

The posterior tibial nerve is most commonly injured at the ankle by entrapment in the tarsal tunnel. More proximal lesions may occur at the posterior knee by severe fractures of the distal femur or proximal tibia, knee dislocations, and soft tissue trauma in the popliteal fossa.

Posterior Tibial Nerve Lesions at the Knee

Clinical Examination and Findings
1. Gait may demonstrate lack of toe off
2. Weakness of or loss of function of the gastrocsoleus, posterior tibialis, and toe flexors
3. Loss of gastrocsoleus and posterior tibialis deep tendon reflex.
4. Sensory loss over plantar surface and lateral border of the foot.
5. Functional loss of ankle plantar flexion, ankle inversion, and toe flexion.

6. Atrophy of posterior calf and foot intrinsics, except the extensor digitorum brevis.
7. EMG examination may show (1) fibrillation potentials and positive sharp waves in the muscles innervated by the posterior tibial nerve and (2) diminished or absent interference patterns of voluntary motor units in the muscles innervated by the posterior tibial nerve.
8. NCV studies may show (1) motor responses reduced in amplitude or absent in the posterior tibial nerve innervated muscles, (2) delay or complete block of the motor nerve conduction velocity across the knee, and (3) medial and lateral plantar nerve sensory responses decreased in amplitude or absent.

Rehabilitation

Pain Management
1. Heat, cold, massage and/or TENS
2. Support hose
3. Lower leg brace with ankle stops if patient is having pain with ambulation

ROM Exercises. Passive to active exercise should begin immediately to maintain ankle plantar flexion, ankle inversion, and toe flexion. Mobilization of the tarsals, metatarsals, and toes may be helpful.

Strengthening Exercises
1. Start strengthening exercises as soon as there is evidence of voluntary muscle activity.
2. Functional motions to be stressed are ankle plantar flexion, ankle inversion, and toe flexion.
3. Electrical stimulation may be beneficial as an early form of strengthening.
4. Avoid overstressing the weak muscles during the strengthening exercises.

Maintaining Muscle Contractility. Use of electrical stimulation can maintain muscle fiber contractility and delay disuse or denervation atrophy. Electrical parameters will vary depending on the status of muscle innervation or denervation.

Limb Protection
1. Counsel concerning foot care and sensory deficit
2. Avoid activities that may compress the nerve

3. Fit with a brace or cane if ambulation is painful
4. Instruct in leg elevation and the use of supportive hose if vascular return is a problem

Posterior Tibial Nerve Entrapment in the Tarsal Tunnel

Pathology
The posterior tibial nerve travels through the tarsal tunnel along with the posterior tibial artery and the tendons of the tibialis posterior, flexor digitorum longus, and flexor hallicus longus. Any structural abnormalities, soft tissue swelling, or space-occupying mass can easily cause compression on the nerve in this space.

Clinical Examination and Findings
1. Weakness in foot intrinsic musculature, except the extensor digitorum brevis
2. Intact gastrocsoleus deep tendon reflex
3. Sensory loss in the medial and/or lateral plantar nerve distributions
4. Gait may be antalgic secondary to pain in toes and sole of foot
5. Possible Tinel's sign over posterior tibial nerve at medial ankle
6. Atrophy of tibial innervated foot intrinsic musculature
7. Patient may describe burning type pain in the sole of the foot, frequently worse at night
8. EMG examination may show (1) fibrillation potentials and positive sharp waves in the tibial nerve innervated foot intrinsics and (2) diminished or absent interference patterns of voluntary motor units in the foot intrinsic muscles innervated by the posterior tibial nerve.[46]
9. NCV studies may show (1) motor responses reduced in amplitude or absent in the foot intrinsic muscles innervated by the posterior tibial nerve, (2) delay or complete block of the motor nerve distal latency with stimulation proximal to the flexor retinaculum, and (3) medial and lateral plantar nerve sensory responses decreased in amplitude or absent. If these sensory responses are present they may demonstrate prolonged distal latencies.

Rehabilitation

Pain Management
1. Heat, cold and/or TENS
2. Contrast baths
3. Foot orthotic

ROM Exercises. Passive to active ankle and toe ROM exercises should be instituted to maintian mobility. Gentle mobilization of the tarsals, metatarsals and toes may prove beneficial.

Strengthening Exercises. Focus should be placed on the foot intrinsics. Electrical stimulation may be helpful in the early stages if tolerated by the patient.

Limb Protection. The patient should be counseled concerning foot care and sensory impairment. Patients should avoid foot wear that would cause compression over the medial foot/ankle.

REFERENCES

1. Thomas P: Clinical features and differential diagnosis. p. 1169. In Dyck P, Thomas P, Lambert E, Bunge R (eds): Peripheral Neuropathy. WB Saunders, Philadelphia, 1984
2. Dyck P: The causes, classifications, and treatment of peripheral neuropathy. N Engl J Med 307:283, 1982
3. Mcleod J, Tuck R, Pollard J, et al: Chronic polyneuropathy of undetermined cause. J Neurol Neurosurg Psychiatry 47:530, 1984
4. Schaumburg H, Spencer P, Thomas P: Disorders of Peripheral Nerves. FA Davis, Philadelphia, 1983
5. Fisher M: Peripheral neuropathies: a common complaint in older patients. Geriatrics 39:123, 1984
6. Thomas P: Selective vulnerability of the centrifugal and centripetal axons of primary sensory neurons. Muscle Nerve 5:S117, 1982
7. Schaumburg H, Spencer P: Toxic neuropathies. Neurology 29:429, 1979
8. Kimura J: Electrodiagnosis in Diseases of Nerve and Muscle: Principles and Practice. FA Davis, Philadelphia, 1983
9. Dyck P, Johnson W, Lambert E, et al: Segmental demyelination secondary to axonal degeneration in uremic neuropathy. Mayo Clin Proc 46:400, 1971
10. Sunderland S: Nerves and Nerve Injuries. 2nd Ed. Churchill Livingstone, London, 1978
11. Stillwell K: Therapeutic heat and cold. p. 259. In Krusen F (ed): Handbook of Physical Medicine and Rehabilitation. 2nd Ed. WB Saunders, Philadelphia, 1971
12. Stillwell G: Rehabilitative procedures. p. 2303. In Dyck P, Thomas P, Lambert E, Bunge R (eds): Peripheral Neuropathy. 2nd Ed. Vol. 2. WB Saunders, Philadelphia, 1984
13. Thomas P, Eliason S: Diabetic neuropathy. p. 1773. In Dyck P, Thomas P, Lambert E, Bunge R (eds): Peripheral Neuropathy. 2nd Ed. Vol. 2. WB Saunders, Philadelphia, 1984
14. Herbison G, Jaweed M, Ditunno J: Exercise therapies in peripheral neuropathies. Arch Phys Med Rehabil 64:201, 1983
15. Cummings J: Conservative management of peripheral nerve injuries utilizing selective electrical stimulation of denervated muscle with exponentially progressive current forms. Journal of Orthopaedic and Sports Physical Therapy 7:1, 1985
16. Arnason B: Acute inflammatory demyelinating polyradiculoneuropathies. p. 2050. In Dyck P, Lambert E, Bunge R (eds): Peripheral Neuropathy. 2nd Ed. Vol. 2. WB Saunders, Philadelphia, 1984
17. Goodgold J, Eberstein A: Electrodiagnosis of Neuromuscular Diseases. 3rd Ed. Williams & Wilkins, Baltimore, 1983
18. Wu Y, Kunz R, Putnam T, et al: Axillary F central latency: simple electrodiagnostic technique for proximal neuropathy. Arch Phys Med Rehab 64:117, 1983
19. Ballantyne J, Hansen S: A quantitative assessment of reinnervation in polyneuropathies. Muscle Nerve 5:S127, 1982
20. Hoppenfeld S: Physical Examination of the Spine and Extremities. Appleton-Century-Crofts, New York, 1976
21. Cyriax J, Cyriax P: Illustrative Manual of Orthopaedic Medicine. Butterworths, London, 1983
22. Benetto M, Markey K: Electrodiagnostic localization of traumatic upper trunk brachial plexopathy. Arch Phys Med Rehabil 65:15, 1984
23. Smith B, Ramakrishna T, Schlagenhauff R: Familial brachial neuropathy. Two case reports with discussion. Neurology 21:941, 1971
24. Weikers N, Mattson R: Acute paralytic brachial neuritis. A clinical and electrodiagnostic study. Neurology 19:1153, 1969
25. Warren J, Gutmann L, Figueroa A, et al: Electromyographic changes of brachial plexus root avulsions. J Neurosurg 31:137, 1969
26. Jaeger S, Read R, Smullens S, et al: Thoracic outlet syndrome: diagnosis and treatment. p. 378. In Hunter J, Schneider L, Mackin E, Callahan A (eds): Rehabilitation of the Hand. 2nd Ed. CV Mosby, St. Louis, 1984
27. Smith K: The thoracic outlet syndrome: a protocol of treatment. JOSPT 1:89, 1979
28. Skurja M, Munlox J: Case studies: the suprascapular nerve and shoulder dysfunction. JOSPT 6:254, 1985
29. Trojaborg W: Motor and sensory conduction in the musculocutaneous nerve. J Neurol Neurosurg Psychiatry 39:890, 1976

30. Spindler H, Felsenthal G: Sensory conduction in the musculocutaneous nerve. Arch Phys Med Rehabil 59:20, 1978

31. Duncan A, Lotze M, Gerber L, et al: Incidence, recovery, and management of serratus anterior muscle palsy after axillary node dissection. JAPTA 63:1243, 1983

32. Berry H, Bril V: Axillary nerve palsy following blunt trauma to the shoulder region: a clinical and electrophysiological review. J Neurol Neurosurg Psychiatry 45:1027, 1982

33. Pasila M, Jarola H, Kiviluoto O, et al: Early complications of primary shoulder dislocations. Acta Orthop Scand 49:260, 1978

34. DiBendetto M: Posterior interosseus branch of the radial nerve: conduction velocities. Arch Phys Med Rehabil 63:266, 1982

35. Echternach J, Levy F: Evaluation of sensory nerve conduction velocity testing of the superficial radial nerve. JAPTA 65:470, 1985

36. Spinner M: Injuries to the Major Branches of Peripheral Nerves of the Forearm. 2nd Ed. WB Saunders, Philadelphia, 1978

37. Wertsch J, Melvin J: Median nerve anatomy and entrapment syndromes: a review. Arch Phys Med Rehabil 63:623, 1982

38. Nakano K, Lundergan C, Okihero M: Anterior interosseous nerve syndromes. Arch Neurol 34:477, 1977

39. Rennels G, Ochoa J: Neuralgic amyotrophy manifesting as anterior interosseous nerve palsy. Muscle Nerve 3:160, 1980

40. Buchthal F, Rosenflack A, Trojaborg W: Electrophysiological findings in entrapment of the median nerve at wrist and elbow. J Neurol Neurosurg Psychiatry 37:340, 1974

41. Liveson J, Spielholz N: Peripheral Neurology Case Studies in Electrodiagnosis. FA Davis, Philadelphia, 1979

42. Subramony S, Wilbourne A: Radicular derivation of sensory action potentials in lower extremity. Arch Phys Med Rehabil 62:590, 1981

43. Johnson E, Fletcher R: Lumbosacral radiculopathy: review of 100 consecutive cases. Arch Phys Med Rehabil 62:321, 1981

44. Dawson D, Hallett M, Millender L: Entrapment Neuropathies. Little, Brown, and Company, Boston, 1983

45. Izzo K, Sridhara C, Rosenholtz H, et al: Sensory conduction studies of the branches of the superficial peroneal nerve. Arch Phys Med Rehabil 62:24, 1981

46. Fu R, DeLisa J, Kraft G: Motor nerve latencies through the tarsal tunnel in normal adult subjects: standard determinations corrected for temperature and distance. Arch Phys Med Rehabil 61:243, 1980

3 Multiple Sclerosis

Mary Jo Given

CHARACTERISTICS OF MULTIPLE SCLEROSIS

Pathology

Multiple sclerosis is a chronic, progressive, demyelinating disease of the central nervous system. It is named for the formation of disseminated scarlike lesions primarily in the central white matter of the brain and spinal cord. These plaques are commonly found in the regions of the optic tracts, third and fourth ventricles, basal ganglia, midbrain, pons, and spinal cord.[1]

The pathological process of the acute lesion is characterized by phagocytosis of the degenerating myelin and oligodendroglial cells. Inflammation and edema are present. Infiltration of lymphocytes and plasma cells occur especially along central venules. Gliosis follows this process with the formation of the plaque.[1]

Epidemiology

The onset of clinical symptoms of multiple sclerosis occurs between the ages of 10 and 50 years in approximately 95 percent of patients. The frequency of multiple sclerosis is slightly greater in females than males with a ratio of three to two.[3] The frequency of multiple sclerosis is significantly greater in whites than in nonwhites, with a ratio of eight to five.[4]

The incidence of multiple sclerosis worldwide is correlated with geographic latitude.[4] The high incidence regions where more than 30 cases per 100,000 are reported are located along the 40° to 60° north latitude and 30° to 40° south latitude. These areas include northern United States, southern Canada, northern and central Europe, southern Scandinavia, eastern Russia, South Africa, and northwestern Australia. Regions of medium frequency with 5 to 29 cases per 100,000 include southern United States, southern Europe, The Mediterranean, northern Scandinavia, eastern Russia, southern Africa, and northwestern Australia. Low frequency areas with rates below 5 cases per 100,000 are found in northern Canada, Mexico, northern South America, northern Africa, and Asia.

The age of critical exposure to a yet unclear risk factor in the environment appears to occur before the age of 10 or 15 years. Individuals migrating between low and high risk regions after the age of 15 retain the multiple sclerosis risk level of the region of their childhood years. Individuals migrating before the age of 15 acquire some risk level of the region of their new residence.[3,4]

The frequency of multiple cases of multiple sclerosis within families averages 6 percent of the multiple sclerosis population.[4] The closer the relationships, the higher the risk among family members. The incidence of multiple sclerosis in identical monozygote twins is 25 percent, 12 percent for fraternal dizygote twins, 1 percent for siblings, 0.5 percent for parents, and 0.3 percent for other relatives.[2] Although high risk families do exist, there is no proof of a definite genetic pattern.

Before the Second World War and British troop occupation in the Faeroes, small islands north of Norway, the incidence of multiple sclerosis there was zero. In the 20 years that followed, the incidence rose to the high range, then remarkably returned to near zero.[4] A similar event was the epidemic of multiple sclerosis in Iceland after the occupation of troops during World Wars I and II.

Etiology

Although the pathogenesis of multiple sclerosis is unknown, hypotheses have been postulated based on epidemiology, virology, genetics and immunology. Geographical distribution and migration research suggests multiple sclerosis is an acquired, latent, persistent, and environmental disease compatible with a virus.[4] Epidemics of multiple sclerosis following the two world wars on the Faeroes Islands and Iceland suggest the disease is transmittable by some environmental agent.[4] Familial clustering of multiple sclerosis suggests some genetic predisposition to the disease.[3,4] There may be an alteration in genetic coding of antigens, which are expressed on the lymphocytes and involved in controlling the immune responses. In laboratory animals, lesions much like those in multiple sclerosis occur after encephalitis, with an immune reaction developing after cerebral injection with myelin basic protein.[4]

Symptoms

Symptoms and signs of multiple sclerosis are highly variable in character, intensity, and duration related to the location, size, and frequency of the lesions.[2,3,5,6] The initial symptoms in the order most commonly reported are weakness or paresthesia of one or more limbs, visual or occulomotor disturbances, ataxia and tremor, and bladder and sexual dysfunction.[3] Onset of symptoms may be sudden, within hours, or gradual, over weeks or months. Clear clinical symptoms may be preceded by vague chronic complaints of fatigue, difficulty in functioning, balance problems, walking difficulty, decreased energy, and emotional stress.

Progression of symptoms is highly variable. Symptoms may completely or partially resolve in a "remission" within days or weeks. This is characteristic of the benign form of multiple sclerosis, comprising about 25 percent of the multiple sclerosis population.[2] A relapse or exacerbation of the original symptom or the development of a new symptom may occur at an interval of months to

years after an initial attack. The average interval between exacerbations in this "relapsing-remitting" form of multiple sclerosis is 18 to 24 months.[2] This form of the disease is present in the majority of patients. Incomplete and variable recovery from successive relapses results in gradual cumulative disability. The levels of disability range from minimal and moderate to significant functional restrictions.

The "chronic-progressive" form of multiple sclerosis is characterized by progressive deterioration with limited remissions. Severe disability or death usually occurs within 5 years. This least common form of the disease is present in approximately 5 to 10 percent of patients.[2]

Individual Signs and Symptoms

Motor symptoms frequently include spasticity and weakness. Extensor plantar reflexes, ankle clonus, and deep tendon reflexes may be exaggerated. Sensory symptoms, in addition to paresthesias, numbness, and tingling, include sensations of constriction, dullness, and pain. Trigeminal neuralgia is reported in 2 percent of multiple sclerosis patients.[7] Lhermitte's sign of an electric feeling down the back to the legs on flexing the neck is present in approximately one-third of patients.[3] Blunting of cutaneous sensation and decreased position and vibration sensations are also present.

The cerebellar signs of ataxia and tremor may also be accompanied by nystagmus, dysarthria, and inability to perform rapid alternating movements. Cerebellar signs are frequently progressive and persistent and are less subject to remission.[3]

Primary dysfunction of the autonomic nervous system may include bladder, bowel, and sexual dysfunction.[3] Frequency, urgency, incontinence, and retention are present as bladder disturbances. Constipation is common in advanced disease, with upper motor neuron abnormalities noted on somatosensory evoked potentials. Erectile impotence and absence of bulbocavernosus reflex occurs in men. Sexual dysfunction in women includes loss of libido associated with decreased genital sensation and lubrication. Partial loss of thermoregulatory sweating has been reported below the face and below the waist, especially in patients with other autonomic system involvement.[3]

Visual disturbances may be present as blurring due to optic neuritis, visual field cut due to scotoma, and eye pain occasionally with generalized headache. Dissociation of eye movements may be seen as diplopia, internuclear ophthalmoplegia, or nystagmus.

Cognitive and behavioral changes of intellectual deterioration and euphoria are correlated with increased severity and longer duration of multiple sclerosis.[3] The misconception that mental changes, especially euphoria, were "very common, if not universal" probably dates back to a 1926 study of unselected patients.[2] Moderate or severe loss of intellectual function and euphoria has been reported in 20 to 25 percent of multiple sclerosis patients.[2,3] Depression, also present in about 25 percent of patients, is not correlated with duration of the illness or severity of the disability.[3]

Other symptoms encountered with multiple sclerosis less commonly are vertigo, tinnitus, deafness, facial weakness, facial pain, and seizure disorders.[7]

Diagnosis

The diagnosis of multiple sclerosis cannot be established with certainty based solely on current laboratory tests. The disease is identified by the pattern of signs and symptoms with the supporting evidence of the test results. It is essential to rule out other demyelinating, neurological, vascular, inflammatory, structural, hereditary, or neoplastic disorders. After differential diagnosis has excluded any other explanations for the neurological disorder, the diagnosis of multiple sclerosis is usually classified as definite, probable, or possible.

Definite Multiple Sclerosis

Definite multiple sclerosis is usually diagnosed on the basis of multiple lesions and multiple occurrences.[2,3,7] The neurological examination must reveal objective evidence of white matter involvement. Examination or history must indicate involvement of two or more separate lesions in the central nervous system and must confirm the occurrence of two or more episodes of neurological abnormalities lasting at least 24 hours and separated by at least 1 month or slow stepwise progression of signs and symptoms over 6 months.

Probable Multiple Sclerosis

This diagnosis is usually made on the basis of either multiple lesions or multiple occurrences. Examination reveals a documented single episode with complete or partial recovery of two or more separate lesions characteristic of white matter abnormalities. There is involvement of only one neurological sign on two or more separate episodes.

Possible Multiple Sclerosis

This diagnosis is based on a lack of objective signs. No more than one lesion can be identified. Two or more separate episodes of symptoms may occur without objective signs.

Laboratory Tests

Laboratory tests enhance the reliability of a diagnosis of clinically definitive multiple sclerosis. The cardinal disturbances, manifest in over 90 percent of patients with definite multiple sclerosis, are one or more abnormalities in the cerebral spinal fluid.[7] These include abnormalities of oligoclonal bands, elevated immunoglobulins, slightly increased protein, or mild mononuclear pleocytosis. Brain scans, using computed tomography (CT) or magnetic resonance imaging (MRI), may enable visualization of white matter lesions.[3] Visual, auditory, or somatosensory evoked potentials provide evidence of conduction abnormalities in the central nervous system, which often are present even before symptoms appear.[3]

Physician Management

The neurologist or internist coordinates treatment for the multiple sclerosis patient. Since the etiology and pathogeneses are yet unknown, medical treatments remain only tentative, directed toward a hypothetical disease process.

Adrenocorticotropic hormone (ACTH) and corticosteroids are widely administered to reduce the inflammatory process in the central nervous system. Double blind studies support the efficacy of ACTH for more rapid recovery from an acute exacerbation of the disease. Side effects include water retention, hypertension, indigestion, insomnia, infection, hemorrhage, and uncontrolled diabetes.[8] Reports on the benefits of the use of ACTH in long-term progression of multiple sclerosis have been inconclusive.[9]

Cyclophosphamide (Cytoxan) when administered with ACTH for immunosuppression in experimental treatment has produced positive results, stabilizing some patients with progressive multiple sclerosis.[10] Side effects include depressed white cell count and cystitis.[8]

Azathioprine (Imuran) has been reported to decrease the progression of multiple sclerosis in some studies but other studies were inconclusive.[8]

Cylosporine A, used for cardiac and renal transplant patients, may prove useful for multiple sclerosis patients.

Plasmapheresis has also been used to remove immune complexes for multiple sclerosis patients with inconclusive results.[8,9]

Many treatments, generally abandoned for lack of proof of their value, have been identified by the International Federation of Multiple Sclerosis Societies.[9] These include diets, vaccines, and other symptomatic treatments.

Pharmacological Agents

Pharmacological agents are directed at management of the symptoms and complications associated with multiple sclerosis. Antispasticity drugs, when carefully regulated, are used to reduce spasticity sufficiently to enable ease of movement without creating weakness or fatigue. These include baclofen, diazepam, and dantrolene sodium.[11,12]

Bladder problems may benefit from treatment with the additional anticholinergics, such as propantheline and or oxybutynin.[3,8]

Bowel dysfunction, mainly constipation, may be treated with mild laxatives.[3,8]

Education and Psychological Management

Education and psychological management of multiple sclerosis requires insightful dialogue with the patient. Informing the patient of the diagnosis of multiple sclerosis prematurely may be detrimental to the patient and affect the insurance status. In many cases where multiple sclerosis is initially suspected, the early diagnosis is never confirmed.[8] It is important for all involved with the patient to be aware of what the patient has been told. When definite multiple sclerosis is the most reasonable diagnosis, most patients are informed.

Patients should be given sufficient information to counter the overly negative image of multiple sclerosis and dispel myths about etiology and prognosis. Systematic studies show that the majority of multiple sclerosis patients remain ambulatory and have minimal shortening of life expectancy.[8]

Kurtzke's 5-year rule suggests that the degree of neurological disability at 5 years from the date of onset will be the approximate neurological function at 15 years in the majority of patients.[13]

Counseling for family planning should be provided as needed. Pregnancy has not been shown to alter the prognosis in multiple sclerosis patients.[14] Patients with multiple sclerosis do tend to have less exacerbations during the 9 months of pregnancy but catch up with more relapses in the postpartum months. The stamina required for child rearing is a greater factor to consider than the pregnancy and delivery.

Patients may wish to obtain current information on multiple sclerosis and may benefit from involvement in multiple sclerosis support groups. It is often recommended that patients join the national and local multiple sclerosis societies.[15] Information can be obtained from the National Multiple Sclerosis Society, 205 East 42nd Street, New York, 10017, USA.

MULTIPLE SCLEROSIS EVALUATION

Comprehensive evaluation provides the physical therapist with the information needed to plan an individualized treatment program for the patient. This evaluation is especially important for the management of multiple sclerosis because the disease is characterized by such high variability in nature, location, and severity of neurological signs and symptoms.

Subjective Evaluation and History

1. Identify the patient's chief concerns by questioning for the nature, location, and onset of the current problems.
2. Review the previous episodes to gain a perspective about the disease progression.

3. Review prior management to determine guidelines for current treatment. Include questions regarding exercise tolerance, heat sensitivity, and benefits or side effects of medications.
4. Review the patient's history for secondary diagnosis or special precautions before planning a fitness and rehabilitation program.
5. Get the patient's own assessment of recent and present functional abilities. Occasionally, there may be inconsistencies in the patient's or family's expectations and the real functional abilities.
6. Determine the patient's knowledge of the disease and assess expectations, goals, and needs for compatability with the condition.
7. Consider the impact of the patient's cognitive and emotional behaviors and attitudes. Note the general impressions regarding a wide range of positive and negative behaviors, such as acceptance, anger, anxiety, cooperation, coping strategies, denial, dependency, depression, euphoria, fear, independence, judgment, memory, motivation, pragmatism, problem solving, resourcefulness, safety awareness, and uncertainty.

Neuromuscular and Musculoskeletal Examination

Muscle tone, length, strength, and timing are all interrelated components of movement. Information about tone, range of motion, strength, and coordination must be combined while examining and treating the patient.

Muscle Tone

Muscle tone is examined by estimating amount of resistance to passive lengthening of the muscle at both slow and fast speeds.

Hypertonus, in the form of spasticity, is often present with multiple sclerosis. Describe the muscle group, intensity, duration, and the positions or activities that increase or decrease the tone. Particular attention should be given to long toe muscles, ankle plantar flexors and invertors, knee extensors and flexors, hip adductors, extensors, and flexors, trunk extensors, shoulder adductors, elbow, wrist, and finger flexors. The intensity of spasticity ranges from mild, which interferes with fast movements, moderate, which interferes with both slow and fast speeds, to severe, which interferes with slow movements and blocks fast movements. The lower limbs are usually more involved than the upper limbs.[3] Moderate to severe maintained lower extremity extensor spasticity may be accompanied by intermittent, involuntary flexor spasms.

Deep tendon reflexes may be exaggerated and brisk. Clonus at ankle and knee can be elicited and the beats counted. Sustained clonus may be noted. Testing positions should be consistent.

Hypotonus, in the form of a floppy or flaccid quality on passive lengthening, although uncommon, may be present in patients where cerebellar lesions predominate or where demyelinization affects the anterior and posterior horn and rami of the spinal cord. Hypotonus is more common in the upper than lower limbs. The deep tendon reflexes may also be decreased.

Range of Motion

Range of motion abnormalities are often related to abnormal muscle forces or chronic postural changes.

Hypermobility or excessive flexibility may be related to chronic abnormal postures. Particular attention should be given to spinal curves, excessive cervical and lumbar lordosis, thoracic kyphosis, knee recurvatum, and supination of the foot and ankle.

Hypomobility is frequently due to spastic antagonists and may progress to a contracture, a permanent disability. Particular attention should be given to all areas where antagonist spasticity is noted, such as toe extension, ankle dorsiflexion, knee flexion, hip abduction and extension, shoulder flexion and abduction, elbow extension and finger extension. For this reason, it may be convenient to perform the passive range of motion and tone evaluations together.

Postural abnormalities, especially those associated with chronic pain, should be evaluated. Particular attention should be given to low back pain. Weakened neck, torso, and leg musculature may result in postural changes in sitting, standing, and walking. Patients may seek treatment for their painful neck, back, weak leg, and general fatigue long before other signs of multiple sclerosis are recognized.

Muscle Strength Evaluation

Muscle strength evaluation can be performed manually, with testing devices or thorough description of observed functional abilities. The patterns of weakness in limbs and trunk commonly seen in multiple sclerosis are noted on Table 3-1. The distribution of weakness may be assymetrical, as monoplegia or hemiplegia, or present as paraplegia or quadriplegia, dependent on the scatter in locations of central nervous system lesions.

The manual muscle test can be used in patients with mild or moderate spasticity. The manual

Table 3-1 Patterns of Muscle Weakness in Multiple Sclerosis

Foot	Intrinsics weaker than long toe muscles with clawing of toes
Ankle	Dorsiflexors and evertors weakness greater than plantar flexors and invertors with drop foot and ankle instability
Knee	Flexors weaker than extensors with back knee in stance
Hip	Abductors and flexors weaker than adductors and extensors with gait swing difficult and lateral lurch or stance phase
Lower Trunk	Flexors weaker than extensors with lordosis over anterior rotated pelvis with back pain
Upper Trunk	Extensors weaker than anterior thoracic and pectoral muscles with kyphosis and round shoulders
Neck	Flexors weaker than extensors with forward head
Facial	Palatopharyngeal weaker than lingual facial muscles with speech and swallow dysfunction
Hand	Intrinsics weaker than long finger muscles with clawing of hands
Wrist	Extensors weaker than flexors with dropped wrist
Elbow	Extensors weaker than flexors with decreased locking for stable extended elbow
Shoulder	Abductors, external rotators, and flexors weaker than adductors, inward rotators, and extensors with decreased arm elevation

muscle grade should be qualified indicating the presence of tone and the limitation of active range of motion. The number of repetitions the patient can perform should be indicated when rapid fatigue impairs function. The degree of movement, coordination, speed, tremor, and ataxia should also be noted.

Quantitative assessment of grip strength can be evaluated using a dynamometer. Isotonic and isokinetic testing equipment, (Orthotron, Cybex, or KinCom) can be used in muscle groups where active resistance is possible. The ability to quantify forces generated at varied speeds as well as ability to change directions, provides valuable information in monitoring and motivating the patient.

In cases where spasticity is severe and voluntary control is minimal, strength can be described in terms of functional muscle patterns with estimates of available strength. Extensor spasticity and strength in lower extremities may be sufficient to enable standing and pivot transfers. Mass flexion of neck, trunk, and lower extremities is used against gravity to roll and initiate sitting from the supine position. The patient may lack sufficient voluntary strength in isolated movements and use underlying tone to enable function. Evaluation results provide essential information useful in the careful regulation of antispasmodic medications.

Sensory Evaluation

Functional vision should be evaluated. Decreased acuity, especially for central vision, is often reported as blurring. Diplopia, or double vision, and nystagmus, the rhythmic beating eye movements, also account for decreased vision in multiple sclerosis. Visual disorders, with temporary increased blurring of vision, may be induced by violent exertion, heat, menstruation, or emotional disturbances.

Proprioception, joint position sense, and kinesthesia, perception of movement, can be assessed by asking the blindfolded patient to reproduce or describe the position or movement passively performed by the examiner. Awareness of vibration can be examined using a tuning fork on bony prominences.

The sensations of light touch, deep pressure, temperature, and pain of the skin should also be evaluated. These sensations are often described as impaired or absent. The skin should be examined for signs of trauma, bruises, abrasions, and wound infections, which may be associated with decreased sensation and coordination. Skin over bony prominences of the body should be examined for pressure sores associated with decreased sensation and decreased mobility. Special note is given to the ischium, sacrum, trochanters, knees, ankles, heels, shoulders, and elbows.

Pain should be identified and evaluated. Musculoskeletal pain may be associated with spasticity, spasms, and chronic posture problems. Dysesthesia, paresthesia and causalgia may represent alterations in cutaneous sensation. Segmental nerve root pain can be identified by its distribution. Diffuse electric feelings passing down the back to the legs on neck flexion is not uncommon.[3] Discomfort due to limb edema may be associated with circulatory changes, immobility, or water retention.

Functional Evaluation

Examine the patient's ability to perform functional activities essential for daily living. In many settings, the functional evaluation of gross movement skills is performed by physical therapy; whereas fine motor activities, such as speech, feeding, swallowing, hygiene, self-care, dressing, and homemaking are reviewed by the combined efforts of speech therapists, nurses, and occupational therapists. It is important to consider the effect of fatigue on functional activities. The patient's performance early in the day may be stronger than at the end of the day. Function may also be influenced by respiratory status. Diminished diaphragm and abdominal excursion may result in shortness of breath, weak cough, and decreased volume.

1. Bed mobility includes rolling to sidelying, prone, supine, and assuming sitting. The patient's tolerance of these positions due to pain, skin pressure, or contracture should also be considered.
2. Functional sitting includes the ability to assume and maintain sitting with and without the arms supporting.
3. Functional standing includes the ability to assume, maintain, and shift one's weight in standing.
4. Transferring should be evaluated to and from the bed, chair, wheelchair, car, shower, tub, and toilet. Independence in toileting includes comments on bowel and bladder continence, ability to arrange clothing and collection devices, and self-hygiene. Amount of assistance and special transfer equipment should be noted, such as slide board, rails, safety benches, and hydraulic lifts.

Consider the patient's methods of mobility and gait. Gait evaluation should include the need for assistance, either by people or walking aids, as well as the distance, time, and deviations observed. Walking aids include various types of canes (straight, quadripod, Canadian/Lofstrand or quadripose flexible base), walkers (folding, reciprocating, or wheeled), and orthosis (plastic or metal, static or dynamic). Distances and time should be documented and estimated velocity can be calculated.

Deviations, such as footslap, toe drag, ankle inversion, genu recurvatum, lateral lurch, scissor gait, wide base, circumduction, hip hiking, pelvis dropping, increased lordosis, trunk lurching, and diminished arm swing, should be observed from side, front, and back views. A visual inspection of the shoe for excessive wear provides additional information about gait. Ataxia with slowed, irregular foot placement and broad base gait should be noted.

It is also worthwhile to observe ambulation ability on floors, carpets, ramps, curbs, stairs, and outdoors with consideration for inclement weather conditions. The ability to change directions, step to the side or back, turn, and walk slowly or brisk is also important. Consider the need of a parent with multiple sclerosis to sprint quickly to the rescue of a toddler. The ability to run is often neglected in evaluation.

The patient's ability to rise from the floor after a fall often includes the pregait skills of assuming hands and knees, kneeling, and half kneeling positions.

Mobility for distances should be evaluated for the patient with limited ambulation. The patient's ability to manage and propel a wheelchair and the suitability of the chair for the individual's needs depends on such factors as chair type, weight, size, features, and attachments. A motorized three-wheel cart is often used in cases of decreased mobility and endurance. Use of a car with special adaptations, hand controls, trunk lift for chair or cart, or need for special transportation services should be discussed.

A home assessment of the stairs, entry, doorways, hallways, and space for safe maneuverability should be considered.

Goals and Plan of Treatment

Treatment goals and regimen can be prioritized and individualized based on the results of the evaluation. The general areas to consider in treatment are listed.

1. Developing the patient's problem solving skills involves increasing the patient's self-awareness and acceptance, as well as motivating, guiding the patient's decision making regarding his physical needs and abilities.
2. Reducing abnormal tone is accomplished through inhibition of facilitation.
3. Restoring functional range of motion is accomplished through selective stretching and positioning.
4. Strengthening and balancing muscle groups is accomplished through graded exercise.
5. Increasing awareness and compensation for visual and proprioception losses is accomplished by increasing or substituting additional sensory feedback.
6. Increasing functional skills needed to restore more independence requires the simulation and practice of those activities of daily living.
7. Improving gait pattern is accomplished through preambulation exercises, gait activities, and/or assistive devices.
8. Decreasing fatigue requires a program of both rest and aerobic training.
9. Assisting in selecting and securing appropriate equipment.
10. Planning for discharge and long-term care involves consultation with an interdisciplinary team of doctor, nurse, occupational and speech therapists, social worker, psychologist, vocational counselor, and most important the patient and family.

MULTIPLE SCLEROSIS MANAGEMENT

General Principles for Treatment

Graded Exercise

Graded exercise is needed to maintain or increase the body's capacity for normal activities. Inactivity has been associated with detrimental complications including disuse atrophy, contracture, cardiovascular compromise, osteoporosis, thrombophlebitis, respiratory problems, bowel and bladder dysfunction, pressure sores, and depression.[5]

Overexertion has been associated with transient aggravation of symptoms of multiple sclerosis (Uhthoff's phenomenon).[3] Overemphasis of this principle may have resulted in overcautious fitness and exercise management of the multiple sclerosis patient. Although fatigue to the point of exhaustion should be avoided, especially during exacerbations, exercise is essential.

The therapist should observe carefully the patient's reaction to exercise to determine the appropriate amount and pace.[11] Initially, activities should be ordered, alternating restful relaxing activities with more strenuous energy-consuming activities. Signs of fatigue are seen when performance variables, such as power, speed, or distance, drops to 50 percent of the initial best performance. Rest is then indicated.

Aerobic Exercise

Aerobic exercise should be seriously considered for patients during remissions to promote physical fitness and gradually reduce the limitations of fatigue.[8] Patients just beginning a training program should work with the guidance of the physician and or physical therapist. Heart rate is a useful indicator of effective training levels for aerobic exercises. As a general rule, the heart rate for training is calculated by taking 60 to 80 percent of the estimated maximum heart rate, which is 220 minus the patient's age.

Aerobic exercise should be preceded by a period of stretching exercises. Sustained aerobic activity can progress from a few minutes to a half hour. A cool down period of gentle exercise for 10 to 20 minutes should follow the aerobic period. Two to three periods of rest, for 10 to 20 minutes daily, is also recommended.[16]

Vigorous exercise includes brisk mat and floor routines, shallow water calisthenics, walking in water, swimming, brisk walking, stair climbing, exercycling, rowing, pushing a wheelchair, or in cases of minimal dysfunction, jogging. A cool environment for exercise is often necessary.

Some patients may tolerate daily aerobic training or combine a program of two different aerobic activities performed on alternating days. Other patients may perform strengthening and slow-paced resistance exercises on alternate days with aerobic activities only three or four times a week.

Heat and Cold

The effects of heat and cold should be considered in treatment. Exposure to heat, of either increased body temperature or increased heat from the environment, may cause dramatic temporary worsening of neurological symptoms and functional abilities. Heat has been shown to decrease the conduction in demyelinated fibers.[3]

1. Encourage the patient to seek a cool environment, especially for exercise. Air conditioning may be needed.
2. Exercising within several hours of awakening takes advantage of the lower basal body temperature.
3. Exercising in water from 75° to 80°F has the added benefit of rapidly dissipating the heat generated by the exercise.[17]
4. The multiple sclerosis patients can cool down further by a cool shower or bath or cold applications, especially for reduction of tone in spastic muscles.

Muscle Tone

Regulation of abnormal muscle tone is needed to enable coordinated movement. Facilitation of the weak muscle can be accomplished by quick stretch, brisk ice, tapping, brushing, and vibration, although these effects may be only temporary. Application of repeated quick stretch and resistance to other muscles in the same pattern may also facilitate the weaker muscles.[12,18,19]

Inhibition of spastic muscles can be accomplished by slow passive and active stretching through normal range of motion.[19] Local cold applications may provide temporary decrease in tone. The patient may be positioned with the spastic or tight muscle in a lengthened position during cooling, followed by active exercises to the antagonist muscles. Rhythmic rotation, especially at the shoulders, trunk, and pelvis may increase relaxation of spastic muscles and restore mobility.[19]

Another method of decreasing abnormal tone is the use of techniques advocated by neurodevelopmental therapy.[18] It is important to understand that reflex inhibiting postures may provide only a temporary decrease of abnormal tone. Sequencing components of movement patterns may facilitate long-term retention of functioning motor patterns provided practice is incorporated into the therapeutic strategy (see Ch. 9). Using handling techniques, the therapist assists and guides the patient's movements out of spastic patterns in an attempt to inhibit tone. A reflex inhibiting movement pattern in the lower extremity includes hip external rotation, abduction and extension with dorsiflexion, and eversion of ankle and toes. The reflex inhibiting movement pattern for the upper extremity includes scapular elevation and protraction, shoulder abduction and external rotation, elbow extension, wrist and finger extension, and thumb abduction. These positions can be incorporated into active strengthening and dynamic functional movements. Voluntary muscle control can be improved in both agonist and antagonist muscles, while tone is inhibited. Weight-bearing with the body parts on normal alignment is another method of decreasing hypertonus. It is helpful to precede functional skill training with activities to decrease tone.

In cases of severe spasticity, positioning in bed and sitting can also be used to reduce abnormal tone patterns; maintain range of motion; and reduce pain, posture, and skin problems. Mass extension patterns can be decreased by sidelying and erect sitting, while mass flexion pattern benefit from lying in the prone position. The physical therapist should instruct the patient, family, or care giver to perform the activities and assume these positions as needed on a daily basis.

Range of Motion

Range of motion must be maintained or restored through stretching and positioning. Active and passive stretching, can be coordinated with daily efforts to reduce spasticity. Range can be performed in functional positions of standing, half kneeling fourpoint, and sitting, to increase balance in these positions. Special attention is needed to prevent contractures at the hip, knee, and ankle that prevent comfortable bed positioning and disturb posture for standing and walking. An isometric hold of the tight muscle against resistance followed by relaxation and gentle elongation may be of benefit for increasing range.[19]

Splinting or inhibitory casting may be indicated to increase range when sensation is intact but is usually contraindicated if sensation is absent. For contracture resistant to ranging, surgical treatment could be considered if sufficient active movement control remains to assure improved function postoperatively.

Postioning can also be used to maintain range of motion. Prone positioning increases hip extension. A well-fitting chair provides lumbar support and increases ankle dorsiflexion if foot rests are adjusted to provide support to the forefoot. A tilt table with straps at the torso, pelvis, and knee may be useful in reducing ankle knee and hip contractures.

Sensory Feedback

Sensory feedback can improve motor performance. Increasing the patient's use of visual inputs may be helpful in compensating for cutaneous, proprioceptive, and vestibular dysfunction. Patients with decreased sensation of light touch, deep pressure, and pain must be encouraged to visually monitor the manipulation of objects for dexterity and safety. Proprioceptive neuromuscular facilitation advocates visual following of limb diagonal exercises to improve speed, coordination, and muscle recruitment.[19] The patients may benefit from use of a mirror to monitor irregular foot placement in gait, especially if ataxia is present.

In cases of persistent double vision, patching of one eye may reduce difficulty during functional activities. The eye patch should be placed on alternate eyes daily and worn only as needed.

Vertigo associated with occular nystagmus and head and body movements may respond to training the patient to move slowly and have eye movements slightly precede head and body movements to the same direction. Patients with visual difficulties often benefit from home programs that are recorded on audio cassette tapes rather than written and illustrated instructions. The verbal cues on tape often improve timing and coordination of exercises.

Proprioception can be increased through added resistance to movement. Small cuff weights for he wrist (1–2 lbs.), ankle (2–3 lbs.), or the waist (3–4 lbs.) may slightly improve control of movement in patients who present with ataxia as their primary problem. Use of weighted canes, crutches, or walkers may also be helpful. Approximation and rhythmic stabilization also improve proprioception and facilitate contraction of muscles to improve stability at the joint. Patients can be progressed to control multiple joints by assuming developmental positions of increasing postural challenge.

Functional Training

Functional skill can be improved by practicing the necessary components of the skill. Prerequisite components of skilled movements, as seen in the sequence of normal development, include[11]

1. Mobility, which requires flexibility and strength through range of motion
2. Stability, which requires co-contraction of the muscles to hold the joints in position
3. Weight shifting, which requires the ability to shift the proximal body segments over a fixed distal body part
4. Skill, which requires the ability of the distal body part to move freely while the proximal joint provides necessary stability

Although the adult with multiple sclerosis does not need to recapitulate infancy, use of the developmental positions may be beneficial. Selecting a position where the patient can successfully initiate movement, hold against resistance, and balance may enable progression to a more challanging activity.

1. Rolling can be used to increase mobility or resisted to increase head control and trunk

strength needed for improved sitting balance.
2. Lying prone on elbows improves scapular stability beneficial for lateral transfer skills.
3. Balancing movements in the hands and knees position increases weight shifting through the pelvis, which is needed for standing.
4. Kneeling and weight shifting while standing increases the leg and trunk control needed for ambulation.

Keeping the patient as independent as possible for as long as possible is the main goal of treatment. Repeated practice of functional activities is needed to improve the patient's performance, confidence, and endurance. Practice sessions scheduled at times of both maximal performance and moderate fatigue develop necessary compensatory skills for safety. Emphasis should be at the level of difficulty appropriate to challenge the patient but still enable success. Breathing exercises should be incorporated into exercises and activities to maximize function and reduce fatigue and shortness of breath.

Mobility in the Home

Mobility in the home or community needs to be maximized through pregait and gait exercises and use of equipment as needed.

Gait Deviations

Deviations, such as footslap, toe drag, and ankle inversion may be managed by decreasing tone and stretching the plantar flexors and invertors combined with facilitation and strengthening for the dorsiflexors and evertors. In cases of persistent ankle muscle imbalance, an ankle-foot orthosis can be made by an orthotist. A dynamic and flexible brace is appropriate if good knee control is present. A more static orthosis is preferred if spasticity is high or if the knee is weak. In cases of significant weakness throughout the entire limb, an ankle-foot orthosis may provide only limited benefit.

Genu recurvatum may be managed by stretching the soleus and strengthening hamstrings and gastrocnemius muscles. In cases where recurvatum is associated with weak quadriceps, strengthening is also indicated. Orthotics, such as ankle-foot orthosis with a plantar flexion stop or a knee cage limiting hyperextension, may be useful, especially when knee pain is reported.

A drop of the pelvis during swing phase may suggest abductor weakness on the opposite stance leg. Stretching the adductors and strengthening the abductors is indicated. Use of an assistive device, such as a cane opposite the side of greatest weakness, may improve balance and gait. Bilateral support may also be necessary.

Hip hiking to shorten the swing leg can be managed by decreasing extensor spasticity and increasing flexor strength at the hip, knee, and ankle. In the presence of persistent stiffness, hip hiking may be compensatory and useful.

Increased lumbar lordosis may be managed by increasing trunk stability, stretching spine extensors and hip flexor contractures, and strengthening abdominals. Decreased lumbar lordosis benefits from strengthening the spinal extensors.

Posterior or lateral lurching of the trunk is most often related to pelvis alignment and hip strength. Strengthening hip extensors and abductors and stretching of hip flexors and adductors may reduce the deviations.

Ataxia

Ataxia in gait may be improved by activities to increase proprioception and stability in the hands-knees, kneeling, half kneeling, or standing positions. Use of ambulation aids, such as canes; Canadian crutches; or reciprocating, weighted, or wheeled walkers, may provide the necessary additional stability.

Wheelchair

If walking ability is insufficient to meet the functional mobility needs of the patient, a wheelchair should be considered. It is often better for the minimally ambulatory patient to have a wheelchair to enable continued participation in home, family, and community activities. The appropriate selection of a wheelchair considers the patient's build and abilities, life style, prognosis, and home environment.

The type of wheelchair most often selected for persons with multiple sclerosis is a light, durable, stable, standard upright wheelchair, with removable deskrest armrests, and footrests. Reclining chairs may be needed for patients with trunk instability or excessive tone, making upright positioning difficult.

Measurements for seat width and depth, leg

length, seat height, back height, and arm height are taken to assure proper fit. Height of a wheelchair cushion should be considered when taking the measurements. It is useful to refer to the manufacturer's catalogue for specific measuring details. Chairs can then be ordered in standard adult, narrow, tall, junior, or wide sizes.

Many accessories are available and should be considered for the patient's comfort, safety, convenience, and dexterity.

1. Removable desk arms enable slide board lateral transfers and close approach to a desk or table. Adjustable height arms may enable weight shift, chair push ups, and comfort in sitting. "Quad" adapters are available if manual dexterity prohibits control of the small pinlocks.
2. Swinging detachable footrests may provide better foot positioning if heel loops are added. Elevating legs are available if needed. Again, cam spring releases or "Quad" releases make release of leg rests easier.
3. Eight-inch castors with castor locks with "Quad" release increase the stability of the wheelchair when locked, especially during transfers.
4. Pneumatic tires may be desired for outdoor use. Tire rims can be adapted with friction rims of plastic or projections for propelling the chair.
5. Grade aides devices or ramp retarders prevent rolling backward on inclines. This is especially important in negotiating ramps.
6. Antitipping devices may be useful for active patients.
7. Cane and crutch holders and back packs increase carrying convenience.
8. A narrowing device crank mechanism, such as "Reduce-a-width," may be used to enable entry through narrow doorways.
9. A wheelchair cushion and lumbar support may increase comfort during prolonged sitting.
10. Adaptations for the home for stairways, such as ramps or lifts, may be needed.

A battery-powered motorized chair is often selected for the patient with limited endurance but with a significant distance to travel in the home or outdoors. Three-wheeled carts are only practical where architectural barriers, steps, curbs, or steep ramps are not a problem. Due to the substantial weight of the base unit, battery, and seat, which frequently separate, trunk lifts are advisable to ease the car-loading process. Additional useful accessories are double-width wheels to increase the wheelbase and the stability of the cart.

Home Exercise Programs

Exercise programs should be individualized to suit the patient's level of disability, life style, and home and community resources. Two case histories and exercise program outlines are presented here to stimulate ideas for patient care.

Case History One

A 28-year-old woman with multiple sclerosis presented with minimal disability. An evaluation was performed on her third and fourth day in the acute hospital.

Subjective evaluation revealed the current problem, of 2 weeks' duration, to be left foot dragging and stiffness, decreased balance with staggering to the left, and increased blurring of the left eye. Two previous episodes of leg and vision problems had occurred. The first, onset at age 22, began with weakness in both legs that lasted about 4 weeks, resolved completely, but was not diagnosed. A second relapse occurred at age 25 with blurred vision in the left eye and left leg stiffness and weakness. At this time the diagnosis of probable multiple sclerosis was discussed and treatment with corticosteroids was initiated with rapid partial improvement in 1 week. Mild residual left eye blurring and left leg stiffness remained.

The patient was not performing any exercises at that time. Before her exacerbation 3 years ago, the patient complemented her sedentary office work life style with evening runs averaging 3 miles three times weekly. After the second occurrence of symptoms, the patient stopped running due to leg stiffness. The patient's current goals were steady walking, without tripping, and restored fitness. She was undergoing a 10-day series of adrenocorticotropic (ACTH) therapy and reported her vision had already improved. She appeared motivated to exercise as instructed.

The current evaluation revealed mild extensor spasticity in left ankle plantar flexors and knee extensors. Left ankle clonus of six beats and bilateral extensor plantar reflexes could be elicited. Manual muscle tests with grading scale from 0/5 to 5/5 are summarized with weakest areas listed first. The movement quality and range of motion limitations are also listed. The left dorsiflexors, evertors, and knee flexors were grade 3+/5. The left plantar flexors, knee extensors, hip outward rotators, and hip abductors were grade 4−/5. Ataxic quality movement was present in left hip abduction. The left hip extensors, inward rotators, and adductors were grade 4+/5. The right dorsiflexors, evertors, knee extensors, and flexors were grade 4+/5. The right plantar flexors and all hip motions were grade 5/5. Isokinetic testing quantified knee peak torque using Cybex. Torque generated for left knee flexors of 12 ft-lbs, left knee extensors of 40 ft-lbs, right knee flexors of 42 ft-lbs, and right knee extensor of 76 ft-lbs were all significantly below normal strength. Tight left plantar flexors limit dorsiflexion to 5°. Bilateral hip flexor tightness of 15° limited extension and was associated with increased lumbar lordosis in standing. Lumbar kyphosis was noted in prolonged sitting. Trunk extensors and abdominals were grade 4/5. Forward head position and round shoulders were noted with chronic discomfort reported in the neck and upper and medial scapular region. The neck flexors were grade 4/5 and extensors were grade 4+/5. The scapular adductors and upward rotators were grade 4/5. Other bilateral arm strength was grade 5/5, except for slight ataxia and slightly decreased rapid alternating movements noted in the left arm. Left grip strength was 47 pounds; on the dominant right, grip was 60 pounds. Proprioception, vibration, and cutaneous sensation were intact except for fourth and fifth digits of left hand and below the left knee. Vision in the left eye was blurred. The functional evaluation revealed that the patient performed all personal, home, and work activities independently. She ambulated 180 feet per minute, tolerating about 5 minutes, without assistance but with consistent left foot slap, occasional foot drag, and occasional genu recurvatum. An average of two episodes of imbalance were noted for 10 foot tandem walking. Braiding was impaired to the left more than to the right. Single limb stance could be maintained on the left for 4 seconds and on the right for 8 seconds. Running was slowed with rapid fatigue. Negotiating stairs was difficult when controlling descent or ascending with the left leg. The patient reported a feeling of a small bladder with slight increase in frequency but no urgency or incontinence.

In the hospital physical therapy emphasized decreasing tone in the left leg. The posterior calf region was cooled using moist towel ice packs for 15 minutes followed by stretching, especially for the soleus muscle in slight knee flexion. Clonus was decreased after cooling. The dorsiflexors and abductors were given gentle resistance, brisk ice, and repeated quick stretch to facilitate contraction. Balance in hands and knees, kneeling, half kneels, standing were challenged, and a rocker equilibrium board was used to stimulate reactions to an unpredictable and uneven terrain. Patient began practicing exercises suitable for performance at home immediately, so a program was well established before returning home. The emphasis of physical therapy exercise programs for this minimally involved patient included improving symmetry, improving fitness, increasing motivation, and providing education. Initial exercises were performed daily, about 10 of each, with the floor routine in the morning and the standing-walking routine after an afternoon rest period.

1. Hip lift with a lateral shift
   Purpose—Increase hip, knee, and ankle stability necessary for weight shifting
   Position—Lie on back, knees bent, feet flat
   Movement—Raise hips and shift pelvis to the right, to the left, lower
2. Abdominal curl
   Purpose—Support of the trunk
   Position—Lie on back, knees bent
   Movement—Raise head and shoulders to 30°, reaching with the arms toward knees, hold, lower slowly
3. Side leg lifts for hip abductors
   Purpose—To steady hip in standing and walking
   Position—Lie on right side with a slight bend

at the right knee

Movement—Raise the top left leg upward, backward, return to center position and lower, 3 lb weights can be added for extra challenge, repeat on the other side

4. Leg lifts on the stomach

   Purpose—Strengthens spine and hip extensors and knee flexors

   Position—Lie on stomach over a pillow

   Movement—Bend knee slightly and raise the whole leg several inches upward; alternate legs; 3-lb weights can be added for extra challenge

5. Balance on hands and knees

   Purpose—Improves balance and coordination of the limbs and trunk

   Position—Hands and knees, on a firm surface

   Movement—Hold your balance, lifting one leg and the opposite arm, alternate

6. Ankle pull ups and pull outs (Fig. 3-1)

   Purpose—To strengthen dorsiflexors and evertors

   Position—Loop theraband or elastic tubing around a leg of solid furniture, sit with leg straight in front of the furniture with a loop around the forefoot near toes

   Movement—Bend ankle, pulling toes up toward you for pull ups, twist ankle in the direction of the little toe for pull outs. Note: Quick stroke of ice to anterior and lateral calf, frequently facilitates these muscles.

7. Heel cord stretches in standing

   Purpose—Reduce tightness of posterior calf muscles

   Position—Stand with feet parallel and arms at shoulder height on the wall

   Movement—Lean hips forward toward the wall keeping heels on floor

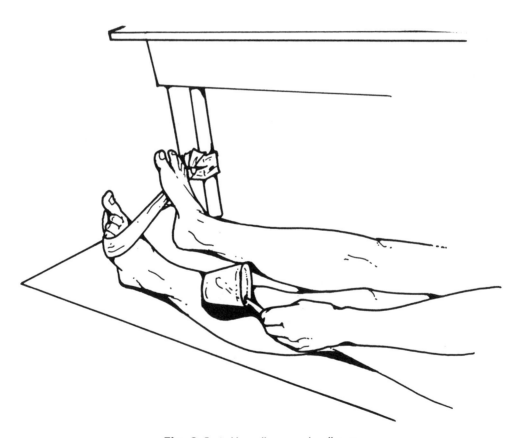

Fig. 3-1 Ankle pull ups and pull outs.

8. Standing lower leg lifts

   Purpose—To improve balance and strengthen knee flexors

   Position—Stand erect holding a counter or solid furniture

   Movement—Bend one knee 90° while keeping the hip straight, lifting the foot and lower leg

9. Bent Knee Walking

   Purpose—To increase knee extensor strength needed to reduce genu recurvatum and knee buckling

   Position—Stand with slight knee bend, about 30°, and heels flat

   Movement—Walk maintaining the knee bend with a heel and toe gait

10. Braiding (Fig. 3-2)

    Purpose—To improve balance and foot placement

    Position—Stand with feet 6 inches apart holding a counter or touching a wall for balance

    Movement—Going right, the left leg crosses forward, the right leg unwinds, the left leg crosses backward, the right leg unwinds, repeat. Going left, the right leg crosses forward, etc.

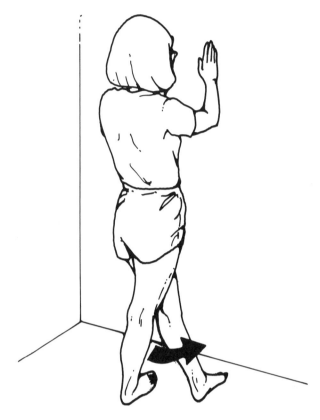

Fig. 3-2 Braiding.

The patient was instructed in posture awareness and encouraged to sit erect with a support to the lumbar area to reduce back discomfort. She was instructed to raise the angle of her reading material at her desk to reduce the forward head problem. She returned to work 3 weeks after the relapse.

An aerobic program of swimming and water exercise three times per week was initiated 4 weeks after the recent exacerbation. The patient monitored her pulse and began with walking tandem and balancing on one foot with eyes open or closed in waist-high water. Stretching exercises were performed for heel cords and hip flexors. Jogging in place was initiated for 1 minute followed by a brief rest and pulse check. A vigorous swim of 100 yards was followed by a second pulse check. Slow flutterkicking with a swim board was then performed for several minutes and a cool down period of 5 to 10 minutes of floating and bobbing finished the 20 to 30 minute session. Endurance was increased by dropping speed and performing an additional lap (25 yds) and rebuilding speed on subsequent sessions. Gradually, over a period of 3 months, swimming endurance tripled. As strength increased, several exercises were eliminated, such as hip lifts and leg lifts on stomach; and the floor routine was performed on days alternating with swimming. Brisk walking for 10-minute periods was added.

Therapy follow-up was provided weekly for the first month and then each month for the second to fourth months. Recheck included review of her exercise record of accomplishments, gait evaluation, manual muscle test of key weakened muscle groups, and Cybex recheck. Patient showed particular pleasure at improved gait, balance, and velocity and improved control and strength of left leg. She continued the routine of stretch and strengthening, alternating with aerobic and endurance activities.

Case History Two

A 41-year-old man was seen with moderate to severe disability. An evaluation was performed in the home. Subjective evaluation revealed the current problems to be loss of his already limited ability to walk even a few steps with a walker and an inability to climb stairs even with maximal assistance. Two weeks before evaluation, the patient had managed stairs with the assistance of his wife and son, to a waiting wheelchair, enabling his commute to work as a radio dispatcher.

The patient reported six prior hospital admissions over the last 10 years since multiple sclerosis was first diagnosed, with increased blurred vision, numbness, spasticity, and weakness in the legs, necessitating increased use of a wheelchair over the last 3 years. He reported general benefit from ACTH, antispasmodics, and physical therapy. The patient reported recurrent relapses about every 12 to 18 months which lasted about 2 months. One extended period of remission, lasting 2.5 years, occurred after an experimental trial of cyclophosphamide and ACTH. The patient functioned with residual blurred vision and paraparesis. Currently, the patient's chief goals were adapting his home as needed, getting equipment for mobility at work, and resuming limited ambulation.

Evaluation revealed predominant moderate extensor tone bilaterally throughout the legs, with occasional flexor spasms elicited by light touch to feet or passive movement of the legs out of extensor synergy. Bilateral sustained clonus could be elicited. Limited passive range of motion throughout the lower extremities was evident bilaterally in dorsiflexion to $-5°$, kneee flexion to $110°$, straight leg raise to $60°$, hip extension to $-15°$, and hip abduction to $20°$. The thoracic and lumbar spine was hypermobile with kyphosis. The right dominant arm demonstrated mild increased ellbow flexion and finger flexion tone, whereas the left upper extremity was normal. Voluntary movement in both legs was very limited. Bilateral hip adduction and hip, knee, and ankle extension movements were in the $2+/5$ range unless reinforced by a mass extension pattern providing transient increased strength. Toe movements and dorsiflexion were absent bilaterally. Hip and knee flexion were $1/5$ on the right and $2-/5$ on the left. Bilateral

hip abduction of $2/5$ was present only out of the extension pattern. Trunk extensors grade $3/5$, flexors $2/5$ and obliques $3/5$. The right shoulder external rotation, flexion and abduction, elbow extension, and wrist flexors grade $4-/5$. Right intrinsics and lumbricals were $3+/5$, whereas long finger flexors were $4/5$. The left shoulder elbow and wrist were grade $4+/5$, whereas intrinsics and lumbricals were $4/5$. Neck extensors were $4/5$ and flexors were grade $3+/5$. Right facial muscles were slightly decreased in strength. Sensation was most impaired at the feet and ankles where vibration and proprioception were absent. Light touch, pinprick, and temperature were dulled. Vision, although blurred, was sufficient for office work as a dispatcher, which required monitoring calls and checking route sheets. Diplopia was reported with evidence of right lateral nystagmus. Hearing was intact, speech slowed, and scanning with minimal dysarthria. No swallow problems were reported or observed. The functional evaluation revealed independence in bed mobillity using upper extremities to reposition legs as needed. The patient assumed sitting independently with sitting balance dependent on arm support. Sitting balance was poor when unsupported. He required assistance to stand with a walker but once standing, maintained that position using extensor tone. A right static ankle–foot orthosis, used for the last 6 years, continues to provide some ankle and knee stability for transfers and stance. He transferred with a half stand pivot from standard bed and current fixed arm wheelchair, requiring assistance when fatigued. The patient has toilet guard rails enabling toilet transfer but assistance is sometimes needed. Urinary urgency and frequency was reported without daytime incontinence. The patient reported using a urinal at night and at work; he regulated his bowels with diet. The patient had a shower bench with a back support, allowing a lateral transfer in an accessible bathroom. The patient was able to ambulate with a "swing to" gait with a walker for 10 feet in 9 seconds with moderate assist if hip extension was maintained. The patient was using a fixed arm wheelchair with indoor wheels and fixed leg rests. The wheelchair weight of 44 pounds made it difficult for the patient's wife to transport the chair over the stairs or in and out of the car. The patient is independent in wheelchair mobility but, with decreased power and control in his right hand, he has loss of grip when pushing the chair, especially for ramps.

The chief rehabilitation goals for this significantly restricted patient were restoration of recently lost skills, focusing on essential functional exercises, providing aids to mobility, and reviewing compensatory methods to assure safety. Home therapy was recommended and provided until transfer skills were consistent and the necessary equipment was secured, at which time outpatient services near his place of work were provided. Equipment ordered for this patient included a new wheelchair, a 28-inch transfer slide board, and electric stair lift. The equipment was rented with conversion to ownership in 18 months. The patient's gradual progressive disability suggested ownership would be advisable. The wheelchair selected was a lightweight, durable, narrow, adult frame with removable desk arms and swing away footrests with heel loops. Pneumatic tires with ramp retarders were selected for outdoor safety. A spoke protector and friction coating on the hand rim were selected to reduce the danger of loss of grip and injury to the hand in wheel spokes. Straps were attached to the push handles to accommodate the walker, and a back pack was installed. A tempered foam cushion and knit cover was also selected. Access to his home, which has six interior steps, was provided with a stairway chair lift. The patient's vacation home, with two exterior steps, totaling 12 inches, required a 12-foot ramp at significantly lower cost than the stair lift. Use of an external collection device with a leg bag for bladder dysfunction was initiated especially for work. Physical therapy programs were coordinated to follow the patient's daily cool home shower. Rhythmic rotation and stretching preceded handling activities in progression from horizontal to upright postures. Practice of safe slide board lateral transfers were emphasized. Progressive control in standing transfers and stepping, using an anteriorly weighted wheeled walker, was attained. Strengthening, using graded resistance; quick stretch; and selective positioning was reinforced by a supplemental exercise program performed twice daily.

1. Lower trunk rotation (Fig. 3-3)
    Purpose—To sufficiently reduce extensor tone in legs to enable rolling and assumption of sitting
    Position—Lie on back with knees bent; a strap may be used around knees to add control
    Movement—Slow rhythmic rotation of knees to the left and right can be performed using the control strap or with the aid of a home assistant
2. Hip lifts with legs elevated
    Purpose—Maintain essential hip extension for assumption of standing
    Position—Lie on back with legs elevated on a bench or stool with hip and knee at 90°
    Movement—Lift hip, hold, and lower
3. Arm diagonals in rolling (Fig. 3-4)
    Purpose—Increases strength of arm and upper trunk
    Position—Lie on back, clasp hand at wrist
    Movement—Swing arms up and out as you roll to the side return; rest and swing the other way

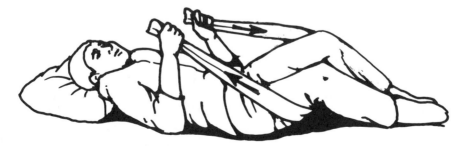

Fig. 3-3 Lower trunk rotation.

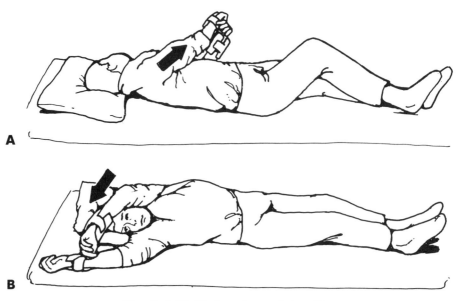

Fig. 3-4 (A,B) Arm diagonals in rolling.

4. Push up
    Purpose—Strengthens arms and shoulder girdle necessary for assuming sitting and transferring
    Position—Lie on stomach, place hands on the firm bed at shoulder level
    Movement—Push straight up, balance on the knees, keeping the back and hips straight
5. Arm diagonals in sitting with trunk control
    Purpose—Increases shoulder and trunk strength, trunk balance, and deep breathing
    Position—Sit erect in chair with spine 1 inch from the back of chair
    Movement—Stretch arms up and out to make a "V"; as the back extends, breathe deeply, fold arms down, and cross them to make an "X" as spine flexes and exhale fully
6. Arm theraband pulls (Fig. 3-5)
    Purpose—Increases wrist and elbow strength
    Position—Loop theraband around the wheelchair push handle, and grasp the end
    Movement—Alternate pulling various directions, forward, upward and, downward
7. Chair armrest push ups
    Purpose—Strengthens shoulder depressors

and elbow extensors and relieves pressure on buttocks in sitting
    Position—Hands on chair arm rests, feet flat on floor, spine erect
    Movement—Push and straighten elbow, lifting the buttocks from the chair
8. Knee extension in sitting
    Purpose—Strengthens knee extensors and stretches hamstrings
    Position—Sitting erect in the chair
    Movement—Straighten knee so that leg is straight. Weights or resistive band may be used to increase strength, and a control strap loop around foot may assist in stretching
9. Heel cord stretch in sitting
    Purpose—Safety during stretch of plantar flexors
    Position—Strap is looped around sole of the shoe (or foot) at the base of the toes
    Movement—Pull back with the arms, pulling toes up toward the body
10. Shallow knee bend
    Purpose—Provides a gentle stretch to the calf and increases knee control
    Position—Stand straight in front of a chair, with arms supported on a walker or solid object

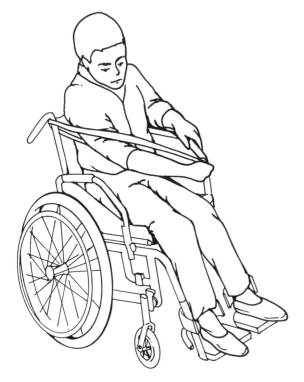

Fig. 3-5 Arm theraband pulls.

Movement—Maintain your balance as you slightly bend the hips and knees, then straighten

An aerobic program of propelling the wheelchair was initiated 2 weeks after beginning home physical therapy. The patient used the local park running track 3 days per week until he returned to work 6 weeks later. Accompanied by his son, who took his father's pulse, the patient slowly wheeled to the track in 10 minutes. The quarter mile was accomplished in 12 minutes while his son performed his casual jog. A slow wheel home and a cool shower was the protocol alternated with days when the visiting home therapist provided exercises. After returning to work, the patient reported that his large office area provided a sufficient endurance challenge and his track wheeling was reduced to 1 day per week, weather permitting. He continues to roll a quarter mile on a "good day" in 10 minutes flat.

Follow-up was provided twice weekly for 4 weeks and once a week for 8 weeks, with emphasis on gait pattern and emergency procedures, such as rising after a fall. A mat program to facilitate movement control within the extensor tone was performed to improve leg flexion. A three-fourths prone position was used to enable hip flexion with abduction for a crawl. Balancing on hands and knees was performed initially over a bolster with maximal assistance and progressed to moderate assistance without a bolster. Trunk balance remained fair and maximal assistance was still required when rising from the floor to the bed or chair in the event of a fall. Gradually, the gait pattern became reciprocal, with better swing through on the left than on the right. The patient was able to walk 25 feet in 20 seconds or less. The patient continues his independent exercises, dividing them into two parts and performing them on alternate mornings due to the priorities of his work and his supportive family.

REFERENCES

1. Adam CWM: The general pathology of multiple sclerosis, p. 203. In Hallpike JF, Adams CWM, Tourtellotte WW (eds): Multiple Sclerosis. Williams & Wilkins, Baltimore, 1983
2. McAlpine D, Lumsden CE, Acheson ED: Multiple Sclerosis A Reappraisal. 2nd Ed. Williams & Wilkins, Baltimore, 1972
3. Matthews WB (ed): McAlpine's Multiple Sclerosis. Churchill Livingstone, Edinburgh, 1985
4. Kurtzke JF: Epidemiology of multiple sclerosis. p. 47. In Hallpike JF, Adams CWM, Tourtellotte WW (eds): Multiple Sclerosis. Williams & Wilkins, Baltimore, 1983
5. Bauer HJ: Problems of symptomatic therapy in multiple sclerosis. Neurology 23:9, 1978
6. Hallpike JF, Adams CWM, Tourtellotte WW (eds): Multiple Sclerosis: Pathology, Diagnosis and Management. Williams & Wilkins, Baltimore, 1983
7. Hallpike JF: Clinical Aspects of Multiple Sclerosis. p. 129. In Hallpike JF, Adams CWM, Tourtellotte WW (eds): Multiple Sclerosis. Williams & Wilkins, Baltimore, 1983
8. Tourtellotte WW: Comprehensive management of multiple sclerosis. p. 513. In Hallpike JF, Adams CWM, Tourtellotte WW (eds): Multiple Sclerosis, Williams & Wilkins, Baltimore, 1983
9. Brown JR: Therapeutic Claims in Multiple Sclerosis. National Multiple Sclerosis Society, New York, 1982
10. Hauser SL, Dawson DM, Lehrich M, et al: Intensive immunosuppression in progressive multiple sclerosis. N Engl J Med, 308:173, 1983
11. Schneitzer L: Rehabilitation of patients with multiple sclerosis. Arch Phys Med Rehabil 59:430, 1978

12. Stockmeyer SA: An interpretation of the approach of Rood to the treatment of neuromuscular dysfunctions. Am J Phys Med 46:900, 1967
13. Kurtzke JF, Beebe GW, Nagler B, et al: Studies in the natural history of multiple sclerosis. J Chronic Dis 30:819, 1977
14. Poser S, Raun NE, Wikstrom J, Poser W: Pregnancy, oral contraceptives and multiple sclerosis. Acta Neurol Scand 59:108, 1979
15. National Multiple Sclerosis Society, 205 E 42nd Street, New York, New York 10017
16. Russell WR: Multiple Sclerosis: Control of the Disease. Pergamon Press, New York, 1976
17. Gehlesen GM, Grigsby SA, Winant DM: Effects of an aquatic fitness program on the muscular strength and endurance of patients with multiple sclerosis. Physical Therapy 64:653, 1984
18. Bobath B: Adult Hemiplegia: Evaluation and Treatment. 2nd Ed. William Heinemann Medical Books Limited, London, 1978
19. Knott MA, Voss DE: Proprioceptive Neuromuscular Facilitation. 2nd Ed. Harper & Row, New York, 1968

4 Spinal Cord Injury

Bill O'Daniel and Betti J. Krapfl

A total program of care for the spinal cord injured patient is best accomplished by a multidisciplinary approach. Single physician management, wherein one physician is thoroughly schooled in the care of spinal cord injuries, is a real plus to facilitate communication between the patient and those members of the multidisciplinary team. Each member of this team (i.e., physicians, physical therapists, occupational therapists, nurses, and counselors) should have a thorough understanding of the specific roles of each discipline and how the program is to be integrated to provide a team approach.

We advocate the functional approach to rehabilitation whereby functional goals for the level of injury are set, and the *daily* program for the patient is designed to work on these specific goals. A patient begins at a basic level, and as progress is made, the daily physical therapy program changes appropriately. This concept negates the older practice of having spinal cord injured patients work on programs such as weight lifting and specific exercise programs from day one to discharge. Because the functional status of patients usually changes during therapy, an ongoing evaluation must be made regarding the patient's response to the program; the program must be updated to meet patient needs. In other words, there must be a graduation from one program to a more difficult one.

PROGRAM PHILOSOPHY

Daily therapy programs should be designed for the normal routines of life. The patient should be required to get up and start moving as if he were going to begin his usual daily routine. Dressing in appropriate clothing, not in hospital gowns, is important. The length of treatment day should be as normal as possible. Monday through Friday treatment is sufficient. As part of their rehabilitation program, patients need to learn how to deal with leisure time on weekends, a normal pattern for most of us. "Weekend therapy" tends only to satisfy a patient's desire to "work harder so as to get well quicker," to be "entertained" and to increase the cost of rehabilitation, as shorter stays do not tend to occur in such situations. A *full* program, five days a week, is sufficient to tax fully the physiological capabilities of the spinal cord injured patient.

When treating several spinal cord injury patients with similar disabilities, activities such as wheelchair skills, mat exercises, and transfer practice can be done as a group. This encourages group interaction and competition in a "fun" way. If the group consists only of paraplegics, fewer personnel are required to teach the needed skills.

One of the most conservative aspects of a rehabilitation program should be that of skin care. With proper skin management a person can (1) participate in a full rehabilitation program (2) have a fulfilling social and personal life, (3) go to school and enjoy most of the same activities as do able-bodied students, and (4) engage in a profession as a dependable, productive employee.

BASIC PRINCIPLES

An estimated 15,000 to 20,000 new spinal cord injuries occur every year. The 1985 annual report for the National Spinal Cord Injury Statistical

69

Center[1] includes the following data:

1. Sixty-one percent of new injuries occurred in patients 16 to 30 years of age; 19.4 percent occurred in patients aged 31 to 45; 14.6 percent occurred in patients over 45; 4.9 percent occurred in patients less than 15 years of age. Eighty-two percent of all spinal cord injuries occurred in males.

2. Motor vehicle accidents accounted for 47.7 percent of all new injuries; falls ranked second at 20.8 percent; acts of violence accounted for 14.6 percent, and sports accounted for 14.2 percent. All other causes equaled 2.7 percent. Overall, 52 percent of the patients had cervical lesions; 34.4 percent had thoracic lesions, and 9.8 percent had lumbosacral lesions; in 2.9 percent of the patients, the type of lesion was unreported.

3. In the neurological impairment category (i.e., level and extent of injury), at admission, 28.1 percent of patients were reported as incomplete quadriplegics; 26.4 percent were reported as complete paraplegics; 24.2 percent were listed as complete quadriplegics, and 17.7 percent were reported as incomplete paraplegics. Unreported were 3.5 percent of the patients. *At discharge,* this order of ranking remained the same; the percentages of neurologically incomplete lesions were slightly higher. In cervical lesions resulting in quadriplegia, the C5 neurological level of lesion occurred most often. In cases of paraplegia, T12 was the most common neurological level of lesion.

Functional Goals for Specific Levels of Spinal Cord Injury

Before planning a treatment program for a person with a spinal cord injury, the therapist should have an understanding of realistic goals for the various levels of injury.

Functional goals are presented that represent efforts by both physical and occupational therapists. Since job responsibilities for physical therapists and occupational therapists differ among institutions, for the sake of completeness, the entire program for functional goals are given.

It should not be assumed that the presented goals for each level of injury will be achieved during the first admission; this will vary according to individual recovery rates. Multiple admissions may be required for some individuals who present numerous problems in addition to their spinal cord injury.

Thirteen criteria have been established, which are pertinent to minimize dependency at each level. Some factors that cause variations in achieving levels of independence are motivation and psychological adjustment, motor and sensory preservation, medical complications, body build, age, family support, life style, education level, and architectural limitations of the environment to which one is returning. It is important to note that although some people are physically capable of performing these various high energy expenditure tasks, such as transfers and dressing, some choose instead to devote their energies to other priorities, such as work or school.

Close team management with overlapping roles and responsibilities among all departments is necessary to allow the person the option of pursuing and achieving all available options. Continued support by the nursing department allows a person to refine and perfect skills on a normal timetable.

The Thirteen Criteria

1. The wheelchair is a mode of transportation for the disabled person. The electric wheelchair has mechanical power, which allows the individual the greatest freedom and mobility. The manual wheelchair requires "patient energy" or assistance if he is unable to propel the wheelchair himself. A standard part of any wheelchair, electric or manual, is a cushion that meets each person's needs to provide optimal skin protection.

2. Wheelchair mobility is the ability to move a wheelchair around within the person's environment, which includes level terrain, rough terrain, curbs, and ramps.

3. A weight shift is the means of relieving pressure from any bony prominences. When sitting, these prominences are primarily the ischial tuberosities and the sacrum. Methods of weight shift are forward lean, side to side, half push-up, and full push-up.

4. Transfers are a means of getting from the

wheelchair to a bed, car, toilet, tub, or floor, etc. It may be done with or without a sliding board. Many methods may be used; transfers must be tailored to the individual's needs.

5. Feeding is the ability to feed oneself with or without equipment.

6. Self-care includes brushing teeth, combing hair, simple bathing, shaving, bowel program, and bladder care.

7. Communications include signature writing, typing, and use of phone and tape recorder. In some cases, an environmental control system is used.

8. Dressing includes dressing and undressing of the upper and lower extremities.

9. Driving includes the actual active driving with hand controls, as well as a process of transportation in the spinal cord injured person.

10. Homemaking includes light homemaking skills, such as independent sandwich making and light housecleaning, and heavy homemaking skills, such as independent top of the stove cooking, housecleaning, laundry, and marketing.

11. Standing means any process that puts almost full weight on the lower extremities. The benefits of standing are that it (1) reverses the sitting curve, (2) improves circulation, and (3) creates psychological well being. Most people like to stand up and face people at eye level. Gaiting is a process of ambulation by any means, including the use of orthoses and/or crutches.

12. Self-padding is a process of providing independent skin protection at night with foam pads and sheepskins. It also includes being able to position oneself in the bed, either prone or supine.

13. Skin check is a process of checking one's own skin for redness with the use of a mirror.

The C1–C3 Quadriplegic

The C1, C2, or C3 quadriplegic is the most expensive level to equip and to provide independence because of the severe motor and sensory loss. This individual will require full-time attendants.

1. Two wheelchairs, manual and electric, are usually required. The manual wheelchair is used when the individual is being transported via an automobile, when the electric wheelchair breaks down, or when an area is inaccessible to electric wheelchairs. The manual chair needs troughs for the arms, high back for head and trunk support, and no wheelrims.

2. The C1–C3 quadriplegic is dependent in moving the manual wheelchair but is able to propel the electric chair independently on level surfaces using chin or breath controls.

3. Weight shift can be done independently using chin or breath control while in the electric wheelchair. Full recline weight shifting increases skin sitting tolerance, upright endurance, and decreases attendant care. The person requires dependent side-to-side weight shifts while in a manual wheelchair.

4. The individual is totally dependent in transfers. One person should be able to complete transfer but must keep the ventilator in mind while developing transfer techniques to and from the bed, tilt table, and car. Several different methods may be used, a sliding board being the primary option.

5. The patient is dependent in feeding.

6. He is dependent in bathing, hygiene, and bowel program, all of which are most easily done in bed.

7. He is dependent in dressing.

8. Any communication, such as typing, signature writing, using the telephone, tape recorder, game playing, or environmental control systems, must be performed with a mouth stick.

9. He is dependent in driving and must use a van to be transported in the electric wheelchair. He may be transferred into a car, otherwise.

10. He is dependent in homemaking.

11. He stands on a tilt table.

12. He is dependent in placing his pads for skin protection at night and does not sleep prone because of the ventilator.

13. He is dependent in checking his skin for redness.

The C4 Quadriplegic

The C4 quadriplegic is probably off the ventilator part- or full-time. It is still expensive to equip the C4 quadriplegic for independence in a wheelchair, communications, and feeding activities. This individual will continue to need full-time attendant care but can be left alone for short periods when properly equipped, if he is off the ventilator.

1. This person uses the same type wheelchairs as the C1–C3 quadriplegic but can use a wheelchair with a lower back due to the fair to good head control and increased scapular mobility. This allows more visibility of the environment.
2. Wheelchair mobility is the same as for the C1–C3 quadriplegic.
3. Weight shifts are the same as for the C1–C3 quadriplegic.
4. Transfer techniques are the same as for the C1–C3 quadriplegic; however, more options are available because of the absence of the ventilator.
5. He is sometimes able to feed himself with varying success, with the aid of mobile arm supports.
6. The person is dependent in bathing and bowel program, which are most easily done in bed. He has variable success with self-care activities using a mobile arm support.
7. He is dependent in dressing.
8. Typing can be accomplished with mobile arm support or a mouth stick. All other communication activities must be performed with a mouth stick or an environmental control system.
9. He is dependent in driving. Transportation is the same as for the C1–C3 quadriplegic.
10. He is dependent in homemaking.
11. He can stand on a tilt or standing table.
12. He is dependent in self-padding.
13. He is dependent in checking his skin for redness.

The C5 Quadriplegic

The C5 quadriplegic has increased mobility and independence because of a motor picture, which allows hand-to-mouth activities. The weak C5 quadriplegic is a person with grade 3+ or less biceps and grade 3 or less around the shoulder girdle. The strong C5 has grade 3+ or stronger biceps with moderate weakness around the shoulder girdle. The C5 quadriplegic continues to require attendant care in the morning and afternoon for activities of daily living and transfer activities. This individual will also require minimal assistance during the day in activities, such as emptying his leg bag. He can be completely independent, however, during the day with proper equipment.

1. The weak C5 quadriplegic still needs a slightly higher wheelchair back, but a strong C5 can use a back of regular height. The manual wheelchair has quadpegs. The type of electric wheelchair will depend on the method of weight shift.
2. The electric wheelchair may be propelled by a joystick. Propelling the manual wheelchair for any distance may be limited because of fatigue. The introduction of lightweight manual wheelchairs may alter the fatigue problem.
3. Weight shift is variable from independent to totally dependent from side to side.
4. Transfers require moderate to maximal assist. The person may or may not be able to help with balance and some push. One assistant is able to do bed, car, and commode transfers. A floor-to-wheelchair transfer can be accomplsihed by one assistant for the person who is not overly large or spastic. (See High Quadriplegic Transfers—"Beach")
5. Feeding is done with mobile arm supports if the person is a weak C5 or with a brace if he is a strong C5.
6. The individual is able to brush his own teeth with a brace but is usually dependent in shaving and combing his hair. He is dependent in bathing.
7. The strong C5 can dress his upper extremities with varying success. The weak C5 is dependent in all dressing.
8. Typing, phone use, writing, and tape recorder use are performed independently with equipment.

9. The individual is dependent in driving. Transportation is either via a van and lift or through manual transfer to an automobile.
10. He is dependent in homemaking.
11. He can use a standing table.
12. He is dependent in self-padding.
13. He is dependent in checking his skin for redness.

The C6 Quadriplegic

The C6 quadriplegic is the first level to have a muscle and sensory picture that allows varying degrees of independence. The assistance from an attendant varies from person to person, depending on activity level, endurance, and motivation. The individual may be able to live alone with morning and evening attendant care. However, few C6 quadriplegics become totally independent and live alone without attendant care.

1. The wheelchair should have a regular back height and adaptations such as quad releases on the armrests, quad pegs, caster locks, grade aids, and brake extensions. With a properly equipped wheelchair and lightweight cushion, the patient is more easily able to perform transfers, body positioning in the chair, and maneuvering on varying terrains. Lightweight manual wheelchairs are providing the opportunity for greater independence.
2. The person can be independent in wheeling on level terrain, 6° ramps, and going down curbs backwards but is dependent in maneuvering on rough terrain.
3. Weight shifts vary from partial to total independence using side-to-side or half push-up methods.
4. Some people may become independent transferring with a transfer board to and from the bed, car, portable commode, and infrequently, to a chair sitting in a tub. Others vary from total dependence to moderate or minimal dependence because of the aforementioned physical and medical factors.
5. The individual is independent, feeding himself with or without equipment.
6. Simple hygiene is accomplished independently with equipment. Bathing assistance sometimes is needed for washing feet and buttocks when he is sitting on a portable commode or a chair in the shower. Bowel program is usually accomplished on a portable commode. The person may be able to do digital stimulation with a dil stick but may need more assistance with the clean up.
7. The individual is independent in upper extremity dressing and undressing. Success with lower extremity dressing and undressing varies.
8. Communications are independent with adaptive equipment.
9. He is independent in driving a car or a van with a lift.
10. He can be independent in light housekeeping and sandwich making.
11. He will use a standing table or stall bars.
12. A C6 quadriplegic will rarely become independent in self-padding with adaptive equipment.
13. He has varying success in checking his skin for redness with a mirror.

The C7 Quadriplegic

A C7 quadriplegic is the first level with the potential of living totally alone without attendant care. The goals the average C7 quadriplegic might attain are as follows:

1. The manual wheelchair is equipped with plastic-coated or regular rims or quad pegs.
2. Wheelchair mobility is independent on all terrains except extremely rough terrain. Independence going up and down curbs will depend on the height of the curb.
3. Weight shifts are independent, side-to-side, or full push-up.
4. Transfers are usually accomplished independently, with or without a sliding board to and from the bed, elevated toilet seat, and the car (including putting wheelchair in/out of the car). A well-coordinated C7 quadriplegic may accomplish floor-to-wheelchair and tub transfers with assistance.
5. Feeding is independent.

6. Simple hygiene is independent. Fingernail care is independent. Bowel program is independent with dil stick and equipment. Bathing is usually independent.
7. Upper extremity and lower extremity dressing and undressing are independent.
8. Communications are independent with or without adaptive equipment.
9. Driving is with hand controls.
10. The individual is independent in homemaking and cooking, except for heavy housekeeping.
11. Standing is accomplished in stall bars.
12. Self-padding is independent but very difficult. He is able to get prone from a sitting position, as well as prone to supine on a double bed.
13. He may be able to check his skin for redness independently with an adapted mirror.

The C8 Quadriplegic

The quadriplegic at the C8 level should be able to live completely independently.

1. The wheelchair has regular or slightly lower back height with minimal adaptations (i.e., caster locks).
2. The individual is able to do a full push-up weight shift independently.
3. The C8 quadriplegic is independent in wheeling on regular and rough terrain and in doing wheelies and curbs.
4. He is independent in bed, car, toilet, shower chair, and sofa transfers. He may have varying success with floor to wheelchair and tub to wheelchair transfers.
5. He is independent in feeding himself.
6. He is independent in self-care, including bowel program on padded elevated toilet seat.
7. The individual is independent in dressing and undressing.
8. The C8 quadriplegic is independent in all forms of communication.
9. He is independent in driving a car. There is no need for a van; the person is independent in getting the wheelchair in and out of a car.
10. He is independent in homemaking except for "spring" cleaning.

11. The person can get up and down from standing in stall bars independently.
12. The C8 quadriplegic is independent in self-padding and is able to roll from supine to prone and back independently.
13. He is independent in checking his skin for redness with a mirror.

The Paraplegics

A quadriplegic requires minimal adaptve equipment. He will have varying success with ambulation with knee-ankle-foot orthoses (KAFO) and crutches. For the purpose of this discussion we have chosen three levels of paraplegics: T4, T10, and L2. These groups represent levels without abdominal musculature, with abdominal musculature, and levels with some lower extremity muscle preservation.

1. A lightweight wheelchair is used with minimal adaptations (i.e., caster locks).
2. The individual is able to do a full push-up weight shift independently.
3. He is independent wheeling on regular and rough terrain and independent in doing wheelies and curbs.
4. The T4 paraplegic is independent in all transfers, including floor to wheelchair and tub to wheelchair, although he may not choose to be. He may be able to transfer in and out of pickup trucks and jeeps. The T10 paraplegic should be able to transfer to and from most surfaces. The L2 paraplegic should be able to transfer to and from all surfaces.
5. The paraplegic is independent in feeding.
6. The T4 paraplegic may still require a padded elevated toilet seat for bowel program. T10 and L2 paraplegics may require a padded toilet seat only for the bowel program.
7. He is independent in dressing and undressing.

Patient Evaluation

A thorough assessment of the spinal cord injured patient is vital. This valuable information will serve as the tool for

1. Establishing a neurological baseline
2. Planning the entire treatment program, including setting goals

3. Documenting neurological return
4. Documenting neurological loss
5. Charting progress from initial evaluation, to discharge, to re-evaluation in ensuing years

Establishing a Neurological Baseline

In establishing a baseline of information, the following tests should be performed

1. Sensory Test: light touch, pain, and proprioception
2. Tone
3. Manual muscle test (Motor)
4. Range-of-motion test
5. Functional check out: bed mobility, wheelchair, transfers, ambulation.
6. Physical therapy evaluation form

Sensory Test

Performing a sensory test in a consistent manner is essential to maintain accuracy, especially if another therapist must do the testing the next time. Set standards and stick to them.

Sensory testing should include light touch, superficial pain, and proprioception. Always establish the normal area with the patient (above the level of lesion).

Light Touch. Use the distal pad of a finger and lightly touch each dermatome in the body. Throughout the test, continue to compare "impaired" responses to the normal dermatome. Patients will often want to "pass" the sensory test. They see it as a pass/fail situation. Be careful in explaining the necessity for establishing exactly where they cannot "feel." One method of performing a more accurate test is having them close their eyes until the test is completed. Another method is to alternate touching/not touching in a dermatome. Consistency is the key.

Superficial Pain. Superficial pain is tested by a sharp object (i.e., safety pin). Again, it is necessary to document an accurate picture. One must distinguish between sharp and dull. If light touch is preserved, the patient might say, "I can feel that, yes." Retouch them with a pin in a normal dermatome and ask if the sharp sensation is the same. If not, then pinstick is absent or impaired in that particular dermatome. Usually, if one portion of

a dermatome is absent or impaired, then the entire dermatome is also impaired. Areas of hypersensitivity within a dermatome may be present. This is considered impairment and should be noted on the test form. Also be sure to document any inconsistency of responses for future references.

Proprioception. Proprioception or position sense should be tested in the following manner:

1. Upper extremities. Test the four fingers by positioning each finger in a flexed or extended position. Ask the patient to respond "up or down." One error means absent proprioception.
2. Lower extremities. Position the great toe in an up/down position. Ask the patient to respond "up or down;" one error is considered absent proprioception. The ankle, knees, and hip joint can likewise be tested (i.e., in an up/down or bent/straightened position).

Sensory tests are easily interpreted if standards are used consistently. They can be color coded for ease of recognition. For example, black striped equals impaired, completely shaded equals absent, and white equals normal.

Tone

Spasticity or tone is generally assessed by documenting the pattern exhibited (flexor or extensor, full body, lower extremities, or upper extremities). A description of these patterns, as well as comments on severity, will suffice. Spasticity that interferes later on with functional activities should also be documented.

Manual Muscle Test (Motor)

Manual muscle testing often can be an enigma to some therapists. With repeated practice, however, it can become an exciting challenge. See Table 4-1 for functional muscle innervation levels. In dealing with the spinal cord injured patient, assessing muscle strength at initial evaluation, interim periods, at discharge, and re-evaluation is an absolute must. The spinal cord injured person may not be able to assume "testing positions." Therefore, portions of the test may be performed with the patient sitting in a wheelchair, supine, and/or on an elevated mat. An adjustable height treatment table is, of course, ideal.

Table 4-1 Functional Muscle Innervation at the Levels of Spinal Cord Injury

Spinal Level	Muscle Innervation
C1–C3	Sternocleidomastoid—P
	Spinal accessories—P
	Upper trapezius—P
	Diaphragm—P at C3 only
C4	Middle trapezius—P
	Anterior, middle deltoid—Tr
C5	Deltoids—F
	Biceps—P
	Rhomboids—P
	Shoulder internal / external rotators—P
C6	Wrist extensors—P/F
	Triceps—Tr
	Latissimus dorsi—Tr/P
	Forearm pronators—F
C7	Triceps—P/F
	Wrist flexors—P/F
	Finger flexors—Tr/P
C8	Intrinsic: finger / thumb—T/P
	Extrinsic: finger / thumb—T/P
T1–T10	Intercostals—Segmental innervation
T6–T12	Abdominals—Segmental innervation
L2	Quadratus lumborum—F
	Sartorius—P/F
	Iliopsoas—P/F
	Quadriceps—Tr/P

Tr = Trace muscle innervation; palpable only.
P = Partial muscle innervation.
F = Full muscle innervation.

The muscle test is a source of communication. One should adhere to strict interpretation of the grade definitions. Consistency in subsequent tests is important. Significant changes can only be interpreted appropriately if therapists use the same standards of muscle grading.

For a *functional program,* the strength of a muscle is the important fact to document. Partially innervated muscles can be hypertrophied to a strength level approaching or measuring that of a fully innervated muscle. If lack of muscle mass has influenced the grade, put an asterisk by that grade. Below, in the comment section, put an asterisk with the date by it. Note your comments on muscle mass (i.e., lack of normal muscle mass indicates partial innervation).

Patients must go full range against gravity before a resistance grade can be given. Resistance is usually given near or at the end of the range. By definition, range means normal range of motion. If the patient cannot go through full normal range due to joint and/or contracture problems, grade the strength through patient's range, put an asterisk, and comment below on range.

If every therapist adheres to the same standards, consistency and expertise (with much practice) will be developed. As with sensory testing, color coding not only highlights immediately what the motor strength is but also establishes what needs to be worked on. We use a red pen for all grades to and including 3 (fair). They are not *functional* against gravity. For fair plus (3 +) and above, we use black pens. (A blue pen usually does not copy well; thus medical records being copied for legal purposes, etc., will be of poor quality.)

Range-of-Motion Test
Document as WNL (within normal limits) or record actual ranges for any exceptions. Standard range-of-motion testing procedures should be used in your assessment.

Functional Checkout
Probably one of the most practical documents the therapist can achieve is the functional checkout. One should know first the functional neurological levels of the patient (i.e., the motor and sensory test). Next, the therapist should know what reasonable goals to expect for this level of function. A test to document the level of function for the patient should logically follow before a rehabilitation program begins, to document *the reason* for doing the program. Finally, functional changes should be documented to justify the program.

A functional checkout method is shown in Figure 4-1. Goals are set. The first actual testing should not be done until the patient is mobilized, that is, out of bed and able to participate in the program. Obviously, in cases of higher levels of quadriplegia, mobilization would not affect the initial evaluation. In cases of lower levels of quadriplegia and in paraplegia, however, the early assistance required for functional activities should be documented, as this will usually change by discharge to independent or independent with equipment. The example shown has enough columns to document initial, discharge, and first follow-up testing. The follow-up testing demonstrates how much of the training was retained on a practical level. Overenthusiastic

PHYSICAL THERAPY FUNCTIONAL CHECKOUT

KEY:
- 0 - Dependent
- 1 - Assisted - physical
- 2 - DO NOT USE
- 3 - Assisted - physical & equipment
- 4 - Assisted but does not do
- 5 - Independent with equipment
- 6 - Independent with equipment but does not do
- 7 - Independent
- 8 - Independent but does not do
- 9 - Not applicable

Name_____

Date Onset_____ Age_____

Unit No._____ Dr._____

Injury_____
Level   Partial / Complete

		Anticipated Goals				COMMENTS
	Date					
	Therapist					
BED	Turning Side-Side					
	Turning Supine-Prone					
	Supine - Sit					
	Self Padding					
	Skin Check					
WHEELCHAIR	Weight Shift					Standard WC / Power drive
	Frequency Weight Shifts					
	Cushion Type					
	Hours Sitting Tolerance					
	Propel Smooth Terrain					
	Propel Rough Terrain					
	Open and Close Doors					
	Do Wheelie					
	Do Curbs					
	Do Ramps					
TRANSFER	In and Out Of Bed — WC / WALK					
	On and Off Commode or Raised Toilet Seat — WC / WALK					
	In and Out Shower-Bathtub — WC / WALK					
	In and Out Car — WC / WALK					
	Put Wheelchair In and Out of Car					
	To and From Sofa — WC / WALK					
	Down To and Up From Floor — WC / WALK					
GAIT	Type Braces					
	Doff and Don Braces					
	Wheelchair to Standing					
	Smooth Terrain					
	Rough Terrain					
	Stairs					
	Ramps					
	Falling					
STAND ONLY	Method					
	Frequency					
	Duration					
SUMMARY	Activities Requiring Attendant Care Daily					

Use reverse side for additional comments

Fig. 4-1 Example form for functional checkout.

therapists may insist on certain levels of function for quadriplegia that may not be reasonable for the actual home situation. As the physical therapist gains experience in this area, a more practical approach should be considered (i.e., accepting less than full independence in patients who may choose a different life style at home due to age, size, family situation, financial considerations, environmental barriers, etc.) At best, setting functional goals for some quadriplegics early on is an educated guess that improves with experience. For some patients, more than one admission to the rehabilitation program may be required to meet the appropriate goals originally set.

Once the therapist sets the goals and does the initial functional checkout, a program can be designed for treatment. This is called the *functional approach,* that is, the functional activity the patient needs to learn becomes an integral part of the daily treatment program. The therapist is required to evaluate the patient daily regarding response to the treatment program and modifications that may be necessary. This procedure develops a "customized" program for each patient; requires one-on-one physical therapist involvement; fully uses the *evaluation skills* of the therapist; and helps to prevent monotonous, routine exercises that are done day-one to discharge for no reason. By this procedure patients graduate from one task to another during the program so that at discharge, if goals were well set, the patient is not doing the same daily program as when it was initiated.

Physical Therapy Evaluation Form

When specific evaluation forms are used for testing, this recorded information does not need to be repeated in the therapist's notes. The notes should be condensed for ease of reading, saving time and for clarity.

SPECIAL PROBLEMS SEEN IN SPINAL CORD INJURIES

Autonomic Nervous System Dysfunction

In spinal cord injury levels T6 and above, the dysfunction of the interrupted autonomic system can lead to serious disturbances of blood pressure.

Orthostatic Hypotension

Orthostatic hypotension (postural hypotension) can occur when initially changing from the supine to sitting or standing position (i.e., to a wheelchair or tilt table). Because of the altered function of the autonomic nervous system, the blood pressure is lowered in the upright position. Blood tends to pool in the pelvic region and/or the lower extremities. This pooling results in lightheadedness or fainting. The symptoms of pooling can be alleviated by the use of full-length elastic hose and an abdominal binder and by coming to the sitting or standing position gradually. Should postural hypotension occur while sitting in a wheelchair, an attendant should grip the push handles, putting one foot on the tilt bar, thus tilting the wheelchair backward until the patient's head and upper body are nearly horizontal to the floor. This maneuver will increase the blood pressure and relieve the hypotension. Gradually return the patient to the upright position once the symptoms have passed.

Over a period of time as the spinal shock phase passes, the body tends to accommodate the blood pressure changes and postural hypotension resolves.

Another problem related to postural hypotension that may occur as a result of lowered blood pressure is a decrease in the amount of urine produced by the kidneys. When sitting or standing, there may be little or no urine noticed in the collection bag (if an internal or external catheter is in place). After reclining the patient, this collection bag may fill quickly as a result of the increase in blood pressure. Care should be exercised to drain the collection bag once it begins to fill.

Autonomic Dysreflexia (Hyperreflexia)

Autonomic dysreflexia (hyperreflexia) is a "mass reflex" syndrome occurring in spinal cord lesions to a large extent at or above the T6 level. Milder symptoms can occur in lesions down to and including T10. The exact etiology is not clear. Hyperreflexia occurs when noxious visceral or cutaneous stimuli are introduced into the body below the level of lesion. These stimuli give rise to afferent impulses into the spinal cord, which stimulate the sympathetic portion of the autonomic nervous system. This results in spasms and narrowing of the blood vessels, which in turn causes an increase in blood pressure. In the intact spinal cord, the noxious stimuli are reduced or eliminated by the regulatory discharges from the baroreceptors in the carotid artery and via the splanchnic outflow to the aorta. In lesions of T6 or above, the descending controlling stimuli have lost their efferent loop, resulting in "the mass reflex" syndrome. The increase in blood pressure is picked up via the baroreceptors in the carotid artery; the brain signals the heart to slow down and the blood vessels above the level of lesion to dilate. Because the modulating signals cannot reach the splanchnic outflow, which would affect the aorta, the blood vessels in the lower extremity remain constricted. The lack of this input into the aorta results in an overall increase in the blood pressure. Pilomotor erection and diaphoresis also occur. Clinical symptoms include headache, sweating (above the level of lesion), nasal stuffiness, "goose pimples," blurring of vision, hypertension, bradycardia or tachycardia, ventricular premature beat, and Horner's syndrome.

In spinal cord injuries, the most common cause of autonomic dysreflexia is overstretching of the bladder. If an indwelling catheter is used, the overstretch may be the result of (1) a blockage or kink in the catheter or drainage tubing, (2) a leg bag or drainage bag that is completely full, (3) a defective or incorrectly attached leg bag, or (4) cystitis.

Changing a catheter or irrigating the bladder may also trigger an episode of autonomic dysreflexia.

If an indwelling catheter is not used, autonomic dysreflexia may result (1) if the bladder becomes overextended due to excessive filling without sufficient voiding or (2) if bladder inflammation from infection is present. Voiding, itself, may trigger autonomic dysreflexia on occasion. Bladder spasms, stones, and infections often increase the susceptibility of autonomic dysreflexia.

Another possible cause of autonomic dysreflexia is a bowel that is full of stool or gas. Any stimulus to the rectal area, such as digital stimulation during a bowel program or rectal examination, can trigger a reaction. Hemorrhoids increase the chance of occurrence.

Skin irritations, wounds, or anything that would normally be painful, such as decubitii, burns, etc., are other sources of autonomic dysreflexia.

Preventing autonomic dysreflexia is very important. Patients should take the following precautions:

1. Patients using an indwelling catheter should be monitored daily to make sure there is no grit inside the catheter. The catheter and drainage bag should be kept empty.
2. Keep the catheter and drainage bag empty. Continue to take the anticholinergic medications as prescribed.
3. A patient on an intermittent catheterization program should catheterize as often as needed to prevent overstretching of the bladder.

Hyperthermia/Hypothermia

Due to the altered state of the autonomic nervous system in spinal cord injuries, the temperature of the body has an increased tendency to fluctuate according to the temperature of the environment. The higher the level of injury, the greater the tendency of fluctuations in temperature.

Hyperthermia

Hyperthermia refers to an elevation in body temperature, which may occur from being outdoors on a hot day, sitting in a hot car, being covered with too many blankets indoors, etc. One or more of the following symptoms may indicate hyperthermia:

1. Skin feels hot and dry and appears flushed
2. Feeling of weakness.
3. Dizziness
4. Visual disturbances
5. Headache
6. Nausea
7. Elevated temperature
8. Irregular, weak, and rapid pulse

Prevention of hyperthermia when exposed to an overheated environment is important. The following preventative measures are suggested:

1. The patient should become familiar with how long he can remain asymptomatic in an overheated environment.
2. The patient should drink lots of fluids.

3. The patient should wear protective, lightweight clothing.
4. The patient should wear a hat.
5. When outdoors, a patient can mist himself by using a spray bottle that contains a mixture of half water and half alcohol or plain water.
6. The patient should rest more often in hot weather.
7. When indoors, the patient should limit the amount of clothing worn and the number of blankets used.

If hyperthermia occurs, decrease the body temperature by removing the cause or moving into a cooler environment, using a fan, or sponging or misting the body with tepid water. The patient should drink cool fluids. If body temperature rises above 102° and cannot be lowered within 30 to 60 minutes, a physician should be called. Untreated hyperthermia can lead to loss of consciousness and convulsions.

Hypothermia
Hypothermia refers to a decrease in body temperature. It can occur when a spinal cord injured person remains in a cold environment too long. One or more of the following symptoms may indicate hypothermia:

1. Cold skin
2. Shivering
3. Decreased body temperature
4. Decreased blood pressure, pulse, and respiration
5. Confusion

Dressing warmly and limiting the amount of time spent in a cold environment are excellent preventive measures. Warm socks (preferably wool) should be worn during cold weather. If hypothermia occurs, warming the body can be done by

1. Removing oneself from the cold environment
2. Adding more clothing or blankets
3. Using a warm shower or tub bath (The patient should be sure to dress warmly afterwards so evaporation does not occur and cooling recur.)
4. Wrapping the extremities in warm, moist towels

Skin problems can occur with hypothermia, so the skin should be checked closely. In untreated cases of hypothermia, sleepiness, drowsiness, and even death can occur.

Spasticity

Spasticity, due to hyperactive reflex patterns below the level of lesion, is common in varying degrees after spinal cord injury. Normal reflex activity becomes hyperactive after spinal cord injuries because of the loss of the modulating influences from the brain. Hyperactive reflexes, as seen in spinal cord injuries (without associated brain stem or cerebral involvement), are usually tonic/clonic in nature. They can be flexor, extensor or a combination of the two. *Rigidity,* when seen in spinal cord injuries, usually indicates the possibility of an associated brain stem or head injury. These hyperactive reflexes can be stimulated by sensory input, such as nociceptive stimuli, light touch, proprioception, and maneuvers that trigger the tonic stretch reflex (i.e., quick change in position of the body and/or extremities). Nociceptive stimuli may manifest as bladder irritation, decubitus ulcers, fractures, bowel problems, restrictive closing, etc.

Spasticity is not necessarily detrimental to the spinal cord injured person. Many times a minor degree of spasticity helps the patient achieve a functional activity. The pumping action of the spasticity also helps to maintain improved circulation. In addition spasticity will help to forestall the effects of disuse atrophy to the muscles involved.

Severe spasticity, however, can interfere with functional activities, such as transfers, dressing, driving, sleeping, ambulation, and personal hygiene. Drugs, such as Valium and Lioresal, are used with varying degrees of success on an individual basis. In cases where the spinal cord injury is complete and functional activities are significantly affected, a neurosurgical procedure exists that helps to significantly decrease spasticity in the lower extremities. This procedure is called a percutaneous selective posterior-sensory radio-frequency thermal rhizotomy. In this procedure needles are inserted into the intervertebral foramen onto the nerve roots after they exit from the spinal cord (Fig. 4-2, 4-3).

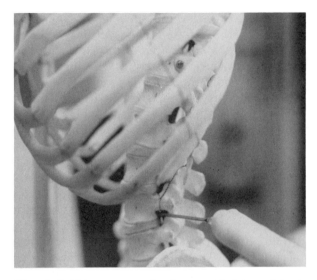

Fig. 4-2 Rhizotomy needle placement in intervertebral foramen.

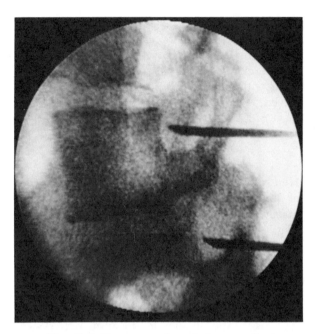

Fig. 4-3 Fluoroscopy lateral view, needles in intervertebral foramen.

Radio-frequency current is used to disrupt the function of the small and intermediate sensory fibers (Fig. 4-4). This will affect the A-delta and C pain fibers and the I-A sensory fibers of the gamma loop. Thus, nocioceptive stimuli and the tonic stretch reflexes will be reduced or eliminated. This will significantly reduce spasticity in most cases. Other sensory stimuli that can also cause

spasticity problems that are currently difficult to control are light touch and proprioception. In cases of incomplete spinal cord injury when impaired or normal pain sensation is present, there is another neurosurgical procedure called a micro-

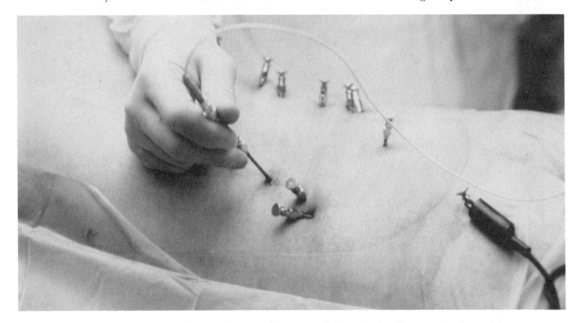

Fig. 4-4 Rhizotomy needles in place; probe inserted through needle to make thermal lesion.

rootlet rhizotomy, wherein the small and intermediate sensory fibers are surgically sectioned. This requires an open surgical procedure, whereas the percutaneous radio-frequency rhizotomy is done without open exposure of the tissues involved.

Heterotopic Ossification

Heterotopic ossification (HO) is the development of abnormal bone in soft (nonskeletal) tissue, primarily in the region of the hip and knee joints (Fig. 4-5)

It occurs in many spinal cord injured individuals and may develop within a few days after the injury occurs or several months later. The cause of heterotopic ossification is unknown, but it occurs only below the level of injury. Rapid onset of heterotopic ossification is signaled by an increased swelling of the hip or knee and an increased warmth or redness overlying the swelling. Loss of range motion in the affected joint becomes obvious. Swelling occurs in the area of the HO; and there may be an increase in spasticity, swelling of the entire leg, and elevated temperature.

Most patients with heterotopic ossification experience no significant functional limitations. However, in a minority of patients, the HO may result in major losses of range of motion, thus affecting the patient's functional status. Examples would include sitting postural problems due to a loss of hip flexion range and loss of knee flexion range, which may necessitate the use of an elevating leg rest.

The physical therapist working the acute phase of spinal cord injury must be alert to swelling in the thighs and losses of range of motion in the hips or knees without any apparent cause. When this occurs the physician should be notified so that the necessary medical testing can be performed to determine whether heterotopic ossification is oc-

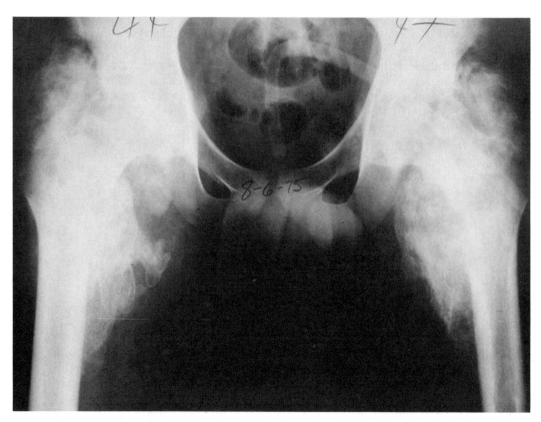

Fig. 4-5 Heterotopic ossification; x-ray of hips.

curring. Currently, a medication called Didronel* is available that has shown success in either slowing down or arresting the process in its early stages.

The unilateral loss of flexion range of motion in a hip will necessitate a re-evaluation of the cushion being used. An explanation of this problem is dealt with under the section titled Cushions.

Post-traumatic Cystic Myelopathy

Post-traumatic cystic myelopathy (spinal cord cyst) is a collection of fluid within the spinal cord that can create progressive damage to the spinal cord, resulting in progressive neurological changes. Spinal cord cysts occur in 5 to 10 percent of spinal cord injuries. They may develop any time from months to years postinjury. The signs and symptoms of spinal cord cysts may include one or more of the following:

1. Significant or major loss of pain or temperature sensation and/or muscle function (above the injury level)
2. Increased sweating or development of an unusual sweating pattern (i.e., sweating only when lying on one side or another or sweating only when in a specific position)
3. Increased spasticity
4. Pain
5. Autonomic dysreflexia (hyperreflexia)
6. One pupil appearing larger than the other (alternating Horner's syndrome)

Hyperhydrosis (marked abnormal sweating) and increased spasticity without other cause, such as decubiti, bladder infection, etc., usually indicate the presence of cystic myelopathy.

Changes in sensation or muscle function may develop gradually. The patient may note that it is more difficult to do some of the functional activities, such as holding items, dressing, change in balance, or burning occurring in areas where previously there had been normal sensation.

Physical therapists should thoroughly educate their patients regarding their neurological status (i.e., their motor and sensory functions) and encourage them to contact physicians should changes occur indicating a loss at a later time. It is imper-

---

* Proctor and Gamble, Cincinnati, OH

ative for a physical therapist to document accurately the sensory and motor levels in the acute phase of the patient so that tests will be available for comparison at a later time. When at all possible, it is advisable to have the same therapist re-test a patient at a later time to determine if significant changes have occurred.

Current neurosurgical techniques to relieve the cyst via drainage tend to maintain the status quo and prevent a further deterioration.

REHABILITATION PROGRAMS

Halo Vest Protocol

The guidelines used at Craig Hospital for treating patients in a halo vest for cervical stabilization are presented in this section. It should be emphasized that all functional activities, with the exception of wheelchair propelling on smooth terrain indoors, requires the presence of a spotter.

1. Lifting—Three-man flat lift into a tipped chair, tilt table, or bed. Remember, top man holds jacket—not metal uprights (Figs. 4-6 and 4-7).
2. Handling—To come to sitting, have spotter hold across shoulders to bring to sitting. Do not hold metal uprights.
3. Transfers—Patients in halo may be transferred after instruction by therapist. Must have hands-on spotting (Fig. 4-8).
4. Weight Shifts—Usually done side-to-side. Patients may or may not assist. Spotters should be present. Have casters *locked forward* and chair *locked*. Be aware of skin protection for insensitive skin (Fig. 4-9).
5. Padding—Tilt table should have standard padding to clear bony prominences. Place a pad or towel under the halo apparatus to prevent it from puncturing the tilt table and to allow for sliding (Fig. 4-6). The bed should have standard padding on stomach, back or sides, above and below bony prominences. When on side, make sure the bottom area is not pinched by the halo jacket.
6. Sitting—Always wear a seatbelt and place it at high chest level. Make sure posterior uprights are not caught on back upholstery.
7. Wheelchair handling—Indoor smooth terrain

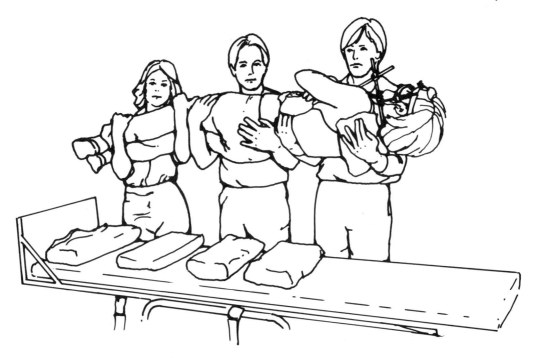

Fig. 4-6 Three-man flat-lift. Patient in halo vest. Notice hand positions and padding placement. A fourth person could be used to ventilate a patient with an Ambu-bag.

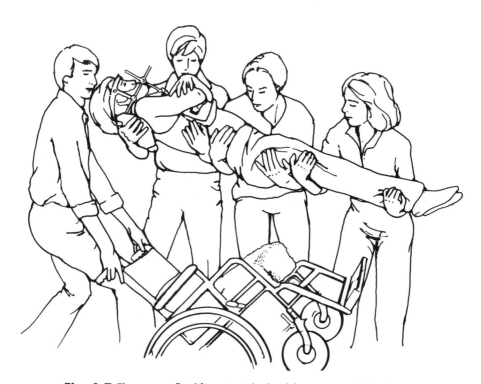

Fig. 4-7 Three-man flat lift to tipped wheelchair; patient in halo vest.

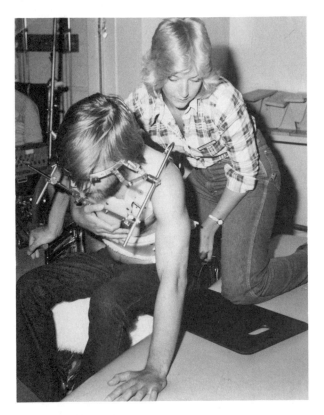

Fig. 4-8 Transfer of patient in halo vest with a spotter.

A ventilator-dependent quadriplegic who is referred to physical therapy may still have medical problems that prevent participation in a full program. An early program may consist of being on a tilt table one or two times a day for an hour. The individual may still have IVs, will probably be on a large ventilator, and may not be able to vocalize because of the tracheostomy.

Mobilization Program

To get this person up on the tilt table and transport him to the physical therapy department is a major undertaking. He is flat lifted by three people to a tilt table (see Fig. 4-6). He may need the assistance of a manual resuscitator during the transfer. Although transporting the individual to the department often requires more time than is actually spent in therapy, it is still important to transfer the patient. Exposure to this patient care atmosphere may be the patient's only diversion from the hospital room. Therapy also provides a reason to wear personal clothing, another psychological

may be independent. All other chair skills should be done with a spotter.

8. Mat work—Should be done on elevated mat. Must have a spotter. Spotters remember to hold jacket—not uprights.
9. Standing—Tilt table is the usual method. Standing table may be used as indicated. Stalls bars are not used.
10. Outings and passes—Will be decided by the treating physician and team members.

Quadriplegic C1–C4

Specific Activities for Ventilator Dependent Quadriplegics (C1–C3)

In addition to upper and lower extremity paralysis, the ventilator-dependent quadriplegic will be unable to breathe without the aid of a ventilator. Difficulty with communication is compounded by the sight and sound of the ventilator.

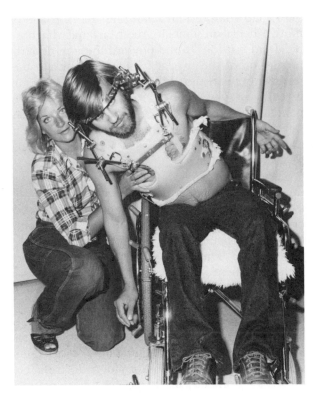

Fig. 4-9 Assisted weight shift. Patient in halo vest.

boost. Finally, the physical therapy setting provides the patient an opportunity to become acquainted with other patients and staff members.

The tilt table provides the ventilator-dependent quadriplegic with a different viewpoint of his surroundings. He no longer needs to spend 24 hours a day observing the ceiling and faces towering over him. The tilt table also increases his ability to tolerate the upright position, thus preparing him for sitting in the wheelchair. The therapist can carry out range of motion while the patient is on the tilt table.

Progressing a high quadriplegic from an *early program* to a *full program* varies according to the individual's medical status. Variables that influence this progress in a wheelchair include (1) the degree of hypotension, (2) skin tolerance, and (3) overall tolerance to the wheelchair. As a person progresses to a full program, transporting him to the department becomes a less complex process. The use of the portable ventilator, as well as the individual's increased sitting tolerance, makes the transport process easier and requires less staff. The portable ventilator is much quieter and can be strapped onto a lap board on the chair (Fig. 4-10). It allows more wheelchair mobility, both around the hospital and outside. In the physical therapy department, one of the first activities worked on is the transfer onto an elevated mat. After the technique is perfected, variations can be used to transfer the patient to/from a bed to the wheelchair. When setting up the transfer, the wheelchair is set at a slight angle to the elevated mat and the ventilator is placed on the mat.

Since the quadriplegic remains on the ventilator during the transfer, it is important to have ample tubing. After positioning all the equipment, good body mechanics and sliding board are used to transfer the patient. The procedure requires only one person. The transfer can be accomplished with the patient's feet on the floor (Fig. 4-11). The preferred method however, is to have the patient's feet up on the mat (Fig. 4-12). The spotter can be in front or behind the patient. Throughout the process the individual is taught how to instruct someone else to transfer him. These instructions should include simple directions for a safe transfer, as well as good body mechanics for his attendant's protection.

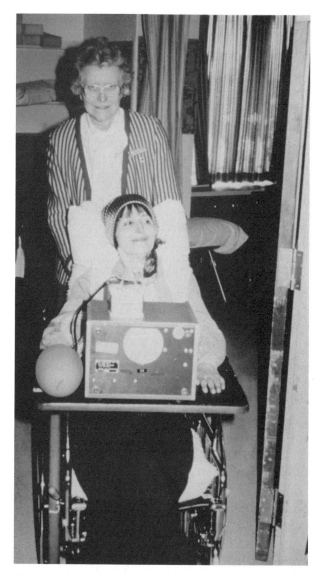

Fig. 4-10 Ventilator-dependent quadriplegic. Transport to physical therapy using a portable ventilator.

Mat Activities

Once the patient is on the mat, the emphasis of the exercise program will be on such activities as attaining the long-sitting position through stretching the individual's hamstrings, vestibular stimulation, strengthening the neck muscles, and practicing transfers. The ventilator-dependent quadriplegic has frequently been in bed for a longer period of time than other spinal injured patients. His hamstrings are usually tight, prohib-

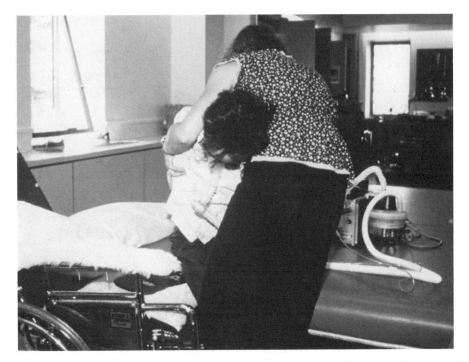

Fig. 4-11 Ventilator-dependent quadriplegic. One-man assist transfer to mat, feet on the floor.

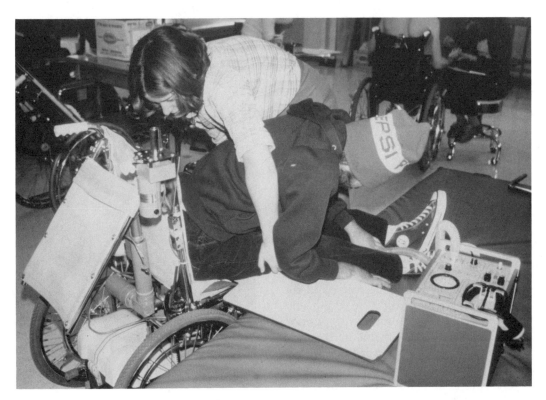

Fig. 4-12 Ventilator-dependent quadriplegic. Preferred alternate transfer to mat. *Feet up* placement of transfer board.

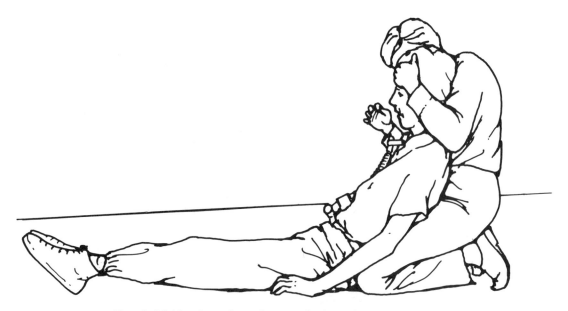

Fig. 4-13 Ventilator-dependent quadriplegic. Long sitting on mat.

iting him from long sitting. By stretching the hamstrings to establish the long-sitting posture (i.e., 110° hip flexion with the legs straight), the patient can work toward a balance point for ease of transfer (Fig. 4-13).

Vestibular stimulation is another area of emphasis during the mat program. The individual is leaned first to one side and then to the other to increase his body awareness. (Fig. 4-14)

Isometric exercises for strengthening the neck muscles are done to gain head control and for assistive breathing in an emergency. Functional activities using the neck muscles may include using a mouth stick for communication and operating a Sip'n Puff wheelchair.

Bed Transfer

Transfer into and out of bed is the next area of emphasis. The best method varies from individual to individual according to size, spasticity, and the person in the family who is going to be responsible for the transfer. In addition to the sitting position transfer, (see Figs. 4-11 and 4-12), another possible method is a flat transfer using two or three sliding boards. One is placed under the shoulders (Fig. 4-15), the other under the hips. If a third one is used, it is placed under the heels.

Individuals who have experienced postural hy-

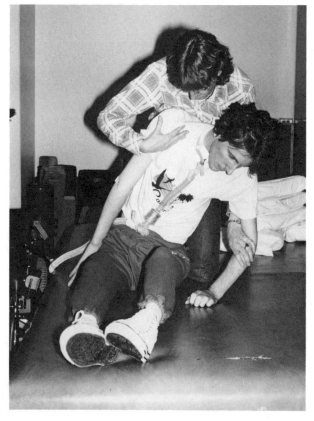

Fig. 4-14 Ventilator-dependent quadriplegic. Vestibular stimulation by leaning side-to-side.

potension when quickly assuming a sitting position may prefer a flat transfer. Some situations (i.e., size of the patient and/or attendant) will require the use of a mechanical lift for all transfers. Developing the most functional transfer method requires a lot of time and practice.

Wheelchair Maneuvering

Wheelchair training should introduce the patient to the wheelchair and its removable parts. He should learn to instruct others in handling and maneuvering the wheelchair. Exercises can be done to strengthen the patient's neck musculature in the sitting position. Independent mobility is offered to the high quadriplegic through the use of an electric, reclining wheelchair (Fig. 4-16).

Examples of possible drive controls for this chair include a chin control or a Sip'n Puff control (see Fig. 4-16). The chin control requires more strength and endurance in the neck to operate. The Sip'n Puff control is activated by sipping or puffing into a tube. Occupational therapy traditionally is involved in ordering and training the high quadriplegic with this equipment.

Since skin protection is vital to the high quadriplegic, the ability to do a weight shift independently is important. The ability to recline the wheelchair provides a needed weight shift. It also provides the individual with an opportunity to rest without having to transfer back into bed (Fig. 4-16).

The respirator will fit on an extended tray on the back of the chair. It will be equipped with three batteries, two giving power to the chair and the other one providing power to the respirator (Fig. 4-17).

The therapist should stress the need for daily transportation. The size and weight of the electric reclining wheelchair necessitates the use of a van to transport it. Aluminum ramps or mechanical built-in lifts can be used. The ventilator-dependent quadriplegic can be transported in a car when

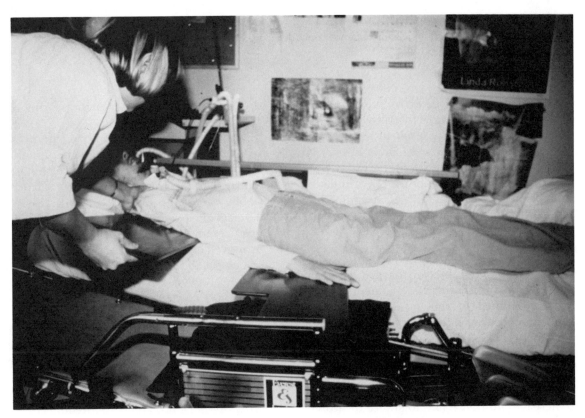

Fig. 4-15 Placement of transfer board under shoulders.

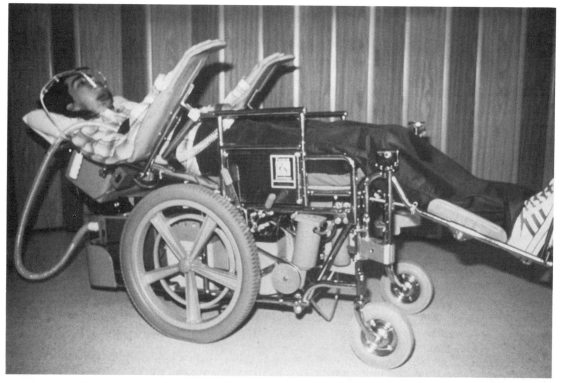

Fig. 4-16 Ventilator-dependent quadriplegic. Reclined with Sip'n Puff control.

using his manual wheelchair. In this case, the ventilator and its battery are first lifted onto the car seat. A sliding board is used to transfer the individual. The manual wheelchair is lifted into the trunk or back seat. Harness-style safety belts are used during transportation of the ventilator-dependent quadriplegic, both in a car and/or in a van.

Mat Program

The goals and philosophies of the mat program for the C4 and the ventilator-dependent quadriplegic are outlined in this section. These mat activities are encouraged for persons with this high level of physical dependency.

Functional Goals

The functional goals of the mat program are

1. To increase endurance and tolerance to sitting
2. To develop an awareness of balance
3. To strengthen the innervated musculature

through active exercises; weight bearing on arms
4. To gain and maintain mobility of the neck, trunk (especially rotation), and the upper and lower extremities (without overstretching the hamstrings and the back such that balance and stability are compromised)
5. To provide a variety of active and passive postures and movements to increase the sense of movement and to decrease the patient's fear of being handled

Progression of Program

Initially, the individual begins a gentle mat program in supine, sitting, and sidelying. A gentle side-to-side rocking motion is found helpful for the apprehensive individual in sitting or lying (see Fig. 4-14).

Using a full length mirror during sitting activities assures the person of the support he cannot feel. It also allows the therapist to monitor the patient's facial responses. Isometric neck exercises are in-

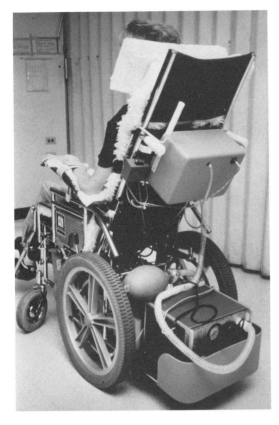

Fig. 4-17 Wheelchair with respirator and batteries on rear tray.

dicated in this early stage. Incorporating passive reaching and rotational movements during the mat activities can replace the traditional extremity range of motion.

Once a trust level is established between the person and therapist, more variations and postures can be undertaken, depending on the individual's medical condition. (Fig. 4-18)

The patient must be taught to use neck and shoulder muscles for balance. If the neck strength is adequate, it is important to teach the patient how to right the head in a fall. Weight bearing through the passively placed hands and/or elbows is found helpful in maintaining range, facilitating stability, and decreasing the pain of an immobile joint.

When appropriate, the prone position, position on knees and elbows, and activities on a therapeutic ball and/or bolster are included (Figs. 4-19 and 4-20). A high quadriplegic on a ventilator can also be treated on the therapeutic ball.

It should be noted that not all of these activities are appropriate or indicated for all patients. The person's body size, age, anxiety level, neck strength, joint range limitations, and spasticity all are influencing factors in determining the type of mat program best suited for the individual. However, the presence of the ventilator is not auto-

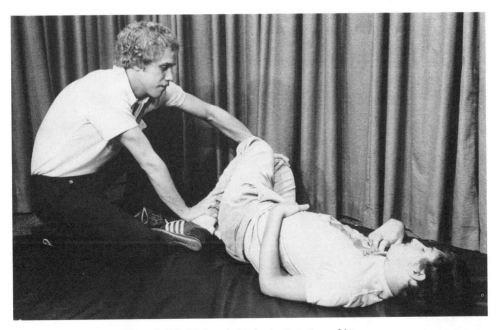

Fig. 4-18 High quadriplegic. Rotation of hips.

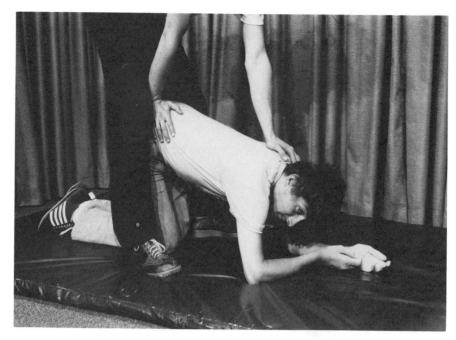

Fig. 4-19 High quadriplegic. On elbows and knees.

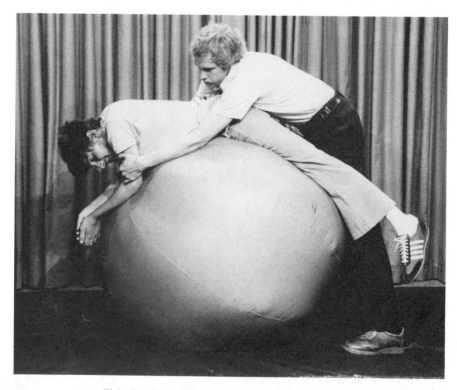

Fig. 4-20 High quadriplegic on therapeutic ball.

Table 4-2 Mat Exercises for C4 and Ventilator-Dependent Quadriplegic*

<table>
<tr><td valign="top">

1. Long sitting
   A. Stretching and Mobility
      1. Reach hands toward toes
      2. Hands under knees, rock from one elbow to the other
   B. Balancing—Righting with head and shoulders
   C. Strengthening
      1. Isometric neck exercises forward, backward, and sideward
      2. Keeping the chin tucked
   D. Breathing—Exhale slowly when reaching hands toward toes; inhale slowly as the person is brought back up with arms over head

II. Supine
   A. Mobility—Legs to chest (as in backward somersault); rotate side-to-side, keeping shoulders flat; person can rotate head opposite to direction of hips
   B. Strengthening
      1. Isometric neck extension into the mat
      2. Isotonic neck flexion, straight up and diagonally

III. Sidelying
   A. Mobility and Strengthening
      1. Lift head off of mat (lateral flexors)
      2. When being rolled supine to side, tuck the chin and lift the head
      3. When being rolled side to supine, push the head backward (helps desensitize shoulder pain by gently rolling on it)

</td><td valign="top">

IV. Prone
   A. Mobility
      1. Position the arms in flexion above the head
      2. Position the arms in abduction and external rotation
   B. Strengthening
      1. Prone on elbows
         a. Neck exercises as above in Sitting
         b. Shift weight from elbow to elbow using head movement
      2. With pillow under the chest, raise and turn head side-to-side (pillow under forehead may be necessary)

V. Knees and elbows—Strengthening and vestibular stimulation neck exercises as above in Sitting

VI. On therapeutic ball and/or bolster
   A. Strengthening, mobility and vestibular stimulation
      1. On knees with forearms on ball in weight-bearing position, do neck exercises as in Sitting position
      2. Sitting on bolster in riding fashion, do similar exercises as in long leg sitting; this position loosens adductor spasticity
      3. Lying prone over top of ball or bolster, rock back and forth

</td></tr>
</table>

* It is emphasized that this selection of activities is not always appropriate for all patients. It does provide a variety of sensory stimulation for these quadriplegics who, because of their level of lesion, experience severe sensory deprivation. Such activities demonstrate to the person and his family that movement and handling need not be feared.

matically a contraindication for any or all of the activities.

Specific Activities
See Table 4-2 for a list of various exercises.

Dependent Transfers

Transfers for the complete C4 and ventilator-dependent quadriplegics (C1–C3) most often require the use of one sliding board, sometimes two, depending on the method and type of transfer. These dependent transfers are safely performed by one person or spotter (as referred to here). The method of transfer depends on a number of factors including the patient's anxiety level, body size, neck strength, balance, comfort level (of the tracheostomy site in particular), tightness of the hamstrings and the back, and spasticity. The body mechanics of the spotter and the type of transfer are also determining factors when considering the method of transfer.

Several basic principles listed here should be remembered to perform any transfer safely and efficiently.

1. Follow good body mechanics.
2. Plan ahead. Clear the area of obstructions and put necessary objects close at hand. Be sure the ventilator is strategically located to allow for enough tubing length for the excursion of the transfer.

3. Stabilize the transferring objects. Caster locks are helpful in preventing the wheelchair from turning away.
4. Explain to the person what is to be accomplished. This encourages the individual's participation and learning so that he can verbally instruct anyone in the transfer.
5. Consider skin protection. When placing the sliding board under the ischial tuberosities, be sure to push it down into the transferring object rather than against the ischial tuberosities (Fig. 4-21). Be sure to move the hips forward of the rear tire so that the buttocks do not scrape the tire during the transfer.
6. Lean the person as far forward over the knees as possible with the arms crossed in the lap. This helps unweight the hips and makes the slide easier. The ventilator hose can be secured with rubber bands to prevent it from falling off the trachea.
7. The hips should lead first. The shoulders should be rotated away from the direction of rotation of the hips. This also helps unweight the hips and make the slide easier.
8. Avoid pulling on the clothes or the catheter tubing.
9. Do not pull on the person's arms to bring him to sitting. It is best to lift from behind the shoulders.
10. Standing in front lessens the fear of falling but makes it more difficult to bring him to sitting or to lay him down.
11. Positioning the feet up on the transferring surface increases balance.
12. Positioning the feet down on the footrests or floor unweights the hips more than with feet up.
13. When doing a shower/commode chair transfer, covering the sliding board with rip-stop nylon material allows for a better slide for the bare bottom. A towel under the buttocks also helps.
14. When doing a car transfer, it is sometimes easier to pull the hips from inside the car rather than to push them in from the outside.

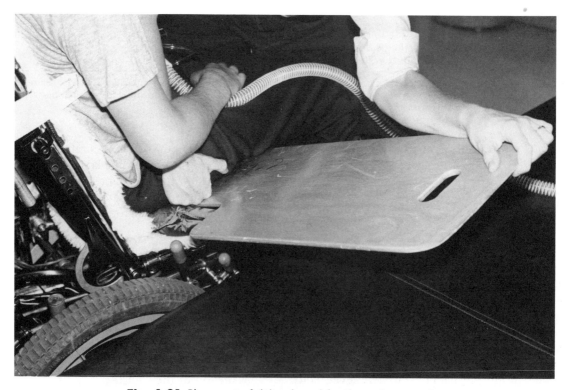

Fig. 4-21 Placement of sliding board for dependent transfer.

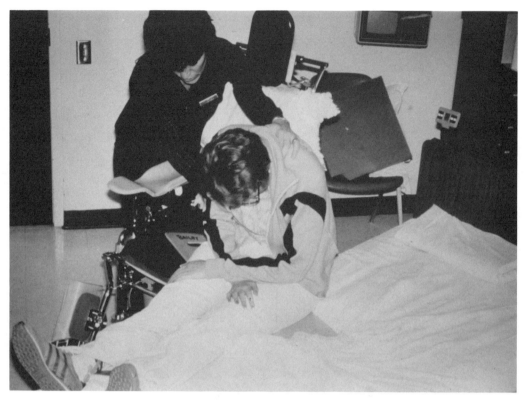

Fig. 4-22 Dependent transfer. Sliding patient on transfer board.

The types of transfers routinely considered are

1. Wheelchair to bed. Begin by placing the wheelchair at an angle to the bed. Remove footrests, sit patient upright, position patient's legs either up on the bed or with feet on the floor. Lean patient slightly away from the bed and place sliding board under the ischial tuberosities (See Fig. 4-21). Position patient firmly onto the transfer board. Slide patient over onto the bed (Fig. 4-22).
2. Wheelchair to couch
3. Wheelchair to car. The procedure is similar to the wheelchair-to-bed transfer. Additional considerations would be three optional feet positions: (1) both feet in car, (2) one foot in car and one foot out of car, or (3) both feet out of car (Fig. 4-23). Feet positioning will vary depending on the type and size of car, patient size, and amount of spasticity.
4. Bed to commode (usually not for ventilator-dependent persons)
5. Wheelchair to airplane seat. Because of the fixed armrest on the aisle seat, a transfer board cannot be used. Proper body mechanics are especially critical when *lifting* a ventilator-dependent person (Fig. 4-24).
6. Wheelchair to floor (beach). Other transfers are considered according to the person's needs (bath bench, water bed, etc.). An alternate method to *sitting* bed transfers is a *flat* transfer into the reclined wheelchair. The manual wheelchair can be used to tip the person to the floor rather than lift him. These two methods are described more specifically.

Flat Bed to Wheelchair Transfer
This transfer is an option for someone who cannot tolerate the upright position or for a spotter who cannot handle the person sitting. The reclined wheelchair is placed flush to the bed with one board placed under the shoulders and one under the hips. The person is then slid over gradually. (See flat transfer for ventilator-dependent quadriplegic.)

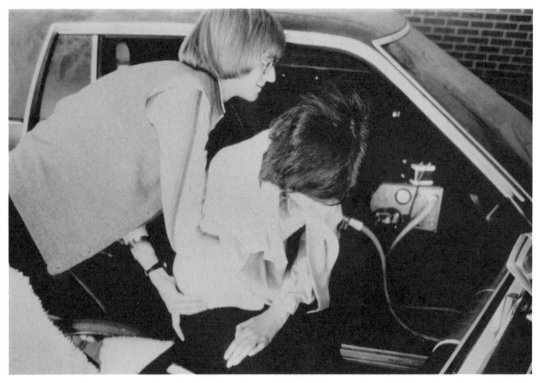

Fig. 4-23 Ventilator-dependent transfer. Note: Portable ventilator is placed on seat; patient's feet are out of car. Attendent is sliding patient into car on transfer board.

Floor (Beach) Transfer

Due to the module and batteries on the power wheelchair, *only the manual wheelchair* is suitable for the floor transfer. One spotter can safely tip the person into a wheelie and lower the wheelchair over backwards. For heavier person, two spotters may be needed to tip the person and wheelchair from the floor. Following is a brief outline of the steps for this procedure.

To the Floor
1. Lock rear wheels.
2. Place the ventilator on the floor out of the way, to the side. Remove the ventilator tray and backpack (Fig. 4-25A).
3. Take the patient's feet off the footrests and let them dangle. (This prevents the knees from falling into the person's face when the wheelchair is tilted back.)
4. Tip the wheelchair into a wheelie position and gradually lower the wheelchair all the way to

the floor so that it rests on the push handles. (Fig. 4-25B)
5. Remove the seat belt and release the brakes.
6. Flex the knees close to the chest and slide the wheelchair forward out from under the person's back.

Up From the Floor
1. Tip the wheelchair backwards to the floor.
2. Bring the patient's knees to his chest and slide the wheelchair as far under his back as possible. (His hips do not need to be flush against the cushion because he will slide down as the wheelchair is brought upright.)
3. Hook the knees over the front of the seat with the feet dangling (not on the footrests). Adjust cushion properly.
4. Fasten seat belt. Lock large wheels and the casters.
5. Kneel behind the person to support the head and shoulders on your lap. Lift the wheelchair

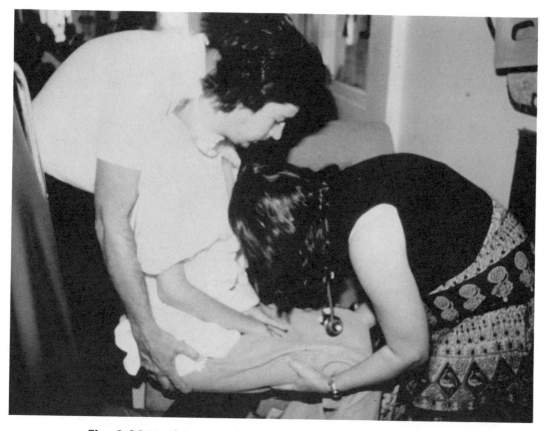

Fig. 4-24 Ventilator-dependent transfer to airplane seat: lifting patient.

up by the handgrips by going from kneeling to half kneeling, and then to standing.

6. Adjust the person into proper sitting position.

Exposing the person to as many variations in movement and position is felt to be very important for his total well-being. The high level quadriplegic experiences extreme sensory deprivation. Getting onto the couch or into the car for the first time after an injury can be very meaningful to the individual. On the other hand, the family situation, home accessibility, individual needs, etc. all have an influence on what transfers will realistically and practically be carried on at home. It is emphasized that a sliding board transfer can be safely done by one spotter. However, there are times when families choose to lift the person (either manually or by using a mechanical lift) for expediency rather than transfer him. During family instructions all methods for moving the person are explored to determine the best ways for both the individual and his family.

Dependent Wheelchair Handling Instructions

The following instructions are designed for those persons who will be handling the wheelchair of the disabled individual who is *dependent* or unable to give complete verbal or physical assistance. Before discharge, the therapist should demonstrate, teach, and practice these handling skills with the patient.

Remember that these are general, basic instructions and the therapist will "individualize" the handling skills. Items to be considered that might necessitate changes in these instructions include (1) type of wheelchair (i.e., a recline wheelchair with a high back, elevating footrests); (2) body size

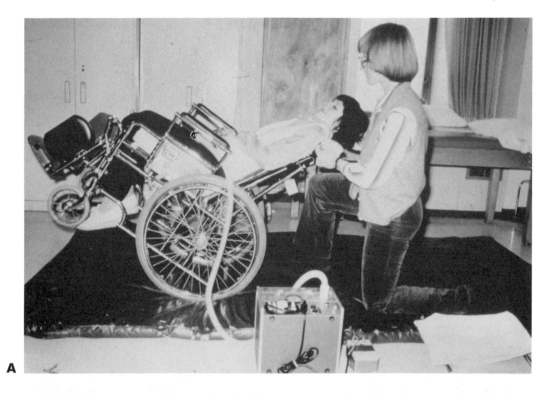

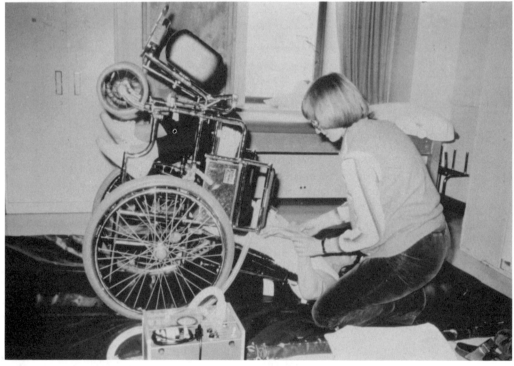

Fig. 4-25 **(A)** Ventilator-dependent transfer to floor. Tilt wheelchair/spotter's position. **(B)** Ventilator-dependent transfer to floor. Patient on floor.

and weight of the disabled person, and (3) body size, weight, and basic motor skills of the person assisting the patient.

The person handling the wheelchair should assume a basic position during certain activities known as the *classic spotter position,* which allows the safest protection from injury or strain of the assistant's own body, especially his back. This position also provides the greatest mechanical advantage and the least energy expenditure, allowing the safest control of the wheelchair and the disabled person.

Classic Spotter Position

The assistant, or spotter, places hands on the wheelchair push handles. The spotter turns sideways, moving his hip or thigh into the back of the wheelchair and spreading his feet comfortably apart for a wide base of support (Fig. 4-26).

Before any wheelchair handling activity, the spotter must make sure that the disabled person is correctly positioned in the wheelchair and appropriate straps and seat belt are secure. All wheelchair parts should be firmly locked in place.

These handling skills require practice and sometimes more muscle power than one person can provide. The spotter should plan ahead and request the assistance of other persons if attempting wheelchair handling on/or over any unusual or unfamiliar surfaces. The spotter should be able to give the necessary instructions to those assisting him.

Concrete to Concrete Curbs. The terrain is solid and basically even. The front casters will not get stuck or dig into the surfaces.

Up: The spotter pushes the wheelchair facing *forward* to the curb until the front casters are a

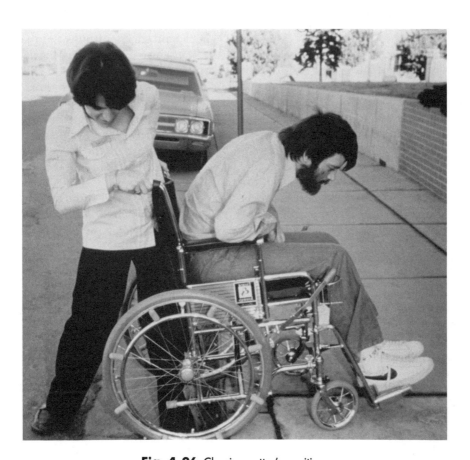

Fig. 4-26 Classic spotter's position.

few inches from the curb. With his hands on the hand grips and one foot on a tip bar of the wheelchair, the spotter pulls back on the hand grips and pushes down on the tip bar, balancing the wheelchair on the rear wheels (wheelie position). The spotter rolls the chair forward until the rear tires touch the curb. By placing his foot on the tip bar, the spotter gently lowers the front casters on the top of the curb (Fig. 4-27A). The spotter assumes the *classic spotter position* and rolls the wheelchair up and over the curb (see Fig. 4-26).

Down: The spotter approaches the curb with the wheelchair facing *backward* to the curb. The spotter assumes the *classic spotter position,* with one foot on the curb under the wheelchair and the other below, or both below depending on the spotter's height. The spotter eases the wheelchair's rear wheels down the curb. (see Fig. 4-27A.) The spotter then places a foot on the tip bar, places the wheelchair in the wheelie position, turns the *wheelchair sideways,* and then eases the front casters down.

Uneven Terrain/Curbs. The terrain is soft or loose and basically uneven. The front casters will get stuck or dig into the surfaces if allowed contact.

Up: The spotter approaches the curb with the wheelchair facing *backward* and balanced in the wheelie position. The spotter assumes the *classic spotter position* with one foot on the lower surface and the other foot up on the curb or both feet on the curb, depending on the spotter's level of comfort. The spotter must have his knees bent and keep his back straight. He then tips the wheelchair back and pulls the rear wheels up and over the curb (Fig. 4-27B). Once up the curb, the spotter holds the wheelie position and pulls the wheelchair backward until the uneven area is cleared and then eases the front casters down.

Down: The spotter approaches the curb with the wheelchair facing *forward* and balanced in the wheelie position until the rear wheels come to the edge of the curb. The spotter assumes the *classic spotter position* with one foot on the lower surface under the wheelchair, the other foot up on the curb, or both feet on the curb, depending on the spotter's level of comfort. He then tips the wheelchair back and eases the rear wheels down the curb (see Fig. 4-27B). Once down the curb, the

spotter holds the wheelie position, turns, and pulls the wheelchair backward until the uneven area is cleared and then eases the front casters down.

Stairs. A long or steep set of stairs is a dangerous and difficult obstacle for the person assisting a disabled person in a wheelchair. Avoid these stairs. When necessary, a set of stairs that are short, sturdy, and wide can be safely managed by one or more persons. It is best to use the following technique rather than removing the disabled person from the wheelchair and carrying that person up or down the stairs.

Up: The spotter approaches the stairs with the wheelchair facing *backward* and then balances the wheelchair in the wheelie position. The spotter assumes the *classic spotter position* with one foot up on the next one or two steps (depending on height and safe positioning of spotter) and the other foot on the step or surface just above that of the wheelchair. The spotter must have his knees bent and keep his back straight. He then tips the wheelchair back and pulls the rear wheels up and over the step until the rear wheels touch the higher step (Fig. 4-28).

Care must be taken to hold the wheelchair securely in the wheelie position back against the higher step while the spotter moves the foot from under the wheelchair and up one step. The spotter can then reposition the other foot up one step and is once again in position to pull the wheelchair up the next step.

Continue up the stairs in this manner—pull, stop, reposition, pull—until at the top of the stairs. Remember to hold the wheelie position and turn the wheelchair sideways to the stairs before easing the front casters down.

Down: The spotter approaches the stairs with the wheelchair facing sideways to the stairs and then balances the wheelchair in the wheelie position. He turns the wheelchair to face *forwards* to the stairs. Holding the wheelchair in this position, the spotter assumes the *classic spotter position,* placing one foot on the step just below the wheelchair. The spotter must have his knees bent and keep his back straight, placing the other foot up on the higher one or two steps (depending on height and safe positioning of spotter). He then tips the wheelchair back and eases the rear wheels down

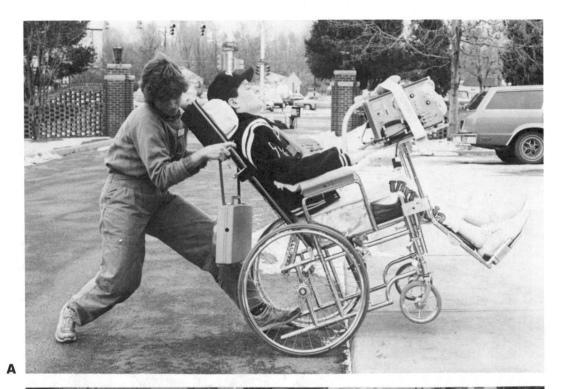

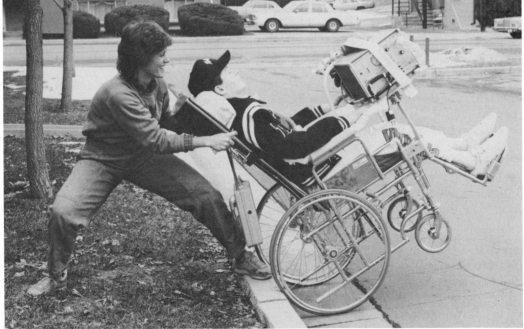

Fig. 4-27 (A) Curbs: front casters on curb. **(B)** Curbs: up curb to grass, backwards.

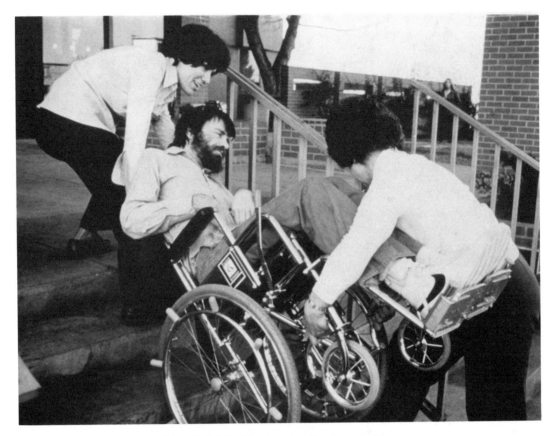

Fig. 4-28 Up/down stairs: Spotter's position.

the step, letting the wheelchair slide down his leg until the rear wheels touch the lower step. The spotter must hold the wheelchair securely in the wheelie position back against the lower step while moving the higher foot down one step. The spotter can then reposition the other foot to the step just below that which the wheelchair is on. Continue down the stairs in this manner—ease down, stop, reposition, ease down—until at the bottom of the stairs. Remember to ease the front casters down.

Ramps. If the inclined surface is solid and basically even but has a *steep grade,* it is best to use the following technique:

Up: The spotter approaches the ramp with the wheelchair facing *forward* and places the front casters up on the ramp (using the motions of the wheelie position). The spotter assumes the *classic spotter position,* spreading his feet comfortably for the steepness of the incline. The spotter then pushes the wheelchair forward sidestepping his feet to keep the hip in continuous contact with the back of the wheelchair (Fig. 4-29). The spotter must stop, holding the wheelchair against the hip and repositioning his feet. Continue up the ramp in this manner.

Down: The spotter approaches the ramp with the wheelchair facing *backward* and assumes the *classic spotter position.* Remember to keep the hip in continuous contact with the back of the wheelchair and sidestep with feet, easing the wheelchair down the ramp. It may be necessary to stop and reposition the feet with each rollback of the wheelchair. Continue until down to the bottom of the ramp, get the wheelchair in the wheelie position, turn the wheelchair sideways, and ease the front casters down.

Rough Terrain. If the surface is uneven, and/ or loose, the front casters will get stuck or dig into

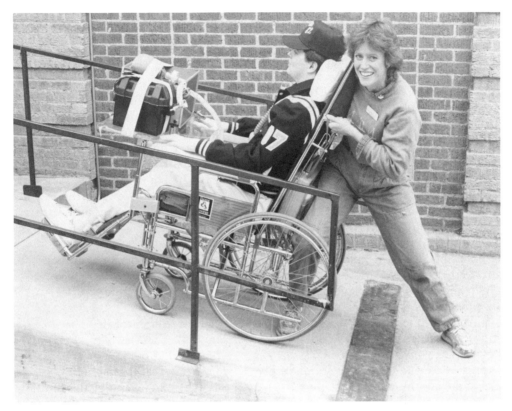

Fig. 4-29 Ramp.

the surface if allowed contact. To avoid this contact, pull back on the push handles and push down on one tip bar to balance the wheelchair on the rear wheels (wheelie position). Once in the wheelie position, the wheelchair can be pulled more easily *backward*, rather than pushed forward over the grass, gravel, stones, etc.

Comments. If at any time it appears that the spotter is losing control of the wheelchair and the disabled person, it is best to force the wheelchair to tip over backwards rather than frontwards or sideways. The disabled person will then not run as great a risk of being completely flipped out of the wheelchair. This is especially important to remember when handling the wheelchair up and down stairs.

When it is necessary for one or two additional persons to assist the spotter in handling the disabled person in the wheelchair, the following guidelines are recommended:

1. The primary spotter takes the initiative to give instructions to those assisting. Discuss what each is to do *before* starting the task.
2. The additional persons should be reminded of "knees bent and back straight" body mechanics.
3. The additional persons should hold the wheelchair frame rather than holding any removable parts of the wheelchair.
4. The additional persons may not be in a position mechanically appropriate to push or pull, but may best assist by holding the wheelchair position so that the top spotter can reposition his feet.
5. The additional persons should avoid pulling or pushing on the rear wheels of the wheelchair, unless there are two assisting that can time the push or pull to allow for even rolling of both wheels.

Quadriplegia C5–C8

At Craig Hospital stabilization is usually accomplished soon after the accident by means of a halo vest.

After all evaluations are completed, the therapist designs a treatment program based on the goals set in the functional checkout (See Fig. 4-1). If there are no associated injuries, the quadriplegic patient at the C5–C8 level (in halo vests) can begin a *mobilization program* immediately.

Mobilization Program

Tilt table standing is one of the first activities of the program. Full-length support hose and an elastic abdominal binder, towel binder, or corset can be used to help offset early symptoms of orthostatic hypotension. The patient should be taken to the physical therapy department if possible. This introduces the patient to a friendly environment where socialization with other patients can begin. While on the tilt table, the patient can begin upper extremity range of motion and exercises. Early during the adjustment period of the upright position, the therapist must monitor the patient's pulse and blood pressure. Dizziness is an early sign of hypotension. Should the patient faint, lowering the tilt table immediately will reverse the hypotension. By carefully monitoring the patient's vital signs, the physical therapist can usually avoid this "passing out" syndrome. This will help build patient confidence in the therapist. The therapist should gradually increase the maximal angle of the tilt table to 65°. Patients vary in the number of days required to reach the maximal adjustment to the tilt table.

Several days after beginning the tilt table, or sooner if possible, one can begin sitting the patient in a recliner wheelchair. The same precautions against hypotension (i.e., abdominal binder and support hose) are appropriate. A 45° angle from a full supine position is a good place to begin in the wheelchair. Increase the angle daily according to the patient's tolerance. Once the full upright position is attained without hypotensive symptoms, a switch to a regular upright wheelchair can be made.

During the early phase of wheelchair sitting, *weight shifts* should be performed every 15 minutes.

In a recliner wheelchair, this is done by fully reclining the wheelchair for 1 to 2 minutes. The buttocks area (i.e., ischial tuberosities) should be inspected after 15 mintues. If there is no problem with redness, resume sitting for 15 more minutes. The ischial tuberosities should be inspected again. Thirty minutes is the usual maximal time for the first time up in the wheelchair. Patients can increase their daily sitting time in 15 to 20 minute increments if the skin in the ischial area is maintained. When one stays in the semireclined position for 15 minutes or longer, the sacral area should also be inspected for undue pressure.

Weight Shifting

After the quadriplegic "graduates" to an upright wheelchair, weight shifts can be accomplished by one of the following methods:

Forward Weight Shift

1. The brakes on the rear wheels of the wheelchair should be locked.
2. The front casters should be locked forward so that they extend under the footrest of the wheelchair. Locking the casters to the front prevents the wheelchair from flipping forward during the weight shift.
3. The seatbelt is removed and the patient bends forward, laying his chest on his thighs and his head on his knees, with his arms dangling beside his lower legs. A spotter should remain in front of the patient.
4. The patient maintains in this position for 1 to 2 minutes, shifting weight and pressure to his legs and to the front of his wheelchair, allowing pressure relief off of his buttocks.
5. The patient may require assistance in locking the wheelchair, bending forward, and most especially in coming back up to the proper sitting position after the weight shift. One can offer assistance in coming back to the sitting position by standing beside the chair, holding the patient with one arm across his chest, and pulling the patient upright toward the back of the chair.
6. A patient is often independent in this type of weight shift with the use of *arm loops* on the back of his wheelchair. Initially, some assistance may be needed to place and or to

remove the arms from the loops and in resuming the upright position.

Side-to-Side Weight Shifts

1. The brakes on the rear wheels of the wheelchair should be locked.
2. The casters should be locked forward.
3. The person assisting with this weight shift should place a chair beside the wheelchair, facing the same way as the patient.
4. The seatbelt, as well as the arm rest and brake extension on the side next to the assistant should be removed.
5. The assistant leans the patient forward just enough for his back to clear the metal upright of the wheelchair back and then pulls the patient toward him, allowing the patient's elbow to rest on the assistant's thighs, and the patient's back to rest on the assistant's chest. One arm of the assistant is used to cradle the patient across the chest under his arms. The lean should be enough to the side so that all pressure and contact with the cushion on the *opposite* side of the buttocks is relieved. This

can be checked by the assistant by reaching behind the patient's back with his free arm to feel under the patient's opposite buttocks. (Fig. 4-30)

6. This position is maintained for 1 to 2 minutes, and the assistant replaces the patient to the proper sitting position in the wheelchair as follows: Support the patient with the cradling arm and stand up. Lean the patient back to the sitting position.
7. The weight shift is not complete until the same procedure is accomplished on the opposite side, thus relieving pressure to both sides of the buttocks.
8. The patient is often independent in this type of weight shift by hooking his hand or wrist behind the push handle of the wheelchair. Initially, he may require assistance in hooking his hand or wrist and guarding in assuming the upright position.

Tilt Back Leg Lift Weight Shifts

1. The brakes on the rear wheels of the wheelchair should be locked.

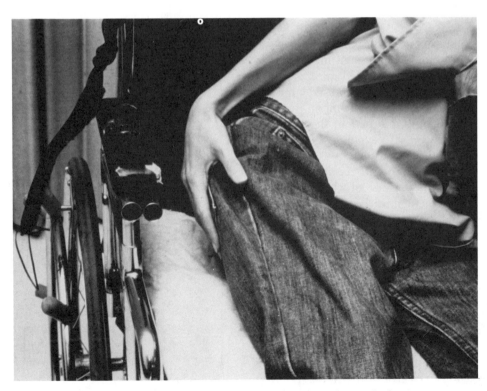

Fig. 4-30 Weight shift showing relief of pressure from ischial area.

2. This weight shift requires the assistance of two persons, one to tilt the wheelchair back (best done with the assistant sitting). The other assistant (standing) then lifts and holds up each leg from 1 to 2 minutes. This assistant holds the leg under the knee and the ankle, flexing the leg, allowing pressure to be shifted to the patient's back and off his buttocks on each side.

Push-Up Weight Shift (for the C7–C8 Quadriplegic)

1. The brakes on the rear wheels of the wheelchair should be locked.
2. The person assisting with this weight shift should be concerned with the patient's balance as he attempts to do a push-up with his hands on the armrest of the wheelchair. By placing your hands on the patient's shoulders, one will give the patient that added stability and confidence to lift his buttocks off the cushion and hold that position for 1 to 2 mintues. Initially, the patient may attempt the push-up with his elbows on the armrest and may need the balance assistance.

Progression

A mat program usually begins the same time as the tilt table program. A three-man lift is used to transfer the patient to the elevated mat.

Once the patient has been mobilized and has been sitting 3 to 4 hours daily in an upright wheelchair, the therapist and patient should begin discussing the type of wheelchair to be ordered for home use. As there is usually a 4 to 6 weeks time lag between ordering and receiving the patient's wheelchair (in the *best* of circumstances), this piece of equipment must be ordered as soon as possible so that the patient will have the wheelchair before discharge. Lightweight wheelchairs have proven to be satisfactory for the C6–C8 high quadriplegic, and in some cases, even for the strong C5 quadriplegic.

The tilt table program is usually discontinued once the patient has reached full tolerance to the upright wheelchair. Some quadriplegics prefer to continue a standing program for psychological reasons. For the C5–C6 quadriplegic, this can be best done by using an electric or hydraulic standing table. A C7–C8 quadriplegic can use stall bars (Fig.

4-31). Standing tables and stall bars are rarely used by quadriplegics after discharge.

If family members are on location during the rehabilitation program, they should be involved with the program from the beginning. Having them observe and participate as appropriate will help to relieve the anxieties about the quadriplegic loved one. Appropriate home instructions and

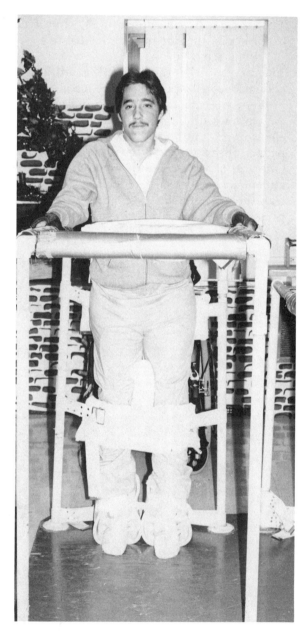

Fig. 4-31 C7–C8 quadriplegic standing in stall bars.

practice can be done as part of the ongoing program. This will prevent a last minute rush of instructions for the family at the time of discharge. If family members cannot be present throughout the program, at least 1 week should be allowed for *all disciplines* to teach home instructions adequately.

Remember, the functional approach to rehabilitation means *practicing daily* those skills needed to reach the maximal independence possible for the level of quadriplegia. As independence is gained, time becomes available for discharge planning.

The average time for a rehabilitation program should to 10 to 12 weeks, including the acute period if there are no associated injuries to delay full participation in the rehabilitation period.

Mat Procedures

Purpose

The purpose of mat procedures is to

1. Introduce the patient to exercises and proper body mechanics for functional activities (i.e., transfers, dressing, wheelchair activities)
2. Gain maximum balance, coordination, and endurance
3. Strengthen for functional activities
4. Stretch the hamstrings to a functional length (i.e., 110° of straight leg flexion)
5. Gain maximum efficiency from the respiratory system

Program

The following mat program offers examples of exercises for long sitting, supine, and prone positions.

Long Sitting. For stretching and mobility, the patient should

1. Reach with hands toward toes. Hold the position, then sit back up and repeat the procedure. Care should be taken to prevent the patient from stretching his back. Intrinsic back tightness will be important to the quadriplegic for maintaining balance in the sitting position.
2. With legs separated, he should reach with both hands toward the right foot, then to the center, then toward the left foot.

3. With arms under knees, the patient should lean forward with his nose toward his knees.
4. With arms hooked under his knees, he should rock from one elbow to the other.

The following exercise is to promote balancing.

1. The patient should raise arms out to the sides (shoulder level), reach forward, back out to the sides, forward, up, forward, back to the side, forward and down.
2. Circle arms forward and then backward
3. Try to clap hands with palms forward, and then backward.
4. Alternate arm motions (i.e., one arm forward and one arm backward; then reverse the procedure).
5. Raise arms out to the sides (shoulder level), rotate head and trunk to the right, back to the center, then to the left.
6. Raise arms frontward (shoulder level, elbows slightly bent), lean back as far as possible without losing balance; slowly bring the elbows backward and the head forward without losing balance. Modify this exercise by first turning to the right and then to the left.
7. Ball playing.

This exercise is designed to strengthen muscles.

1. Place hands slightly behind hips (the distance varies depending on the degree of elbow flexion desired). Fingers should be pointed outward. Bend elbows, hold the position, and then straighten the elbows.
2. Place hands by hips with the fingers slightly bent and pointing backward. Tuck chin on chest and push up to relieve weight from the buttocks by depressing shoulders.
3. While leaning on left elbow, place right arm under the left leg and attempt to move leg out to the side. The patient should resume the sitting position and repeat the exercise with the left arm and right leg. Reverse the procedure to move the legs together. (Modification: Place the elbows between the legs and attempt to separate them by pushing out with the elbows.)
4. Go from sitting position to supine and then back to the sitting position (Figs. 4-32A and B).

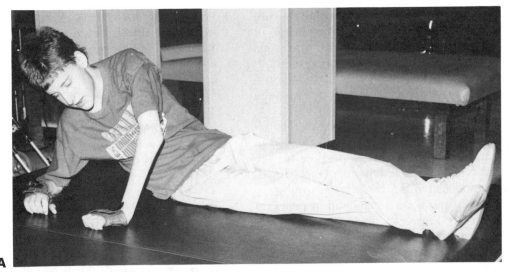

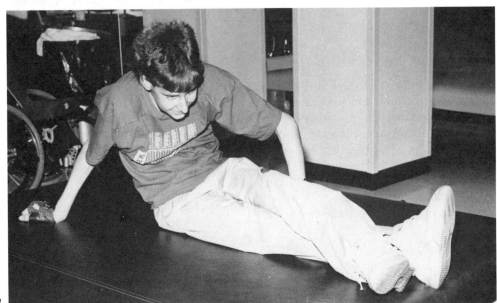

Fig. 4-32 (A) Up on one elbow. **(B)** Up on one hand, pulling on leg with other arm.

The following steps outline a typical weight-shifting exercise.

1. Do a sitting push-up, then shift the weight to the right, back to the center, to the left, and back to the center.
2. Place both hands on the mat to the right side. Unweight the left hip by leaning into the arms. Do push-ups from this position. (Modify the push-ups by using only the right forearm.) Repeat and reverse direction.
3. Place the left hand by the right knee (inside or outside) and the right hand by the right buttocks. Rotate head and shoulder down and around to the right as you push the hips to the left. Repeat in the opposite direction. (The lower the head, the higher the lift.)
4. Do sitting push-ups, forward and backward.

The following breathing exercise should be performed to a specific count.

1. Inhale through the nose.
2. Breathing in slowly, raise arms, with elbows slightly bent, above head.
3. Hold this position.
4. Reach down toward toes, slowly breathing out through mouth.

Supine. The following steps outline a stretching-strengthening exercise.

1. Reaching forward, with hands toward toes, raise head and shoulders from mat and then lower them. Try to raise head and shoulders to the right, to the center, and then to the left.
2. Lateral bending—With the arms by the sides, elbows bent, dig head into the mat toward the right while reaching with the shoulders and right hand toward the right knee to form a "C" with the body. Return to the center position. Repeat to the left side.
3. The arms should be at the sides. Bend elbows and press into the mat along with head to form an arch in the back. (Modification: Press the elbows into the mat, arch the back, and raise the head.)
4. Place hands under the hips, palms up. Raise buttocks by pressing the elbows into the mat. (Modification: As above, but with the head raised.)
5. Place the arms out to the sides, shoulder level. Press elbows into the mat and raise head and shoulders. (Modification: Press harder on one elbow to shift weight to the other side. Reverse the procedure.)
6. Rolling or turning—Cross legs at ankles.
7. Pull up knees and roll from side to side. This may require assistance.

A typical breathing is described in the following steps.

1. Place the arms by the sides.
2. Inhale through the nose while raising arms.
3. Exhale through the mouth while lowering the arms.
4. Continue to exhale by raising the head and shoulders from the mat.

Prone. In the prone position, the following exercise is designed to strengthen the upper extremity, neck, and back.

1. Place arms by sides. Raise the head, shoulders and arms. Turn head from side to side.
2. With the arms out at shoulder level, raise head and arms. Rock side to side.
3. Place hands by shoulders with palms down, elbows bent. Push on hands and raise head and shoulders. Shift weight from the right to the left.
4. Place hands beside hips with palms down, fingers toward the feet and elbows bent. Keeping the head down, roll the shoulders together forward, and push on the hands to lift trunk off the mat.
5. Place hands at sides with palms up. Pinch shoulder blades and elbows together while raising head.
6. Do push-ups.
7. Prone on elbows. Rock side to side.
8. Place one arm down at the side; the other, up above the head. Switch arms, as if in swimming, back and forth.

Transfers

In transfers, skin protection is the number one priority. Stabilizing the wheelchair and the other transferring object are important to the quadriplegic because he will push against those objects.

When teaching the transfers to a patient, one should demonstrate to the person what is to be done, how assistance will be given and how he will be protected. The patient should have already experienced pretransfer activities on an elevated mat to prepare him for the actual transfer techniques.

Basic Transfer to and from a Mat Table or Bed
1. Position the wheelchair.
2. Put the patient's feet up on the mat or bed first. (This presumes the hamstrings have been sufficiently stretched to 110°—straight leg raising.) The patient may use a leg loop or his arm to lift the leg up on the mat/bed depending on his strength. (Fig. 4-33A) Having the legs up provides balance. The

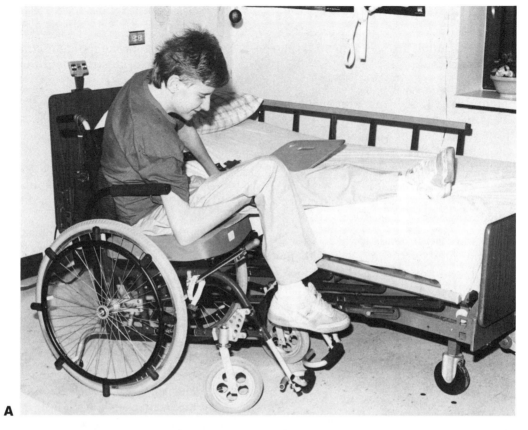

A

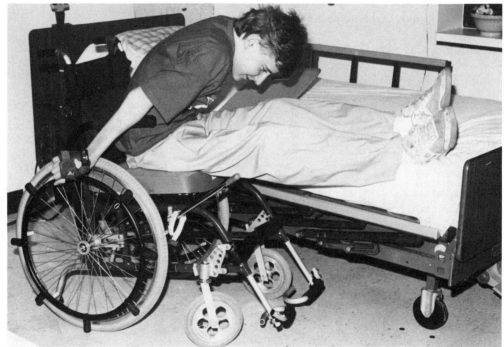

B

Fig. 4-33 (A) Transfer: Patient using his arm or a leg loop to lift the leg to the bed. **(B)** Mat/bed transfer. Patient pushing forward on tires. (*Figure continues.*)

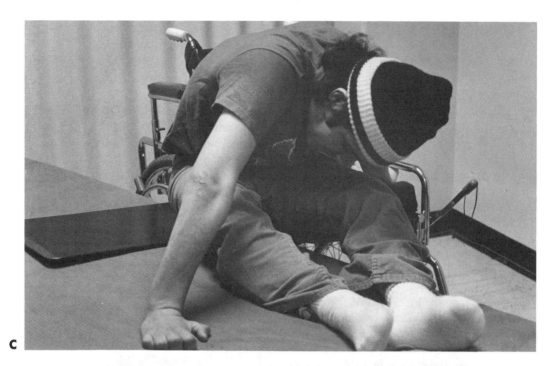

C

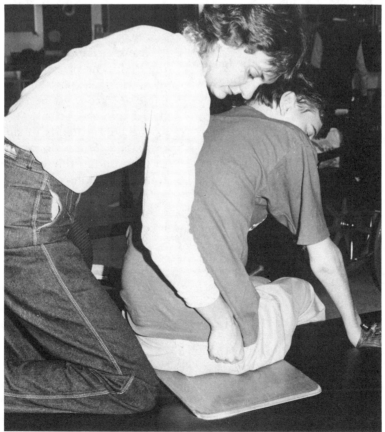

D

Fig. 4-33 (*Continued*). **(C)** Quadriplegic transfer technique showing hand placement and shoulder rotation. **(D)** Quadriplegic transfer. Therapist assists with waistband.

111

patient should not lean on the leg being lifted. This adds further weight and makes the activity more difficult. If using a leg loop, use the deltoids, *not* the biceps. This keeps the knee from bending. Place a pillow on the wheelchair footrests in case a foot slides off the mat or bed.

3. When using a transfer board with a cutout, place the board so that the cutout goes around the wheel. Be sure to push it down into the cushion and not into his ischials. Also be sure the board is *under* the ischials and *not* the thighs. As he slides forward he would slide the board out from under himself if the board is not well placed.

4. Slide the patient forward in front of the tire, to avoid hitting it. This is done by leaning him forward over the knees and having him push off from the tires (Fig. 4-33B).

5. Place the hands so that the arms are externally rotated and the elbows are straight. Do a shoulder depression or a rocking motion, sliding sideways toward the mat or bed. Some people use a push-pull method with the biceps (i.e., push on one arm and pull on the other). The hands must be well stabilized on the mat. The person will slide in an arc depending on where the arms are placed, so be sure the hips stay in front of the tire. Remember the hips should lead first. The shoulders will be rotated away from the direction the hips are going. This unweights the hip that is sliding (Fig. 4-33C).

6. Once on the mat or bed, remove the transfer board.

To give assistance in these transfers, the therapist will want to be behind the patient and the wheelchair. The therapist's outside hand will be by the patient's outside shoulder, to keep him from losing his balance forward or sideways. The therapist's other hand is on the waist band or pants pocket to help the patient slide if he needs the help. It is also a good position to keep him from hitting the tire (Fig. 4-33D).

The following transfers can be done a variety of ways according to the person's strength and abilities. Not all people will be able to do them.

Because they are more difficult they require repeated practice, as well as assistance initially.

Portable Shower/Commode Chair Transfers

Transfer to a Portable Shower/Commode Chair from the Bed with Minimal Assistance or Independently. The transfer board can be covered with rip stop nylon fabric; this helps the patient's bare skin slide easier and provides more skin protection.

1. Position the shower/commode with the brakes locked; place the sliding board under the buttocks; slide the patient onto the shower/commode using the same basic method used for a bed to wheelchair transfer, remembering proper body mechanics. Hand holds are a little more precarious due to the hole in a commode seat.

2. Once on shower/commode, remove the transfer board and place the feet on the footpedals.

Transfer from a Portable Shower/Commode to the Bed. The placement of the board is often the most difficult part of this entire transfer and extreme care must be taken to avoid forcing the board into the ischials. This could easily happen as the bottom tends to sink into the hole of the commode. Some people place the board in the section under the commode seat. Others slide forward on the commode seat out of the hole before placing the board. Some patients can get enough shoulder depression to lift up onto the board once it has been placed as close to the hips as possible, though still not under them (Fig. 4-34A).

The size of the hole in the commode seat makes a signifcant difference in the ability to place the transfer board. Smaller holes are great for transferring and board placement but should not be so small that it is difficult for the bowel program to be done.

Transfer to a Portable Shower/Commode Chair from the Bed Requiring Moderate to Maximal Assist

1. Position the commode with the casters locked (if available).

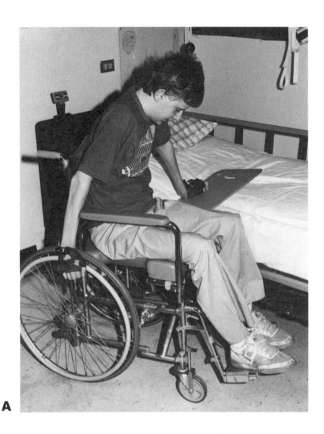

Fig. 4-34 (A) Transfer from shower/commode wheelchair to bed: Hand placement, shoulder depressions. **(B)** Sliding patient to shower/commode wheelchair, using towel.

A

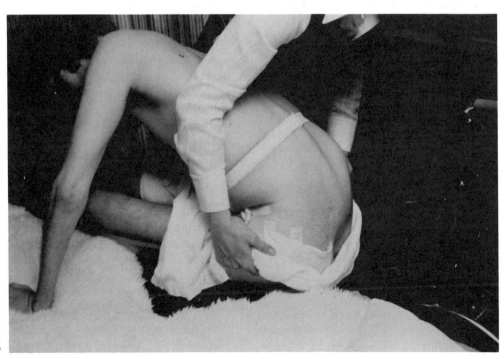

B

2. Place a towel or sturdy pillowcase directly under the hips and the thighs of the person to be transferred. This will be the sliding surface and will also give the spotter something to hold on to.
3. First sit the person up and place the board under the hips. (If the board is placed and the person then brought to sitting, the person may slip off the board in the process of coming to sitting.)
4. Begin sliding onto the shower/commode chair using the towel as a means of helping the person slide. It will be vital that proper body mechanics by both parties be used. Be sure to unweight the hip toward the shower/commode chair (Fig. 4-34B).
5. Once on the shower/commode chair, the board can be removed and the feet placed on the footrests. The towel can be removed by leaning the person forward over his knees, supporting the patient's shoulder, and pulling out the towel with the spotter's other hand.

Transfer from the Portable Shower/Commode Chair to the Bed with Moderate to Maximal Assist

1. Position the shower/commode chair next to the bed. Place the towel under the person's hips. This can be a difficult maneuver depending on whether the person's hips have slid down into the hole. Have the person do a side lean as in a side-to-side weight shift. This unweights one hip so the towel can be slid under the hip through the commode seat hole. Have him lean the other way to pull it up through the other side. If the commode has an opening on one side, pull the towel up through that side last. Be sure the towel is under the hips and thighs and is cradling the testicles.
2. Place the transfer board under the hips. *Be sure not to dig the board into the ischials.* The towel should help prevent this possibility.
3. Place the feet up on the bed and proceed with the transfer using the basic transfer techniques.

Tub Transfers

Transferring to a tub is accomplished easier if one uses a chair or shower bench in the tub. A transfer board covered with nylon also makes this transfer

easier. Try to use a transfer board shorter than the one the patient normally uses.

1. Position wheelchair along side of the tub and lock all brakes.
2. Place the board appropriately. Put tub-side leg into the tub and the other foot as close to tub as possible.
3. Slide into the tub chair. Once balanced, bring the opposite leg into the tub. Get positioned in the chair for showering.

When getting out of the tub chair or shower bench into the wheelchair, skin safety is again of the utmost importance.

1. Dry thoroughly. Position the wheelchair and remove the cushion. One could use an old cushion that won't be damaged by water. Place the board *under* the hips if possible; if not, then as far under as possible. A strong shoulder depression lift will be needed to get up onto the board.
2. Place the wheelchair-side leg on the footrest and the other one as close to edge of the tub as possible. Slide the patient out of the tub into the wheelchair using good transfer techniques.
3. Once in the wheelchair, bring the leg out of tub, position it and remove the transfer board.

As mentioned before, these transfers will not work for all quadriplegics, but they represent some of the more common approaches. The best way to find out if they will work is to try them. Practice with clothes on and a regular transfer board at first and then progress to practicing with bare skin and a covered transfer board. Successful transfer with clothes does not guarantee success without clothing.

Car Transfers

Getting into the Car on the Passenger Side. This transfer can also vary according to the person's strength, size, body mechanics, and the type of car. The level of independence will vary as well. The following describes the procedure for a C5 or weak C6 quadriplegic.

1. Position the wheelchair at an angle with the door open, so that the front of the rear tire is

even with the front part of the car seat back. Place the patient's feet into the car on a plastic bag if the person's legs tend to spasm in extension. The bag helps the feet slide.

2. Place the transfer board as in the bed transfer.
3. Slide the patient forward in front of the tire; then slide him into the car using basic transfer techniques.
4. Once in the car, remove the transfer board and position the patient accordingly.

Getting out of the Car on the Passenger Side. To get out of the car on the passenger side, reverse the preceding procedure. Some therapists use a technique wherein the feet are on the ground rather than in the car to transfer in and out. This requires more balance and more pivoting when moving to avoid the wheelchair tire. The transfer can then be done using the wheelchair and the inside dashboard as pushing and pulling surfaces. This technique can also be used when the patient is transferring into the driver's seat as the steering wheel can be used to assist him in the transfer.

Another foot placement is that of one foot in the car and one foot out. This can be used going either into or out of the car. Try all techniques and use what works best for that particular individual. (For a strong C6 and a C7 quadriplegic, the preceding steps are done more or less independently. (Fig. 4-35A and B)

Putting the Wheelchair into the Back Seat of the Car. It is easier to lift a standard manual wheelchair by the front end rather than in the middle. It is also easier to lift low on the wheelchair, moving it around the pivot point (rear wheels).

1. Unlock the nearest brake, flip up the footrests, and push the wheelchair away from the car; this puts the rear wheels in a better position to pull in.
2. Lift the front end by the footrests and rotate the wheelchair so that the *footrests are on the ledge.* Unlock the remaining brake (Fig. 4-36A).
3. Scoot over in the seat, flip the front seat forward, and pull the rear wheels up by pushing down on the footrests. Be sure to push straight down to avoid tipping the wheelchair sideways (Fig. 4-36B).

4. The rear wheels should now be up on the ledge. Roll the wheelchair in by lifting up on the footrests and pulling the chair in (Fig. 4-36C). Be sure the wheelchair push handles are inside the car. Push the wheelchair sideways onto the back seat.
5. Flip front seat back, and close the door.

Removing the Wheelchair

1. Open the door, flip front seat forward, and pull the wheelchair to the upright position. Roll the rear wheels onto ledge. One may need to use one hand to roll the rear wheels back via the rim and the other hand on the footpedals. Push down on them to lift the rear wheels.
2. Lower the rear wheels to the ground by stabilizing the wheelchair by the footrests.
3. Flip the seat back, and scoot the entire car seat back. Scoot over in the seat and pivot the wheelchair around until all four wheels are on the ground. Open the wheelchair seat by pushing straight down on the nearest front seat corner, which unweights the opposite rear wheel.
4. Lock the nearest brake. Flip the pedals in place. Reassemble the wheelchair, then transfer, swinging the hips first.

Once the patient is proficient in removing the wheelchair, he can begin eliminating steps to increase speed and efficiency, while still maintaining safety. The patient can eliminate the following steps: (1) moving the seat of the car, (2) removing the armrest, (3) locking the front casters, and (4) locking the brakes.

Comments

1. Avoid using any chrome part of the car, such as window or gutter, as a hand hold. Chrome can be very hot in the summer and cause burns.
2. Hot seats in summer can burn insensitive skin. (*Fabric upholstery* usually solves this problem)
3. Air conditioning and fresh air vents can allow frost bite on the feet.
4. With long distance travel, remember to do weight shifts and to use a good cushion.
5. Don't sit on wire seat "coolers."

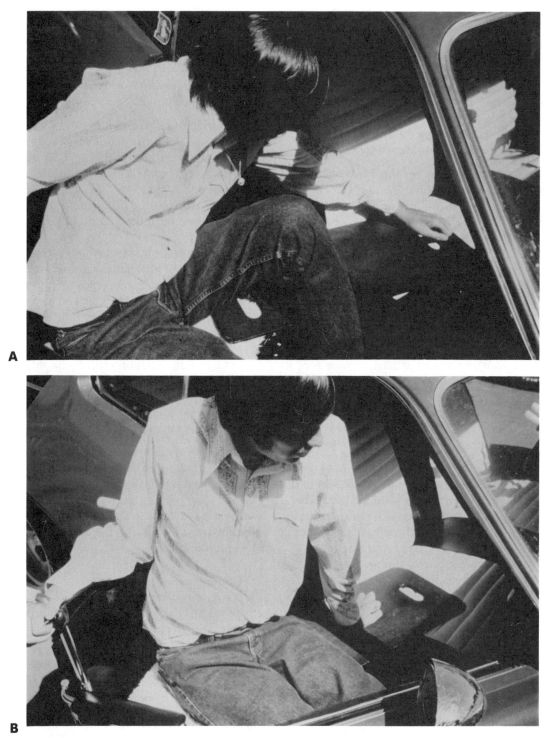

Fig. 4-35 (A) Placing transfer board independently. **(B)** Sliding across transfer board.

Fig. 4-36 (A) Wheelchair placement on door ledge. **(B)** Pivoting wheelchair on door ledge by pushing down on footrests. **(C)** Pulling wheelchair into the car.

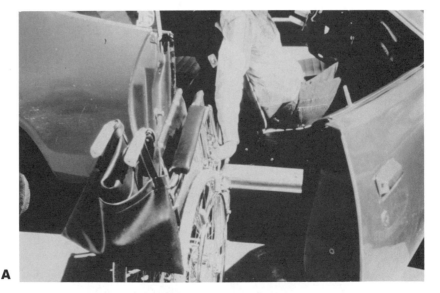

A

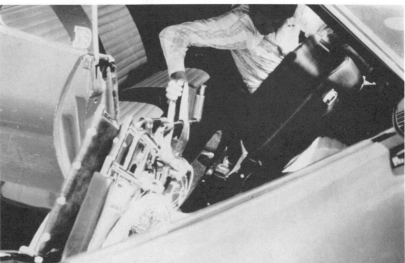

B

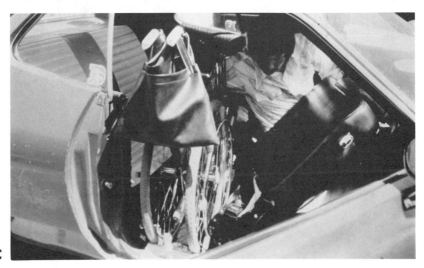

C

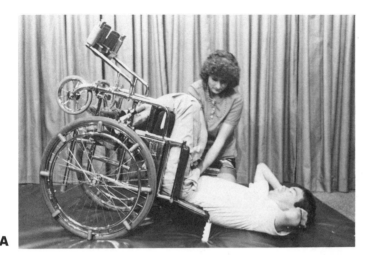

A

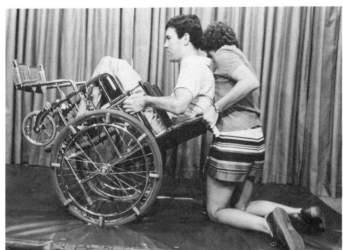

B

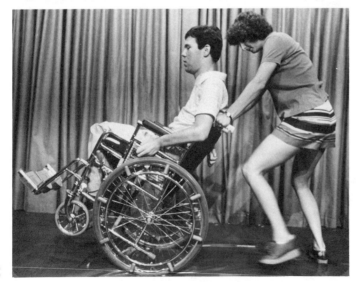

C

Fig. 4-37 (A) Placing both legs over the seat. **(B)** Continuing to lift patient; assistant upright on knees. **(C)** Assistant in standing position.

Beach Transfers

The purpose of this floor-to-wheelchair transfer is to provide a mechanism for assisting a C5–C8 quadriplegic up from or down to the floor, beach, or grass. This allows him to participate in practical activities, such as exercising, sun bathing, rafting, snow skiing, picnics, and playing with children or family on the floor or in the backyard at home. Refer to the following figures for examples and instructions: Figure 4-25A and B for getting a quadriplegic down to the floor and Figure 4-37A through C for getting a quadriplegic up from the floor.

Wheelchair Activities

No matter what the level of a person's injury, he will encounter obstacles to the wheelchair when outdoors. The first obstacle he will probably encounter is a curb. For a discussion of curb handling for the C5 quadriplegic, see dependent wheelchair activities under C1–C4 quadriplegics. A C6 quadriplegic will most likely need help going up and down curbs. (See up/down curbs in Section C1–C4 quadriplegics). Most C7–C8 quadriplegics are able to go down curbs independently. Those with only fair balance must lock their casters forward, once in position, to back down the curb. They must then lean forward as far as possible with the chest on the knees. They must roll slowly backwards toward the edge of the curb, until the rear wheels roll off evenly.

Once the rear wheels are down, those who have locked their casters must unlock them. If they have come down a small curb, they can sit up in the wheelchair. They must then pivot the chair around so the front casters come off the curb. One rear wheel must remain next to the curb to keep the foot pedals from hitting the curb as the chair pivots around. Once the front casters drop off the curb, there will be a jolt, so the person must watch his balance. (See curbs and other wheelchair activities under the Section Paraplegia).

For help on rough terrain, the quadriplegic's assistant can put him in a wheelie position and pull him backward through the roughest ground and possibly push him through the minimally rough ground.

The area of greatest difficulty for all people in wheelchairs is steps/stairs. It is always best to find two people to help a quadriplegic to go up the stairs. The person who is in back of the chair is the primary pulling person and the person in the front of the chair is the pushing and braking person. When possible, the person in the wheelchair should also help. The person in the back must tip the wheelchair back into a wheelie position. He must have a firm grip on the push handles, preferably with a thumb and forefinger on the chrome part of the handle, just in case the hand grip pulls off. The person in back is the coordinator of the team and calls the "pull" signal. He assumes a stance with legs far apart on the steps, hips and knees bent, back straight. He will pull with his arms straight.

The person at the bottom is a pusher and the braker. He should hold securely to any nonremovable part of the wheelchair that he can grasp to provide adequate brakes for the wheelchair (Fig. 4-38). The person in the wheelchair will pull back on the wheels on the "pull" signal. (See Fig. 4-39 for an example of one person assisting a C6–C7 quadriplegic going up the steps.)

When all persons are ready, the back person calls "pull." Everyone pulls or pushes the wheelchair up the stair on the rear wheels, keeping the wheelchair in the wheelie position. On "hold," the person in the front keeps the wheelchair wheels firmly against the back of the step while the back person repositions himself, possibly tipping the wheelchair down momentarily in the process, keeping feet apart and back straight. Then everyone should be ready for the "pull" signal again, continuing in this pull and hold fashion until at the top of the steps. When safely and completely on the landing, the front wheels can be lowered to the floor.

To go down the steps, the process is reversed, except that now everyone acts as brakes. The top person again gets more of the work, but the person at the bottom should lighten his load considerably. The wheelchair is tipped into a wheelie position, with everyone holding onto the chair as they did when going up. When everyone is in position, the rear wheels are taken slowly toward the edge of the step. The chair is slowly lowered down to the next step on a "down" signal. On "hold" signal, the bottom person again holds the rear wheels

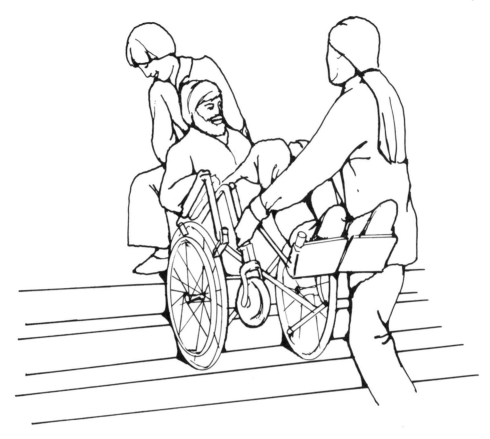

Fig. 4-38 C7–C8 quadriplegic: two-person assist on steps (stairs).

firmly back against the step, while the top person repositions into a position of good body mechanics. This sequence continues until the team is at the bottom of the steps where the person is again on level terrain. If the quadriplegic is a very large person, it is always good to use three people to help—one in back and two in front.

Paraplegia

Stability of the Spine

Surgically, instrumentation and fusion is performed to provide spinal stability. Postoperatively, a Jewett hyperextension brace is used to (1) remind the patient and all those working with him that a bony injury has occurred and (2) to prevent excessive trunk flexion and extension. Patients are usually allowed to perform all activities that can be physically accomplished while in the brace, *except falling* (i.e., no brace ambulation for 6 to 12

months and no actual practice in unassisted falling backward in a wheelchair).

If surgery is not performed and bed rest is prescribed for stability for approximately 12 weeks, physical therapy activities are limited to the tilt table (if physician approved), bilateral upper extremity strengthening with weights and/or pulleys, and bedside range of motion to the lower extremities.

Paraplegics who have undergone instrumentation and fusion and are in a Jewett or similar-type back brace, and those who have completed the required bed rest, can begin mobilization on a tilt table. Paraplegics without functioning abdominal muscles will respond better to the upright position early on if the patient uses an abdominal binder and support hose. The tilt table is used as a tool to get the patient out of his room and to lessen the effects of orthostatic hypotension. Wheelchair sitting can begin simultaneously. An upright wheelchair is used. Dizziness can be relieved by tilting the wheelchair backward until symptoms have resolved. After the first 15 minutes in the wheelchair, the ischial area should be inspected; if redness is absent (a pink coloration is acceptable), an additional 15 mintues can be spent in the sitting position. Increase the sitting time to 20 minutes once or twice a day as tolerated.

Push-up weight shifts are taught immediately. For safety reasons, remember to lock the wheelchair. Balance in doing a pushup will vary depending on the level of paraplegia; the therapist should assist as appropriate until the weight shift can be done independently. Weight shifts should be done every 15 to 20 minutes.

A three-man lift from a tilt table/stretcher or sliding board transfer from the wheelchair can be done to transfer the patient to an elevated mat.

As in the case of quadriplegia, the therapist and patient should discuss and order the appropriate wheelchair for home use. Lightweight wheelchairs are preferred by most patients. Few adaptations (i.e., caster locks) are required.

Family participation and home instructions are similar to those stated in the section Quadriplegia; C5–C8.

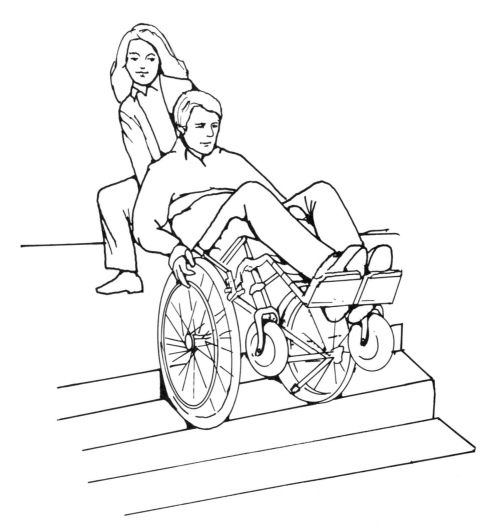

Fig. 4-39 C7–C8 quadriplegic: one-person assist on steps (stairs).

Jewett Brace Protocol

Indications for a Jewett Hyperextension Brace

All patients with instrumentation and fusion should be immobilized in a Jewett brace for a total of 4 weeks. Incomplete injuries with questionable fixation should be immobilized for as long as 8 weeks, depending on the physician's recommendation.

Activity Level

1. Activities that tend to produce pain should be restricted, especially trunk flexion and rotation.
2. Patients are allowed to do all activities while in the Jewett brace except for falling. They can participate in indoor and outdoor wheelchair skills including curbs and wheelies; however, after a safe method of falling is taught, patients should not participate until out of the Jewett brace and at least 3 months postinjury or postsurgery.
3. The brace should be worn at all times when the patient is up.
4. Most transfers are allowed while the patient is in a Jewett brace, with the exception of a wheelchair to and from the floor and putting the wheelchair in or out of a car. These transfers often cause extreme trunk flexion and rotation, as well as excessive pain.
5. Unilateral wall pulleys are allowed.
6. No swing-through gaiting is permitted before 4 months, preferably 6 months, postsurgery.
7. Driving is not permitted while still in a Jewett brace.

Mat Activities

Any of the quadriplegic mat activities listed previously under quadriplegic are appropriate. In addition, the following exercises are recommended.

Sitting

Stretching Mobility

1. With legs together and the arms at shoulder height, twist to the right, then to the left, reaching the left arm behind the back as far as possible. Then reverse.
2. With the legs straight, reach for the ball of the foot from the outside of the foot and bring the toes towards the knees (i.e., ankle dorsiflexion).
3. While long sitting, slowly bend a knee, bringing the sole of the foot toward the opposite thigh (do not force this movement).
4. Cross both legs and stretch forward slowly.
5. While side sitting, walk the hands to the right, then to the left.

Balancing

1. Play catch with one or two balls in all positions of sitting (i.e., long sitting, side sitting, cross-leg sitting.
2. Practice balancing with the eyes closed.

Strengthening

1. Place the fist at the hips and do a shoulder depression to take pressure off the buttocks, then wiggle the trunk and buttocks side to side. Try using two push-up blocks, then one block and one fist. Try a push-up with the legs crossed.
2. With both hands to one side by a hip and knee, take the pressure off both buttocks as you lift.

Transferring

1. With hands at the hips, do a shoulder depression and tuck the head to scoot backward. Then do a shoulder depression and raise the head to scoot forward.
2. Scoot while in a side-sitting position.
3. Practice continuous rolling the length of the mat, keeping the feet on the mat.
4. Move the legs and feet to the right, then to the left in a circle.
5. Practice the floor-to-wheelchair transfer.
6. Practice getting on the knees in front of a wheelchair, then doing push-ups (have a spotter for this activity).

Supine

Stretching—Strengthening

1. Place the hands under the hips, lift the head and press the elbows into the mat bracing up on the elbows as if coming to a sitting position. Do many repetitions.
2. Do pull ups with a spotter.
3. Get up on the elbows and do elbow push-ups.
4. Get to the sitting position, then place one hand under a knee, bringing the knee to the chest.

Then rock backwards to the supine position. Rock backward and forward; then rock side to side, always holding the knee. Then repeat holding both knees.

Sidelying
1. With one leg crossed over the other and lying on the mat, turn and do sideways push-ups.
2. In the same position, twist the trunk.
3. Try to lift the trunk off the mat using the arms for balance only.

Prone
Upper Extremity and Back Strengthening
1. Place the hands at shoulder level with the fingers pointing inward. Push up with the hands, straighten the elbows. Try making a circle with the body while in the push-up position.
2. With the hands at the sides, lift the head, shoulders, and arms while first reaching for the left then the right foot.
3. Hands at shoulder level, do a push-up, going only half the way down; then shift to the right and to the left.
4. Push up on the hands, then walk the hands forwards, backwards and sideways.
5. With the palms down at the hips and the elbows slightly bent, tuck the head; push to the mat, trying to lift the stomach from the mat.

Hands and Knees
While prone, tuck the head, push with the arms and get on hands and knees. Assume the side-sitting position with the hands to one side, from this position get up to the hands and knees.

Balancing and Strengthening
1. Shift the weight from the right to the left side, as well as back and forth (do not sit back on the feet).
2. Tuck the head and raise the back using the abdominal muscles.
3. Push up, then clap the hands.
4. Try balancing on one hand; shift the weight in a small circle.
5. Crawling, move the legs with your hand, forward and then backward.
6. Reach diagonally back across the body while you look at the ceiling and twist the trunk.

Transfers

Generally, paraplegics should be independent in transfers to and from a bed, car, toilet, shower, commode chair, sofa, and airline seat. Bathtub (i.e., to the bottom of the tub) and floor transfers are more difficult and success will vary. Factors that can alter the success of all transfers include weight, age, associated medical problems, life style, and motivation. The physical therapist should *attempt to teach all* transfers *deemed appropriate* for the patient. The patient will choose whether to continue to perform the transfers after discharge. Patients will modify their transfers by trial and error after discharge. It is important that *basic techniques* have been taught upon which the patient can later develop personal modifications.

The therapist should keep in mind a few basic principles, which should be emphasized when teaching transfer techniques. For maximum safety, the skin must be completely protected. At no time should the patient bump any part of his insensitive skin. The patient must be reminded that he can damage tissues and cause a potential pressure sore. An additional safety measure is to stabilize the object to which the person is transferring. Lock the brakes on the wheelchair. Always remember that the patient may have poor balance and strength at first.

Basic Instructions
1. Lock the brakes, lock the front casters forward, position the chair, and remove the armrest and place it in the rear armrest hole. (Some armrests can be lifted or swung out of the way.)
2. Demonstrate exactly what you want the person to do. Remind him of all the precautions.
3. Tell the patient how you will protect him in terms of skin and potential falling.
4. The person must lift his hips forward of the wheelchair tire (Fig. 4-40A and B).
5. With feet still on the footpedals, the patient should place one hand on the remaining armrest and the other on the surface to which he is going, well away from where he will land (Fig. 4-41A and B).
6. To *lift* across, the patient should use a duck-and-lift method. To duck, the patient brings head and shoulders down toward the knee

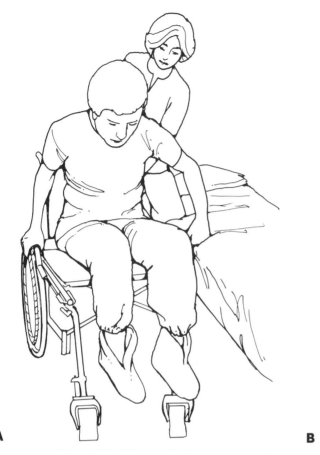

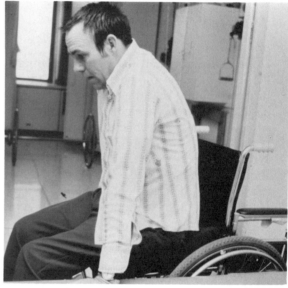

A   **B**

Fig. 4-40 (A) Paraplegic transfer. Hips forward of tires, assisted. **(B)** Paraplegic transfer. Hips forward, independent.

opposite the direction of transfer. This counterrotation shifts weight forward over the knees so that less weight is over the hips. To lift, the patient stays in the duck position and lifts hips over to the transferring object. Being in a forward duck position makes the arms longer in relation to the trunk, making it easier to get a high lift. If feet are placed correctly, they can act as a pivot point and assist with balance (Fig. 4-42).

7. Once the hips have completed the transfer, the patient is ready to reposition the legs. If not safely in position on the object to which he transferred, the patient must scoot back. If transfer was done to a bed or elevated mat, the patient must lift the legs to this object. One method is to lean onto the arm already on the mat or bed for more balance. The other arm is

used to lift the leg nearest the bed or mat (Fig. 4-43).

Try to discourage the patient from using his pant leg because this will increase the chance of losing control of his leg. He should lift his leg either under the knee or preferably under the gastrocnemius or ankle. After that leg is safely on the bed or mat and straightened out, the patient can lift the other leg by the same method. Give as much assistance and guidance as needed.

To assist the person in the early stages of learning, the therapist should be in a position to protect himself and the patient. He can most safely do this by being behind the patient and the wheelchair. One leg should be up on the mat or bed and the other on the floor either between the wheelchair tire and the bed or straddling the tire.

The therapist's outside hand will be on the patient's outside shoulder, in front, because the patient would most likely fall forward if he loses his balance. The other hand should hold the patient's inside pocket or waistband of his pants. This is used to help lift the patient if he gets too close to the tire or if he doesn't lift far enough onto the bed or mat. The therapist should be careful not to pull the patient's pants into the crotch. The therapist may be required to give moderate assistance at first. If the patient is very large, the therapist may want an assistant to stand in front in case the patient should lose his balance. If the patient is heavy and weak the therapist may also need to assist in lifting him. It is vital for the therapist to use good body mechanics.

Toilet Transfers

1. Begin by teaching the transfer to an elevated toilet seat. Progress to a padded toilet seat if appropriate.
2. Teach without the use of a grab bar; the patient may not have one at home. Use a toilet seat as a hand hold (Fig. 4-44).
3. Emphasize pushing down on the toilet seat when transferring, not away, especially with the portable seats, which are a little less stable than the bolt-on type.
4. For balance on the toilet seat while doing the bowel program, the patient should lean on the wheelchair, sink or whatever stable object is next to the toilet. The foot position can make or break the balance. Place the feet on the

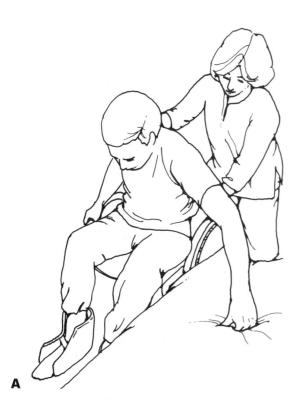

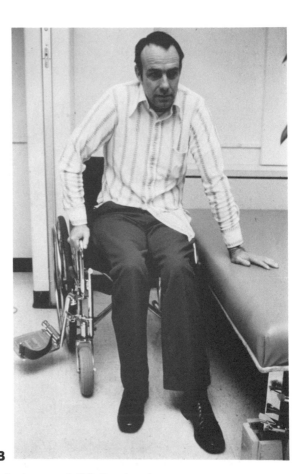

Fig. 4-41 (A) One hand on armrest; one hand on bed, assisted. **(B)** One hand on armrest, one hand on elevated mat, independent.

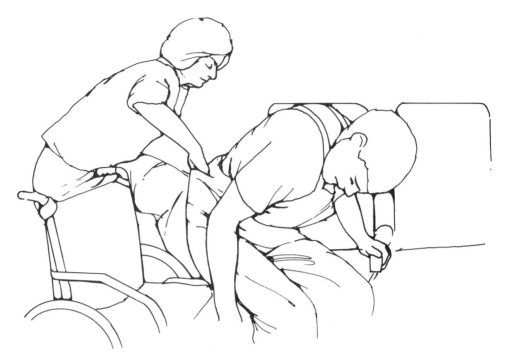

Fig. 4-42 Duck-and-lift transfer, assisted.

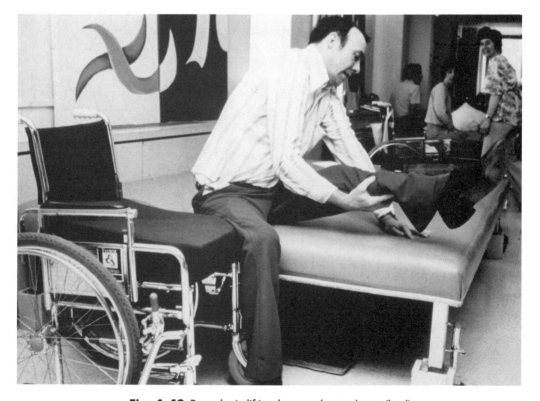

Fig. 4-43 Paraplegic lifting leg on elevated mat (bed).

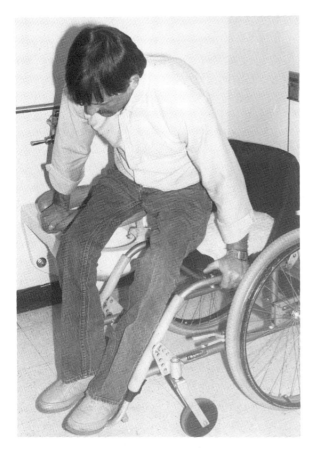

Fig. 4-44 Paraplegic transfer to elevated toilet seat, independent.

floor, footpedals, or a stool, whichever provides the best balance.

Car Transfers

A two-door car is preferable for car transfer because it allows the wheelchair to be pulled into the back seat. In addition, the door is larger, allowing more room in which to work. With a four-door car, the wheelchair must be pulled in the front seat. A split front seat is required so that the paraplegic can load and unload the wheelchair.

The technique for a car transfer is the same as for a bed transfer except that the patient must bridge a larger gap. The choice of transferring on the driver's or passenger's side of the car will depend on where one parks, be it a busy street or a small parking lot, etc. It can also depend on (1) placement of hand controls, (2) length of legs, (3)

seat adjustment, and (4) type of wheelchair (fixed axles or quick release axles).

If the seat is too far forward to allow driving when the wheelchair is in the back seat, the back seat of the car may have to be removed to allow more room for the wheelchair.

Transferring into the Car on the Passenger's Side
1. Make sure the seat is all the way back.
2. Position the wheelchair and lock with the casters in the backward position. Place the armrest on the back seat within reach.
3. Transfer in, using the seat as a hand hold. Swing the hips over first. Avoid the tendency to go head first into a car; this makes for an unsafe transfer and poor body mechanics. Bring the feet in last. (Some paraplegics find it easier to put their feet into the car first, and then transfer.) (Fig. 4-45)

Transferring into the Car on the Driver's Side. The major difference on this side of the car is the steering wheel, which the patient will have to avoid hitting; however, a steering wheel that tilts alleviates this problem. Some patients actually prefer this method because they use the steering wheel for pushing and pulling during the transfer (Fig. 4-46).

Putting the Wheelchair in and out of the Car. Please refer to the section on Quadriplegia C5–C8 in Chapter 3 for detailed instructions on this technique. The basic technique will be appropriate for paraplegics as well. With the advent of lightweight wheelchairs, quick-release axles, and folding versus rigid frames, new parameters affect the techniques for putting the wheelchair in and out of the car. It would be prohibitive in this text to list all the details with each variation of lightweight wheelchair. Figures 4-47 and 4-48 demonstrate optional methods.

Tub Transfers

To get to the bottom of the tub:

1. Fill the tub first. This prevents burns on the feet caused by inadvertently turning hot water on insensitive skin. Test the temperature of the water on the back of the hand. Have towels within reach. Place a cushion in the

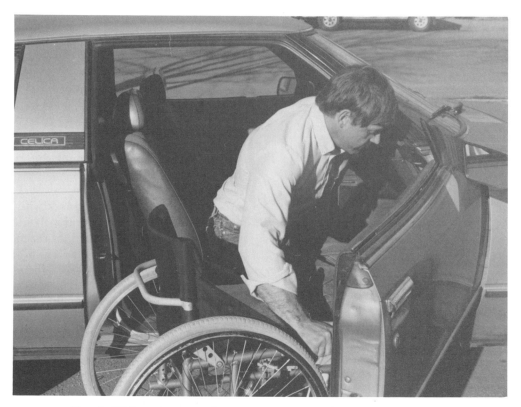

Fig. 4-45 Paraplegic transfer to car, passenger side. Hips in car, head out.

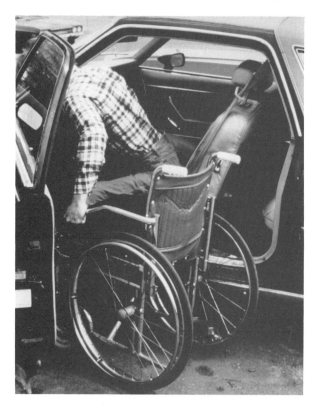

Fig. 4-46 Transferring hips into car, driver's side.

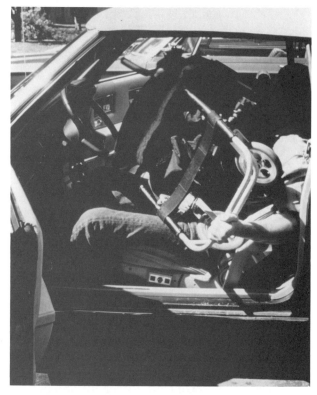

Fig. 4-47 Lifting lightweight wheelchair into car.

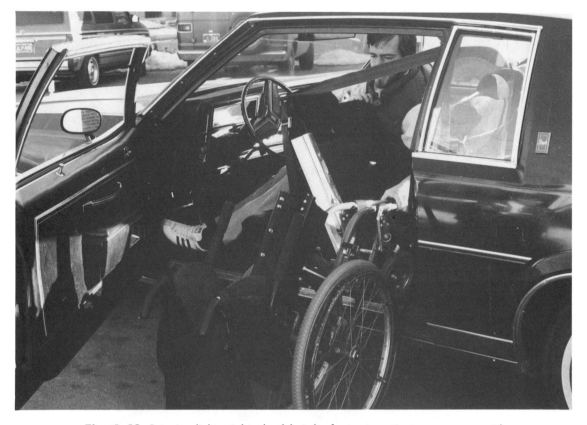

Fig. 4-48 Gripping lightweight wheelchair by footrests, patient on passenger side.

bottom of the tub. Can use a Bye-Bye Decubiti cushion filled with water and air.

2. Pull the wheelchair facing the side of the tub. Swing the pedals back and put the feet over ledge of the tub. Lock the brakes with the wheelchair next to the tub; casters should also be locked (Fig. 4-49A).

3. Scoot forward to the edge of the seat. Hold onto armrest with one hand and tub ledge with the other hand. Transfer onto the tub ledge. Hand holds for this may vary according to the lift and balance.

4. Position the legs to the side toward faucets. Hold onto the armrest or the ledge of the tub with the hand closer to the faucets, and position the other hand on the ledge on the opposite side of the tub. Do not use the soap dish for transfer. It is not stable or meant to have any weight borne on it. Pivot the hips out over the cushion and ease down into the tub (Fig. 4-49B).

To get out of the tub:

1. Drain the tub, dry thoroughly, remove the cushion from the wheelchair, and put a dry towel in it. Dry the edge of the tub well. Some people put a wet towel on the tub ledge for added friction. This works very well and gives a more stable sitting position.

2. Place the faucet-side hand on the wheelchair side of the tub ledge and the other on the back tub ledge. Lift the hips up onto the ledge using a "duck and lift" technique. The legs may or may not need to be positioned before lifting.

3. Position the legs once on the ledge. Place one hand on the wheelchair arm and the other on the tub ledge. Lift hips to the wheelchair seat. Many people prefer lifting straight up and leaning backwards. Be careful not to drag the sacrum on the wheelchair. Try to do a shoulder depression and lift hips first, if possible.

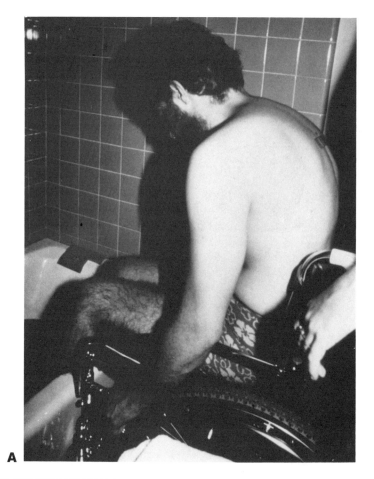

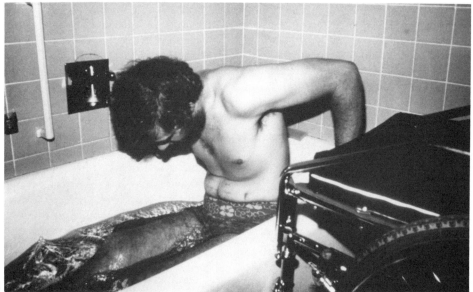

Fig. 4-49 (A) Locking wheelchair. **(B)** Patient lowering himself into bathtub.

4. Reposition in the wheelchair; finish drying and dressing. Depending on bathroom architectual barriers and whether or not the wheelchair has removable footrests, the technique for transferring into the tub may vary.

These techniques are only guidelines. Some people are fearful, for a variety of reasons, of transferring into the bottom of a tub. Often people prefer taking showers. In such cases, it is quite easy to place a *folding chair* or *bath bench* in the tub. With a flexible shower hose one can shower quite well.

Floor Transfers
Transfer from the Wheelchair to the Floor
1. Position wheelchair, lock the casters facing backwards, and swing the footrests away.
2. Scoot to the edge of the wheelchair. Position the feet back slightly.
3. Hold onto the armrest with one hand and place the other hand on the floor about where the knees would land. When one hand is positioned, place the other one on the floor as well. (Fig. 4-50)
4. Gravity will help pull the hips down. Bearing most of the body weight on the arms will keep the knees from hitting the floor too hard. The patient will thus be in an all-fours position. (The all-fours position is a good one to practice on a mat to develop the necessary control.)
5. By moving one hand out to the side to control the hips, move into a side-sitting position.
6. The above technique can be used for a one-man assist to transfer a C6 or lower quadriplegic onto the floor. The patient must lock his elbows once the hands are on the floor. The assistant should control the hips. Protect both the hips and the shoulders to the floor position.

Transfer Back into the Wheelchair
1. Remove the cushion; the patient positions himself side sitting. When he is up on his knees he should be facing the center of the wheelchair.
2. Come to the knees by *pushing* up, mostly with the hip-side hand and by pulling or stabilizing with the other hand on seat by the opposite

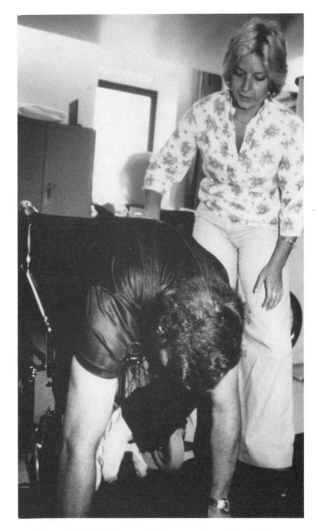

Fig. 4-50 Easing self down to floor, hands first.

armrest. *Do not pull on the back of the wheelchair;* it could topple over onto the patient.
3. After assuming the kneeling position, let the chest rest on the wheelchair seat. Position the hands with one hand on the lower part of the armrest and one on the upper part of the armrest (not the forearm) (Fig. 4-51A).
4. Assume the vertical position. Push straight down with both hands until both arms are straight and the hips are above wheelchair seat height. Do not lean forward and put chin over the wheelchair back. This tends to produce a poor position mechanically, and the hips will

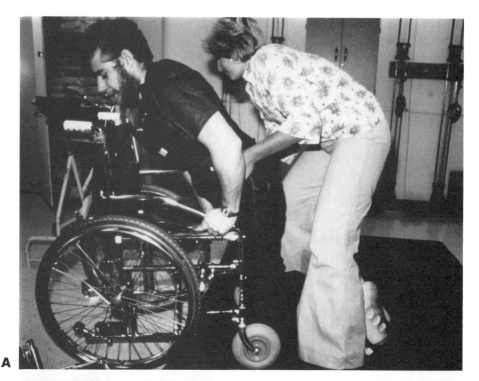

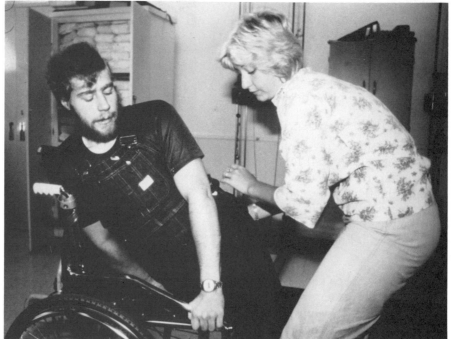

Fig. 4-51 (A) Pushing down, one arm on armrest, one on seat. Lifting hips above seat height, assisted. **(B)** Further trunk rotation with one hip onto seat.

not be high enough. *Once in a pushed up position do not let go or move hand positions.*

5. Rotate or pivot toward the downhill arm (Fig. 4-51B). Lower oneself and position oneself in wheelchair. The therapist should help stabilize the person's hips when he is kneeling and lifts at the waistband if needed.

Transfer onto the Floor using a Forward Pivot

1. Position the wheelchair with the casters back and the footrests swung away.
2. Scoot forward to the edge of the wheelchair seat. Position legs out to one side.
3. Place the arm on that particular side on the armrest or wheelchair seat. Put the other hand down on the floor, slightly forward so the patient won't sit on it.
4. Swing the hips out to the side, away from the wheelchair so the hips won't hit on any wheelchair part (Fig. 4-52).
5. Lower the hips to the floor easily, landing squarely on the bottom.

Transfer Up in Wheelchair Backwards

1. Position the wheelchair, remove the cushion, lock casters back. Put the patient in a position in front of the wheelchair with hips slightly to the side with legs at an angle outwards. Cross the legs so that the chair-side leg is on the outside or on top.
2. Put the chair-side arm on the seat next to the armrest and the other hand by the hip, as close as possible. Lift the hips up into chair by using the duck-and-lift technique. This must be used to avoid hitting the sacrum or the hips on the wheelchair front or under the seat. Once the hips are in the chair, the upper body must be lifted. *Do not push on the legs to get up, as your knee or hip can be dislocated.*

Getting up from the floor is a difficult maneuver to learn and requires a lot of strength. Both methods have been described, as one method may be easier for someone than the other. These methods are difficult to learn, and neither the

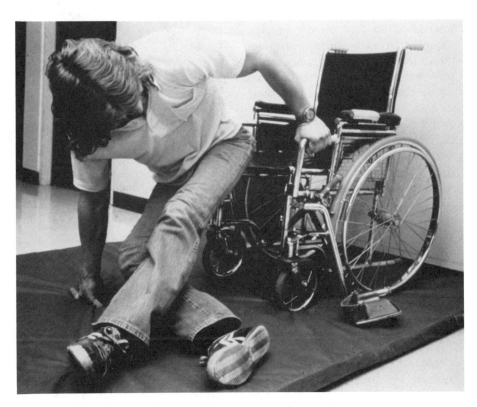

Fig. 4-52 Duck head, swing hips to floor.

patient nor the therapist should become discouraged; they must keep practicing. That in itself will help develop the strength and the skill.

Other transfers are not described here because they are all variations of the original technique using the same basic principles. Other transfers that may be needed or taught are those to couches, restaurant booths, airline seats, theater seats, high examining tables, pickups or jeeps, or swimming pools. It may be necessary to transfer to other chairs without locks or that have rolling casters to get into otherwise inaccessible bathrooms (Figs. 4-53, 4-54A and B).

Wheelchair Activities

Beginning Instructions—Patient Responsible for Timing

Up and Down Curbs: Concrete to Concrete. To maneuver up, the patient approaches a curb in a wheelchair. When the front casters are a few inches from the curb the patient begins instructions to the assistant. The assistant's hand should be properly placed on the push handles; the assistant should push down with his foot on the tailpipe and place the wheelchair in a wheelie position. The assistant then turns sideways with his hip to the back of the wheelchair with his feet at least one foot apart or spread comfortably. (This body position is the *classic spotter position* and will be referred to throughout the text) (see fig. 4-26). The patient rolls the wheelchair forward while the assistant maintains the wheelie and walks sideways to the curb. When the rear tires touch the curb, the assistant gently lowers the front casters to the top of the curb by facing the wheelchair back and placing his foot on the tailpipe to control the movement. The assistant reassumes the classic spotter position. The patient leans forward in the wheelchair with his hips fully back into the chair and places his hands on top of the tires; he will call the instruction "push" when ready (Fig. 4-55). After wheelchair is fully on the curb and stable, the patient sits up and continues to wheel over the smooth terrain.

To maneuver down, the patient rolls the wheelchair toward the curb. He turns the chair so that the wheelchair faces away from the curb. He requests the assistant to place his hands properly

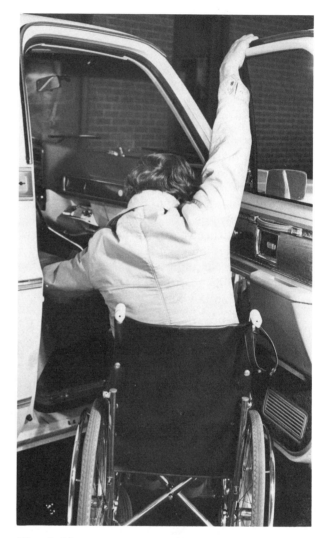

Fig. 4-53 Paraplegic: Pick-up truck transfer, pulling on door with one hand, shoulder depression with other arm on trunk seat.

on the push handles and to assume the classic spotter position with one foot under the wheelchair on the curb. The other foot should be below or both feet should be below, depending on the assistant's height. Patient leans forward in the wheelchair and places hands on top of the tires. Patient shouts "Let's go!" They ease the wheelchair down the curb and the patient sits up. The assistant places a foot on the tailpipe, putting the wheelchair into a wheelie position and turns the wheelchair sideways, then eases the wheelchair out of the wheelie position.

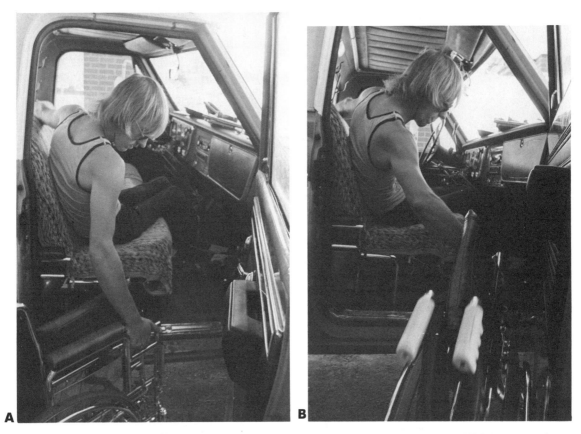

Fig. 4-54 (A) Paraplegic: Wheelchair into truck, folding wheelchair. **(B)** Lifting wheelchair into truck.

Up and Down Curbs: Uneven Ground. To maneuver up uneven ground, the patient approaches a curb in a wheelchair. Before the wheelchair is off uneven surface the patient instructs the assistant to tip the wheelchair to the wheelie position. The patient and the assistant push the wheelchair up to the curb in the wheelie and place casters on the top of the curb. The assistant assumes the classic spotter position. Proceed as described in maneuvering over the curb.

To maneuver down uneven ground, the patient proceeds in the same way as described for going up, but after the wheelchair is on the ground, the patient is tipped into a wheelie. The assistant pulls the patient back into the wheelie position until the wheelchair is on even surface. Then the wheelchair is let down slowly from the wheelie position, and the patient continues on the even surface.

Up and Down Curbs: Concrete to Grass. To avoid dumping the patient out of the wheelchair by hanging up the front casters, one should try the following techniques. To maneuver up, the patient approaches a curb backwards. He instructs the assistant to put him into the wheelie position. The assistant should assume the classic spotter position with one foot on the concrete and the other foot up on the grass, depending on what is a comfortable position for the spotter. The spotter should keep his knees bent and his back straight. The patient places his hands on top of the tires and calls, "Pull." Both the spotter and patient pull simultaneously (Fig. 4-56). Once on the grass the patient and assistant move backward in the wheelie position until uneven area is cleared. The assistant then gently lowers the front casters to the ground.

To maneuver down, the patient approaches a

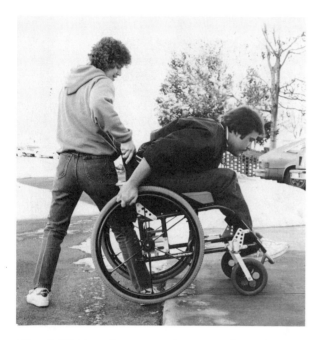

Fig. 4-55 Paraplegic. Up curb—patient leans forward in wheelchair; assistant is sideways with hip to wheelchair.

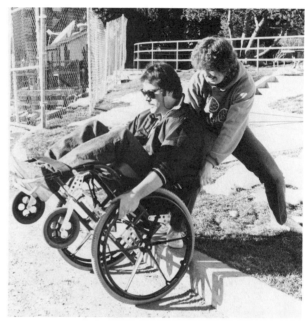

Fig. 4-56 Patient and assistant pull simultaneously up curb.

curb frontwards. The patient is tipped into the wheelie position and pushed until the back wheels come to the edge of the curb. The patient has his hands on the wheels to act as a brake. The assistant has his feet spread apart with his knees bent and his back straight. The assistant should ease the wheelchair over the curb in the wheelie position. He should then turn the wheelchair sideways and lower the patient out of the wheelie position.

Up Steps/stairs

The classic spotter position should be assumed with the patient in a wheelie. The therapist (spotter) has one foot up on the next step (or the next two steps depending upon the safe positioning and height of the spotter) and one foot on the step or sidewalk near the wheelchair.

The spotter then proceeds to pull the wheelchair up over the step with or without the assistance of the patient as was described under the discussion on maneuvering curbs. Some paraplegics will have enough strength to roll the wheelchair up to the next step without assistance. The spotter should maintain the wheelchair in a wheelie position and

hold the wheelchair into the step, while the patient changes his hand position (Fig. 4-57).

The patient should always instruct the spotter and coordinate the timing. Verbal instructions from the patient could be as follows:

1. "I'll pull." The spotter may also have to help pull.
2. "You hold and I'll change hands."
3. "I'm holding."
4. "Tip the wheelchair forward." This allows the spotter to move his feet to the next step.
5. "Move your feet."
6. "Tip the wheelchair backward."
7. "I'll pull," etc.

Repeat this procedure until at the top of the stairs.

Down Steps/stairs

Classic spotter position is assumed with the patient in a wheelie. As already described, the patient is in charge of the verbal commands. Descending the stairs is accomplished in the same manner as was explained under going down curbs. Appropriate

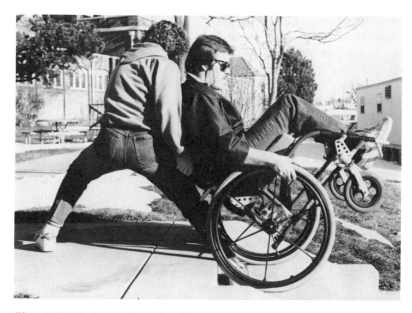

Fig. 4-57 Patient pulling wheelchair up step; assistant maintains wheelie.

verbal commands by the patient to the spotter include the following:

1. "Let's go." The patient and the spotter roll the wheelchair down the step.
2. Patient and the spotter both pull back on the wheel slightly once the rear axle is over the edge of the step, and the spotter helps maintain the wheelchair in the wheelie position.
3. "You hold the wheelchair into the step and I'll change my grip."
4. "I'll hold; tip the wheelchair forward a bit; move your feet; tip the wheelchair backward." The spotter repositions his feet with the nearer foot either directly under the step the wheelchair is on or on the next step up from the wheelchair, depending on personal comfort. His other foot is spread apart, even as much as two steps away from the wheelchair.
5. Repeat the process until at the bottom of the steps.

Rough Terrain

Put the wheelchair into a wheelie position and pull the patient backward. The patient should do most of the work pulling backward on the wheels, with the spotter being responsible for maintaining the wheelie.

Ramps (Steep)

To maneuver up, assume the classic spotter position with the wheelchair in a wheelie position. The patient has his hands on the tires. Place the front casters on the ramp. Lower the wheelchair to the ramp. The patient leans as far forward as possible and makes sure the hips are all the way back into the wheelchair. The spotter leans his hip into the wheelchair with his feet spread apart and back straight. He may have to adjust his feet for the steepness of the incline. Patient gives these instructions:

1. "Push." The patient and spotter push simultaneously. The spotter moves his feet while pushing to keep his hip continuously in contact with the back of the wheelchair.
2. "You hold." The spotter holds the wheelchair while the patient readjusts his hands on top of the tire.
3. Repeat this procedure until at the top of the ramp.

To maneuver down, the patient and spotter are in the same position as described for maneuvering up, with the patient leaning forward in the wheelchair, his hips all the way back into the chair, and the spotter in the classic spotter position with his feet spread apart. Both the patient and the spotter allow the wheelchair to move slowly down the ramp while they both maintain control of the speed. The spotter maintains continuous contact with his hip into the wheelchair as they ease the wheelchair to the bottom of the ramp. Alternatively, the patient and the spotter allow the wheelchair to move slowly down the ramp one step at a time for the spotter (Fig. 4-58). The spotter continually readjusts his feet so that he is one foot length distance from the wheelchair. This is repeated until they are at the bottom of the ramp.

Wheelies

The patient should place his hands on the wheels, with his head and shoulders relaxed. He should roll forward easily, then backward, and then forward quickly (this provides the momentum to "pop" the wheelie). The patient should work initially on maintaining the wheelie in place. The spotter should have his hands under the push handles while the patient pops a wheelie himself so that the patient can "feel" his balance point. If the patient tends to overbalance in the backward position, the spotter can quickly grab the push handles and prevent a fall. When the patient can maintain a wheelie position, he is ready to attempt various intermediate skills.

Up Curbs. With the spotter in position, the patient should pop a wheelie and approach the curb. There are two methods to pop a wheelie when approaching a curb: (1) sideways or parallel to the curb, and (2) facing the curb head on (Fig. 4-59). For steep curbs the patient may have to have his casters locked.

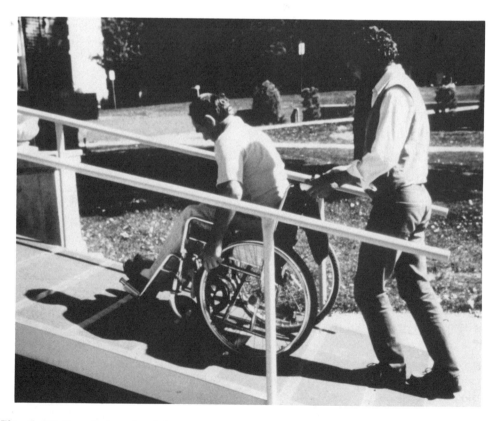

Fig. 4-58 Paraplegic assisted down steep ramp; patient letting tires slide through hands slowly; assistant guiding wheelchair evenly.

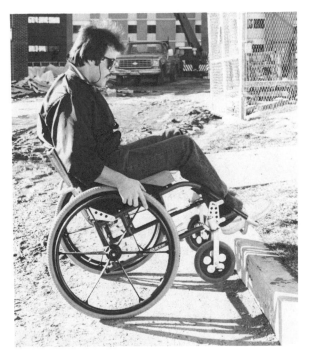

Fig. 4-59 Paraplegic popping wheelie facing curb.

Down Curbs. Begin with small 2-inch curbs. The patient should be able to go to the curb independently. The patient should turn the chair and come up to the curb backward. Coming down the curb, the patient pulls back on one tire and pushes forward on the other tire to turn the chair sideways to the curb.

Maintaining and Moving in a Wheelie. The patient pops a wheelie with the spotter and works on balance. Progress to independence in maintaining the wheelie position. Once it is felt the patient no longer requires a spotter in a wheelie position, the patient must be taught how to fall properly. Once he is able to maintain his balance, the patient relaxes his hand and lets the tire move through his fingers forward and backward in a seesaw fashion. The patient should then learn to gradually roll the wheelchair forward and backward slowly. This should be tried first on smooth terrain. Progress to slightly inclined sidewalks, going down in a wheelie. Then progress to grass, steeper inclines, gravel, dirt, roads, alleys, etc.

Falling and Getting Up from a Fall. In the physical therapy department, use mats or large pillows to practice falling. The patient should then pop a wheelie, tuck his head forward, place one forearm across his knees to prevent them from hitting him in the face, and allow himself to go over backwards (Fig. 4-60). The emphasis should be on the patient maintaining the head tucked position to prevent banging the head. To get up from a fall the patient should roll to the side and out of the wheelchair. He should then set the wheelchair back up, lock the brakes, and transfer back into the wheelchair. A more difficult method to get up is to remain in the wheelchair. The patient should lock the brakes, put one hand on the tire and the other behind the chair on the floor. He should pull back on the tire as he simultaneously pushes from the floor with his hand, with the head tucked forward. He should rotate his head toward the hand on the tire to give some momentum. This should be practiced first with a spotter (Fig. 4-61).

Down Curbs in a Wheelie. The patient should pop a wheelie and slowly approach the curb to the edge. Once the rear axle goes over the curb, the patient should slowly pull the rear tires back to the curb and maintain the wheelie position. To avoid traffic on a busy street, the patient should then turn the wheelchair to the side and let himself out of the wheelie position. If coming down a curb

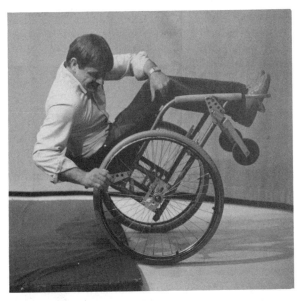

Fig. 4-60 Paraplegic falling on mats; ducking head; protecting knees.

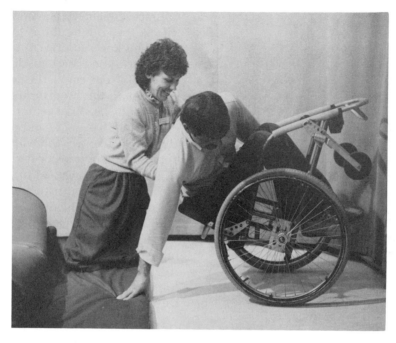

Fig. 4-61 Paraplegic: Up from fall; head rotating toward hand on tire.

on a hill, the patient should turn first into the hill, then turn the chair down the hill. This activity should always be done with a spotter until satisfactory progress is made for independence.

Advanced Wheelchair Techniques

Independent Wheelies Going Down Inclines. Start on shallow inclines with the patient in full control of the wheelchair. Have the patient move forward in a wheelie. Work for full control on all grades of inclines.

Independent Wheelie on Rough Terrain. Begin with a spotter at first then progress to independent activity (Fig. 4-62).

Downstairs in a Wheelie. This activity should be taught to well-coordinated patients only. The procedure is the same as for an independent down curb in a wheelie. When the wheelchair is over the first step and the rear tires are resting on the second step, the patient should immediately and smoothly pull the rear tires back into the first step (Fig. 4-63). If the patient pulls back too fast, he is likely to fall backward out of the wheelie and bounce back down the steps. The patient should

get his balance in the wheelie position, then proceed to the next step. The therapist should spot the patient until he and the patient both feel confident in the technique.

Escalators. The procedure to ascend and descend an escalator is very simple, providing adequate instructions, demonstration, and initial assistance are given. Most paraplegics are able to ride escalators independently; quadriplegics may do so with an assistant.

To ascend an escalator:

1. The patient should roll his wheelchair to the up escalator. The therapist should stand directly behind the wheelchair with his hands on the push handles.
2. The patient should lean forward slightly and place both hands on the black rubber handrailing on each side of the wheelchair. (The hand grasp should be light.) The motion will cause the wheelchair to roll forward off the escalator platform on to the steps. As this occurs, the rear wheels will end up on one step lower than the front casters (Fig. 4-64). It is

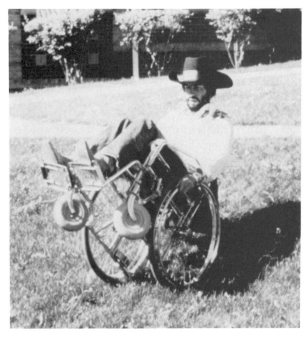

Fig. 4-62 Paraplegic: independent wheelie on steep, rough terrain.

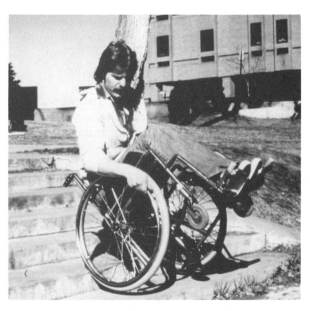

Fig. 4-63 Paraplegic: independent wheelie downstairs.

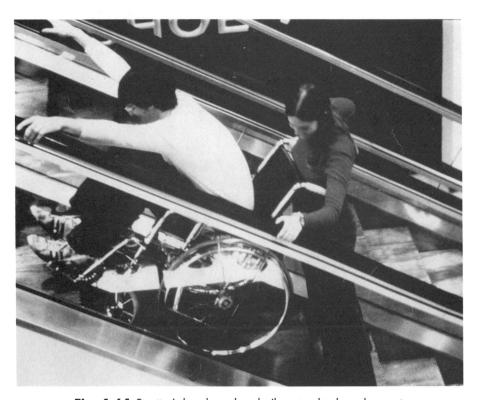

Fig. 4-64 Spotter's hands on handrail; rear wheels on lower step.

extremely important for the patient to remain in a *forward position* with his weight over the front axles. If not, he could tip over backward. The therapist should continue to assume the classic spotter position, being careful not to apply downward pressure on the push handles.

3. At the top of the escalator the patient should prepare to get off by quickly sitting up straight in the wheelchair. At the same time, he should gently but firmly push off the escalator hand

railings. This simple motion will cause his wheelchair to roll off the escalator platform. At this point, he should place both hands on his wheelchair rims and roll safely away from the escalator.

To descend an escalator:

1. The therapist stands behind the wheelchair with hands on the push handles. The patient rolls his wheelchair backward onto the escalator platform.

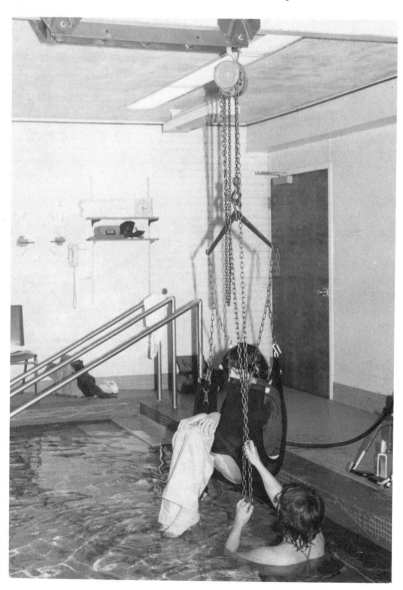

Fig. 4-65 Pool: manual ceiling lift and lift sling.

2. Leaning forward, the patient again places both hands on the escalator hand rails. This motion allows the rear wheels to drop down onto a lower step; the front casters, a higher one. (Often the front casters will not actually touch the step.)
3. At the bottom the patient quickly pushes off from the handrail. This is enough to roll his wheelchair backward across the escalator platform.
4. With both hands on the wheelchair rims, the patient then wheels free of the escalator and turns his wheelchair around.

Therapeutic Pool

The use of a pool program as part of physical therapy rehabilitation has proved invaluable, especially for patients with incomplete spinal cord injuries. However, even patients with complete injuries are exposed to this segment of therapy and can use the skills appropriately in the future.

Size of a pool will depend on what the facility can accommodate. The pool should have a deeper end for actual swimming and a more shallow end with graded steps and handrails.

Regular swimming pool equipment should be present. A few additional options should be considered including

1. A manual ceiling lift and lift sling (Fig. 4-65).
2. Stretcher (Fig. 4-66)
3. Floaters
4. Kick boards
5. Life vests

Water temperature varies with the needs of the physical therapy program, but a temperature of

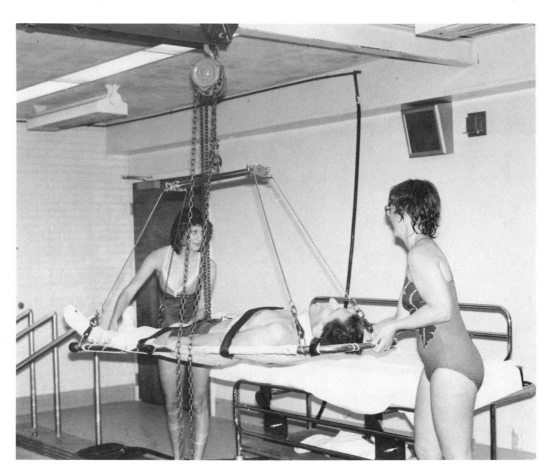

Fig. 4-66 Pool: stretcher for putting patient in pool.

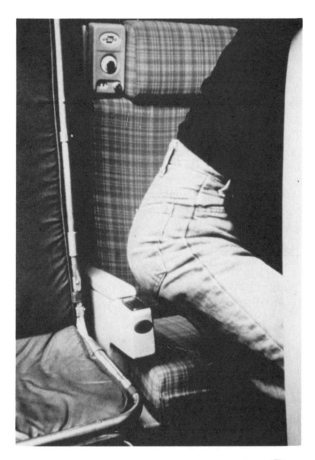

Fig. 4-67 Paraplegic transfer to airplane seat.

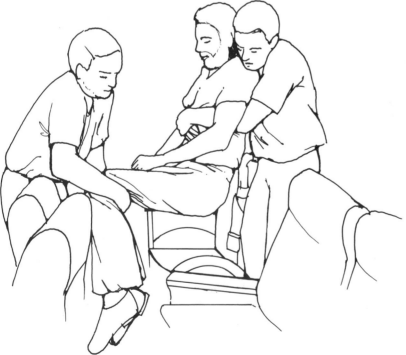

Fig. 4-68 Quadriplegic being lifted to airplane seat.

95°F works well. The therapist should monitor the temperature.

Objectives for pool therapy are to

1. Increase strength and endurance
2. Decrease pain
3. Decrease spasticity
4. Increase range of motion and stretching
5. Improve coordination and balance
6. Expose the patient to swimming strokes
7. Increase breath control and lung vital capacity
8. Teach mobility activities, such as treading water with upper extremities, rolling over in water face down, face up, etc.
9. Prepare the patient for possible recreational swimming
10. Gait training (The buoyancy of the water often allows gait training earlier than is possible out of the water.)
11. Graduation to dry land programs when appropriate

Airline Transfers

One of the main reasons for rehabilitation is to assist the spinal cord injured person in regaining mobility in today's world. For various reasons, a large segment of the able-bodied population chooses airline travel as a means of travel. The spinal cord injured population should also be able to choose air travel. For this reason, the rehabilitation program should be devoted to teaching the patient methods of getting on and off an airplane.

The spinal cord injured person should arrive at the airport in plenty of time to check baggage, go through security (usually by a special route because the normal gates are too narrow to permit a wheelchair), and arrive at the boarding gate in

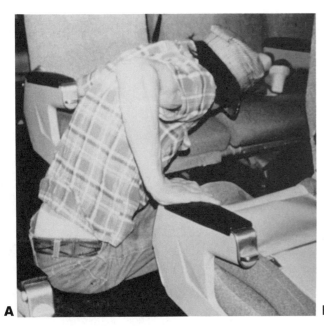
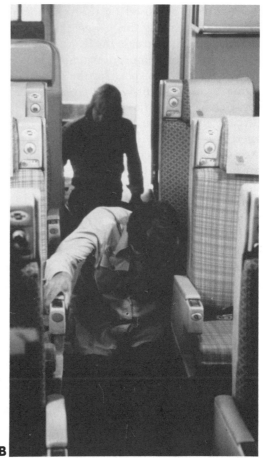

Fig. 4-69 **(A)** Paraplegic transferring to aisle on floor. **(B)** Paraplegic scooting down aisle to chute.

time for the usual preboarding. It is wise to let the airline know in advance that one is traveling by wheelchair and will need assistance in boarding.

Airlines vary in regard to their policy of transporting batteries with an electric wheelchair. Some airlines refuse to carry wet cell batteries. When it is imperative to travel with electric wheelchair and have it operational at the airport on arrival, one should take along a new battery that has not yet been activated. Upon arrival at the destination, one can then activate the battery. Always check with the airline before traveling to find out their policy regarding batteries.

Unless the spinal cord injured person is traveling first class, most often an aisle chair will be needed to transport the traveler down the narrow aisle of the coach section. The typical transport aisle chair is almost *vertical* in back configuration, a position unfamiliar to most patients with spinal cord injuries.

Safety straps are used by the transporting attendant. Experiencing this *upright* position during rehabilitation can help ease the fear and uneasiness of the spinal cord injured patient who will be experiencing this transport for the first time.

Transfer to the airplane seat from a wheelchair or aisle chair can be hazardous, especially due to the fixed arm rest on the aisle seat of most airplanes.

Access to airplane seats for teaching transfers is most helpful. A paraplegic can usually make the transfer without difficulty after a few practice sessions (Fig. 4-67). Quadriplegics who require transfer boards for the usual transfers are best lifted into the seat by airline attendants (Fig. 4-68).

Placement of a sliding board and executing a transfer across the board are generally forestalled by the fixed arm rest and narrow working space. The need to be lifted by usually inexperienced personnel emphasizes the importance of teaching the quadriplegic how to direct others in lifting transfers as needed (See "Self-Instructs" under Program).

If a planned evacuation emergency becomes necessary, the paraplegic can get from the seat to the aisle and scoot to an evacuation chute unassisted (Figs. 4-69A and B). He also should be able to position himself and slide down the chute

independently if necessary (Fig. 4-70). A quadriplegic will need to be lifted and dragged with only the heels touching the carpet to the chute (Fig. 4-71). He can go down the chute in a supine position if two people are at the bottom to catch him and carry him from the site.

The spinal cord injured traveler in a manual wheelchair should insist on staying in his own wheelchair as far as possible when boarding. This will help underscore to airline personnel the importance of the wheelchair to the traveler. The disabled passenger should remind airline personnel that he will need his own wheelchair immediately upon leaving the plane. He should not be expected to retrieve it from the baggage claim

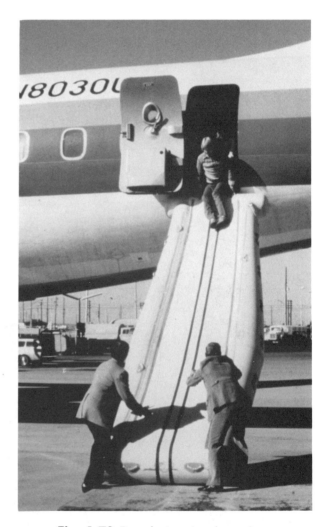

Fig. 4-70 Paraplegic going down chute.

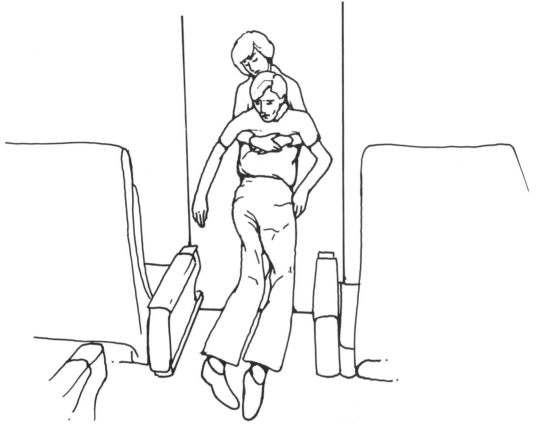

Fig. 4-71 Quadriplegic being dragged to chute.

area. Gentle reminders to the flight attendants when approaching the destination can be helpful.

Functional Electrical Stimulation

The use of functional electrical stimulation (FES) in spinal cord injuries is rapidly becoming one of the most sophisticated and challenging areas for treatment. Although the use of therapeutic electrical stimulation for upper motor neuron lesions is not new, the technologies and the devices themselves are everchanging. FES is becoming more prevalent both in research and in clinical application. It is assumed that the reader has a basic background in electrophysiology. Basic physical therapy textbooks on electrotherapy are good resources for review. This discussion will deal with FES use for upper motor neuron lesions of spinal cord injury.

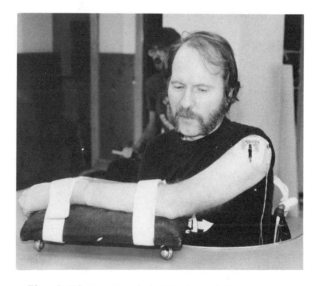

Fig. 4-72 Functional electrical stimulation: isotonic contractions of upper extremity deltoids.

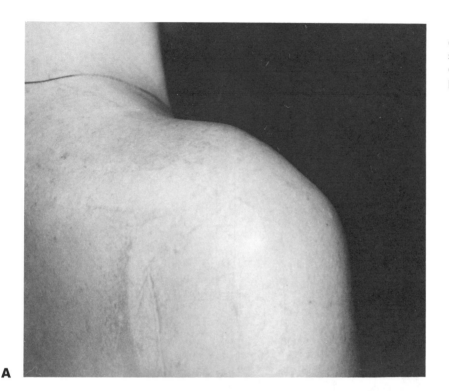

A

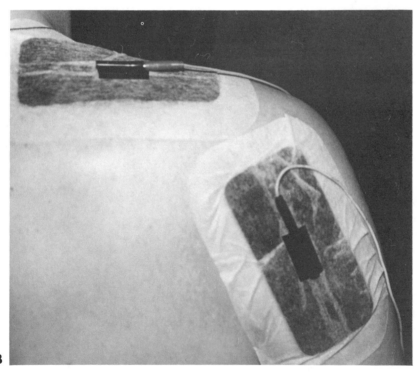

B

Fig. 4-73 **(A)** Functional electrical stimulation: shoulder subluxation. **(B)** Functional electrical stimulation: shoulder properly aligned.

Patient Selection for FES

In spinal cord injuries, candidates for FES must demonstrate an incomplete upper motor neuron lesion. The therapist should understand that a spinal cord injury can produce both upper motor neuron and lower motor neuron lesions (i.e., the spinal cord and the nerve roots at the level of injury can be affected). When choosing a candidate for FES, a functional goal should be established (e.g., wrist extensors for an incomplete C6 quadriplegic, elbow extensors (triceps) for an incomplete C7 quadriplegic, etc.). These areas often exhibit selective peripheral nerve root damage in addition to the spinal cord lesion. Denervated muscles do not respond to functional electrical stimulation. A quick check with a faradic/galvanic stimulator will decide this issue. If a response to the faradic current is achieved, then using an FES unit for functional gains may be appropriate.

In incomplete spinal cord injuries, the rationale for using FES on a nonfunctioning muscle could be for the biofeedback effect. This would be appropriate for a muscle at a critical level, such as wrist extensor for C6, the triceps for C7. In cases of both acute and long-term injury, a poor (2) grade muscle seems to be ideal for a trial with FES.

The Uses of FES

Strengthening

Disuse atrophy can be reversed by using FES. The quality of the initial contraction elicited will depend on the length of time that has elapsed since the injury occurred. In the case of a long-standing injury, the therapist should not be discouraged if there is only minimal contraction in a muscle. In such a case, strengthening atrophied muscles will require time. The therapist should observe to see if there is full recruitment, (i.e., increasing stimulus until there is no further muscle contraction). Additional current will serve no useful purpose and could increase the chance of a skin reaction. Subjective quality of the contraction and amount of current required should be documented to assess

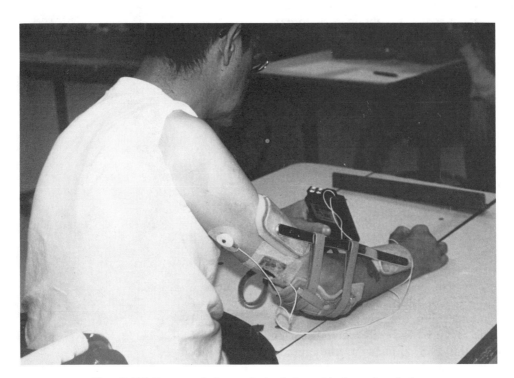

Fig. 4-74 Functional electrical stimulation with dynamic splinting.

progress. Isometric or isotonic contractions can be used with the FES unit. Isometric contractions permit full recruitment without joint motion.

Studies have suggested that a program of 10, 10-second full recruitment isometric contractions with 50-second rest periods can increase muscle strength significantly.[2] Isotonic contractions, with or without the use of weights, can be performed according to standard exercise protocols (Figs. 4-72 and 73A and B).

It is recommended that full range of motion not be done with FES and weights because the chances of tissue damage may be greater with stress at the end of the range when using resistance.

Thorough evaluation of the muscle being treated and the methodology of documentation of progress can not be overstressed. Objective measurements should be used including manual muscle testing, strength measurements (tensiometer), active range of motion, etc.

Re-education

FES appears to have a biofeedback effect (i.e., motor/sensory reintegration) in some patients. Often only one or two treatments to nonfunctioning muscles are needed to obtain a voluntary contraction by the patient. Once this voluntary response occurs, the FES program becomes one of selecting the best method of strengthening.

Dysfunction may be the result of spasticity in the antagonistic muscle. Often the use of FES in the agonist muscle will result in a decrease in the antagoinist interruption. Reciprocal inhibition is often the reason for success in these cases.

Inhibition of Spasticity

Through reciprocal inhibition, spasticity may be decreased and/or eliminated in antagonistic muscles by using FES to agonist muscles. Trial and error seems to be the best method to follow.

Increase Range of Motion (Stretching)

Again, reciprocal inhibition seems to account for success when stretching spastic, contracted muscles. This can be accomplished either by using a dynamic stretching splint and applying FES to the agonist muscle (Fig. 4-74) or in weight-bearing positions with the FES applied to the agonist muscles (i.e., using a tilt table to stretch gastrocnemius with FES to the anterior compartment muscles).

Electrical Bracing

FES can be used in specific cases as a substitute to bracing (Fig. 4-75). If there is no retention of training with FES, and continuous FES is required for proper function, then the decision is based on patient preference and practicality of conventional

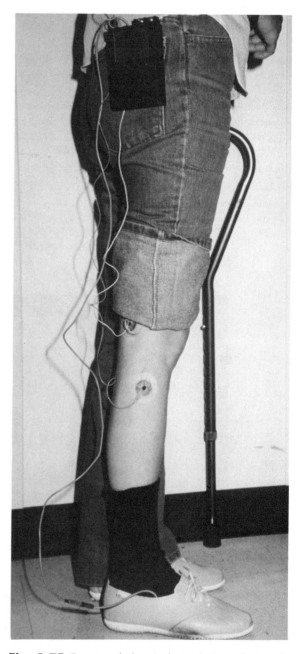

Fig. 4-75 Functional electrical stimulation substitute for bracing.

bracing versus electrical bracing. If there is some voluntary function in the muscle receiving FES, strengthening and re-education may require long-term use of the FES unit.

Re-Evaluation

Annual re-evaluations (or as advised by the physician) are important. The current medical status of the patient is reviewed by the physician, with special attention given to the bladder and the kidneys. The physical therapist will repeat motor and sensory testing. When possible the same therapist should do the repeat testing to enhance consistency. In situations where the testing indicates an improvement in motor function, *upgrading* in *functional skills* may be appropriate. When testing indicates a *loss* of sensory and/or motor function, the therapist should notify the attending physician. A spinal cord cyst may have occurred, requiring the attention of a neurosurgeon. Equipment checkout and repairs can also be completed during re-evaluation.

BRACING

Philosophy

The consideration of whether to brace the complete spinal cord injury above the L2 motor level is controversial. Certainly one of the first and greatest concerns the spinal injured person has is whether he will be able to walk again. As time begins to pass during the early rehabilitation phase and the completeness of the injury becomes more apparent to the individual, the question of some type of ambulation outside of a wheelchair is still paramount in the minds of the majority of paraplegics.

One approach from medical professionals is to deny braces to paraplegics above the L2 motor level on the basis of poor long-term use at a functional level. Other arguments against the use of braces are the high energy expenditure requirement and the cost of training. These professionals tend to emphasize acceptance of wheelchair independence as the ultimate goal for the spinal cord injured paraplegics. We believe, however, that consideration should be given to fitting par-

aplegics and in exceptional cases, C7–C8 quadriplegics with KAFOs. We advocate the Scott-Craig (Scott Orthopedics, Inc., Denver, CO) orthosis due to its design, which provides a mechanism for balance (Fig. 4-76). The design incorporated into the shoe and solid ankle provides a stable base of support. In Figure 4-77A and B, the sole of the shoe has been removed to show (1) the longitudinal plate, which provides anteroposterior stability; (2) transverse metatarsal plate, which provides mediolateral stability; and (3) a double stirrup with a short strut, which provides attachment to the ankle joint.

Through adjustment of the double action ankle component, the center of gravity of the individual can be moved to provide an optimum balance state. The *adjustable, double action ankle joint* allows one to control the amount of dorsi-flexion and plantar flexion range. This makes a significant

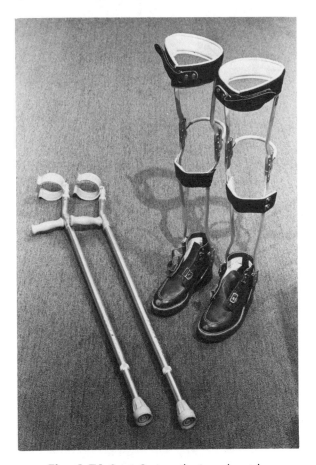

Fig. 4-76 Scott-Craig orthosis and crutches.

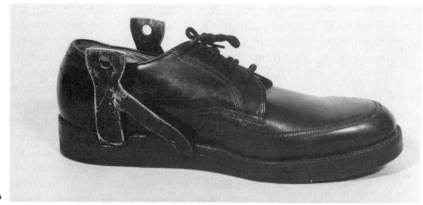

A

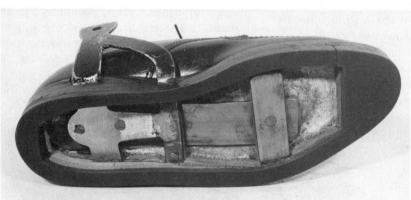

B

Fig. 4-77 (A) Scott-Craig shoe setup. **(B)** Sole removed.

difference in the immediate success of an ambulation program outside of parallel bars and probably increases the chances of long-term use. One of the greatest fears a paraplegic must overcome immediately is the fear of falling. Being in a state of complete balance without the use of crutches, as can be accomplished in the Scott-Craig KAFO, tends to alleviate to a great degree this problem much earlier than when one uses a flexible orthosis (Figs. 4-78A and B).

Due to the balance capability of this orthosis, energy requirements when doing a swing-through gait are decreased, that is, when in the stance phase of gaiting, the orthoses balance the patient, thus freeing his arms for crutch position changing without a lot of energy expenditure for balancing.

The Scott-Craig orthosis allows the paraplegic to experience ambulation on a trial basis before the final decision is made regarding bracing. We believe that the paraplegic deserves the option of trying ambulation with bracing; moreover the de-

cision not to brace based on the difficulty and higher energy requirements is much more appropriate when it comes from the patient himself after having had a trial experience.

The emphasis on eventual outcome for bracing is important. At the L1 and above complete motor level of injury, it is the exception rather than the rule that postdischarge, a paraplegic will continue being a *functional gaitor* (i.e., use his KAFOs exclusive of a wheelchair). However, a significant psychological point to remember is that many paraplegics do maintain the ability to use the KAFOs in a functional manner whenever they choose to do so; they can ambulate in all normally encountered situations.

The *majority* of paraplegics above the L2 motor level will use the Scott-Craig orthoses for *exercise ambulation only*. The importance of being able to do this, from the patient's standpoint, cannot be overemphasized. Long-term follow-up surveys have also indicated a strong personal feeling by

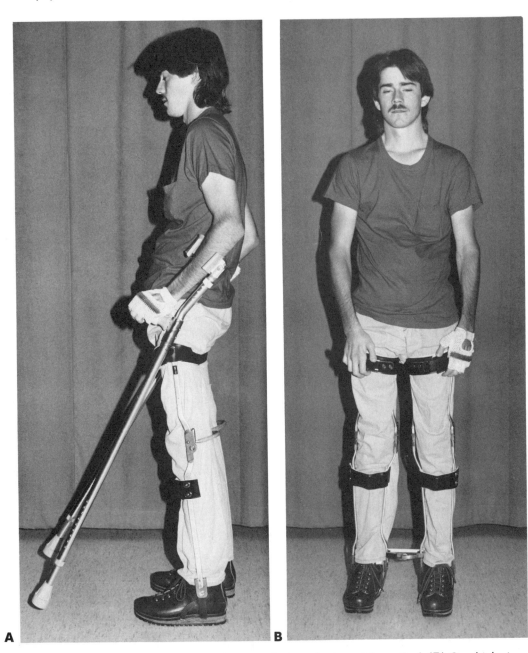

Fig. 4-78 (A) Quadriplegic balanced in Scott-Craig orthosis, crutches raised. **(B)** Quadriplegic balanced in Scott-Craig orthosis, standing without crutches.

these patients that the option to try bracing, even in the face of eventually not using them for various reasons, is very psychologically important to them.[3] This tends to confirm the point that spinal cord injured people need to be involved in the decision-making process regarding ambulation.

Patient Selection

To emphasize the need for patient involvement in the decision process for ambulation is not to de-emphasize the importance of patient selection criteria. Obviously, some circumstances make ambulation a more practical goal from the onset. Before pursuing trial braces with the patient, the following criteria should be considered.

1. The patient should be independent in all self-care areas appropriate for his level of injury.
2. The patient must have orthopaedic clearance for gaiting. This normally occurs 6 to 8 months postinstrumentation and fusion.
3. The patient must be willing to spend the necessary 4 to 6 weeks in the program and to work 5 full days a week on gaiting.
4. The patient must have sufficient funding for all necessary equipment (braces and crutches) and for the gaiting program itself. Funding should be preauthorized before starting a program.
5. The patient must be in good general health and without excessive absenteeism from therapy due to illness.
6. The patient should have adequate range of motion at the hips (at least 5° to 10° of hyperextension), full extension of the knees, and at least 5° to 10° of dorsiflexion in the ankles. If the patient is close to the required ranges, a stretching program may be carried out concurrently with the gaiting program.
7. The patient's skin should be free of pressure sores, especially in those areas that have potential contact with braces.
8. The patient should participate regularly in a standing program at home if the program is delayed for any reason, such as instrumentation and fusion. This home program is necessary to maintain the range in the hips and ankles, thus preventing any delay in the bracing program once it has been initiated.
9. The patient should express an understanding of the limitations of gaiting, including the higher energy consumption in functional versus exercise usage. The patient also should have realistic expectations.

Patients with severe spasticity will be considered on an individual basis, since spasticity decreases the likelihood of potential ambulation and increases the potential for skin breakdowns. The patient's weight and body type will also be considered. In general, overweight patients do not do as well and probably are not appropriate for long-term, extensive programs.

After the patient's trial with temporary braces, and before the patient's custom fit braces are ordered, the following criteria should be met:

1. The patient must express continued willingness to work as demonstrated through regular attendance and effort in the therapy sessions.
2. The patient must be able to doff/don the temporary braces independently.
3. Balancing the patient in the braces should appear feasible.
4. The patient should be independent getting up and down from a wheelchair to the parallel bars and in gaiting in the parallel bars. He should have the strength and endurance to ambulate several lengths of the parallel bars without rest.
5. The patient must have assumed responsibility for skin check after using the temporary braces.
6. The patient must have exhibited good judgment in the safe use of the braces.

After a successful trial period, the orthotist measures the patient and the KAFOs are made. During this time the ambulation program is continued in the trial orthoses. Much training can be accomplished before the patient's actual orthoses arrive.

Balancing Technique

The process of balancing begins with a thorough evaluation of the patient. Special attention should be given to the following areas:

Range of Motion

Contractures or tightness of the low back, hips, knees, or ankles will affect the patient's ability to balance and walk. Contractures of the hips and knees can be caused by heterotopic ossification, as well as muscle tightness. Tightness of the low back or hip flexors will prevent the necessary lordosis and hip extension needed for balancing in the KAFOs. Tightness of the iliotibial band, which is not uncommon in the low level paraplegic (T12–L1), will not allow for the proper amount of hip adduction, thereby causing excessive weight-bearing on the medial aspect of the shoes. Tightness of the hamstrings will prevent locking of the brace knee joint, and ankle plantar flexion contractures of more than the neutral position will not only cause the heels to pull out of the shoes, but will also cause excessive pressure on the leg under the anterior tibial band. If the tightness in any one of these areas is greater on one side than the other, it will result, when standing in the braces, in a compensatory rotation of the pelvis and trunk, thus affecting the balancing technique.

Range of motion in the ankle joint should be measured with the knee extended. Five to ten degrees of passive dorsiflexion range is usually required to keep the heel in the shoe during push-off phase of ambulation.

Do not set the ankle joint of the orthosis in more dorsiflexion than is present in passive dorsiflexion range; this would cause the heel to rub the shoe and/or pop out of the heel counter if low quarter shoes are worn. One good way to stretch the heel cord is to use a tilt table in conjunction with a functional electrical stimulation program to the anterior compartment at least 1 to 2 hours per day. Once the heel cord is stretched, even in the presence of spasticity, a solid ankle orthosis, if worn consistently, usually will maintain the stretch.

Muscle Function

In the absence of functioning abdominals or back extensors, a greater lordosis occurs, thereby making it necessary to balance the patient in more ankle dorsiflexion than the patient with some functioning abdominal and back extensor musculature requires. Unilateral preservation of trunk and hip musculature will cause trunk and pelvic rotation.

Spasticity

Excessive, intermittent, or constant abdominal and hip flexor spasticity will cause the patient to jackknife when balancing or gaiting. More spasticity on one side than the other may cause trunk rotation or the shooting forward of one leg ahead of the other.

Scoliosis

Scoliosis, either functional or structural, may lead to trunk and pelvic rotation with consequent unequal weight-bearing on both extremities.

Leg Length Discrepancies

Leg length discrepancies may be apparent or real and related to the range of motion, to a scoliosis, to a pelvic obliquity, or to a displaced healed fracture of the lower extremity. The amount of lift compensation is best determined when the patient is in *his* KAFOs and is in the standing position.

The KAFOs should be checked before fitting on the patient. Will they stand balanced on their own? The KAFOs arrive from the orthotist with the pins in the double Becker (Becker Orthopedic Appliance Co., Troy, MI) ankle joint screwed down to set the KAFOs at 5° of dorsiflexion. The most probable cause of imbalanced orthoses would be a rocker-bottom surface of the soles of the shoes. The soles have to be perfectly flat from the heel to the metatarsal bar; from the metatarsal bar to the toe, the sole surface should be slightly concave. Second, check to see that both KAFOs have been set in the same amount of dorsiflexion. This can be done by placing them parallel to each other and viewing them from the side to see if all four uprights are parallel. Dorsiflexion can also be checked with a fluid goniometer.

Another means of checking for the proper amount of initial dorsiflexion would be to drop a plumb-bob from the top of the lateral uprights. The bob should fall just anterior to the lateral orthotic ankle joint and not more than 1 to 1.5 inches forward of this point.

From the back, determine if both braces have the same contour from the floor to the top of the brace. If one brace tilts more medially or laterally than the other brace it may indicate that one shoe has a higher medial or lateral sole buildup than the other.

Each shoe should be in about 7° of external rotation. When the medial sole angle is placed on a straight line, the lateral sole edge should flare out approximately 7° from this straight line.

The contour of the anterior tibial band and the posterior thigh band should be checked for equal concavity. If the concavity of the bands on both KAFOs is not equal, the result may be excessive hip or knee flexion or extension in one brace as compared with the other. By checking these factors before fitting the patient with the orthoses, any balancing problems can be eliminated.

Orthoses are adjusted in the following manner: To set them in more dorsiflexion, the anterior screws must be loosened with a rachet wrench or an Allen wrench. Then the posterior screws must be tightened to push the pins within the channels down, thereby bringing the toe up or the orthosis forward on the stirrup (Fig. 4-79).

To set the KAFOs in more plantar flexion, the process is reversed. The posterior screws should be loosened and the anterior screws tightened down, thus pushing the toe down. The ankle joint should be checked in both instances to make sure the screws are down firmly so that the joint is *solid*. Keep in mind that a minor adjustment, one fourth to one half turn of the Allen wrench at the ankle joint, causes a major anterior or posterior displace-

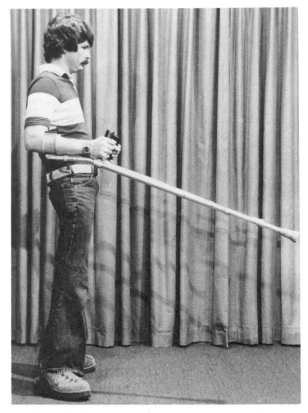

Fig. 4-80 Paraplegic balanced in his Scott-Craig orthosis.

ment at the top of the brace. In essence this changes the patient's center of gravity. Usually only a minor ankle adjustment is necessary to balance the patient (Fig. 4-80).

Once a patient is in the orthoses, the balancing process should begin with the patient standing in the parallel bars wearing a pair of shorts so that the entire trunk and lower extremities can be viewed. First, the KAFOs should be checked for proper fit. The uprights should follow the contour of the legs closely but not cause excessive pressure on the skin. The medial thigh cuff should be 3 inches below the adductor tendon. The top of the upper lateral cuff is 1 inch longer than the medial, placing it 1 to 1.5 inches below the trocanter. The lateral portion of the anterior tibial cuff should be 1 inch below the head of the fibula. Next, determine what adjustments at the ankle joint must be done to balance a patient in his KAFOs. The patient should relax his shoulders by taking his

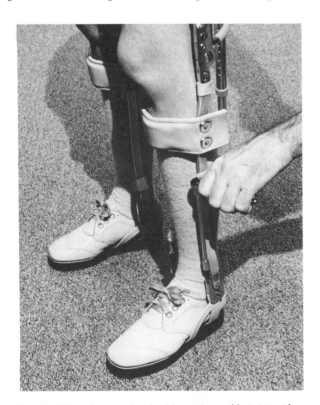

Fig. 4-79 Adjusting the double action ankle joint with a rachet wrench.

hands off the bars and placing them down by his sides. This allows the patient's pelvis to go into a posterior pelvic tilt, thereby sagging into the support provided by the posterior thigh and anterior tibial band. The therapist should be standing in front of the patient to prevent a loss of balance or to determine the direction of the loss of balance should it occur. The therapist is then ready to make the necessary adjustment to balance the patient. If the patient is falling forward, the adjustment for balance has to be made into plantar flexion as previously described. If the patient is falling backward and jack-knifing at the hips, an adjustment into dorsiflexion has to be made. A loss of balance to one side with rotation of the pelvis would indicate an apparent or real leg length discrepancy, which must be compensated for with an entire sole lift. The height of the lift is determined by placing lift boards under the sole and then checking for balance. When an adjustment is made on *one upright* of a KAFO, an equal adjustment must be made on the *other upright* to keep them parallel. *Failure to have both uprights parallel will result in a rotational stress force on the knee joint of the KAFO.* In cases where there is unequal spasticity of the lower extremities, a spreader bar may be necessary to insure equal stride length (Fig. 4-81). All adjustments in balancing should also be checked out in the gaiting process to determine if the balancing continues step to step.

A majority of patients with fairly recent injuries and the absence of contractures and deformities can usually be balanced easily by the aforementioned process. For those individuals who present balancing problems, a more in-depth analysis of the balancing process must be performed. This analysis may result in the addition of parts to the basic KAFO to compensate for problems and to achieve balancing.

A basic principle for achieving balancing is stretching out of contractures to a minimum. Another principle to bear in mind is that the floor or sole of the shoe is the focus point of the forces disbursed throughout the braces. Therefore, analysis should begin with the position of the shoe or foot in the shoe. It has been found that corrections made here may solve problems present more proximally at the knee or upper thigh. Good, firm, quality arch supports to correct excessive prona-

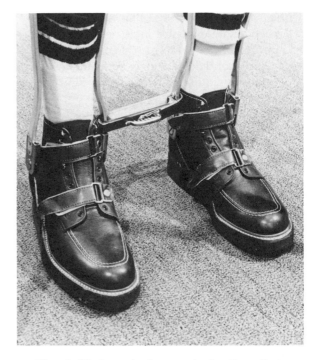

Fig. 4-81 Spreader bar attached to Scott-Craig orthosis.

tion of the foot may correct the following proximal problems:

1. Rubbing of the medial malleolus and medial upright, thus eliminating the need for T-*straps*
2. Medial rotation of the tibia causing medial condyler pressure on the knee joint, thereby eliminating the need for a medial condyle pad
3. Knee hyperextension in the brace, seen especially at heel strike or toe off, thus eliminating the need for posterior calf band. If the heel cords are excessively tight or spastic, boots or high top shoes can prevent the heel from pulling out of the shoe. Vibram (Qualaug Rubber Co., N. Brookfield, MA) soles on the shoes can prevent slipping on wet or slick surfaces. Medial or lateral T-straps may be necessary if malleolus pressure cannot be corrected with arch supports. Additional padding added to the medial or lateral aspect of the anterior hinged tibial band may be necessary for more equal distribution of tibial pressure or to correct the medial or lateral

tibial condyler pressure. This padding would also eliminate excessive knee flexion. If arch supports do not correct tibial condyler pressure, condyle pads may be needed. As previously mentioned, sole lifts or adjustments at the ankle joint usually compensate for pelvic rotation caused by heterotopic ossification, scoliosis, or minimal contracture deformities. In high level paraplegics, a trunk corset with metal stays may be necessary to decrease excessive lordosis and to provide the necessary trunk stability for balancing.

When balancing of the patient in his KAFOs is achieved, gait training can proceed.

Gaiting Techniques

After a patient is balanced, a demonstration and short practice session of the basic principles of gaiting should take place in the parallel bars. Gaiting should then progress to the use of forearm crutches outside of the bars to prevent the buildup of a false sense of security that the bars provide.

Good crutch-KAFO ambulation using a swing-through gait pattern simulates normal walking to a great extent because it is continuous, without halting movements or frequent rest periods. It is also smooth, with forward progression taking place within a minimum of vertical displacement. Finally, stride length is consistent and trunk movement is minimal. The accomplishment of a good gait pattern will depend on the neurological level of the patient, as well as the gaiting instruction.

The first factor to consider is crutch type. Forearm crutches with front opening cuff allow maximal use of the principle of balance without crutch support in the braces. Any type of axillary crutch encourages support and balance to come from the crutches rather than from the KAFOs. A forearm crutch with side opening, as opposed to front opening cuff, allows the proper support between hand and forearm in the lifting phase.

The second factor to consider is crutch length. The crutch should be adjusted to allow a 15° to 20° bend of the elbows with the shoulders relaxed when the crutches are placed 6 to 8 inches diagonally forward and outward from the toe of the shoe. This corresponds to the height of the greater trocanter. A longer adjustment of the crutches will

cause a greater vertical displacement with consequent greater energy expenditure. It will also result in either an abnormally long or short step. If it is an abnormally long step, it will cause a buildup of momentum, resulting in a halting gait pattern, frequent need for rests, and possible loss of balance. If it is an abnormally short step, it will result in a swing-to rather than a swing-through gait pattern, which is more energy consuming because it does not use the principle of balance. At first the patient may feel the need for greater crutch length to get a lift, but this compromise will lead to an unstable gait pattern later. Good crutch-KAFO ambulation should be smooth, with the feet barely skimming the floor; to achieve this, the initial attention to proper crutch length is important.

The next factor to consider is the instruction. The basic instructions are lean, lift, and relax. With the crutches placed forword about 8 to 10 inches, the patient should lean forward, leading with the pelvis, into the support of the extended arm on the crutch. Forward flexion at the waist should be avoided because it may cause the patient to jack-knife and fall backward. Forward flexion also causes extensive anteroposterior displacement of the trunk. The lift is accomplished by depression of the shoulders, which in combination with the lean results in the swing-through phase. The lift is done without unnatural or excessive head movement and should not be excessively forceful or fast because this will cause either too long or too short a step and too hard an impact on heel strike. The lift should provide a long, smooth, equal stride. The lift should be of equal strength on both crutches to allow the stride of both legs to be equidistant. To accomplish equal stride length, shoulder relaxation must also be simultaneous. After heel strike has taken place, the patient should relax the shoulders. This will allow the solid ankle joint to rock the patient forward to foot flat and to allow for balancing while the crutches are brought forward. Timing of shoulder relaxation must be exact. Too early relaxation will produce insufficient push to get from heel strike to foot flat, resulting in loss of balance backward. If pushing is prolonged, it will cause continued forward progression of the body and need of throwing crutches forward to prevent a forward fall. The patient would not have the momentary relaxation and balance needed for a smooth gait and for energy conservation. To continue shoulder relaxation and consequent balancing, the crutches should be brought forward by bending of the elbows or circumduction of the crutches. Bringing the crutches forward by elevating the shoulders causes loss of balance because it flexes the upper trunk forward on the pelvis and legs. Both crutches should be brought forward simultaneously to allow for shoulder relaxation and balance.

Next to be considered is the therapist's technique in assisting the patient during crutch-KAFO ambulation instruction. The use of good body mechanics is necessary for the safety of the patient and therapist. For the therapist to use his leg strength to the maximum, he must be close behind and slightly to the side and in step with the patient, with one hand on the patient's shoulder, the other hand grasping the patient's opposite back pants pocket (Fig. 4-82).

To correct a patient's loss of balance, the therapist needs only to push the pelvis forward and the shoulders back and to ask the patient to relax. In the initial stages of gait training, the patient may need help with lifting the legs, but when help in achieving balance is needed, lifting should stop because it prevents the patient from achieving balance by causing trunk flexion.

As gaiting ability and balance progresses, less assistance should be given to allow the patient to feel his own loss of balance and what is needed to regain it. This is achieved first by taking the hand support away from the shoulder and later from the pelvis. Walking closely behind the patient will give the confidence to gait without assistance.

While gaiting is progressing on smooth surfaces, instruction should also begin in getting up or down from a wheelchair or sofa; getting in and out of a car; gaiting on inclines, stairs, curbs, and grass; and getting up from a fall. These techniques vary from patient to patient, usually according to the neurological level, but all use certain basic principles.

Getting Up or Down from a Wheelchair

To get up or down from a wheelchair, two techniques may be taught: straightforward and back-

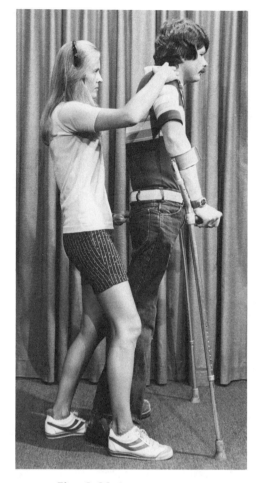

Fig. 4-82 Spotter's position.

ward or rotation. The straightforward and backward method is possible with a Scott-Craig brace because of the bale lock mechanism.

The Forward and Backward Method

After locking the braces, the patient should place the crutches perpendicular to the floor with crutch tips just behind the front caster. With a quick, forceful straight down push involving head ducking, then extension, the vertical lifting swings the legs under the trunk. When the vertical position is attained, shoulder relaxation should occur to allow balance while bringing the crutches forward (Figs. 4-83A and B). The therapist spots the patient by standing at the side of the wheelchair with one hand on the patient's shoulder, the other on the patient's opposite back pants pocket. Thus, the

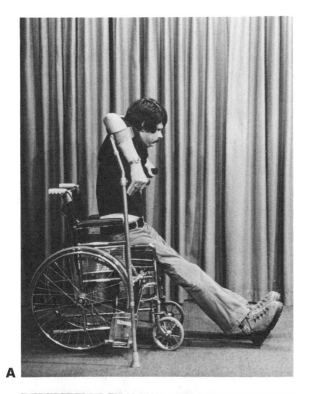

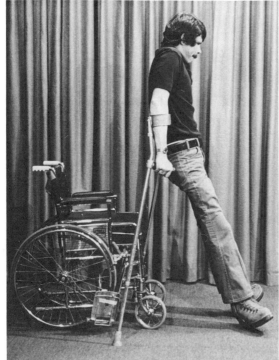

Fig. 4-83 **(A)** Placement of crutches. **(B)** Patient comes to standing.

therapist can assist with the lift and with the balancing. The reverse technique is used for sitting down backwards. Standing about 6 inches in front of the wheelchair, the patient places both crutches back just behind the front casters, bends slightly forward at the waist, and lowers himself slowly while bending the elbows. The bale locks of the KAFOs will unlock as they catch on the cushion of the wheelchair.

Another means of coming to standing straightforward is by pushing off on the wheelchair armrests, which have been reversed (if desk arms are used) and put in the highest position. This method requires a wheelchair with adjustable type armrests. Before pushing off, the patient should slip his hands through the forearm cuff of the crutches so that he can bring his crutches forward with elbow flexion and then grasp the hand grip. To sit, the process is reversed.

The Rotational Method

The rotational method of standing involves first locking the braces then rotating the body in the chair so that the patient is sitting primarily on one buttock. The legs are crossed, taking care that the bale lock of the crossed leg does not unlock. To prevent unlocking requires either sufficient trunk rotation or the placement of the heel of one shoe on the toe of the other shoe. The push to standing is accomplished with one crutch placed perpendicular to the floor in front of the front caster of the wheelchair while the other arm is pushing on the opposite armrest. The other crutch needs to be placed nearby so that it can be reached after the patient is up and balanced. The reverse rotational process is used in getting from standing to sitting. The rotational standing method is used primarily for getting off a low sofa.

Gaiting on Inclines, Stairs, Curbs and Grass

Ascending and descending stairs is taught both forward and backward using a crutch and a rail or both crutches (Fig. 4-84). To go forward with either one or two crutches, the crutches are placed on the step above; then with a slight forward lean, the patient depresses the shoulders and straightens the arms to get sufficient lift to land above. Shoulder relaxation, resulting in balancing, must occur quickly after landing to prevent further pushing,

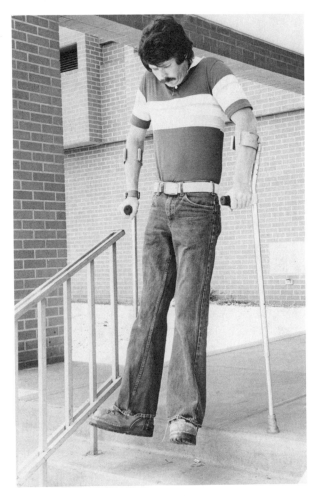

Fig. 4-84 Paraplegic going down stairs forward or going up backward.

crutch and handrail. The crutch is placed on the step above and the other hand placed on the rail at the same level. In this position, the lift is then accomplished with shoulder depression and elbow extension. Immediate relaxation and balancing is needed to then bring the crutch up to the next step. Descending stairs backwards is taught for the patient having a fear of looking down a flight of stairs. The crutch near the forward edge of the step and the hand on the rail are on the same step as the patient. With shoulder depression, elbow extension and head ducking, the legs are lifted to the step below.

Stair climbing requires experimentation by the therapist and patient to determine the best crutch placement on the steps and to determine the best method for the individual patient. The therapist is best able to assist the patient from behind in both ascending and descending process.

Curb climbing is accomplished in the same way as stair climbing, except that two crutches are used. When ascending a small curb, the patient may prefer to keep both crutches down, do a lift and balance, and then bring the crutches up. Higher curbs require this slight forward lean provided by placing both crutches up on the curb first. To descend small curbs, the crutches may be placed down first. On higher curbs, for those patients without functioning back extensors, it will be necessary to keep the crutches up on the curb; otherwise, it is difficult to place the crutches down first without a fast, hard, forward flexion of the trunk on the pelvis. The methods of ascending and descending inclines will depend on the degree of incline. Slight inclines will allow the use of a swing-through gait pattern similar to that used on smooth terrain but with a few minor changes. Going down a slight incline requires a longer stride to advance the crutches before gravity pulls the trunk forward. A longer stride is accomplished by placing the crutches less far forward than usual and holding the lift longer. Going up a slight incline requires a closer crutch placement and a shorter stride to decrease the backward gravitational pull on the pelvis while bringing the crutches forward.

Steeper inclines require the use of a swing-to gait pattern rather than the swing-through. When ascending a steep incline, the body weight is maintained on the forward crutches and the toes of the

which would cause a loss of balance forward. In this balance position, the crutches are brought forward to the step above. Descending stairs forward requires a slight forward lean and shoulder depression on the crutches, which are on the same step as the patient. After landing on the step below, the patient should relax his shoulders and balance. For the patient without functioning abdominal muscles, descending stairs is accomplished by first placing the toes of the shoes over the edge of the step. Then with shoulder depression, there should be a head ducking, then extension to provide momentum for swinging the legs forward.

Ascending stairs that are open or that have a lip is accomplished most easily backward, using one

braces. The solid ankle joint does not allow for a foot-flat phase (Fig. 4-85).

To gait on a slope or sidewalk that slants down on one side the patient must put the downhill crutch in front of the uphill crutch, which will cause the downhill leg to swing farther forward than the uphill leg. This will allow better balancing while bringing the crutches forward.

Getting Up from a Fall

Getting up from a fall is very difficult, and only a few patients reach a level of competence to complete this maneuver independently. To get up, the crutches should be placed with the forearm cuffs near the knee joint. Directional placement of the crutches is determined by experimentation. From the prone position, the patient needs to push up and walk the hands backward until the feet are flat; then, while balancing on the feet and one hand, the patient picks up one crutch by the hand grip. This crutch is brought forward to form a tripod with the feet so that the other crutch can then be picked up and brought forward. With both crutches in position, the patient can then come to a vertical position by walking the crutches backward until he is balanced.

Progression

Four to six weeks is usually required to develop the necessary skills and confidence leading to continued use of the braces at home.

In general, once the patient has learned gaiting skills well and uses the KAFOs regularly, an ankle-foot orthosis (AFO) polypropylene can be substituted for the metal AFO (Fig. 4-86A and B). This is accomplished by cutting the uprights of the lower portion of the metal KAFO and attaching the polypropylene AFO to the metal uprights. Using the polypropylene AFO allows the patient to change shoes more conveniently. The drawback with the polypropylene AFO is that one loses the ability to adjust the balance of the patient in the manner that is possible with the double action adjustable metal ankle joints. We recommend that the paraplegic retain the metal lower portion so that it can be used in an emergency should the polypropylene AFO break. The lower the neuro-

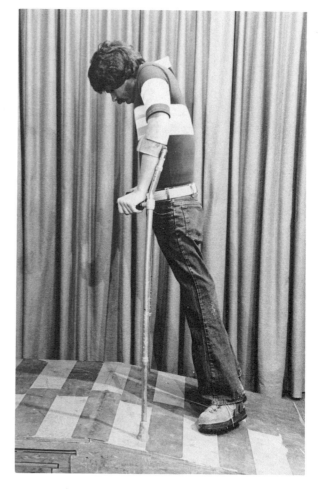

Fig. 4-85 Paraplegic going up incline.

logical level of the paraplegic, the greater the success with the polypropylene AFO attachment; these patients tend to regain a sense of balance in more than one position over a period of time.

Use of Scott-Craig Ankle-Foot Orthosis

An AFO is appropriate for patients with spinal cord lesions that result in no useful motor function distal to the knee but good grade quadriceps and good medial lateral knee stability. Crutches or a walker must be used for hip support. Reverse action of the latissimus dorsi can act on the pelvis as a substitute for weak or nonfunctional gluteus medius. A double action ankle joint and a full sole plate in the shoe are required to give full control

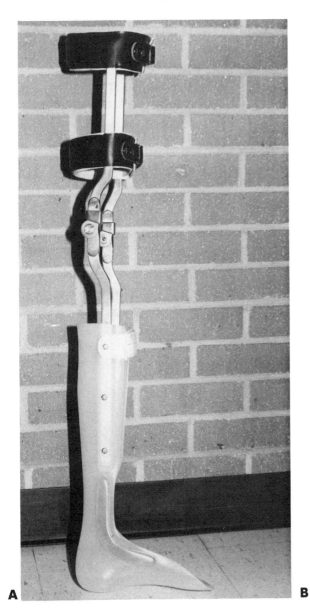

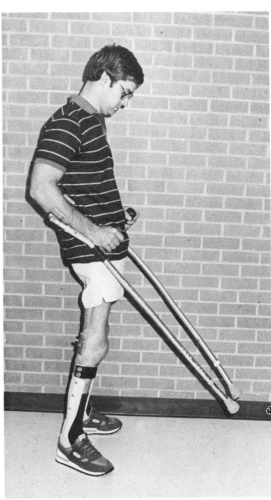

Fig. 4-86 (A) Side view of Scott-Craig polypropylene KAFO. **(B)** Paraplegic balanced in Scott-Craig polypropylene KAFO.

of the knee (Fig. 4-87). With the adjustable ankle, dorsi and plantar flexion stops can be adjusted and fixed to assist weak quadriceps or to prevent recurvatum. To assist weak quadriceps, the ankle joint will be adjusted to maintain the knee in a neutral position. To prevent recurvatum, slight dorsiflexion or the neutral position can be used.

Use of Polypropylene AFO

In the presence of a flail ankle, good skin, and no severe clonus, a polypropylene AFO can be used (Fig. 4-88). The disadvantage of this orthosis is the lack of adjustability as is found with the Scott-Craig AFO. If good knee stability is present, i.e.

good grade or better quadriceps and medial/lateral knee stability, a trial in a polypropylene AFO should be done. If recurvatum occurs, one can attempt to reshape the polypropylene into more dorsiflexion by first heating the orthosis. Only slight changes are possible, however, with this type of orthosis. An easier solution is to add the appropriate heel lift on the shoe that is needed to accentuate knee flexion and thus prevent recurvatum. In situations where proprioception in the knee joint has been lost due to the injury, many patients will overextend the knee joint strongly to reduce the fear of the knee buckling, which could result in a fall. In this situation it is hard to control the recurvatum problem with a polypropylene AFO.

It should be remembered that in cases of active ankle function in incomplete injuries, the polypropylene AFO generally will not allow use of the

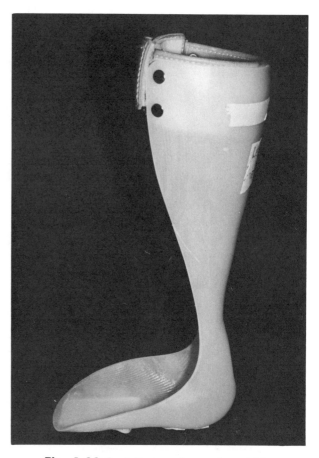

Fig. 4-88 Scott-Craig polypropylene AFO.

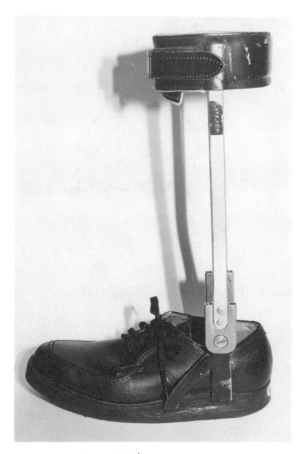

Fig. 4-87 Scott-Craig AFO.

active motions. The therapist should then decide whether knee control or the use of the functioning musculature is the most important element in bracing.

When measuring for the polypropylene AFO, the patient's shoe type should be considered. That is, will there be a heel, and if so what height will it be? Changing shoes with varying heel heights will affect the control of the knee joint. A high heel with the polypropylene AFO accentuates knee flexion; a lower heel accentuates extension.

If recurvatum cannot be controlled by the Scott-Craig double action AFO or a polypropylene AFO, one should use a standard Scott-Craig KAFO with a free knee, allowing for knee flexion in the swing phase, but preventing recurvatum during the stance phase.

SKIN MANAGEMENT

One of the most conservative aspects of a rehabilitation program is skin care. With proper skin management a person can (1) participate on a full rehabilitation program; (2) have a fulfilling social and personal life; and (3) go to school or work as a dependable, productive employee. Failure to care for the skin can result in devastating complications.

Skin sores or reddened areas can be prevented by the following measures:

1. Weight shifts (See descriptions in Ch. 3, the section on C5–C8 quadriplegia programs.)
2. Skin inspection. Routine skin inspection every morning and evening must be a way of life. It can be done with the aid of a hand mirror or with an assistant (Fig. 4-89), but it is the patient's responsibility to know the condition of his skin.

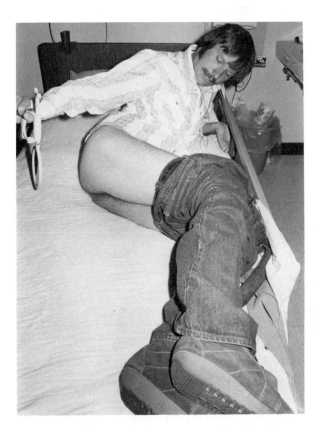

Fig. 4-89 Quadriplegic using a mirror for skin inspection.

3. Cushion inspection. A cushion for the wheelchair is essential. Whether an air, foam, gel or water cushion is used, be sure the ischials are not "bottoming out." There should be a 1 to 1¼-inch space between the ischials and bottom of cushion. There also needs to be even weight distribution along both thighs from ischials to just proximal (2 to 3-inches) to popliteal fossa.
4. Positioning/padding in bed. Use a turning schedule that does not allow redness to appear on bony prominences. Depending on the body type, one will tolerate a turning schedule of 2 to 5 hours (turning from side to back to side). The length of time can be gradually increased by 30-minute increments in a given position if redness does not occur. The only exception to this schedule is *sleeping prone*. Usually one can safely lie prone for up to 8 hours by using proper padding. Sleeping prone at night is very important for two reasons: Patient and attendant or family member can sleep uninterrupted for 8 hours, lying prone straightens hips and prevents tightness at hips and knees. (Fig. 4-90A through C for an example of a C7 quadriplegic independently positioning his pads and rolling prone.)

Padding

The following three diagrams and instructions illustrate side, back, and prone positions of sleeping with appropriate padding.

If you need further protection from developing red spots, cover pillows or pads with sheepskin. Adjust padding according to individual needs based on skin checks.

Warning: Do not substitute folded towels or blankets for foam padding or pillows. These can be too firm and can cause skin breakdown.

Side Position Padding (Fig. 4-91A)

1. Head—Small, foam support under head. Size of foam depends on individual comfort. Cover support with materials that are not irritating to your skin.
2. Back—Support behind back to maintain side position. Be sure bottom hip is pulled back to prevent rolling backwards on sacrum.

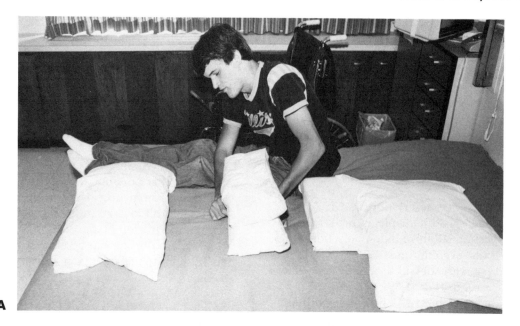

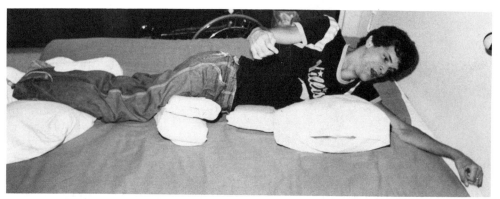

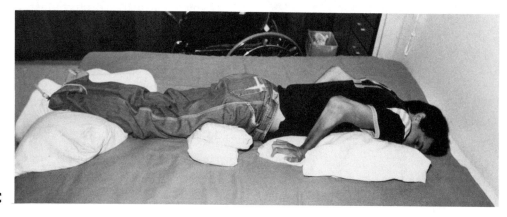

Fig. 4-90 (A) Quadriplegic positioning pads in bed. **(B)** Rolling onto position pads. **(C)** Quadriplegic rolled onto position pads.

Place pillow behind back

place pad between legs

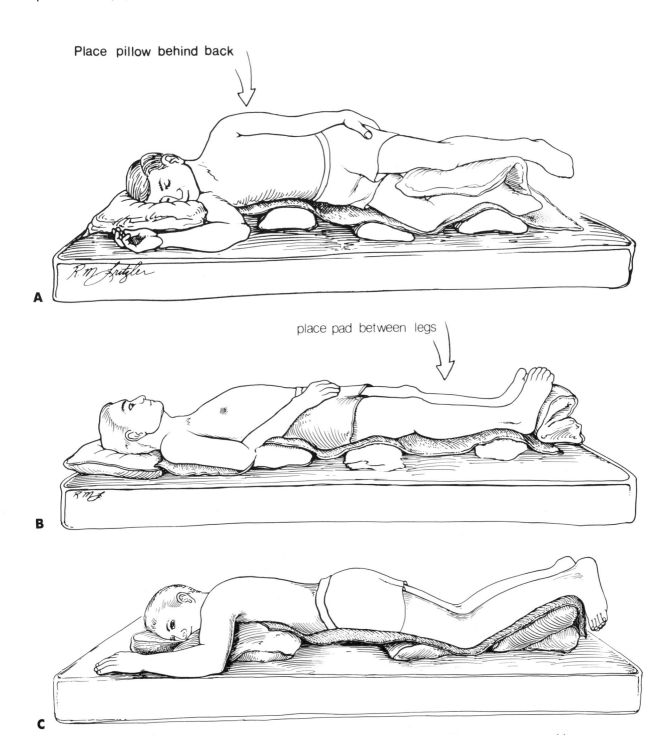

Fig. 4-91 **(A)** Side position padding. **(B)** Back position padding. **(C)** Prone position padding. (Courtesy of Craig Hospital Publications Department, Englewood, Colorado.)

3. Hips—Pad placed above and below the trochanter (hip). When pads are placed correctly, a flat hand can be slid between body and bed to be certain that pressure has been relieved. If the pressure has not been relieved, an additional pad can be added.
4. Ankle—Pad placed above the lateral malleolus (ankle joint).
5. Between lower legs—Pillow placed lengthwise between legs to prevent pressure on the knees and ankle joints. *Do not have legs directly on top of each other.*

Back Position Padding (Fig. 4-91B)

1. Head—Small, foam support under head. Size of foam depends on individual comfort. Cover support with materials that are not irritating to your skin.
2. Back—Place pad under lower back to provide elevation of the sacrum, relieve pressure on sacral area and relieve muscle tiredness in the back.
3. Knees—The bend at the knee is a natural curvature. Use a pad above the popliteal space (area behind the knee). Pad must not be in the popliteal space.
4. Ankles—A small pad is necessary at the back of the heel to relieve tension on the calf of the leg. Also, the heels must be off the bed to prevent skin breakdown.
5. Feet—A soft foot support is placed to allow simulation of weight bearing on the ball of the foot.
6. Between lower legs—Foam pad or pillow placed between the knees to prevent possible breakdown at the knee and ankle joints.

Prone Position Padding (Fig. 4-91C)

1. Head—Small, foam support under head. Size of foam depends on individual comfort. Cover support with materials that are not irritating to your skin.
2. Chest—Use one or more pillows according to comfort.
3. Thighs—Foam pads placed above the knees to prevent redness. May need two layers if too much pressure on knees.

4. Shins—Pad(s) or pillow(s) under shins to elevate feet high enough to avoid pressure on toes (helps prevent ingrown toenails). An alternative is to allow toes to hang off the end of the bed. Feet should be at a right angle to the leg as per illustration.
5. Between knees—Pad placed between knees to keep knees and ankles apart so that pressure sores do not develop.

EQUIPMENT

The technology in durable medical equipment is constantly changing. The equipment that is mentioned in the following pages is to suggest what equipment is available to the clinician and guidelines for its use. By publication, it is likely that other equipment will be on the market and it is important for the practicing clinician to stay informed about new equipment and its availability and incorporate it into their practice when appropriate.

Cushions

When the patient is first mobilized from the bed to the wheelchair, a cushion should be placed in the wheelchair. There are three basic types of wheelchair cushions: air, foam, and gel. Many variations and combinations of these categories are available.

The following is a representative list of available cushions.

1. BBD* (Bye-bye-decubiti)—Air cushion; inexpensive; lightweight, sheepskin cover; available in various sizes from pediatric to adult. Some people have excellent results with this cushion and use it for years.
2. Roho*—Air cushion; lightweight; fairly expensive, but gives excellent skin protection; one of the best cushions on the market; usually has very low ischial pressure readings; cover makes it more compact without compromising or increasing pressure on the ischials. A large variety of sizes is available. In addition, a variety of spacing and sizing of the actual air cells in the cushion is available. It

---

* See Appendix 4-1—Cushion Manufacturers.

also comes in regular and low profile heights. Some patients have initial difficulty with an air cushion affecting their balance, and thus function. However, if redness on the ischials prevents them from building up skin and/or sitting tolerance in the wheelchair, then the Roho is an ideal cushion to use.

3. Jay*—Floite cushion. It is fairly heavy (5 pounds) for quadriplegics to lift in and out of the wheelchair. It is expensive, gives excellent skin protection with low pressures on the ischials, has a cover, and provides good balance and sitting position in the wheelchair. At present available sizes are limited.

4. Foam—Many different foam cushions are appropriate for spinal cord injured patients. Examples include AKROS*, combination foam and a compartment or bladder of water within, T-foam*, a dense foam that conforms to the patient's body, and Stainless*, which has laminated layers.

No matter what type of foam cushion is chosen, it must have at least 1 to 1¼ inch thickness between the ischials and the bottom of the cushion. (See section on Skin Management.)

Foam cushions tend to wear out within 6 to 9 months, even if they are rotated in the wheelchair. To alleviate any skin problems, the therapist should order at least two to send home with the patient.

Foam does provide a solid sitting base for the patient. Another advantage is the option of being able to cut out relief areas for bony prominences, such as the ischials.

Problem Solving with Cushions

Pelvic obliquity and ensuing unequal pressure on one ischial tuberosity can be the result of heterotopic ossification in the hips, unequal spasticity in the hip flexors, scoliosis, and unilateral amputations. When this situation exists, the therapist should re-evaluate the wheelchair cushion. We have found that the following procedures provide solutions in some cases:

---

* See Appendix 4-1—Cushion Manufacturers.

1. Use a double manifold Roho cushion and increase the air pressure on the ischial side receiving the most body pressure. Reduce the air pressure in the lesser weight-bearing side of the cushion. This will tend to equalize the ischial pressures if the spine and pelvis are still flexible. If this is not successful, a custom Roho can be designed; consult Roho, Inc.

2. If using a Jay cushion, a custom cushion can be ordered that channels most of the Floite material to the higher pressure side.

3. When using a foam cushion, a wedge of high density foam can be placed under the high pressure side, lateral border. In addition, a small wedge can be cut out of the lateral border of the low pressure side with a sharp knife or electric knife.

If these solutions are ineffective, consult your local orthopaedic service for custom seating systems.

Considerations and Criteria for Manual Wheelchairs

The therapist must consider several criteria when assessing the patient's present and long-term needs. Although each patient will be evaluated individually some *common factors* should be considered.

Levels of Injury

C5 Quadriplegia—No Wrist or Hand Function, No Abdominals, No Truck Balance ± Spasticity

1. Back height—Usually requires an increased back height
2. Chest strap
3. Quad pegs
4. Caster locks
5. Anti-tippers
6. Stability of the armrests

C6–C8 Quadriplegia—Partial Wrist and Hand Innervation, No Abdominals, No Trunk Balance, ± Spasticity

1. Back height—May begin with standard (16-inch) back height and then eventually lower the height
2. Chest strap
3. Quad pegs or dipped rims

4. Caster locks
5. Ability to load in a car
6. Anti-tippers
7. Stability of the armrests

High Paraplegia T1–T7,—No Abdominals, No Trunk Balance, ± Spasticity

1. Back height—Usually can have a standard or lower back height
2. Possible chest strap
3. Caster locks
4. Ability to load into a car
5. Anti-tippers
6. Stability of armrests

Midrange Paraplegia T8–T11—Partial Abdominal Innervation, ± Spasticity

1. Caster locks
2. Anti-tippers

Low Paraplegia T12–L4—No Essential Required Options

Posture

A high quadriplegic usually requires a full reclining wheelchair with head rest. If spasticity is a problem, body positioners are usually attached to the wheelchair back as appropriate.

The typical C5–C8 quadriplegic tends to slump in the wheelchair, especially with the more popular lightweight wheelchairs and lower back heights. In this slumped position the quadriplegic has the balance to do activities with his arms without the use of a chest safety belt. Quadriplegics tend to refuse the use of a chest-height belt because it (1) requires unfastening to do forward position activities, and (2) is not aesthetically pleasing. An additional complication in the newer lightweight wheelchairs is the soft back, which tends to stretch quickly, adding more sag to the upper trunk and accentuating round shoulders.

Creativity is required to resolve these problems. We recommend the following methods for quadriplegics:

1. Use of a Jay* cushion provides good seating support.

---

* See Appendix 4-1—Cushion Manufacturers.

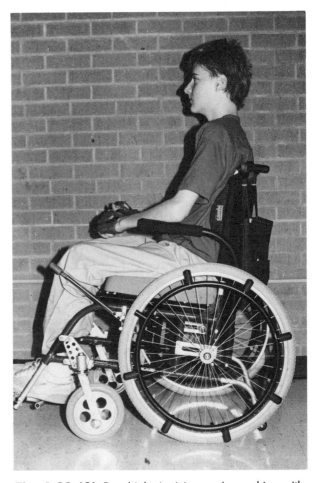

Fig. 4-92 (A) Quadriplegic sitting on Jay cushion with Combi pad.

2. Use a Combi* lumbar pad. This creates a lordosis in the lumbar spine, which reverses the sitting sag kyphosis (Fig. 4-92).

If the back height of the wheelchair is two to three fingers width below the inferior tip of the scapula, the above mentioned techniques tend to provide the quadriplegic with an overall better sitting posture.

Depending on the level of paraplegia, sitting posture is usually a problem of the loss of the normal lumbar lordosis. This is accentuated by the use of a wheelchair with a low back height and one with a soft back material that sags. The higher the level of paraplegia, the greater the problem. Higher levels of paraplegia should have a back height two to three fingers width below the inferior tip of the scapula. The use of the Combi lumbar pad tends to reverse the kyphosis problem.

Many who have been paraplegics for several years or longer report nonspecific back pain. We have found that this problem is relieved by the use of the lumbar pad. There is usually an immediate relief of symptoms once this pad is used.

Previous Experience

Recently injured patients require equipment with additional safety features, such as

1. Caster locks
2. Anti-toppers
3. Increased back height
4. Chest strap
5. Firm armrests

At re-evaluation, the patient's preference should guide equipment choice. Patients know what they need. Eliminate some options if requested.

Life Style—Sedentary Versus Active

A patient's life style will help determine equipment type such as

1. Axles—Movable versus nonmovable
2. Wheels—Mag versus spoke
3. Wheelchair—Folding versus rigid. Although more cumbersome, rigid chairs are more durable because there are fewer parts to break.

Body Type—(Large, Tall or Short)

Considerations of body type include

1. Frame size
2. Armrest with skirt guards or wet weather guards to prevent hip abduction
3. Rigid chair (for heavy person)
4. A top-heavy person can stretch out the upholstery on a folding wheelchair.

Coordination

Poor coordination might indicate a need for more safety features, such as caster locks, safety belt, higher back, or stationary arms.

Home-Work Situation

A small house or work area may require the use of swing-away footrests to get up to a desk or a bath tub. Armrests to sit on or a more formal looking chair may be required.

Patient Preference

Try many wheelchairs and pick what the patient prefers. The ultimate decision is usually up to the patient. Peer pressure is a factor.

Many manual wheelchairs are available on the market today, from the standard ones to the lightweights. Some of the wheelchairs we have found successful over a number of years with many spinal cord injured patients include*

1. Quickie: I, II, and III
2. Rolls 500: Rigid, Fold, and ATS (Invacare)
3. Everest and Jennings
   a. Rigid–Lightening
   b. Fold–Ultralight
   c. Sportsman
   d. Active duty lightweight
4. X-L Rigid

Miscellaneous Equipment

Accessories

Hand protectors include such items as wheelie mitts and gloves. These are used to protect the skin, as well as to give added friction for propelling the wheelchair.

Plastic coated rims are warmer to the touch than bare metal and provide a textured surface for grasp.

Standing Devices

Hydraulic or electric standing tables are used in the early mobilization process for quadriplegics. Occasionally, a patient will request such a device for home use. These devices are especially good for stretching tightness in the hips, knees, and ankles, which tends to occur from long-term sitting in the wheelchair.

---

* See Appendix 4-2—Wheelchair Manufacturers.

Stall bars can be constructed from used pipe at a nominal cost. Low level quadriplegics and all levels of paraplegia can use this device safely and independently. We strongly encourage the use of stall bars for those paraplegics who will be returning at a later time for a gaiting program to prevent contractures that would interfere with subsequent bracing and ambulation.

Bathroom Aids

A shower/commode wheelchair is useful in a roll-in-shower and will fit over a standard toilet bowl. Castor locks and quad pegs are adaptations for the quadriplegic patient.

A portable elevated toilet seat is useful for travel. A side opening provides an area for doing a bowel program.

A padded bath bench is useful, both for quadriplegics who can transfer easily and for paraplegics who prefer not to transferto the bottom of a tub.

ACKNOWLEDGMENTS

The authors would like to acknowledge the significant contributions to this material by specific former staff members: Beverly Parrott, R.P.T.; Maggie Mueller, O.T.R.; and Marilyn Greb, R.P.T. In addition, the past and present physical therapy staff has been responsible for developing and implementing many of the concepts presented.

Our sincere thanks to Carol Wickham and Suzanne Warchal, our devoted secretaries, for their patience and many hours spent typing and retyping the manuscript.

We wish to gratefully acknowledge the many hours Marcia Jensen, staff photographer, spent in organizing and taking photographs and in copying slides.

REFERENCES

1. Stover SL, Fine PR, Go BK, et al: National Spinal Cord Statistical Center, Annual Report 3, 6, 1985
2. Babkin D, Timtsenko N (eds): Electrostimulation: Notes from Dr. Ym Kots (USSR) Lectures and Laboratory Periods. Presented at the Canadian-Soviet Exchange Symposium on Electrostimulation of Skeletal Muscles, Concordia University, Montreal, Quebec, Canada, December 6–15, 1977
3. O'Daniel WE, Hahn HR: Follow-up usage of the Scott-Craig orthosis in paraplegia. Paraplegia 19:373, 1981

Appendix 4-1
Cushion Pads

Akros Cushion
Akros Manufacturing, Inc.
36 West Street
Gloversville, NY 12078

Bye-Bye Decubiti Cushion
Ken McRight Supplies, Inc.
7456 South Oswego
Tulsa, OK 74136

Combi Lumbar Pad
Jay Medical, Ltd.
805 Walnut
Boulder, CO 80302

Jay Cushion
Jay Medical, Ltd.
805 Walnut
Boulder, CO 80302

Puritan-Bennett Corp.
10800 Pflumm Road
Lenexa, KA 66215

Roho Cushion
Roho Incorporated
P.O. Box 658
Belleville, IL 62222

Stainless Cushion
Stainless Medical Products
9389 Dowdy Drive
San Diego, CA 92126

Temper Foam (T-Foam) Cushion
Edmont-Wilson
1300 Walnut Street
Coshocton, OH 43812

Appendix 4-2
Wheelchairs and Accessories

A-Bec Mobility, Inc.
Sunrise Medical Company
20460 Gramercy Place
Torrance, CA 90501

Becker Orthopedic Appliance Co.
635 Executive Drive
Troy, MI 48083

Everest and Jennings, Inc.
3233 East Mission Oaks Boulevard
Camarillo, CA 93010

Invacare Corporation
899 Cleveland Street
Elyria, OH 44036-2125

Lumex, Inc.
100 Spence Street
Bay Shore, NY 11706

Qualaug Rubber Co.
North Brookfield, MA 01535

Quickie
Motion Designs
2842 Business Park Avenue
Fresno, CA 93727

X-L Wheelchairs
4950 D Cohasset Stage Road
Chico, CA

Scott Orthopedics,Inc.
1100 E 8th Avenue
Denver, CO 80218

Wheelchair Gloves
Jesse Woodhouse
824 Santa Fe
Springfield, CO 81073

5 Facial Paralysis and Other Neuromuscular Dysfunctions of the Peripheral Nervous System

Richard Balliet

Our present knowledge concerning the neuromuscular retraining of facial paralysis and other peripheral nerve dysfunctions is based on less than a decade of research from around the world. During this time the treatment and measurement of facial dysfunction has become a significant new specialty in rehabilitation. Although this chapter emphasizes the treatment of unilateral facial paralysis, the general logic that is presented is also applicable to bilateral facial paralysis (e.g., Möbius's syndrome) and to other peripheral nerve dysfunctions. A small section at the end of the chapter has been included on specific details pertaining to peripheral nerve dysfunction.

One reason that neuromuscular retraining of facial paralysis is relatively new is that there are apparently no simple therapy procedures for this problem. It will probably never be possible to have a successful "cookbook" or "handout-sheet of exercises" approach to facial retraining because each patient has a unique muscle function profile and intervening psychosocial response to the condition. Also, as will be seen in this chapter, caution should be used because there is reason to believe that many seemingly benign retraining methods may actually be contraindicated. In addition, some conditions, such as hemifacial spasm,[1] and certain diplegias, such as blepharospasms,[2] are not treatable behaviorally because of extensive neuroanatomical involvements (e.g., nerve entrapment). Therefore, this chapter offers basic research re-

sults and associated logic that can be applied in the "general problem solving" of the many combinations of facial dysfunctions. The understanding of "why" certain procedures are used is essential to use these techniques to their greatest extent and to develop even more effective retraining strategies. Ultimately, however, the effective use of this chapter will depend primarily on the therapist's creative application of this information to the individual patient and the patient's accurate compliance with self-training program at home.

INJURIES TO THE PERIPHERAL NERVOUS SYSTEM

Neuroanatomy

The peripheral nervous system consists of the cranial and the spinal nerves from the point that they exit the central nervous system (CNS) to where they terminate at connecting muscles and organs. Listed are the cranial nerves that are directly associated with motor performance:

Oculomotor (III)
Trochlear (IV)
Trigeminal (V)
Abducens (VI)
Facial (VII)
Glossopharyngeal (IX)
Spinal Accessory (XI)
Hypoglossal (XII)

175

The olfactory (I), optic (II), and acoustic (VIII) nerves are not considered to be true nerves; rather, they are CNS fiber tracts that have very poor postlesion regeneration capacity. With the exception of the olfactory, optic and a portion of the spinal accessory, all of these nerves leave the CNS at the brain stem where the motor nuclei reside. The 31 pairs of spinal nerves consist of the following:

1. 8 Cervical (C1–C8)
2. 12 Thoracic (T1–T12)
3. 5 Lumbar (L1–L5)
4. 5 Sacral (S1–S5)
5. 1 Coccygeal (C)

These nerves exit the spinal cord dorsally as sensory roots and ventrally as motor roots. They join peripherally at cervical, brachial, and lumbosacral plexuses that branch into nerve trunks and terminate at their respective distal destinations.[2]

It is possible to have any of these nerves involved in some form of motor, sensory, or tropic disorder. However, most peripheral nerve lesions that are seen acutely, postacutely and/or postsurgically in clinical rehabilitation usually consist of either facial nerve (CN VII), brachial plexus (C5–T1) or injuries to the various nerves of the extremities (C5–T1; L1–S2). These lesions may have various etiologies, including the following:

1. Congenital
2. Traumatic
3. Neoplasm
4. Toxicity
5. Viral
6. Bacteriological
7. Unknown degenerative/functional

Classification of Nerve Injury

All nerve injuries are not the same. Resulting injuries may be classified relative to differing prognoses. The following discussion specifies five levels of axon and related structural damage, as well as resulting function in ascending order of severity.[3] Although functional outcomes relative to the face are described, similar results may occur in the injury of other peripheral nerves. In these definitions, Wallerian degeneration is defined as a traumatic or ischemic injury that stops the flow of

axoplasm down the nerve fiber, which results in the nerve dying distally.

First Degree Injury

1. Minor compression, where the nerve is completely preserved
2. No Wallerian degeneration
3. Intact endoneurial sheaths
4. Only temporary physiological (ischemic) conduction block at point of trauma
5. Intact conduction above and below lesion
6. Spontaneous and full recovery of function

Second Degree Injury

1. Moderate compression, where the nerve is basically preserved
2. Small amount of Wallerian degeneration
3. Intact endoneurial sheaths
4. Temporarily damaged nerve fibers
5. Intact conduction above and below lesion
6. Spontaneous complete or incomplete recovery of nerve axons that regenerate within their own endoneurial tube
7. Incomplete recovery requiring neuromuscular retraining

Third Degree Injury

1. Severe compression, where the nerve is only partially preserved
2. Wallerian degeneration
3. Severely damaged endoneurial sheaths
4. Temporary and/or permanent loss of continuity corresponding to the damage of differing nerve fibers
5. Scar tissue crosses nerve bundles, blocking the advance of regenerating axons
6. Spontaneous cross-wiring of regenerating axons that are no longer contained in their original endoneurial tubes. Dysfunction may include (1) motor and sensory confusion resulting in low motor function and associated or disassociated neuralgia and discomfort, (2) low-threshold and high-threshold motoneuron disordering resulting in poor slow/fine motor control and rapid fatigue, or (3) synkinesis as manifested by involuntary or inappropriate motor function resulting in dyscoordination and low function.

7. Neuromuscular retraining may significantly increase function

Fourth Degree Injury

1. Very severe damage; nerve is only preserved as mangled tissue
2. Wallerian degeneration
3. Destroyed endoneurial sheaths
4. Temporary and/or permanent partial loss of continuity corresponding to damage of differing nerve fibers
5. Scar tissue crosses nerve bundles, blocking advance of regenerating axons
6. Spontaneous cross-wiring of regenerating axons is limited because of extensive debris and scarring resulting in extreme dyscoordination or no function.
7. Neuromuscular retraining should be used only after surgical excision of tissue debris and subsequent anastomosis (i.e., conversion to a third degree injury) (surgical methods are described under fifth degree injury).

Fifth Degree Injury

1. Nerve completely severed
2. Surgery required to reconnect nerve
3. At best, with microsurgery to clean and appropriately reconnect nerve bundles, an "upgrade" to a third degree injury can be expected. Neuromuscular retraining can then be used to facilitate increased function.

Surgical Methods[3–5]

Anastomosis of the Same Nerve. This nerve union is only possible if there is sufficient nerve remaining and if the union is relatively distal to the CNS. Under these conditions, retraining can result in a good functional outcome.

Anastomosis with Nerves from Another Motor Nucleus. A unilateral hypoglossal–facial (CN XII –CN VII) nerve anastomosis to restore facial function is a typical example of this procedure. Part of innervation to the tongue is sacrificed in order to normalize facial tone. It is possible to partially or almost completely retrain a motor nucleus to have a different function, thus resulting in fair to good motor control.

Nerve (Cable) Graft. Typically, the venous cuff of another nerve is used to splice together the two ends of a completely sectioned nerve. Fitted over the end of each piece, it acts as a bridge to allow the nerve to grow across the center of the tube formed by the cuff. Retraining can result in a good functional outcome.

Anastomosis with Healthy Portion of the Same Nerve. In unilateral facial paralysis, this would involve an anastomosis to the normal facial nerve on the other side of the face through the use of a bridging nerve graft. It is currently not clear if, even with retraining, this procedure can result in a good functional outcome.

Plastic Surgery. In cases of extensive nerve trauma, muscle transplants (slings), or tendon transplants in the case of the extremities, may be used sometimes to help restore facial appearance. Because of the often limited kinematics and range of motion associated with such procedures, it is not always possible to restore voluntary control; it may only be possible to help normalize tone.

FACIAL PARALYSIS REHABILITATION

Incidence of Diagnoses

There are no national or international statistics on the incidence of facial paralysis. It is clear, however, from the collected works presented recently at the Fifth International Symposium on the Facial Nerve that there are tens of thousands of patients with this affliction.[6]

Most statistical reports come from individual clinics that tend to specialize in certain types of patient. The largest general patient classification estimate has come from the diagnosis of 4,149 cases of facial paralysis between the years 1968 and 1983 at the Facial Research Department in Amsterdam, Holland.[7] These data compare favorably with that of others (Mark May, personal communication) and is presented in Table 5-1.

In this population more than half of the facial paralysis patients have been diagnosed to have a Bell's palsy and, therefore, are most probably viral in origin. At least 90 percent of these people will have good recovery without any intervention. The remaining patients will have relatively more severe involvements. They will also be more likely to require surgery and/or suffer from some amount

Table 5-1 General Facial Paralysis Classification Estimate[7]

Etiology	Percent
Bell's palsy	53.6
Operative trauma	13.0
Diabetes, hypertension, infection, etc.	11.0
Rare etiologies	6.5
Herpes zoster	5.9
Endotemporal and extratemporal trauma	5.8
Otitis media	4.2

of postacute facial dysfunction requiring some amount of facial retraining.

Anatomy and Kinesiology

The anatomy of the face provides an integral working structure that helps determine the exact amount and angle of facial expression. It is clear, however, that there is a high interindividual variability in muscle angle, size, and position, as well as high intraindividual variations, including asymmetries and the nonformation of certain muscles, such as the risorius.[8] In addition, there are differing patterns of muscle innervation (activity) during the production of various facial gestures and efforts,[8] including the basic sounds used in speech.[9–14]

Knowledge of the anatomical origins and insertions of the muscles to either bone or tissue is essential to understanding facial kinematics and functional assessments. The following discussion describes these relationships, as well as the corresponding nerve branches.[15–16] In addition, Figure 5-1 can be used to picture interactive effects. Note that the facial muscles which are more involved in maintaining basic tone, and are not significantly involved in facial expression, are not included (e.g., tensor tarsi, platysma, and buccinator).

Frontalis

Anatomy

The frontalis muscle is composed of two thin sheets of muscle fibers moving in a somewhat lateral direction up the forehead. There are no bone attachments: The end points of the muscle combine with muscle fibers of the orbicularis oculi at the eyebrows and the aponeurotica, which covers the top of the head. Galea aponeurotica separates these two bands of muscle.

Function

The frontalis acts to wrinkle the forehead but also to pull up the orbicularis oculi and the procerus.

Facial Nerve Branch

The facial nerve branch is the temporal nerve.

Corrugator

Anatomy

The corrugator is a small muscle that is diagonally directed (downward and medially) at the medial end of each eyebrow. It connects to the medial portion of the frontal bone and runs through the frontalis to its end point attachment to the skin.

Function

The corrugator muscle pulls the skin between the eyebrows medially toward the nose, thus causing wrinkling in this area.

Facial Nerve Branches

The facial nerve branches of the corrugator muscle are the zygomatic and temporal nerves.

Procerus

Anatomy

The procerus is a small muscle lying between the medial ends of the corrugator muscles. It blends with the inferior medial ends of the frontalis and is attached on the other end at the nasal bone/cartilage junction of the nose.

Function

The procerus pulls the medial portion of the eyebrows down toward the nose, thus wrinkling the upper portion of the nose.

Facial Nerve Branches

The temporal, zygomatic, and buccal nerves are the facial nerve branches of the procerus muscle.

Orbicularis Oculi Superioris and Inferioris

Anatomy

The upper and lower portions of this wide, flat muscle encircle the eye and act as a sphincter to cause eye closure. The palpebral ligament attaches the medial corner of the muscle to bone. The

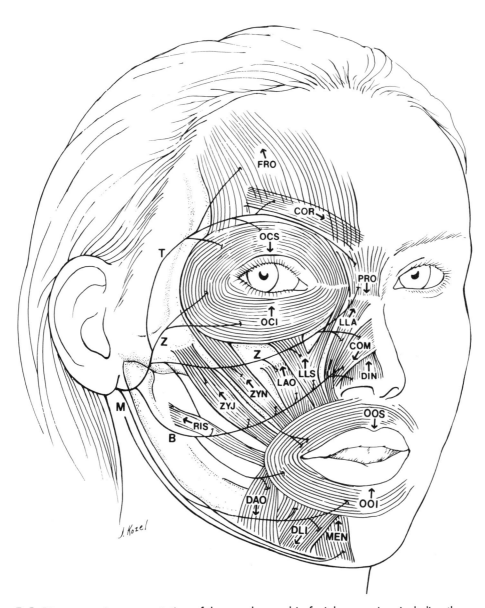

Fig. 5-1 Diagrammatic representation of the muscles used in facial expression, including the associated branches of the facial nerve. Frontalis (FRO), corrugator (COR), procerus (PRO), orbicularis oculi superioris (OCS), orbicularis oculi inferioris (OCI), dilator naris (DIN), compressor naris (COM), levator labii alaeque nasi (LLA), levator labii superioris (LLS), levator anguli oris (LAO), zygomaticus major (ZYJ), zygomaticus minor (ZYN), risorius (RIS), orbicularis oris superioris (OOS), orbicularis oris inferioris (OOI), depressor anguli oris (DAO), depressor labii inferioris (DLI), and mentalis (MEN). Facial nerve branches: temporal (T), zygomaticus (Z), buccal (B), and mandibular (M).

superior and inferior muscle fibers combine at the lateral corner of the eye. Between these points, the inner muscle fibers help form the eyelids; the outer muscle fibers cover the orbital cavity and the bony orbit. The superior muscle fibers combine with the frontalis and the corrugator medially but are only attached to fascia laterally.

Function

Most eye closure involves primarily the orbicularis oculi superioris. The orbicularis oculi inferioris is also involved in the eye closure of children and young adults.

Facial Nerve Branches

The temporal and zygomatic nerves are these muscles' facial nerve branches.

Dilator Naris

Anatomy

This muscle originates at the nasal notch of the maxilla and ends in the skin of the outer portion of the nostril.

Function

The dilator naris enlarges the nostril.

Facial Nerve Branches

The zygomatic and buccal nerves are the facial nerve branches.

Compressor Naris

Anatomy

This muscle originates at the canine eminence above and lateral to incisive fossa of maxilla and ends in the aponeurosis.

Function

The compressor naris draws the edge of the nose towards septum and compresses the nostrils.

Facial Nerve Branches

The compressor naris' facial nerve branches are the zygomatic buccal nerves.

Levator Labii Alaeque Nasi

Anatomy

This small muscle originates at the maxilla next to the nasal notch and travels behind the nose and inserts into the medial portion of the orbicularis oris superioris and connecting skin.

Function

The levator labii alaeque nasi lifts the medial portion of the upper lip and the nose.

Facial Nerve Branches

The facial nerve branches of the muscle are the zygomatic and buccal nerves.

Levator Labii Superioris

Anatomy

Similar to the levator labii alaeque nasi, the levator labii superioris originates in the maxilla next to the nasal notch but also above the infraorbital foramen and from the cheek (zygomatic) bone. It inserts into the skin around the nose, the lateral part of the upper lip including skin, and the orbicularis oris superioris and the skin of the nasolabial groove.

Function

The muscle opens the nostril and raises the upper lip in a lateral direction.

Facial Nerve Branches

The facial nerve branches are the zygomatic and buccal nerves.

Levator Anguli Oris

Anatomy

This muscle is similar to the levator labii superioris except that it elevates the lateral portion of the upper lip and the corner of the mouth. It originates just below the infraorbital foramen and inserts into muscle fibers comprised of the orbicularis oris, depressor anguli, and zygomaticus.

Function

This muscle elevates the upper lip.

Facial Nerve Branches

The facial nerve branches are the zygomatic and buccal nerves.

Zygomaticus Minor and Zygomaticus Major

Anatomy

These muscles originate from the zygomatic bone and insert diagonally into the side of the cheek at the corner of the mouth; muscle fibers intermingle with those of the orbicularis oris and depressor anguli oris.

Function

These muscles draw the mouth both backward and upward.

Facial Nerve Branches

The zygomatic and buccal nerves make up the facial nerve branches.

Risorius

Anatomy

This muscle originates from fascia over the masseter just behind the midcheek area and inserts into skin and the orbicularis oris at the corner of the mouth.

Function

The risorius muscle pulls the corner of the mouth backward and slightly upward.

Facial Nerve Branches

The facial nerve branches are the zygomatic and buccal nerves.

Orbicularis Oris Superioris and Inferioris

Anatomy

The upper and lower portions of this muscle encompass the mouth and are the oral sphincter. The insertion ends of the muscles around the mouth blend into its circumference. It extends up to the nose and to the fold of skin between the lower lip and the chin.

Function

The orbicularis oris is unique because it consists of three sets of muscle fibers that can be differentially contracted. These functions include lip protusion, lip contraction, and lip compression. Acting usually as an antagonist, but also sometimes an agonist, all or part of these functions are involved in most facial expressions.

Facial Nerve Branches

The facial nerve branches of the muscle are the zygomatic, buccal and mandibular nerves.

Depressor Anguli Oris (Triangularis) and Depressor Labii Inferioris

Anatomy

The origin of these muscles is at the mandible; insertions are at the lower corner of the mouth and lip and in the orbicularis oris and skin. These muscles are often woven together from the midline area to the lower lip.

Function

These muscles pull down the corner of the mouth and area of the lower lip.

Facial Nerve Branches

The facial nerve branches are the mandibular and buccal nerves.

Mentalis

Anatomy

These are cone-shaped muscles (point down) that help form the chin. Their origin is in the area between the lower lip and the bottom of the chin; the insertions are into the skin of the chin.

Function

The mentalis help raise and protrude the lower lip. They may appear as the sides of a dimpled chin or as just two small mounds.

Facial Nerve Branch

The mandibular nerve is the facial nerve branch.

Assessment: Facial Nerve Grading Systems

Similar to upper and lower extremity disorders, it is essential for the therapist to be able to assess accurately the patient's facial retraining outcomes. Although numerous subjective methods exist to assess a patient's facial function, currently there are no objective tests.

The 1984 International Assessment Scale and Associated Optional Scale Recommendations

In 1984, all of the existing facial nerve grading systems were evaluated at the Fifth International Symposium on the Facial Nerve in Bordeaux[17] (Table 5-2). At that time it was decided to adopt a new gross scale, which summarized the best features of the existing scales and used only 6 grades (I–VI); this new scale was adopted as a tentative International Scale.[18] This relatively gross evaluation system is based on the John House Scale.[19] Facial function, as measured in terms of percentage of normal activity, is used for comparison purposes to other scales and is not part of the

Table 5-2 1984 International Assessment Scale: Recommended Gross Scale[17]

	Grade I	Grade II	Grade III	Grade IV	Grade V	Grade VI
General Description	*Normal* (100%) Normal facial function in all areas	*Mild Dysfunction* (99–75%) Slight weakness noticeable only on close inspection.	*Moderate Dysfunction* (75–50%) Obvious, but not disfiguring difference between two sides; no functional impairment; noticeable, but not severe synkinesis, contracture and/or hemifacial spasm.	*Moderately Severe Dysfunction* (50–25%) Obvious weakness and/or disfiguring asymmetry.	*Severe Dysfunction* (25–1%) Only barely perceptible motion.	*Total Paralysis* (0%) Loss of tone; asymmetry; no motion; no synkinesis, contracture, or hemifacial spasm.
At Rest		Normal symmetry and tone.	Normal symmetry and tone.	Normal symmetry and tone.	Possible asymmetry with droop of corner of mouth and decreased or absent nasal labial fold.	
Motion		Partial to normal movement of forehead. Eye closure normal with minimal and maximal effort.	Slight to no movement of forehead; ability to close eye with maximal effort and obvious asymmetry.	Slight to no movement of forehead; inability to close eye completely with maximal effort; asymmetrical movement of corners of mouth with maximal effort.	No movement of forehead; incomplete closure of eye and only slight movement of lid with maximal effort; slight movement of corner of mouth.	
Secondary Defects		Very slight synkinesis may be observed on close inspection. No contracture or hemifacial spasm.	Patients with obvious, but not disfiguring, synkinesis, contracture and/or hemifacial spasm are grade III, even if voluntary motor abilities are grade II.	Patients with synkinesis; mass action and/or hemifacial spasm severe enough to interfere with function are grade IV, regardless of degree of voluntary motor ability.	Synkinesis, contracture, and hemifacial spasm usually absent.	

scale. It was also recommended that the assessment should consist of an average of three observers, excluding the person involved in the treatment.

In addition, symposium members recommended that two optional assessments could also be used. The first is a subjective estimate of function as determined by the patient; the second is a precise clinical analysis of each muscle group by the examiner.

It should be noted that the exact methods to facilitate voluntary and/or spontaneous facial movements involved in this or any other grading scale have not been standardized and vary depending on the examiner. The scale, however, is sufficiently gross that interexaminer reliability is thought to be relatively significant.[18]

Subjective Gross Estimate of Function as Determined by the Patient[18]

The patient evaluates his own facial handicap in terms of overall percentage of functional ability. This percentage is useful in assessing results relative to patient satisfaction. This score should be compared to the International Scale; for example, grade III (average observer assessment) would have reasonably good agreement with a 60 percent patient assessment score.

General Directives of a Detailed Clinical Assessment of Each Muscle Group by the Examiner[18]

The method of this analysis is determined by the examiner. It is recommended, however, that at least six voluntary movements be evaluated:

1. Frowning
2. Eye closure
3. Flaring nostrils
4. Smiling
5. Whistling
6. Pouting of lips

The final evaluation score should be an averaged functional score, which may or may not have weighted components, and should be expressed as a percentage between 0 and 100. Secondary defects, such as hemifacial spasm, contraction, synkinesis, tearing, etc., should be assessed separately from the voluntary movements associated with each muscle group and included in the overall percentage to classify the patient's function as one

of the six International Assessment Scores, grades I–VI.

The University of Wisconsin Facial Paralysis Clinical Assessment Scale

The previous optional 1984 International Assessment II guidelines are very general and can be complied with in many different ways. Indeed, it is possible to create an assessment that is almost infinitely detailed and complex. Unfortunately, there is an inversely proportional relationship between the detail of a scale and its reliability, and therefore, its utility. What is most important is that it fulfills its user's requirements to provide an operational and modifiable definition of facial performance.

The following University of Wisconsin Assessment Scale (Fig. 5-2) may be used to fulfill the above optional 1984 International Assessment II requirements. It is based on anatomy as is diagrammatically depicted in Figure 5-1. This method of assessment may be too extensive and time consuming for the average user. It is presented in its entirety as a working model so that any part of it can be used clinically.

Estimates of Volitional Movement, Spontaneous Movement, and Resting Tone

Sample instructions to facilitate volitional movements are given in Table 5-3. Spontaneous movements or more emotional facial responses can be assessed over time while observing the patient during casual conversation, or they can be contrived through the use of the suggested spontaneous movement instructions, which are also listed in Table 5-3. *It is important to note that these sample instructions must be used in a manner that does not violate the precautions mentioned in the section entitled General Indicated and Contraindicated Retraining Strategies.* Compliance with *both* of these directions is essential to facilitate selective motor control and reduce unwanted synergy patterns.

Volitional movement, spontaneous movement and resting tone assessments should be graded from 0 to 100 percent relative to the patient's uninvolved side as a standard (Table 5-4). This is not possible in the case of the bilateral facial paralysis patient or in the case of the unilateral paralysis patient who is suspected of inhibiting

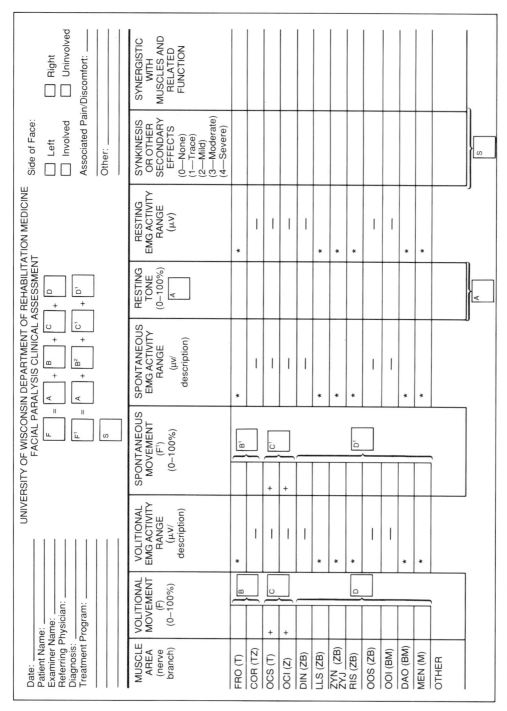

Fig. 5-2 University of Wisconsin Department of Rehabilitation Medicine Facial Paralysis Clinical Assessment. Facial muscle areas: frontalis (FRO), corrugator (and procerus) (COR), orbicularis oculi superioris (OCS), orbicularis oculi inferioris (OCI), dilator naris and alaeque nasi (DIN), levator labii superioris and levator anguli oris (LLS), zygomaticus minor (ZYN), zygomaticus major (ZYJ), risorius (RIS), orbicularis oris superioris (OOS), orbicularis oris inferioris (OOI), depressor anguli oris (and depressor labii inferioris) (DAO), and mentalis (MEN). Facial nerve branches: temporal (T), zygomaticus (Z), buccal (B), and mandibular (M). EMG readings are in microvolts [µV] using surface electrodes. EMG description may include some estimate of control or fatigue. Typically the maximal number of muscle areas examined are no more than six [*]. Eye closure percentages are relative to millimeters of closure. A, B, B¹, C, C¹, and S are assessment summary scores used in the calculation of a gross summary score that can be compared to other scales. [+] Eye closure is graded 10 mm opening = 0 percent, 5 mm opening = 50 percent, 0 mm (closed) = 100 percent, etc.

Table 5-3 Suggested Facial Facilitation Instructions

Muscles(s)*	Volitional Movements	Spontaneous Movements
FRO	Raise forehead	Act surprised (but *not* terrified)
COR	Bring eyebrows together	Express doubt
OCS	Gently close eyes	Sleep
OCI	Gently close eyes concentrating on lower lids	Look very perplexed
DIN	Flare nostrils	Inhale deeply while opening nostrils (as if upset)
LLS	Raise upper lip to show upper gums	Show your "buck teeth"
ZYN	Show incisor tooth (or teeth)	Snarl(s)
ZYJ		
RIS	Pull corner of mouth back horizontally	Sneer/Smile
OOS	Protrude lips	Kiss/Whistle
OOI	Protrude lips	Kiss/Pout/Whistle
DAO	Turn corners of mouth downward	Frown/Pout, be unhappy
MEN	Raise and tighten chin	Firm pout, be spoiled

Frontalis (FRO), corrugator (and procerus) (COR), orbicularis oculi superioris (OCS), orbicularis oculi inferioris (OCI), dilator naris, and alaeque nasi (DIN), levator labii superioris (and levator anguli oris) (LLS), zygomaticus minor (ZYN) and zygomaticus major (ZYJ), risorius (RIS), orbicularis oris superioris (OOS), orbicularis oris inferioris (OOI), depressor anguli oris (and depressor labii inferioris) (DAO), and mentalis (MEN). *NOTE: This list should not be given to patients. It is for therapist use only (see precautions under Section IIID.).*

affect on his or her uninvolved side. In cases like these, the uninvolved side of the face should be evaluated on an additional assessment sheet. Pre-trauma photographs from the patient's home photo album can be used for comparison purposes to help give estimates of the individual patient's facial tone and spontaneous volition.

Estimates of hypertonicity or hyperactivity are difficult to quantify subjectively. Only gross estimates are possible. These should be indicated by percentages that are less than 100 as estimated by apparent dysfunction. For example, a mild amount

of hypertonicity would be graded between 70 and 90 percent. A small notation (e.g. "70 + %") next to the indicated percentage would be helpful for future reference.

Volitional, Spontaneous, and Resting Electromyographic Measurements

Electromyographic (EMG) evaluations are optimal. Typically no more than six muscle areas are examined (see Fig. 5-2, boxes marked*). However, if possible, it is recommended that surface electrode EMGs be performed within the same session.

Table 5-4 Suggested Clinical Muscle Grading System.*

Descriptor	Percent	Volitional or Spontaneous Movement*	Tone*
Normal	90–100	Excellent movement with only minor deviations when tired or under stress	Excellent with only minor droop when tired
Good	70–90	Mild weakness within normal limits under ideal conditions, but may become moderate when tired or under stress	Small droop under ideal conditions; moderate droop when tired
Fair	40–70	Moderate to severe weakness, which is severe when tired or under stress	Moderate to severe droop that will always be severe when tired
Poor	10–40	Small amount of movement can be seen upon excitation and ideal conditions.	Small amount of tone; that is only apparent when not tired
Trace	1–10	Just noticeable movement that can be seen only when excitation is "stopped"	Just noticeable tone
Zero	0	No movement apparent	None

* Estimates of hypertonicity or hyperactivity should be down-graded to correspond to apparent dysfunction (See text).

Facilitation of the six areas is achieved as previously explained (see Table 5-3).

Ideally, the EMG should present the patient with a feedback signal that is rectified and integrated; a low end sensitivity of 0.2 μV over a bandpass of 20 to 1,000 Hz/100 msec integration is recommended. A normal resting tone at these frequencies is typically less than 1.5 μV.

Synkinesis or Other Secondary Effects

Synkinesis is defined as involuntary or inappropriate motor function usually associated with another volitional motor action, thus resulting in dyscoordination. Synkinesis of a muscle area is grossly rated with five categories (zero to four) as it appears to interact with another muscle area under various gesture conditions:

0—None
1—Trace
2—Mild
3—Moderate
4—Severe

Other secondary muscle effects, including tics, spasms, etc., can be specified as required.

Summary Percentage of Function Scores: F, F', and S

The scores for volitional movement and spontaneous movement as related to resting tone can be averaged and weighted relative to importance and then added, thus providing a single average score that may be compared to other assessment scales, including the 1984 International Assessment Scale. This system is an extension of the Janssen Assess-

ment Scale,[20,21] which has been shown to have the highest reliability of any clinical assessment.[19]

Volitional Movement Relation to Resting Tone Score: F. The total scores of four primary volitional movement (including basic tone) factors from Figure 5-2 are weighted by the assignment of a maximum percentage value and total 100 percent when added together, if each is at a maximum value. The four factors are shown in Table 5-5.

Spontaneous Movement Relative to Resting Tone Score: F'. The previous computation is a standard method because it involves asking the patient to make isolated movements on command. Perhaps, more important than this is the evaluation of how the patient performs spontaneously. The column spontaneous movement in Figure 5-2 can be used to make this determination. The same resting tone scores that were used in the computation of the total volitional movement relative to resting tone (A) are used. Total Spontaneous Movement relative to resting tone can be computed as shown in Table 5-6.

Synkinesis/Second Effects Score: S. All of these assessments are concerned with estimates of the patient's ability to selectively excite the face; they do not include estimates of inhibition (i.e., synkinesis, tics, or other unwanted behaviors). In practice, however, these factors are very important to patient outcomes and are in many patients at least three-fourths of what is trained—or actually "untrained." No reasonable method has been found to subtract a synkinesis score from either volitional

Table 5-5 Volitional Movement Relative to Resting Tone Score: F*

Factor	Maximum Possible Percentage
A = Resting Tone [(Total of up to 12 Resting tone Scores/12) × .3]	30
B = Volitional Movement of the Forehead [Total score of (FRO + COR/2) × .1]	10
C = Volitional Movement of Eye Closure [Total score of OCS only × .3]	30
D = Volitional Movement of the Mouth [(Total of DIN, LLS, ZYN, ZYJ, OOS, RIS, OOI, DAO, MEN/8) × .3]	30

* Therefore, the total possible Volitional Movement Score including Resting Tone is equal to:

$$F = A + B + C + D = 100 \text{ Percent}$$

Table 5-6 Spontaneous Movement Relative to Resting Tone Score: F'[a]

Factor	Maximum Possible Percentage
A = Resting Tone [(Total of up to 12 Resting tone Score/12) × .3]	30
B = Spontaneous Movement of the Forehead [(Total score of FRO + COR/2) × .1]	10
C = Spontaneous Movement of Eye Closure [Total score of OCS only × .3]	30
D = Spontaneous Movement of the Mouth [(Total of DIN, LLS, ZYN, ZYJ, OOS, RIS, OOI, DAO, MEN/8 × .3)]	30

[a] Therefore, the total possible Spontaneous Movement including Resting Tone Score (F') is equal to:

$$F' = A + B' + C' + D' = 100 \text{ Percent}$$

[b] See Fig. 5.1 for definations of abbreviations.

or spontaneous facial function; therefore, it is computed as a separate score. As previously explained, each muscle group is individually assessed from 0 to 4 (i.e., no to severe synkinesis). Because a single synergy pattern of one muscle in varying locations can greatly disturb a patient, the *highest* value recorded over all muscles evaluated is used as the total "synkinesis" score. Since the synkinesis associated with either volitional or spontaneous muscle function is similarly gross, only *one* S value is used to represent either assessment condition.

Table 5-7 International Assessment Grade Compared to The Wisconsin[18a]

International Assessment Grade	Wisconsin Assessment Percentage
Grade	Score (F, F')
I	100
II	75–99
III	50–75
IV	25–20
V	1–25
VI	0

[a] Because the Wisconsin Assessment separates out synkinesis and the International Assessment does not, patients with a disproportionately high amount of synkinesis relative to volitional muscle control may not equate well. The relatively small range used in the International Assessment must assume that when synkinesis occurs it is within certain typical limits. If it is disproportionately high, a higher score must be assigned despite a possibly high amount of volitional control. In addition, the Wisconsin Spontaneous Movement Score (F') may not have a good correlation with the International Assessment Score because the International Assessment Scale does not usually represent spontaneous movements.

Therefore, total synkinesis, including other secondary effects, is equal to:

$$S = \text{Highest Synkinesis Score (0–4)}$$

Comparisons of F or F': The International Assessment Scale. As a final recommendation, either F or F' score can be approximately equated to the International Assessment Scale with the conversion factor[18]: (see Table 5-7).

Indicated and Contraindicated Retraining Strategies

The following general information is crucial to performing facial retraining in a manner that will promote new function but not promote synkinesis or other secondary effects. *This information is essential to both the EMG sensory feedback and general mirror and awareness retraining described later in this chapter.*

Electrotherapy May Not Be Clinically Effective

Galvanic and faradic (electrical stimulation) electrotherapy involves the application of electrical current of a particular waveform and frequency at varying intensities. It is applied with either two large electrode pads or a small, localized hand applicator electrode to approximate motor point sites. The number, duration, and intensity of applications are determined by the experience of the particular therapist. Application may be continued for weeks or even years in home treatment by the patient.

Electrotherapy has been used for decades to treat peripheral nerve injuries. Often combined with general "mirror exercises," electrotherapy has become a standard method for treating facial paralysis. It has been theorized that this artificial source of electrical stimulation passively reduces or reverses muscle atrophy so that reinnervation can occur naturally. The assumption is made that nerves will not reinnervate when connected to severely atrophied muscles and that severe atrophy occurs in a matter of days or weeks. Despite its frequent use, however, there are currently no definitive studies to indicate that electrotherapy is actually clinically effective. In fact, there may be reason to believe that electrotherapy is contraindicated.

A recent United States Public Health Service assessment of electrotherapy for the treatment of facial nerve paralysis resulting from Bell's palsy concluded that there is no evidence that electrical stimulation is clinically effective in the treatment of facial paralysis.[22] Specifically, although nerve conduction and muscle contraction occur, the reduction of circulatory stasis, increased muscle and nerve nutrition, and the reduction of atrophy have not been proven. The report concludes that the treatment may only help in some cases because it acts to demonstrate to the patient that his muscles still "work," thus helping reassure the patient and maintain his motivation and confidence in the treatment.

Although it can be argued that electrotherapy acts as a placebo and generally helps motivate the patient while the nerve heals, there is evidence to indicate that electrical stimulation may selectively inhibit or delay onset and rate of reinnervation, as well as collateral reinnervation.[23] There is also evidence that in general, electrical activity in neural circuits may prevent further neurite outgrowth and negatively influence the consolidation of functional circuitry.[24] More specifically, it appears that "direct muscle stimulation inhibits the expected terminal sprouting in a partially denervated muscle . . . [however] the same pattern of activity in [normally] innervated muscle fibers alone does not seem to inhibit sprouting."[25]

In studies where electrotherapy was found to have a somewhat retarding effect on atrophy, morphological changes were confined to type 2b and 2c fibers, which are associated with relatively fast and gross motor activity and are also readily fatiguable. By contrast, the more desirable type 1 fibers, which are fatigue resistant and are associated with relatively slow, fine motor control, have been shown to atrophy much faster than normal under electrotherapy.[23]

These results raise doubts about the clinical efficacy of electrotherapy. It would seem that relatively more active therapeutic training strategies (e.g., EMG and specific mirror feedback methods), which have been demonstrated to be successful in the retraining of late, postacute patients, are potentially more advantageous to the patient. Specific training does require the "active" participation of both the therapist and, in particular, the patient. Currently, however, there is no known "passive" method, such as electrotherapy, that will be of benefit to the neuromuscular retraining of the facial paralysis patient. The patient's "active" involvement is essential to optimal recovery.

Facial Retraining Strategies Must Attempt to Control Only Specific Muscles

Nonspecific or relatively gross facial exercises are often given to patients.[26,27] There is, however, good reason to believe that in many patients with peripheral nerve injury, such instructions are either useless or contraindicated. For example, the following instructions *should be avoided*:

1. Open mouth widely
2. Move lower lip side to side
3. Move eyes up, down, right and left
4. Broad laugh
5. Puff out cheeks, mouth closed
6. Upper lip against upper incisors
7. Close eyes tightly

The first two instructions can do little but train compensatory movements by way of the masseter muscle(s). The third only trains eye movements. The fourth through seventh would seem to be most appropriate, but they may be the worst because they have the potential to promote inappropriate motor control in patients with severe nerve injuries.

Unfortunately, instructions such as these probably promote mass movement and synkinesis in facial patients with severe nerve injury because they are gross enough to facilitate many different muscles to contract, not just the few required for proper motor control. This conclusion is based on several studies that have attempted to define the anatomical and physiological guidelines for locating the specific muscles involved in orofacial and mandibular control.[8–14,28]

The most pertinent study was reported by O'Dwyer et al.[13] as recalculated by Balliet.[28] O'Dwyer et al. simultaneously recorded electromyographic amplitudes of nine facial muscles in six normal humans using hook-wire electrodes; concurrently, nine facial gestures thought most likely to facilitate certain isolated muscle activity were performed. Figure 5-3 represents their combined data recalculated relative to the percentage that each muscle actively participated in the formation of each gesture.[28] Although substantial intersubject differences were apparent, only two gestures were found to promote relatively isolated muscle control. Only the "unilateral snarl" produced mainly levator labii superioris activity and "depress corners of mouth" produced mainly depressor anguli oris activity; all of the other gestures generated activity in many different muscles besides the supposed targeted muscles (gray bars). The patterned contraction of many different muscles was associated with most of the relatively gross gestures that subjects performed. Balliet[28] concluded that all gestural instructions are not equal in their effect. It seemed apparent that because neurologically involved facial patients have a predisposition to the problem of synkinesis and mass action, gestural instructions associated with the relatively more isolated muscle control should have a much greater opportunity for facilitating functional motor control.

The use of retraining strategies involving relatively gross gestures, of course, are not a problem for normal people with problems, such as age-related sagging facial muscles, because their basic motor control is not abnormally patterned. Relatively gross training strategies, however, are probably not suited for the neurologically damaged patient who has had CN VII fiber damaged and, therefore, does *not* have normal patterning. This would include any patient suffering from at least a third degree injury, where the endoneurial

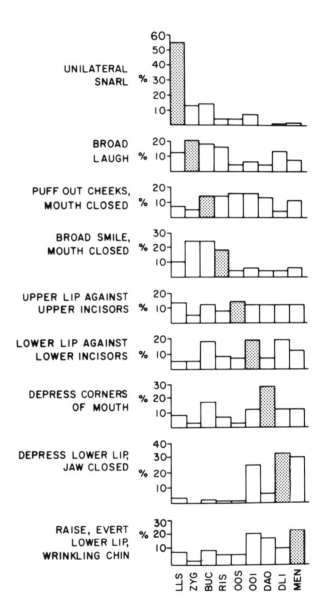

Fig. 5-3 Relative facial muscle activity (%) for various facial gestures as recalculated from O'Dwyer et al.[13] Targeted muscles for each gesture are indicated by gray bars. Facial muscles: levator labii superioris (LLS), zygomaticus minor/major (ZYG), buccinator (BUC), risorius (RIS), orbicularis oris superioris (OOS), orbicularis oris inferioris (OOI), depressor anguli oris (DAO), depressor labii inferioris (DLI), and mentalis (MEN). (From Balliet,[28] with permission.)

sheaths of the nerve fibers have been damaged, thus causing cross-wiring and inappropriate function to occur (e.g., the severe Bell's palsy, compression injury, or anastomosis patient).

This is particularly a problem after the anastomosis of differing nerves such as a CN XII–CN VII anastomosis where, in addition to cross-wiring at the peripheral nerve anastomosis, the proper motor nucleus is no longer connected to the distal nerve. Without selective muscle (or muscle group) retraining, the CNS will usually not be able to reorganize itself, so that part of the CN XII motor nucleus can control the face in a manner disassociated from the way it previously controlled the tongue. As a result, relatively gross retraining strategies will typically result in relatively gross motor control (e.g., hypertonicity and mass movement). Instead the CNS of the severe nerve injury patient must be given optimal information in the form of selective muscle exercises, which will have to optimize the chances to develop selective motor control and, thereby, reduce the chances of dyskinesis and synkinesis.

Retraining Must Emphasize Slow, "Tonic" Muscle Control

Unlike patients with relatively mild pressure or entrapment nerve injuries that do not destroy the basic structures of the nerve, patients who have undergone complete nerve transections with surgical reunion have been shown to have severe disorders in normal motor unit recruitment.[29] These patients do not demonstrate an orderly and additive recruitment in the size and voltage of their motor units as has been normally found to occur.[30,31] Smaller, slower, weaker, and fatigue-resistant motor units are not necessarily recruited before larger, faster, stronger, and more easily fatigued motor units, thus resulting in a lack of slow, fine control and the promotion of poorly controlled, jerky and easily fatigued motor control.

Facial exercises should not encourage fast, automatic or "reflexive" gestures; which are associated with poor control and are more susceptible to fatigue. Alternatively, special care should be taken to give facial instructions and exercises that are extremely slow, distinct, and nonemotional (i.e., slow twitch or tonic muscle activity). This kind of instruction will be much more likely to promote appropriate facial movements that can be slowly controlled with minimal muscle fatigue. Similarly, a patient cannot be expected to isolate muscle activity while relaxing the rest of the face unless the methods of facilitation and practice are slow. Relatively rapid facial movements (Fig. 5-4A) will at best inappropriately reinforce the existing compensatory movements. Typically, these movements can cause more primitive reorganization to occur (e.g., co-contractions, mass action, and synkinesis).

It is recommended that any EMG or therapeutic exercise procedure (e.g., mirror and/or general awareness) should ideally consist of either two or three basic volitional "innervation" components.* Since no data currently exist describing motor unit recruitment in the facial muscles, these suggestions are based on electrophysiological studies that have investigated related subjects, including patterns of normal muscle activity,[30,31] motor unit recruitment of the extremities,[32–35] and clinical studies that have extensively described facial paralysis retraining procedures.[21,28] The following is a description of these basic components.

A Component—Very Slow or Tonic Innervation

Steady muscle contractions should increase at a constant velocity or at a constant acceleration (Fig. 5-4, Graph 2) and not as rapid phasic movements (Fig. 5-4; Graph 1.). This (A) component can be used during initial training or during subsequent instruction. During initial training, only small movements or contractions should be made (typically 5 to 30 μV).

B Component—Fast Phasic and Hold Innervation

Once the slow "Tonic" component is accomplished (e.g., no associated dyskinesis or synkinesis), a muscle innervation strategy of a faster (time constant) and a higher level of activity can be added until a maximum level is reached and held for a short period of time (Fig. 5-4C). This second

---

* The term innervation is defined as the amount of volitional effort as indicated by EMG muscle activity or as observed in actual movement and refers to comparisons between the same muscle groups.

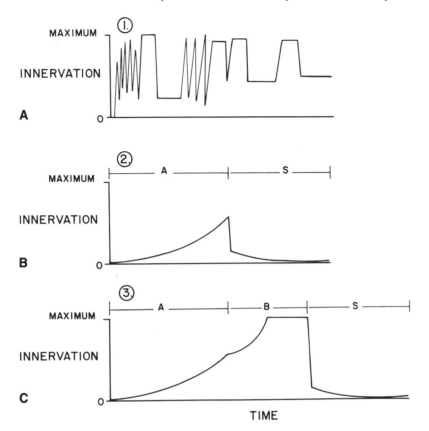

Fig. 5-4 Idealized retraining strategies. Innervation is defined as position and/or integrated EMG. **(A)** #1 poor retraining strategy of rapid "phasic" movements. **(B)** #2 and **(C)** #3 superior retraining strategies involving slow tonic control. See text for description of A, B, and S components. Note that time period for #3 is relatively longer than #2 to allow for complete relaxation after long sustained maximum contraction. Total time period is typically between 5 and 15 seconds.

component should be either reduced or discontinued immediately if synkinesis, dyskinesis, or fatigue become apparent. New and correct motor control cannot be programmed under such conditions; instead, an inappropriate program will be trained.

S Component—Fast Release or Stop Innervation

Whether using the A component, B component, or both, there should always be an abrupt stop for fast release component (Fig. 5-4B, C). This (S) component helps facilitate fast and selective motoneuron inhibition and control. This inhibitory stage is often critical for the patient's development of the feelings associated with successful move-

ment. This is because weak muscle contractions and associated movements often naturally occur so slowly that they cannot be seen until volition is abruptly stopped. In addition, without this neuromuscular strategy, hypertonicity will be perpetuated; motoneurons (and related CNS control mechanisms) must be trained to turn off, as well as turn on.

Finally, it is important for the patient to completely relax between each attempted trial or muscle contraction. The re-establishment of the low end of the tonic range (equivalent to about 1.5 μV at 20 to 1,000 Hz) during each attempted trial will allow the patient to experience the full range of contraction. The complete range must be felt for complete motor control to be developed.

Normalization of the Uninvolved Side: A Question of Balance

It is apparent clinically that the unilateral facial paralysis patient is not normal relative to the amount of innervation usually found in the so-called uninvolved side.[21] For example in post-acute patients, it is typical to find very significant hyperactivity (but usually not hypertonicity) of the uninvolved side, particularly in the area of the zygomaticus major, zygomaticus minor, and levator labii superioris, thus causing a very exaggerated half smile. *This common problem seems to be associated with patients who, despite their disability, do not tend to inhibit their facial movements and/or have previously been involved in exercises where they have been trying very hard to move the involved side by maximally innervating both sides.* These strategies are apparently contraindicated relative to the promotion of normal bilateral facial control. Fig. 5-5 symbolizes this facial balance problem.

In many patients, unless efforts are made to inhibit the uninvolved side of the face throughout retraining, it will apparently receive a disproportionate amount of innervation from the CNS, as

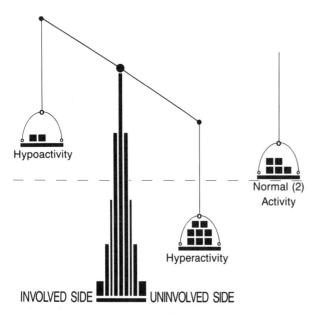

Fig. 5-5 A question of balance: normalization of the uninvolved side of the face. Conceptualization of the reduction of hyperactivity on the uninvolved side of the face to allow the involved, hypoactive side of the face to receive increased activity.

depicted in Figure 5-5 by the hyperactive blocks on the uninvolved side of the balance. Because the involved side is conceivably not receiving the innervation going to the uninvolved side, it will remain relatively inactive, as depicted by the hypoactive blocks. The net result is one of increased imbalance and a worsening of facial appearance (i.e., more than would be the case if only the involved side were hypoactive(paresis). Normal activity, however, can be facilitated (acutely) or reversed (postacutely) by retraining the patient (with EMG, mirror exercises, etc.) in a manner that promotes either equal innervation of both the involved and uninvolved sides, *or* innervation of the involved side followed by innervation of the uninvolved side.

In practice, the first strategy is almost impossible without constant EMG monitoring; a patient using the second strategy may closely approximate the first strategy. Exceptions to this include patients who initially have only small EMG potentials (typically less than 20 μV) and corresponding small amounts of apparent movement on their involved side. In these cases, it is usually much too difficult to "lead with the involved side" or "keep them equal" until a small amount of movement is achieved on the involved side (at least 20 to 30 μV). At this point in training, any method that facilitates the involved side should be used.

The Comprehensive Retraining Program

Over the past 30 years, surgical advancements have been made in the treatment of facial paralysis after traumatic damage to the facial nerve.[6,36] However, the clinical retraining methods for this problem either after surgery, in lieu of surgery, or even after relatively minor cases of Bell's palsy have only become effective in recent years. It is now clear that postacute therapeutic procedures that improve function must produce changes at some level of the CNS and that the brain is extremely plastic if proper sensory inputs are provided during retraining.[37–40]

The literature on the neuromuscular retraining of facial paralysis indicates that the foundation of successful treatment has been the use of EMG sensory (bio) feedback therapy (SFT).[21,28,41–47] This sensory substitution device, when used properly, has consistently demonstrated an ability to increase facial function in postacute patients who seemed to have had paralyzed muscles.

Initially, some patients may have only muscle contractions so small that no movement can be seen or felt. The EMG signals, however, allow the patient to monitor and then correctly facilitate and inhibit their facial musculature. By voluntarily increasing the incidence of appropriate movements, the patient can eventually see and feel these movements, thus allowing the use of specific mirror exercises and other awareness techniques without the use of EMG feedback.

Many other patients with moderate amounts of volition do not require such extremely sensitive sensory feedback information. In these cases the use of a mirror and very specific instructions will usually be more effective because of their simplicity and availability. In either situation, continued practice can develop a new functional neuromuscular program that not only promotes selective voluntary control but also promotes automatic or spontaneous facial movements.

The following outpatient program attempts to optimize all aspects of facial neuromuscular re-education. It can be used in the retraining of facial paralysis patients suffering from any facial paralysis etiology not worse than a third degree nerve injury (see section on Third Degree Injury). Patients having a fourth or fifth degree nerve injury do not have an intact nerve and, therefore, would require facial nerve surgery previous to retraining. This program should be used only as a general guide, not as a rigid procedure. Staying "flexible" with the facial patient is essential to success.

Treatment Environment and Scheduling

A training area where both the therapist and patient can concentrate, as well as discuss personal issues that might arise, is a prerequisite to a successful program. Since the methods in this chapter are expressly aimed at training the patient to train himself at home, the same rules should also apply to the patient's home environment. These factors have been previously discussed in more detail by Balliet et al.[21]

1. A quiet, well lighted, windowed room of at least 120 square feet

2. Adjustable recessed work table approximately 2 × 3 feet with the patient seated comfortably on the shorter side
3. A 12-inch high stand-alone mirror
4. A small nonglare light source
5. Small hand-held compact mirror
6. Sixty to ninety minute session availability
7. Daily to three times per week sessions for 1 to 2 weeks until the patient can conduct program at home
8. In later stages, sessions extended up to 1 time per month

Psychosocial Support: Are We As We Appear?

Facial expression is a primary mechanism by which we are judged. It usually describes if we are happy or sad, serious or whimsical, involved or uninvolved, or if we remember or do not remember. It can relay to others our emotions and our intentions and sometimes our deepest thoughts—despite our efforts to conceal them.

Because of this inherent judgment process, many patients with facial paralysis will keep their face relatively immobile and expressionless. In this way, they believe that they will not accentuate their paralysis, thus appearing even more deformed and ludicrous. Regrettably, this common compensatory strategy will limit the patient's potential for increased neuromuscular function. It may often lead tragically to the inhibition of the patient's natural affect and personality. As a result, many patients consider even a relatively mild incomplete unilateral facial paralysis to be more serious than the loss of an arm because they feel that their face is "who they are."

It is important, therefore, for the therapist to become involved in certain aspects of the patient's psychosocial retraining. The application of this support can be on an individual level or in a support group situation (see the section on Patient Advocacy Groups for Facial Paralysis). Suggested topics include the identification of friends or family members who, since the patient's facial paralysis, are (1) no longer their friends, (2) somewhat negative, (3) have always been supportive, and (4) newly supportive (e.g., a facial paralysis support group or organization); and the identification of positive and negative experiences associated with the patient's facial paralysis (e.g., surgery, experiences with strangers, or work-related problems).

Any of these topics can be discussed not only to allow the patient to vent their feelings, but also to break down barriers and increase trust and respect between the patient and therapist. Patients generally appreciate and find motivational this type of professional caring.

Patient Education

Patients should be taught basic facial muscle anatomy, physiology, and kinesiology, as well as the anatomy of the facial nerve. Basic anatomy pictures (see Fig. 5-1) should be used to visualize the muscles and nerve branches to be selectively inhibited or facilitated. Pictures can also help demonstrate to the patient which muscles are "working" and are also essential to the establishment of specific therapeutic goals.

During the initial visit, patients usually show postural imbalances in both sitting and standing. In sitting, their head may be tilted in the direction of the involved side. They may also use their hand not only to hold their head up but also to hide the involved side of their face from sight. It is necessary to correct these more general postural problems early on in order to increase self-awareness and self-esteem.

Photographic Evaluations

Pictorial record keeping is essential to the recording of both long- and short-term progress.

1. Thirty-five millimeter slides (with relatively high resolution) should be taken routinely and when significant increases in performance occur so that both the patient and the therapist can evaluate long-term progress.
2. Polaroid photographs (with relatively low resolution) should be made for patients so that they will have an opportunity to show their accomplishments to family and friends and receive encouragement.
3. Video tapes of both volitional and spontaneous gestures should be made on the initial visit and at 6-month intervals.

Face Patting (Tapping) Exercise

Facial paralysis patients often inhibit spontaneous expressions of joy and anger. Some patients must even be coaxed to demonstrate the function of their uninvolved side. This inhibition of affect is quite common and unfortunate because this compensatory strategy often contributes to the patients not looking at, attending to, or "feeling" their face.

To get patients to attend to their face, increase their baseline awareness level and start the development of a positive attitude toward their face, they are instructed to pat lightly both sides of the face using their fingers and palms until tingling is perceived a few moments after stopping. Increasing blood flow in this manner may require 30 seconds or up to 20 minutes on the involved side; a lesser amount of time is usually necessary on the uninvolved side.

In cases where synkinesis is apparent, the patient should be instructed to relax the face. EMG monitoring before and after patting can be helpful in reducing hypertonicity and reducing potentially increased synkinesis.

Only in flaccid cases should the patient attempt to cause a mass action response (co-contractions) of the involved side. This should be done while they *secondarily* attempt to co-contract the uninvolved side. This procedure should be discontinued if synkinesis starts to develop on the involved side. At such time, face tapping should only be conducted while the patient is trying to relax the face. It is usually helpful to have the mouth slightly open at the time. Co-contraction should be discontinued if synkinesis or other secondary effects become apparent. The relaxation strategy should then be applied. The exercise may be repeated several times a day, either by itself or just previous to other facial retraining.

EMG Sensory Feedback: A Sensory Substitution Device

The basis of neuromuscular retraining in very low functioning facial paralysis is therapeutic EMG. Its practical clinical application has been made possible because of recent efforts to design equipment specifically for neuromuscular disability patients.

The following is a description of the procedures

that have been used in the treatment of acute and postacute (more than 1-year postonset) postsurgical facial paralysis patients with varying etiologies.[21,40–46] Additional descriptions of general EMG retraining procedures can be found in Basmajian.[47] *In order to have a complete understanding of this subject, the introductory section and the section on Injury to the Peripheral Nervous System must be completed before reading the following subsection.*

Equipment

The following is a basic description of ideal EMG equipment (e.g., Cordis/Hyperion Bioconditioner II, Miami, Florida; BioComp 2001, Biofeedback Institute, Los Angeles, California):

1. Two or four channels of rectified and integrated (100 msec) EMG
2. Low-end sensitivity of 0.2 μVolts @ 20 to 1,000 Hz
3. High resolution video monitor (e.g., 160 points = X axis; 200 points = Y axis)
4. One proportional audio channel
5. Adjustable threshold lines with binary audio
6. Microsurface electrodes
7. Screen-dump printer to provide hard copy records

Generally one channel should be used to monitor the involved side, while a second channel is used to monitor the uninvolved side at an equivalent site. An additional two channels (on four channel machines) can be similarly used to facilitate or inhibit (e.g., synkinesis) additional areas of the face.

Skin Impedance

It is necessary to minimize electrode/skin interface impedance to monitor very small voltage potentials radiating from the patient's skin and muscles without contamination by electrical noise. Therefore, the electrode/skin impedance of all preparations should be no greater than 10,000 Ω. Skin should be recleaned as required to maintain these levels throughout therapy. The placement of electrodes should be replicated during each retraining session by the use of facial landmarks as specified by Polaroid pictures.

In cases where impedance measurement equipment is not available, a simple test will verify the integrity of a skin preparation. The therapist (another person besides the person that is connected with the electrodes) simply touches any exposed (not painted surface) of the EMG machine. A good connection will be indicated if the EMG feedback response remains constant and does not increase. In a bad connection such touching consistently causes an increased (open loop) response.

Retraining Procedures

The following EMG retraining procedures should be conducted in order. Depending on the patient, certain procedures will be more appropriate than others.

General Body Relaxation Training and Postural Awareness. The patient's basic ability to relax must be examined and, if necessary, brought to within normal limits. This increases the patient's general perception of small sensory inputs associated with the slow, small facial movements required to obtain precise facial control. It should be noted that patients under daily stress and/or moderate to heavy coffee drinkers and cigarette smokers usually cannot relax to normal EMG levels and correspondingly are probably not good candidates for facial retraining until they discontinue these substances.

1. Electrodes are attached to the wrist and/or finger flexors of the dominant hand.
2. The patient should be able to bring EMG readings to below 1.5 μVolts @ 20 to 1000 Hz or 0.75 to 1.25 μV @ 100 to 1,000 Hz within about 2 to 3 minutes.
3. As necessary, either microvolt amplitude or time to achieve a microvolt level approaching the levels in number 2 can be trained in descending steps.

Relaxation of the Uninvolved Side. Many postacute facial paralysis patients demonstrate hypertonicity on the uninvolved side.

1. Initial resting potentials of 2 to 10 μV are typical.
2. As in general body relaxation, specific relaxation of the uninvolved side should be followed until a level of approximately 1.5 μV is obtained.

3. The electrode sites most commonly used are in the area of the zygomaticus or frontalis (see Fig. 5-1).

Improvement of Slow Motor Control of the Uninvolved Side. After a basic ability to obtain normal resting EMG potentials is established, the patient should be trained to make slow, fine movements on the uninvolved side. This ability is relatively unnatural in the repertoire of most facial paralysis patients and of many "normal" patients, as well. Characteristically, these facial movements are relatively fast, gross, and hyperactive. Slow, fine motor control is usually trained in the area of the uninvolved zygomaticus muscles (minor/major), because they are the primary movers associated with smiling (i.e., relatively upward and outward movements of the upper lips and cheeks). Once this new strategy is learned, it can be more easily generalized to other muscle groups (e.g., the orbicularis oris in puckering). The specific method is as follows:

1. Slow, fine (tonic) motor control is trained by having the patient slowly contract the zygomaticus muscle(s) area, as in a closed lip smile. The patient and therapist should observe the corresponding EMG trace with the EMG machine set at a relatively high sensitivity (e.g., full scale screen deflection of 50 μV.)
2. The patient's task is to make these muscles contract over a range of 1.5 to 35 μV for a period of time equalling about 10 seconds to produce a ramp [/] on the EMG screen.
3. Once successful, the patient is then asked to contract these muscles under conditions where EMG machine sensitivity is significantly higher (e.g., full-scale screen deflection of 25 μV).
4. The eventual goal of the training is to produce an approximate 10-second ramp function on the screen over a range of 1.5 to a maximum of about 15 μV.

Establishment of Muscle Potentials and/or Motor Control of the Involved Side. After the patient can demonstrate fine motor control of a selected area on the uninvolved side and knows how it feels to make such small movements, training on the involved side can be initiated. The patient is trained to shift these feelings of initial motor control recruitment (not end point maximal contractions) to the same area on the involved side. The following procedures can be used.

1. The patient observes two traces on the EMG screen. One trace corresponds to the involved side, and the other corresponds to the uninvolved side.
2. As the ramp function is produced by the small facial movement on the uninvolved side, the patient tries to replicate simultaneously the feeling of this movement on the involved side.
3. A slow, successive alternation between the sides can then be employed.
4. The patient should be encouraged to rest every 2 to 3 minutes and to think vicariously about differing motor strategies.
5. In patients with either no or low function, this procedure may have to be repeated for many sessions until (1) a small upward deflection occurs (0.5 to 3.0 μV in the case of some reportedly denervated patients) and (2) the second trace is under consistent voluntary control.
6. The patient's uninvolved side should not be allowed to dominate by a factor greater than about 5:1 (ideally no more than 2:1).
7. If the uninvolved side is allowed to dominate, potential activity on the involved side may not occur.
8. Initially, in relatively denervated cases, co-contractions should be permitted until the point voluntary control can be consistently achieved (10 to 15 μV).
9. These procedures should be continued until the patient can see small movements in a mirror (see Specific Action Exercises). This usually corresponds to 15 to 30 μV.
10. In patients who have suffered relatively severe denervation, recovery may involve only a few relatively large motor units; EMG readings can then be at 100 μV or more before actual movement will be seen.

Retraining of Additional Muscle Groups on the Involved Side. After the patient can move an area of his involved side, similar procedures are used in other areas of the face where no visible movement can be seen. Each additional area is often easier because the same basic motor control skills have been learned during previous training.

1. Whenever possible, mirror exercises (see Specific Action Exercises) should be used when volitional control can be visualized: This will allow the patient the opportunity to practice anytime and anyplace.
2. The exception to the preceding is training that has the goal of reducing synkinesis or overall dyskinesia (see EMG Sensory Feedback).

Reduction of Synkinesis with EMG Retraining. Involuntary/inappropriate facial movements that accompany either a voluntary or spontaneous facial movement can be reduced (but usually not completely eliminated) using two channels of EMG.

1. One channel is placed on the area that has the synkinesis (e.g., #1 the inferior orbicularis oculi) while the second electrode is placed on the muscle area that the patient wishes to control voluntarily (e.g., #2 the area between the zygomaticus major and minor).
2. The patient's task is to make very small volitional movements that do not excite the synergistic muscle. Correspondingly, trace #2 will go up slowly to a low level steady state (e.g., 5 μV) while maintaining trace #1 at a low threshold value (e.g., 1.5 to 2 μV).
3. After this is accomplished, progressively higher criteria levels for trace #2 can be established (e.g., 8 μV) while maintaining trace #1 at the same, low threshold value (e.g., 1.5 to 2 μV).
4. When the ability to voluntarily elevate trace #2 to over about 30 μV is obtained, specific action exercises should be initiated. If required, EMG training can be interspaced with these exercises.

Unusual Retraining Situations. It should be noted that there are no firm rules concerning retraining strategies. Certain patients who have no initial function may not respond to the above

shaping procedures. For example, it is common for initial muscle activity (in the 0.75 to 2.0 μV range) to only occur when the patient tries to make maximum effort mass movement co-contractions of the entire face. In this situation the following procedures can be followed:

1. Mass movements should be used initially in the facilitation of function in a particular muscle area but should be extinguished as soon as possible, so that mass movements, synkinesia, and dyskinesia are not perpetuated.
2. Once some amount of activity of the involved side (usually about 10 to 30 μV) can be seen on the screen, associated mass movements of other muscle groups on the involved side can be extinguished by slowly using the EMG to train neuromuscular inhibition. The EMG is used to monitor both muscle areas. The patient's task is to slowly increase the muscle activity of the desired muscle group while attempting to reduce the amount of mass movement (usually corresponding larger trace) of the synergistic muscle group(s).

General Mirror and Awareness Retraining: Specific Action Exercises (SAE). Mirror and simple awareness practice should be performed at home and in the clinic whenever any amount of function can be seen. When performed properly, such procedures can facilitate very specific changes in function, even in postacute patients. *SAE is used here to separate these retraining procedures from other types of mirror exercises, which are not individually prescribed for the very specific needs of the patient.*

Unfortunately, no simple, definitive list of exercises can be handed to the patient. Therefore, even the suggested facial facilitation instructions (see Table 5-3) should not be given to patients without specific and individualized instruction. Facial exercises should be prescribed not only for hypotonic or hypoactive muscles but also for muscles that are hypertonic or hyperactive, including those demonstrating secondary effects such as synkinesis or mass action.

General indicated and contraindicated retraining strategies have been previously described. In summary, these include the following concepts:

1. Electrotherapy should be avoided.
2. Only selective muscle control should be trained. Simplistic exercises such as trying to smile repeatedly, can promote dyskinesia, synkinesia, and decreased functional abilities.
3. Slow, tonic muscle control must be trained. Relatively fast facial movements reinforce existing improper motor control or may perpetuate dysfunction (e.g., synkinesis).
4. Any amount of hyperactivity or hypertonicity existing on the uninvolved side of the face must be normalized to allow the involved side to make increases in function.

Patients should be trained to be active participants and should be trained to be their own best therapists in order to conduct effective retraining at home. The following general procedures will help facilitate this process

1. Based on volitional movement, spontaneous movement, resting tone and (optional) EMG data the therapists should conduct specific SAE retraining procedures for the areas of dysfunction. These may be used either in the home or clinic.
2. When performed properly, facial retraining practice can be extremely exhausting. Therefore, retraining instructions corresponding to particular muscle functions are only given to the patient a few at a time, so that the patient will not be overwhelmed.
3. Upon each visit and without using notes (notebook) the patient is required to demonstrate each of the retraining strategies. During this time, the following procedures should be followed:
   a. Each instruction should be initially repeated before any facial movement is demonstrated, including precautionary comments (e.g., "this should be done very slowly" or "the right side should always lead the left.")
   b. Only after repeating each instruction should each movement be performed.
   c. After each instruction-movement set is performed, the therapist can make corrections in the repeated instruction set and in the actual retraining procedure.
   d. After each instruction-movement set is completed and corrections are made, the patient should enter the modified instructions in a notebook for future reference during home training.

Patients will always initially perform their exercises improperly.

1. When instructional errors are made, the resulting exercise or procedure almost always promotes dysfunction; it is important, therefore, to stress this fact to the patient.
2. In some patients certain retraining procedures may seem "too hard." Accordingly, if a patient is consistently performing any particular retraining procedure improperly, it should be discontinued temporarily.

The therapist should never give instructions regarding how many times an exercise should be done per day.

1. It is important to emphasize to the patient that he *should not* be doing facial exercises in the usual sense of the word (i.e., the building up of muscles through repetitions).
2. Patients *should* be considered participants in facial retraining and reprogramming of their CNS.
3. *How many times or how long* the patient works per day is *not* that important; rather, it is *how well* the retraining is conducted. One "good" trial per day is better than 1,000 trials done incorrectly.
4. Ideally, the patient should try to perform each trial slightly better than the last and should work as many short duration sessions (1 to 15 minutes) as possible.
5. Patients should never practice when tired or when preoccupied with personal issues.

The therapist should give the patient an approximate return to clinic schedule that is based on estimates of functional abilities and home exercise compliance.

1. This schedule must be periodically reviewed.
2. For example, poor compliance may require the patient to frequently return to the clinic to prevent retraining incorrectly.

Eye Closure: Retraining Specific Action Exercise (SAE). Most mild cases of facial paralysis include some inability to close the eyelids (lagophthalmos), and include the general sagging of the orbicularis oculi inferioris (flaccid ectropion). A Bell's reflex (the eye rolling up) usually occurs instead of or at the same time that eye closure is being attempted, thus giving the patient the false impression that his eye has closed. In addition, the eye usually suffers from a lack of adequate tear film or from tear film that is too watery and insufficient in its viscosity, thus resulting in exposure keratitis and, in severe cases, corneal injury and corneal cataracts. Lubrication drops or ointments must be used to prevent such problems. Surgical approaches to prevent the eye from drying include paramedian lid adhesion, tarsorrhaphy (tuck), as well as the placement of gold weights or wishbone springs in the upper lid. Corneal injuries must be dealt with by conjunctival flap, flush-fitting scleral contact lenses and/or corneal transplants.

We have found that EMG feedback is not the best method to use in the retraining of eye closure. Instead, a very simple behavioral training approach can be readily used by the patient at home.[21] The procedure consists of two basic steps: primary eye closure and additional instructions to maintain a downward eye position.

Primary Eye Closure Instructions

1. The head is centered and held in a slightly downward direction. Compensatory movements of the head must be discouraged.
2. The eye of the involved side fixes on a point that is *medial* and at least *60° below eye level.* The eye must not be allowed to roll up. Patients without experience should use a handheld mirror in their lap (or slightly higher) to maintain eye position (i.e., the involved eye views its own *pupil*, not the white of the eye). Patients who can maintain proper eye position without mirror feedback can simply look at a point on the knee or on the floor.
3. While maintaining the preceding position, the patient attempts to *slowly* close the involved eyelid(s). This process should first include opening the eye to its fullest point and then should be followed by *slow* closure. The movement of the uninvolved eye is ignored.

The rationale for the preceding procedure is that the patient cannot experience his lack of eye closure because he seems to feel it closing. Unfortunately, he cannot differentiate between the eyelid's closure and the feeling of the eye rolling up in a Bell's reflex. Postacute patients typically do not relearn to close the eye unless the difference between these two movements is discriminated. Therefore, it is usually necessary to prove to the patient that when he attempts to close the involved eyelid it has not actually closed. The therapist's verbal commands will not be sufficient sensory information. The patient needs to see his own eye and the eylid closing or not closing. A logical process of elimination is used to facilitate this process.

Additional instructions to help maintain a downward eye position include the following:

1. The patient is instructed to slowly close the uninvolved eye and observe its closure in a hand-held mirror as previously described. The patient will be able to watch his own eye close down to just a fraction of a millimeter before "the lights go out."
2. The patient is then instructed to attempt the same task for the involved eye. The patient is asked to note that he can, at best, only see his lid close a very small amount (i.e., much of the iris is still showing) when the "lights go out."

These steps should be repeated until the patient realizes that his involved eye is rolling up and that it is not fully closed because he does not see it near the point of full closure just before the "lights go out." This process of elimination can also help the patient realize that this mirror technique is a very sensitive method of measuring the degree of eye closure. After this is understood and the procedures are followed, the patient should be able to notice increases in lid closure within a few days of practice.

Stress Integration and Voice Patterning. The key to retraining spontaneous facial movements (i.e., those that do not involve thought or effort) is to encourage the patient to use his new volitional abilities during episodes of spontaneous emotion. Many different methods can be used in the clinic and in home training to facilitate this type of animation. The following are some examples.

1. *Play-acting*—Improvisations involving gestures associated with happiness, fear, sorrow, etc. may be used. If nothing else, such play-acting always causes spontaneous laughter. The therapist encourages the patient to use muscles that will promote smiling, puckering, frowning, etc. under both voluntary and spontaneous conditions.

2. *Exchanging of Jokes*—Jokes may be collected from friends or joke books. The object is for the therapist and patient to try to outdo the other in making the other laugh. The therapist encourages the patient to use his new smiling ability during laughter.

3. *Voice Patterning*—This involves having the patient slowly enunciate words while looking in a mirror. The patient is encouraged to exaggerate the movements of his facial muscles (e.g., pucker, smile, etc.) while minimally moving the jaw.

4. *"Stadium Talk"*—The patient pretends to sit on a bench in a noisy stadium. A friend is sitting on the same side as the involved side of the face, while an enemy is sitting next to the uninvolved side of the face. The patient's task is to look straight ahead and talk at a moderate to high volume out of his involved side to his friend, being careful to open his mouth wide on that side and inhibit all movement on the uninvolved side, so as to not let the enemy hear them. This serves the purpose of encouraging the patient to acquire a consciousness that is associated with talking out of the involved side and inhibiting the usual pattern of talking (with corresponding head turning) out of only the uninvolved side. Eventually, this encourages the use of speech automatically transmitted from the center of the mouth and at a reasonably high level of volume.

Initially, exercises such as these, should be practiced at home, in quiet formal sessions. After the patient has mastered the correct feelings or sensations associated with such gestures, they must be added to the emotional facial gestures made on a daily basis. This second step may seem unreasonable at first, but such "added consciousness" usually becomes much easier and more automatic in 2 to 4 weeks. With time, the new facial repertoire can become automatic, permanent and the new program for his facial behavior. Only when the patient becomes tired or extremely emotional will some amount of dyskinesis and/or synkinesis occur. It should be noted, however, that to a certain degree fatigue affects normal people as well.

Case Studies

The following two postsurgical patients were retrained on a postacute basis with the program described in this chapter. These patients were selected only on the basis of their abilities to comply with instructions. Before retraining, both patients had been involved in extensive nonspecific mirror exercises[26] but had shown no improvement. Some of these results have been previously described by Balliet et al.[21]

Case Study J. B.

History

J. B., a 49-year-old housewife, who had a left acoustic neuroma surgically removed resulting in a complete left hearing loss and injury to the facial nerve, had a complete left facial paralysis at 2 years after the operation. At this time, a left CN XII–CN VII anastomosis was performed. In three subsequent operations to treat lagophthalmos, attempts were made to fit a gold weight in the eyelid and to implant a wishbone spring. None of these operations, however, resulted in full eye closure. At 4 years postanastomosis, the patient's left facial paralysis was assessed and was found to have a moderately severe dysfunction (grade IV = 30 percent total function) (Table 5-8; Fig. 5-6).

A surface electrode EMG, however, indicated hypertonicity on the involved side of approximately 10.0 mV compared to 1.0 mV on the uninvolved side. No movement in the forehead or eyelid was apparent. Diagnostic needle EMG evaluations found no volitional motor units in the area of the forehead. Poor motor control was found in the area of the mouth, thus affecting smile, frown, and pucker. Involuntary (mass) movements in the

Table 5-8 Case Study Results using Janssen Scale.[20]

Patient	Age/sex		Post	Condition		Rest (30%)	Frontal (10%)	Ocular (30%)	Oral (30%)	Total (100%)	International Scale (Grade)
J.B.	49	F	4 years	CNXII-CNVII	Pre:	20	0	0	10	30	IV
				anastomosis	Post:	26	3	22	23	74	III
M.B.	65	F	3 years	CN-VII	Pre:	0	0	0	0	0	VI
				compression	Post:	28	3	21	25	77	II

(From Balliet et al.,[21] with permission.)

area of the orbicularis oculi inferioris, zygomaticus major, triangularis, and mentalis were noted with swallowing and tongue movements (within the mouth) and equaled approximately 90 and 30 μV, respectively.

Treatment Plan

Treatment consisted of three different strategies, which were presented in the following order but with significant overlap. In addition to the general methods described in the previous sections, the following specific EMG program was conducted:

Reduction of Facial Tone on the Involved and the Uninvolved Sides. J. B. was a 10+ cup a day coffee drinker. When she stopped drinking coffee, the hypertonicity on her involved side decreased from 10 μV to about 1 to 3 μV, with typical values at 1.5 μV after 2 to 5 minutes of relaxation. Similarly, her uninvolved side decreased from

about 3 to 5 μV to about 1.5 μV. Periodic reminders were necessary to maintain this level of tone during the treatments below.

Reduction of Facial Movements on Involved Side Associated with Movements of the Tongue (Synkinesis). One EMG electrode set was placed on the middle of the cheek (zygomaticus major area).

The patient then performed progressively larger tongue movements while EMG potentials were kept below 5.0 μV. Very small movements were used in the first two sessions. A warning threshold tone and video monitor set on high sensitivity (full scale deflection = 25 μV) provided feedback. With this method the patient acquired an awareness for the process, which could then be used at home without an EMG. Within about 2 months (three, 1-hour sessions/week), J. B. was able to make large tongue movements, including outside of the

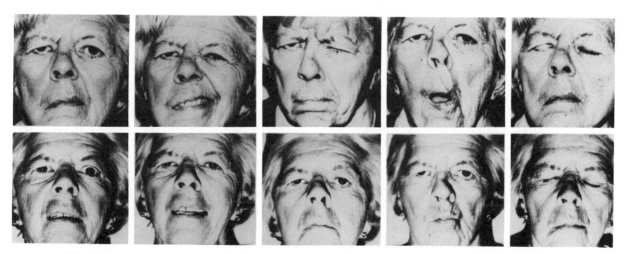

Fig. 5-6 Case M. B. Upper photos are pretraining; lower are of post-training. From left to right: resting tone, smile, frown, pucker, and eye closure. (From Balliet et al.,[21] with permission.)

mouth, without significant synkinesis over an equivalent microvolt range of about 1 to 2 μV.

Similar to the preceding exercise, the patient took progressively larger swallows of water while keeping EMG potentials below 5.0 μV. This proved to be a much more difficult task. After 7 months of therapy, the patient estimated that she experienced a 95% reduction in synkinesis and an equivalent microvolt range of about 1.5 to 15 μV.

The Facilitation of Volitional Control of the Involved Side. EMG facilitation and SAE mirror exercises were used to increase existing function primarily in the areas of the forehead and zygomaticus major. Eye closure exercises were performed. Using the Janssen Scale,[20] it was found that these procedures resulted in a functional increase of approximately 150 percent. The patient was assessed to have moderate dysfunction (grade III = 74 percent total function) (see Table 5-3). EMG potentials corresponded to these changes and synkinesis was significantly reduced. With the exception of the frontalis, the patient felt that she was now functional. She was happiest about being able to eat in public "without her face going off" (synkinesis). These results were acquired with an average of two 1-hour clinic sessions per week and about 30 to 45 min/day of home exercise over a period of 7 months.

Post-Treatment Evaluation

A follow-up evaluation 2 years later indicated that the patient had discontinued her facial exercises, but she had retained all of her functional gains, including spontaneous laughter, frowning, pucker, and eye closure.

Case Study M. B.

History

M. B. was a 64-year-old housewife who had an excision of a right acoustic neuroma and posterior craniotomy resulting in severe compression injury to the facial nerve. Microsurgical inspection showed that only a thin filament of the nerve remained. Three years after surgery, the patient was found to have a right total paralysis (Grade VI = 0 percent total function) (see Table 5-8) (Fig. 5-7). With the exception of a tarsorrhaphy, no further surgery had been performed (e.g., anas-

tomosis) because of potential complications resulting from the patient's age. Stimulation of the facial nerve caused no evoked response. Diagnostic needle EMG examinations indicated only occasional fibrillations and positive waves, with no volitional units in all areas tested (i.e., frontalis, levator labii alaeque nasi, orbicularis oris, or mentalis).

Treatment Plan

Treatment consisted of an initial evaluation, as well as the specific facilitation of certain muscle groups. In addition to the general methods described in the following specific EMG program was conducted:

The Evaluation of Resting Tone and Synkinesis on the Involved and Uninvolved Sides. M. B. was not a coffee drinker and was judged to be a relaxed person. EMG values for her involved side appeared to be denervated at about 0.25 μV; the uninvolved side appeared normal at about 1.0 μV. These EMG readings indicated that the patient's tone was normal and that no exercises would be required for the reduction of tonicity. Synkinesis was also not a problem because no function was apparent on the involved side.

Neuromuscular Facilitation of Hypoactive Muscle Activity on Involved Side. Slow, fine (tonic) control of the uninvolved side was trained in the area of the zygomaticus using EMG (approximately 10 μV over 5 seconds).

The feelings associated with making slow fine movements of the uninvolved side were then transferred to the involved side (corresponding zygomaticus area) through the process of slowly attempting to make bilateral movements. Initially, EMG of the two sides gave feedback regarding the correct initial recruitment strategy of the uninvolved side (up to 100 μV) while only very small differences in EMG potentials (± 0.1 to 0.2 μV over a resting level of 0.2 μV) on the involved side were noted. Using a therapy strategy utilizing a maximal EMG threshold level of 10 μV on the uninvolved side, it took 6 weeks of 1-hour sessions three times per week before M. B. could consistently make volitional EMG potentials of up to 1.0 μV and before she could be sure that she was "really doing something and that it wasn't just the

GOAL ATTAINMENT AGREEMENT

PROBLEM# 3 ;PAGE 1

PATIENT _____ J.P. _____

THERAPIST _____ B.L. _____

DATE _____ 7/18/80 _____

TOTAL DURATION 12 sessions

PERIODIC EXAMS 3x / wk.

GENERAL PROBLEM Weak elbow flexion

ACHIEVED LEVEL 100 %

GOAL (100%) Increase biceps reading from 0-20 mv/sec.

CONDITIONS Support only to arm, no resistance. Triceps must be below baseline of 5 mv/sec. Maximum of 3 trials
per session, 7 repetitions.

HOMEWORK No homework assigned.

RESULTS Achieved 100% at session #10.

FUTURE GOALS Increase arcs of movement 30-90 degrees flexion.

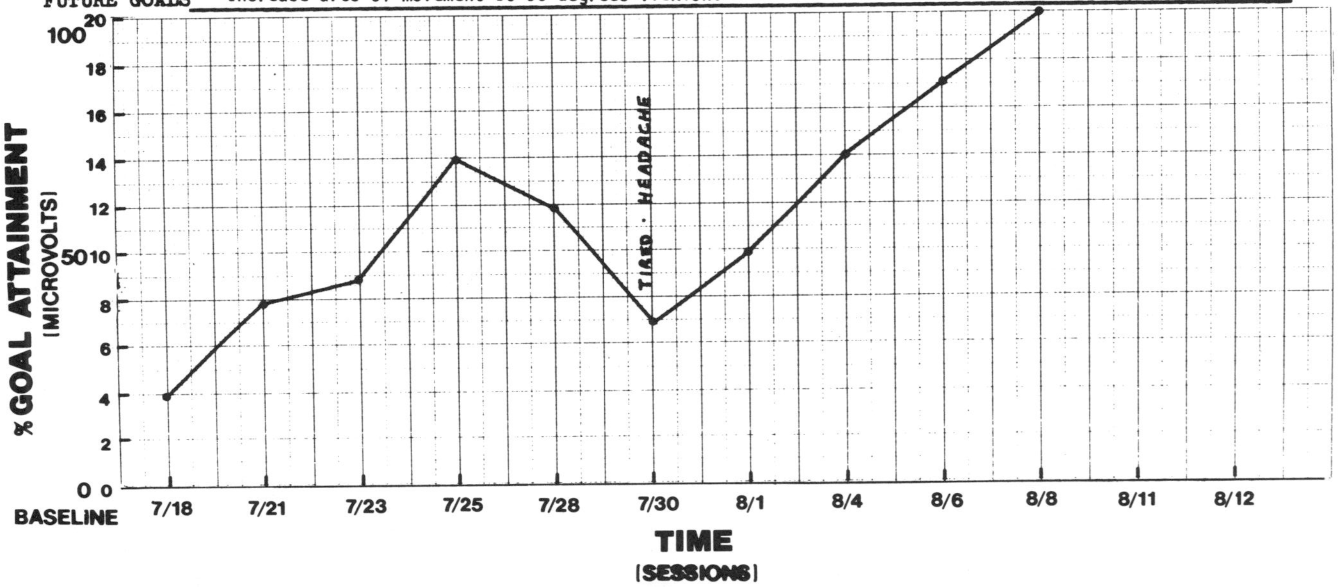

Fig. 5-7 Sample goal attainment record.

machine." The patient reported that at this point she was "sensing, but not quite feeling" her own responses.

After 5 more weeks M. B. could consistently "see" very small contractions in the mirror. In 3 months, she had increased her muscle control to approximately 10 percent out of 30 percent on the Janssen Scale[20] in the area of the zygomaticus (smiling) and the orbicularis oculi superioris (eye-close-using-mirror exercise). At this time, stimulation of the facial nerve caused no evoked response; needle EMG demonstrated insertional activity of all tested muscles in levator labii alaeque nasi, orbicularis oculi superioris, and orbicularis oris superioris with substantially lesser amounts in the mentalis and frontalis. Neither fibrillation potentials nor positive sharp waves were present. Nascent volitional motor units were seen to be under volitional control in similar proportions. Poor to fair recruitment patterns with firing rates of 40 to 50/sec were typical. These results indicated that early recruitment was apparent to a lesser degree even in muscles that were not specifically being trained with the EMG.

Similarly, over an additional 5-month period, EMG and mirror exercises were extended to the areas of the risorius, the levator labii superioris, the frontalis, and the depressor anguli oris.

At the end of 8 months of therapy, M. B. was assessed to have only a mild dysfunction of her right face (grade II = 77 percent total function). This corresponded to a maximum microvolt range of 50 to 90 μV, with the frontalis being movable (up to about 15 μV) but not functional (see Table 5-3 and Fig. 5-6 for details). Although a small amount of general muscle weakness was noted under conditions involving lack of sleep or stress, no synkinesis was apparent. In addition, because of the patient's new eye closure ability, lubrication drops were no longer required to maintain tear film on her involved eye. The patient, however, did not elect to reverse the previous tarsorrhaphy.

Post-Treatment Evaluation

Follow-up evaluations at 2, 3 and 4 years (final evaluation at age 70) found no significant regression. The patient performed about 30 minutes per week of mirror exercises to maintain her overall facial tone. She also reported that she still appre-

ciated being able to kiss her grandchildren and not have them run from her as they had done before therapy.

OTHER PERIPHERAL NERVE DISORDERS

General Acute and Postacute Care

This section presents general methodology to augment the treatment of most peripheral nerve (lower motoneuron) disorders. The assumption is made that peripheral nerve injuries can be similarly classified and that retraining involves similar CNS reprogramming strategies. It is safe to assume that the therapist's ability to retrain motor function and decrease dyskinesis and synkinesis after a peripheral nerve injury depends not only on the severity of the lesion and subsequent healing processes, but also on the neuromuscular retraining of the CNS.

During the acute stage of therapy it is of primary importance that damaged nerves have a chance to heal and that there is no further trauma. Bracing, splinting, slings, and assistive devices should be used as needed. For example, in the common brachial plexus injury, it is important that flaccid paralysis, either resulting from nerve trauma or from stroke and subluxation, be treated with either static or dynamic slings to immobilize the humerus. This allows for healing of the nerves and gives the therapist an opportunity to carefully and systematically build muscle strength and protect against further injury. Numerous schools of thought describe these general procedures and can be used in the rehabilitation of peripheral nerve and CNS injuries.[48]

In the postacute or so-called chronic stage, not only strengthening but also gross and fine motor control can be achieved. In addition, a certain amount of sensation can sometimes be retrained. (A very complete book on upper extremity rehabilitation of peripheral nerves that can also be applied to the lower extremities is "Rehabilitation of the Hand" by Hunter et al.[49])

The following description of general logic and methods can augment most treatments involving peripheral nerve injury, whether it be a brachial plexus injury or an isolated radial, medial, or ulnar nerve injury. The discussion is aimed at the late-acute or postacute stage where most motor control is trained, without the benefit of spontaneous recovery effects.

EMG Sensory Feedback Therapy

As in the previous facial paralysis section, the assumption is made that the problem of motor function retraining is one of information processing rather than necessarily a lack of ability that has resulted from the peripheral nerve injury per se. Although this may not always be true, it is often judicious to make such an assumption. Therefore, the rehabilitation potential of any patient depends not only on the lesion but also on the re-establishment of sensory inputs to the brain that can redirect motor programming.

As previously discussed, we do not recommend the use of electrotherapy to increase function in peripheral nerve injury. Instead, we recommend EMG sensory feedback as an excellent source of specific sensory information. It can be used interactively with other therapy methods to isolate specific functionally related motor control patterns and increase strength and endurance.

Equipment

The same equipment is recommended as previously stated in the facial paralysis section: Electromyographic (EMG) Sensory Feedback: A Sensory Substitution Device.

Evaluation Methods

Standard range of motion and muscle strength tests should be used. In addition, EMG microvolt readings should be recorded from appropriate sites. Particular attention should be paid to consistently specifying the associated method of facilitation, such as resistance, no resistance, quick stretch, position of the extremity (e.g., with or without gravity, supported or not supported) and EMG settings (e.g., scale, bandpass).

It should be noted that intrapatient and even sometimes interpatient microvolt readings may not correlate well with strength or function because motor unit recruitment can be sparse but still indicate relatively large integrated EMG potentials. Therapeutic EMG in effect sums and averages

microvolt amplitudes; it cannot discriminate between a few large motor units and thousands of motor units. For example, any number of motor units may make up a microvolt reading of $100\ \mu V$. If but a few motor units average $100\ \mu V$, function will be poor; but if thousands average $100\ \mu V$, function will be relatively strong.

It is useful to think in terms of reciprocal motor control. It is suggested that a modified functional rating scale be added for upper extremity evaluations (Table 5-9).[50] The table includes EMG agonist-to-antagonist amplitude ratios that we have found to represent typical degrees of motor control, but not necessarily strength. These ratios assume that motor unit recruitment patterns between opponent pairs are approximately equal; however, in some patients this may not be the case. Muscle strength should be graded using standard muscle strength evaluations.

Treatment Environment and Scheduling

The treatment environment is crucial to the patient's success.

1. Treatments should be conducted in a quiet individual room.
2. A minimum of one hour sessions are necessary to provide adequate preparation and treatment line.
3. In postacute or difficult acute cases, training should be conducted daily to three times per week initially, until the patient can conduct the therapeutic exercise program at home without the EMG.
4. When the preceding goals are accomplished, clinic sessions can be dropped to two times per week and eventually less as tolerated.

Goal Attainment Records

Short-term and long-term rehabilitation goals and assessments of progress can easily be presented in a way that is meaningful and motivational to the patient and the therapist. The goal attainment sheet (Fig. 5-7) can be used to quickly and accurately plot subjectively or objectively measured goals. These can be recorded daily at home by the patient or in the clinic by the patient and the

Table 5-9 General Functional Rating Scale[50a]

0 =	Flaccid or constant involuntary synergy/flexion. [1.0:1 EMG agonist/antagonist ratio or worse (antagonist activity higher than agonist)].
	No voluntary movement.
I =	Gross movements through partial range to voluntarily initiate and release movement within present synergy pattern under ideal conditions. [1.1:1 to 2.0:1 EMG agonist/antagonist ratio].
	Slow, gross closing and relaxation of hand to assist in the holding/holding down of objects.
	Volitional, extension synergy used to place arm through sleeve
	Volitional, flexion synergy used to carry handled bag
II =	Beginning to break synergy patterns with isolated voluntary movements through partial range under various task conditions. [1.1:1 to 3.0:1 EMG agonist/antagonist ratio].
	Tasks requiring proximal stability with synergistic distal control
	Hold door open with some synergy
	Extension of elbows for rising from chair
III =	Partially isolated voluntary movements through partial range with some synergy present. [1.5:1 to 5.0:1 EMG agonist/antagonist ratio].
	Upper extremity motion is adequate for most self care tasks with no or slight synergies present
	Tasks requiring gross grasp and release with isolated shoulder and elbow control
IV =	Volition and range within normal limits with reduced function only when fatigued. [greater than 5.0:1 EMG agonist/antagonist ratio].
	Multiple skilled tasks with no significant synergy
	Jebssen hand evaluation[51] 1–2 standard deviations of normal limits

[a] Functional rating of active range of motion of the involved upper extremity in *gravity eliminated position* and the approximate ranges of corresponding agonist to antagonist EMG ratios associated with nonfunctional co-contractions. Representative functional abilities are indicated.

therapist. The results of each session involve the following:

1. Range of motion
2. Repetitions
3. EMG values
4. Other objectives relative to a percentage of the desired goal (0 to 100 percent)

These parameters are plotted on the x-axis, and the number of sessions estimated to complete a single task are plotted on the y-axis. Several goal attainment sheets can be used for different goals that are being simultaneously conducted including (1) finger extension, (2) supination, (3) functional grasp, and (4) other functional tasks.

Methods of EMG Sensory Feedback Therapy (SFT)

Peripheral nerve injuries can cause any muscle or group of muscles to have one or a combination of two basic dysfunctions: (1) flaccidity or extreme muscle weakness; (2) hypertonicity, spasticity and/or synkinesis.

The Facilitation of Flaccid or Extremely Weak Muscles

Flaccid muscles are not the most common problem but are one of the greatest problems encountered clinically, but with therapy weak muscle strength may be initiated. However, these new abilities proceed in a developmental sequence and are usually associated with dyskinesis, synkinesis, and/or other nonfunctional co-contractions. These associated muscle groups may be natural agonists or antagonists and may be located in any region of the body. Often complicating this matter is that the facilitation of very weak muscles seems to require maximum effort. Unfortunately, this effort may also strongly facilitate unwanted synkinesis and/or compensatory movements.

In general, SFT can provide sensory information to the patient concerning very small muscle movements (potentials), which are often not felt or seen by the patient and/or therapist. These correspond to volition resulting from trial and error learning. Often, these EMG potentials can then be brought under weak but consistent control. This activity can then be increased and brought under reciprocal control with other (usually antagonistic) muscle groups and eventually integrated into functional tasks and applied to daily activities.

It is clear that this process involves more than simply the excitation of a particular muscle group. The inhibition of specific muscle groups is also required to facilitate reciprocal and functional motor control. In the situation where lesions are unilateral and an uninvolved side exists, a model of reciprocal innervation on the uninvolved side should be established.

The Reduction of Hypertonicity, Spasticity, and Synkinesis

The assumption is made that hypertonicity, spasticity, and synkinesis involve nonfunctional co-contractions and/or poor reciprocal innervation. As mentioned in the previous section, it is also assumed that such activity will usually, at some point, accompany the return of function. The following is a general description of the overlapping stages of retraining that can be used to facilitate certain muscles and inhibit certain other muscles in a coordinated and functional manner.

When Available, Establish a Model of Reciprocal Innervation on the Uninvolved Side*

1. Decrease activity of the uninvolved extremity to resting level (e.g., 0.5 to 1.5 μV) throughout passive range of motion.
2. Establish reciprocal active range of motion via slow tonic (ramp) control of uninvolved side advancing from relatively low (e.g., 100 μV) to high (e.g., 25 μV) sensitivity ranges.

Establish Inhibition of the Involved Side During Passive Range of Motion.*‡

1. Obtain relative decrease in muscle activity on involved side over shortened static ranges, including minor stress conditions (e.g., intermittent touch).
2. Obtain relative decrease in muscle activity on involved side in progressively more extended static ranges, including minor stress conditions (e.g., intermittent touch).

3. Obtain relative decrease in muscle activity on involved side over *very* slowly increasing velocities.

Train the Selective Inhibition and Reciprocity of the Involved Side During Active Range of Motion*§

1. Develop alternate reciprocal motor control of agonist/antagonistic muscles.
2. Maintain inhibition of the agonist muscle and its antagonist, while simultaneously controlling other muscle(s) of the same extremity.
3. Inhibit spasticity/tone of desired muscle during and after reciprocal motor control of the same muscles.

The Training of Selective Inhibition and Reciprocity

One of the most difficult aspects of reducing hypertonicity, spasticity and synkinesis and other nonfunctional co-contractions is the training of selective inhibition and reciprocity. This section provides further explanation of this process.

These motor control problems are similar because they involve inappropriate muscle activity, which must be inhibited both before and during the retraining of other associated low functioning muscles. The following is a general description of this process.

1. Agonist and antagonist muscles are monitored with the EMG.
2. By trial and error learning, attempts are made to control the reciprocity of these muscles.
3. Initially, a threshold tone may be adjusted to occur if the antagonist muscle exceeds a certain specified level (e.g., 3 μV) during the contraction of the agonist (e.g., 3 to 8 μV). Higher threshold and contraction levels can be used later as ability improves.
4. The patient may concentrate primarily on the excitation of the agonist while in the "corner of his mind" he simultaneously (secondarily) inhibits the antagonist. For example, a patient

---

* Retraining stages are initially conducted under "ideal" conditions (e.g., *gravity eliminated*. Training may be extended to progressively more difficult positions and functional situations as ability improves.

‡ A 70% reduction in activity is recommended before continuing to next sub-stage level.

---

§ A minimum criteria of 2.5 : 1 agonist/antagonist ratio with gravity eliminated should be achieved before continuing to next sub-stage level.

whose fingers go into flexion every time he tries to voluntarily move them would learn to:

a. Reduce the flexion synergy as he also learns to make muscle contractions that cause finger extension (e.g., $1.1:1.0$ to $2.5:1$ μV agonist/antagonist ratio).

b. Initiate only trace movements, that is, movements so small that the fingers are not seen moving (e.g., high sensitivity scale: 2 to 10 μV @ 20 to 1000 Hz).

c. Initiate trace movements that are not associated with general synkinesis and/or co-contractions of an antagonist(s). Under these circumstances the patient should be trained to maintain a relatively low criteria of reciprocity (minimum $1.1:1.0$ to $2.5:1$ μV agonist/antagonist ratio) over an increasingly higher EMG amplitude level (up to 30 to 50 μV). Once this is accomplished, microvolt ratio can then be increased (up to $10:1$ ratios).

d. Progress to more difficult conditions under the same criteria including (1) advancing from gravity eliminated to antigravity; (2) lowering the sensitivity range over increasing microvolt amplitudes; and (3) other functional tasks, such as the gripping or lifting of progressively more difficult objects.

Case Study

The following case study is an example of the successful application of EMG feedback retraining to the neuromuscular dysfunction of a late brachial plexus injury. The methods and associated findings are typical of many peripheral nerve injuries to the extremities.

Case Study H. P. (Figs 5-8 and 5-9)

History

H. P. is a 55-year-old man who suffered a total body burn in an electrical accident, resulting in a left below-the-knee amputation, left brachial plexus injury, and complete upper extremity paralysis. Acute hospitalization followed for a period of just over 4 months. The patient was also seen in occupational and physical therapy on a daily basis. Because of the distance the patient lived

from the hospital, he was periodically admitted for therapy and other related and unrelated medical problems over an additional 6-month period. During this time, the patient's left upper extremity function was at substantially fair to good levels, with the exception of elbow flexion.

Voluntary elbow flexion was either absent or extremely intermittent. At least 90 percent of the patient's attempts at elbow flexion produced only substitution patterns in the shoulder girdle (i.e., external rotation, shoulder elevation while leaving the elbow in extension). Poor volitional control of the brachioradialis and biceps were the major contributors to this problem. Needle EMG examinations demonstrated small numbers of relatively high threshold motor units under voluntary control. At 10 months postinjury the patient was evaluated by our clinic.

Treatment Plan

Treatment consisted of EMG neuromuscular retraining on a one to two times per week basis with the following progressive goals:

If Necessary, Reduce Hypertonicity in Brachioradialis or Biceps Using EMG Feedback. The patient demonstrated 8 to 10 μV in both muscles at resting levels (Fig. 5-10). After the patient eliminated the six (or more) cups of coffee per day from his diet, resting EMG potentials went down to normal at about 1.5 μV within only 24 hours.

Facilitate Brachioradialis and Biceps Muscle Activity with EMG Feedback. Quick stretching and EMG feedback facilitated about 50 to 100 μV of volitional biceps activity in the first 1-hour session. During this time, the patient used the EMG to find "what he had to do to turn on his flexors." Within two more sessions, H. P. rapidly acquired a consistent ability to activate 150 μV of activity in his biceps with only occasional facilitation. In another four sessions, he was able to increase to 175 to 200 μV in his brachioradialis usually without facilitation (Fig. 5-11). This corresponded to no more than about 90° of flexion against gravity *without any additional weight*. At this point, home exercises were prescribed. These involved slow elbow flexion against gravity (i.e., increasing active range of motion without any

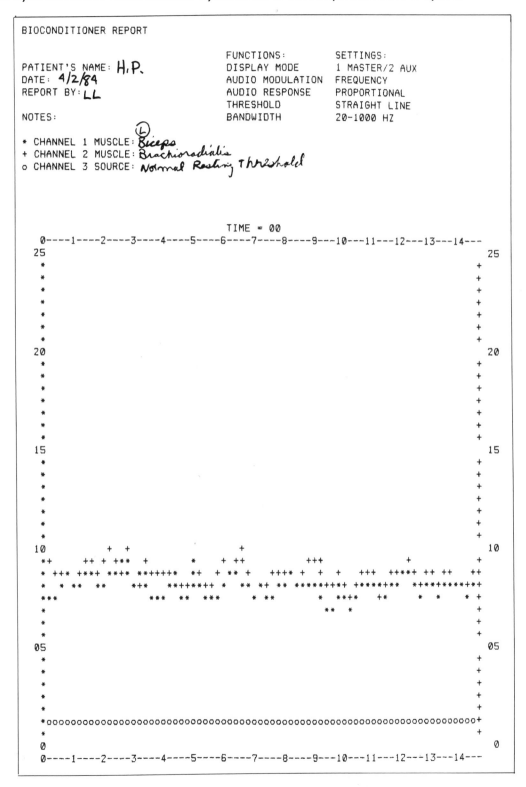

Fig. 5-8 Case of H. P. involved in initial EMG training.

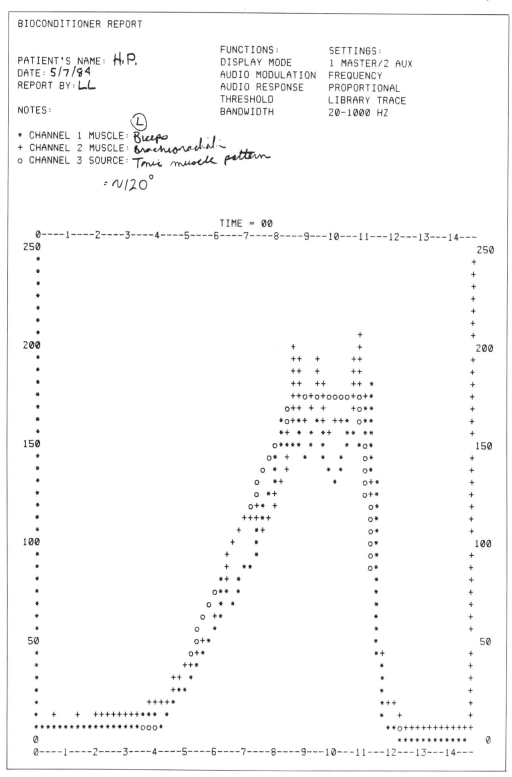

Fig. 5-9 Case of H. P. involved in final EMG training.

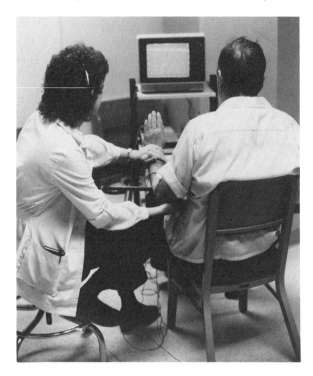

Fig. 5-10 Case H. P. Baseline resting tone of the left biceps (*) and brachioradialis (+) on initial visit. The EMG computer is indicating the "normal" resting tone level of about 1.5 μV/20–1000 Hz (○) for most individuals.

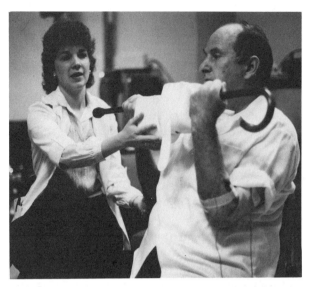

Fig. 5-11 Case H. P. Slow tonic muscle control of the left biceps (*) and brachioradialis (+). The EMG computer is indicating a tonic ramp (○) for the patient to mimic that is equivalent to a rise of 175 μV and about 100° to 120° degrees of active range of motion.

weight. It should be noted that more difficult tasks, such as holding even a 8-ounce object, would cause him to revert back to his old pattern of nonfunctional substitution.

Train Generalizable Functional Abilities Without EMG Feedback. While the EMG activity of the brachioradialis and biceps were being fed back to the patient, progressively more resistance was given, maintaining the same active range of motion. This procedure was begun when a criterion of about 90° to 120° of flexion against gravity (active range of motion without weight) could be achieved without quick stretch facilitation or EMG feedback. This generalization procedure was completed over a period of 4 months of periodic EMG retraining in the clinic (16 sessions) and daily home practice. In both situations, the patient learned to increase, a few ounces at a time, his capacity to lift increasing weight loads until about 10 pounds

could be lifted. Again, care had to be taken not to progress too quickly. Too much weight or too much stretch would cause him to revert immediately to his "old pattern" of shoulder substitution. Retraining with the EMG was clearly helpful, even at the greater weight values. The patient could usually lift 30 to 50 percent more weight with the EMG than without it. The EMG was no longer necessary to maintain his elbow flexion abilities when he could lift 10 pounds over 120° with or without the EMG. This was equivalent to about 250 to 400 μV, indicating that motor unit recruitment had significantly changed because these readings were virtually the same as when the patient had been lifting only his arm against gravity. The patient had been using the EMG as a relative indicator of muscle function and not as an absolute indicator. At this point H. P. was able to generalize independent elbow flexion to any activity, including supination and pronation, as well as wrist and finger flexion and extension.

Post-Treatment Evaluation

At follow-up evaluation 6 months later, the patient had maintained all of his abilities. The only problem during this time involved a nonrelated surgery that required bedrest for several days. During this time his entire left extremity "felt weak," but at home, he was able to slowly increase his function on his own with a series of small weights. It took about 2 weeks to regain his previous level of function. A further follow-up evaluation 4 months later (total of 10 months) showed normal function of the entire extremity.

PATIENT ADVOCACY GROUPS FOR FACIAL PARALYSIS

Two prominent patient-run, nonprofit associations have been organized in recent years to provide information and support for patients with acoustic neuromas and other tumors affecting the cranial nerves. These groups usually have local chapters in the major cities of the United States and Canada. Because many of these problems also affect the facial nerve, these organizations have developed a particular interest in the facial paralysis patient, including the Bell's palsy patient who has residual deficits.

The primary purposes of these groups are to:

1. Provide professionally authorized medical information, self-help aids, and act as an information exchange
2. Promote and support research about the cause and treatment of acoustic neuromas, other cranial tumors, and facial paralysis
3. Provide information, upon request, concerning surgical treatment, neuromuscular rehabilitation, and the alleviation of other postsurgical problems
4. Provide opportunities for patients with similar problems to communicate with each other both in and outside of their region

For information about these groups contact:

1. The Acoustic Neuroma Association of Canada
   P.O. Box 369
   Edmonton, Alberta
   T5J 2J6
   (403) 479-4364 (after 6:00 p.m.)
2. Acoustic Neuroma Association (U.S.A.)
   P.O. Box 398
   Carlisle, PA 17013-0398
   (717) 249-4783

ACKNOWLEDGMENT

Many thanks to Sherry Vike and Jackie Diels, OTR, for their patience in editing this manuscript.

REFERENCES

1. Janetta PJ: Neurovascular contact in hemifacial spasm. In Portmann M (ed): The Facial Nerve. Masson, New York, 1985
2. Chusid JG: Correlative Neuroanatomy and Functional Neurology. Lange Medical, Los Altos, 1982
3. Sunderland S: Cranial nerve injury—structural and pathophysiological considerations and a classification of nerve injury. In Samii M, Janetta PJ (eds): The Cranial Nerves. Springer-Verlag, Berlin, 1981
4. Loew F: History of cranial nerves surgery—introductory lecture. In Samii M, Janetta PJ (eds): The Cranial Nerves. Springer-Verlag, Berlin, 1981
5. Samii M: Nerves of the head and neck. In Omer GE, Spinner M (eds): Management of Peripheral Nerve Problems. W.B. Saunders, Philadelphia, 1980
6. Portmann M: Facial Nerve. Masson, New York, 1985
7. Devriese PP: Prognosis of paralysis. In Portmann M (ed): The Facial Nerve. Masson, New York, 1985
8. Kennedy JG, Abbs, JH: Anatomic studies of the perioral motor system: foundations for studies in speech physiology. In Lass NJ (ed): Speech and Language: Advances in Basic Research and Practice. Vol 1. Academic Press, New York, 1979
9. Ahlgren J: Mechanisms of mastication: a quantitative cinematographic and electromyographic study of masticatory movements in children with special reference to occlusion of the teeth. Acta Odontol Scand, suppl., 44:109, 1966
10. Moller E: The chewing apparatus: an electromyographic study of the action of the muscles of mastication and its correlation to facial morphology. Acta Physiol Scand [Suppl] 280:69, 1966
11. Sussman HM, McNeilage PF, Hanson RJ: Labial and mandibular dynamics during the production of bilabial consonants: preliminary observations. J Speech Hear Res 16:397, 1973
12. Isley CL, Basmajian JV: Electromyography of the human cheeks and lips. Anat Rec 176:143, 1973
13. O'Dwyer NL, Quinn PT, Guitar BE, et al: Procedures for verification of electrode placement in EMG studies of orofacial and mandibular muscles. J Speech Hear Disord 24:273, 1981
14. Abbs JH, Gracco VL: Control of complex motor gestures: oralfacial muscle responses to load perturbations of the lip during speech. J Neurophysiol 51:705, 1984
15. Wafel JH: The Head, Neck and Trunk. Lea & Febiger, Philadelphia, 1974
16. Clemente CD: Anatomy: A Regional Atlas of the Human Body. Urban & Schwarzenberg, Baltimore, 1981

17. House JW: Facial nerve grading systems. In Portmann M (ed): The Facial Nerve. Masson, New York, 1985
18. Portmann M: Conclusions. In Portmann M (ed): Facial Nerve. Masson, New York, 1985
19. House JW: Facial nerve grading systems. Laryngoscope 93:1056, 1983
20. Janssen FP: Over de postoperative facialisverlamming. Thesis. University of Amsterdam, 1963. In Jongkees LWB: Practical application of clinical tests for facial paralysis. Arch Otolaryngol 97:220, 1963
21. Balliet R, Shinn JB, Bach-y-Rita P: Facial paralysis rehabilitation: retraining selective muscle control. Int Rehabil Med 4:67, 1982
22. Waxman B: Electrotherapy for treatment of facial nerve paralysis (Bell's palsy). In: Health Technology Assessment Reports, National Center for Health Services Research. 3:27, 1984
23. Girlanda P, Dattola R, Vita G, et al: Effect of electrotherapy on denervated muscles in rabbits: an electrophysiological and morphological study. Exp Neurol 77:483, 1982
24. Cohan CS, Kater SB: Suppression of neurite elongation and growth cone motility by electrical activity. Science 232:1638, 1986
25. Brown MC, Holland RL: A central role for denervated tissues in causing nerve sprouting. Nature 282:724, 1979
26. Craig M: Miss Craig's Face Saving Exercises. Random House, New York, 1970
27. Daniels L, Worthingham C: Muscle Testing-Techniques of Manual Examination. W.B. Saunders, Philadelphia, 1980
28. Balliet R: Motor control strategies in the retraining of facial paralysis. In Portmann M (ed): Facial Nerve. Masson, New York, 1985
29. Milner-Brown HS, Stein RB, Lee RG, Brown WF: Motor unit recruitment in patients with neuromuscular disorders. In Desmedt JE (ed): Motor unit Types, Recruitment and Plasticity in Health and Disease: Progress in Clinical Neurophysiology. Vol. 9. Karger, Basel, 1981
30. Henneman E, Somjen G, Carpenter DO: Functional significance of cell size in spinal motoneurons. J Neurophysiol 28:560, 1965
31. Henneman E, Samjen G, Carpenter DO: Excitability and inhibility of motor neurons of different sizes. J Neurophysiol 28:599, 1965
32. Hallett M, Marsden CD: Ballistic flexion movements of the human thumb. J Physiol, 294:33, 1979
33. Marsden CD, Obeso JA, Rothwell JC: The function of the antagonist muscle during fast limb movements in man. J Physiol 335:1, 1983
34. Burke RE: Motor unit recruitment: What are the critical factors? In Desmedt JE (ed): Motor Unit Types, Recruitment and Plasticity in Health and Disease: Progress in Clinical Neurophysiology. Vol. 9. Karger, Basel, Switzerland 1981
35. Desmedt JE: Size principle of motoneuron recruitment and the calibration of muscle force and speech in man. In Desmedt JE (ed): Motor Control Mechanisms in Health and Disease. Raven Press, New York, 1983
36. Conley J: New concepts in facial palsy. In Portmann M (ed): Facial Nerve. Masson, New York, 1985
37. Bach-y-Rita P: Central nervous system lesions: sprouting and unmasking in rehabilitation. Arch Phys Med Rehabil 62:413, 1981
38. Bach-y-Rita P (ed): Rehabilitation following brain damage: Some neurophysiological mechanisms. Int Rehabil Med 4:165, 1983
39. Bach-y-Rita P: The process of recovery from stroke. In Brandstater ME (ed): Stroke Rehabilitation. Williams & Wilkins, Baltimore, 1987
40. Bach-y-Rita P, Balliet R: Recovery from stroke. In: Duncan PW, Badke MB (eds.): Motor Deficits Following Stroke. Year Book Medical Publishers, New York, 1987
41. Marinacci AA, Horande M: Electromyogram in neuromuscular re-education. Bull Los Angeles Neurol Soc 25:57, 1960
42. Booker HE, Rubow RT, Coleman PJ: Simplified feedback in neuromuscular retraining: an automated approach using electromyographic signals. Arch Phys Med Rehabil 50:621, 1969
43. Daniel B, Guitar B: EMG feedback and recovery of facial and speech gestures following neural anastomosis. J Speech Hear Disord 43:9, 1978
44. Jankel WR: Bell's Palsy: muscle re-education by electromyograph feedback. Arch Phys Med Rehabil 59:240, 1978
45. Brown D, Nahai F, Wolf S, Basmajian J: Electromyographic feedback in the re-education of facial palsy. Am J Phys Med 57:183, 1978
46. Schram GH, Burres S: Non-surgical rehabilitation after paralysis. In Portmann M (ed): Facial Nerve. Masson, New York, 1985
47. Basmajian JV (ed): Biofeedback: Principles and Practice for Clinicians. Williams & Wilkins, Baltimore, 1983
48. Umphred D: Neurological Rehabilitation. C.V. Mosby, St. Louis, 1985
49. Hunter JM, Schneider LH, Mackin EJ, Callahan AD: Rehabilitation of the Hand. C.V. Mosby, St. Louis, 1984
50. Balliet R, Levy B, Blood KMT: Upper extremity sensory feedback therapy (SFT) in chronic cerebrovascular accident patients with impaired expressive aphasia and auditory comprehension. Arch Phys Med Rehabil 67:304, 1986
51. Jebsen RH: An objective and standard test of hand function. Arch Phys Med Rehabil 50:311, 1969

6 Coma

Sandra C. Brooks

Coma is a nonsleep loss of consciousness lasting for an extended period of time.[1] This condition can result from a wide range of pathophysiological conditions including hematomas, infarcts, hemorrhages, anoxia, and toxins, to name just a few. Regardless of the pathophysiology, the area of the brain damaged by the coma is the brain stem. This damage can be from direct insult, from pressure from above, or from widespread vascular insufficiencies.

SIGNS AND SYMPTOMS

The patient in a coma will be unresponsive to any input including pain. The patient may be seen in a variety of postures from full extension (as in decerebrate rigidity), to flexion of the upper extremities and extension of the lower extremities (as in decorticate rigidity), to asymmetrical posturing. To plan an appropriate treatment program for the comatose patient it is important to differentiate during the assessment whether the patient's unresponsiveness is due to

1. An inability to sense the stimulus
2. An inability to process the stimulus into a response
3. An inability of the musculoskeletal system to respond to the command

This assessment approach requires an in-depth neurological assessment, musculoskeletal assessment, and functional activities assessment.

EVALUATION

Neurological Examination

Neurological examination assesses the patient's ability to sense and process a stimulus. This information will give clues about the level of the patient's neural damage and the particular stimuli that will be more effective in eliciting responses in the patient. On initial assessment, only parts of the examination may be appropriate; that is, cranial nerves (CN) III, IV, VI may be impossible to test in a patient who never opens his eyes, even in response to deep pain. Inability to complete part of the assessment should be recorded, as return of function may allow later assessment of those pathways, nerves, etc.

Although the neurological examination can begin in several different ways, one approach is to start with the cranial nerve assessment. The following equipment is needed to perform the neurological examination of the cranial nerves: vials of different scents, such as ammonia, lemon, or perfume; a pencil or object to track while doing the ocular cranial nerves; and a piece of cotton and a safety pin for the light touch and sharp-dull discrimination. The cranial nerves, associated functions, functional outcomes, and interpretations are listed in Table 6-1.

Olfactory

To test the olfactory nerve (CN I), hold a vial of strong smelling substance such as ammonia under the patient's nose. If there is an aversive response,

Table 6-1 Cranial Nerve Assessment

Nerve	Stimuli	Expected Response	Interpretation
I. Olfactory	Strong scent held near nose.	Facial grimace or head turning	Lack of response may indicate perceptual, processing or motor problems
II. Optic	Test visual fields	Patient should see laterally, superiorly, and inferiorly	Inability to see in a given field suggests damage along a given portion of the ocular nerve/tract
III. Oculomotor	Pupil constriction (CN3) tracking	Both eyes should track vertically and horizontally	Difficulty can help pinpoint brainstem damage
IV. Trochlear	Same as oculomotor	Same as oculomotor	Same as oculomotor
V. Trigeminal	Sensation to forehead, cheeks, and jaw	Facial twitching or other indication of perception of touch	Lack of response may indicate perceptual, processing or motor problems. May limit effectiveness of stimuli to face to achieve oral motor of head orienting.
VI. Abducens	Same as oculomotor	Same as oculomotor	Same as oculomotor
VII. Facial	Observe muscle activity	Facial grimacing, frowning, etc.	Lack of response may be due to a multitude of factors. Damage may give patient difficulty in nonverbal communication.

(continued)

such as turning the head or pulling away, the pathway is intact. Possible causes of nonresponse include

1. Damage to the pathway itself, which could occur during damage to the cerebrum or anterior pole of the temporal lobe
2. Damage to the pathways from the olfactory and limbic system to the motor response areas. (These tracts are also found between the cerebrum and the brain stem.)
3. Damage to the descending motor pathways
4. Damage to the musculoskeletal system preventing expression of the command. This damage may be direct (as in a concussion) or indirect as in immobilization weakness.

Three clinical implications are related to olfactory dysfunction.

1. Damage to this area may affect higher mental skills (secondary to tracts position relative to the frontal lobe) or emotional responses (secondary to connections with the limbic system/temporal lobe).
2. There are connections between the limbic system and the reticular activating system. Input from the reticular activating system is critical to maintain cortical responses (i.e., arouse the patient).
3. The influence of the olfactory/limbic system may be one way to aid the patient to produce active movement via an avoidance response.

Table 6-1 (*continued*)

Nerve	Stimuli	Expected Response	Interpretation
VIII. Auditory	Sound presented to each side	Turning head, facial grimacing	Lack of response may be due to a multitude of factors. Unilateral hearing loss may cause the patient to use asymmetrical postures in response to verbal cues
	Shift patient so center of gravity is not directly over the base of support	Righting and regain center of gravity over base of support.	Lack of response may be due to neurological damage or musculoskeletal factors, such as weakness and joint limitation
IX. Glossopharyngeal	Tactile input to back of throat	Gag	Lack of response may be due to neural damage or muscular weakness
X. Vagus	Same as glossopharyngeal	Same as glossopharyngeal	Same as glossopharyngeal
XI. Accessory	Observe/palpate sternocleidomastoid and trapezius muscles	Muscle contraction	Lack of response may be due to neural or muscular damage or decreased range in the cervical spine or sternoclavicular joint
XII. Hypoglossal	Active movement of tongue	Symmetrical movement of tongue	Lack of response may be neurological or muscular. Damage may lead to difficulty with speech and swallowing

Optic

Cranial nerve II, the optic nerve, is assessed by the patient's ability to see in all parts of the visual field. The optic nerve is traditionally assessed by evaluating visual fields. However, if the patient is not sufficiently aware to assess the nerve in this manner, it can be assessed at a later date. Various visual field deficits can help pinpoint the location of damage. By understanding the area of damage, other deficits exhibited by the patient can be understood and allowances can be made in treatment. For example, in a lesion of the midbrain just posterior to the optic chiasm, (Fig. 6-1), the optic tract may be damaged. The fibers near the tract, which may also be damaged, in the anterior midbrain are the descending corticospinal tract affecting the motor control of the body. A patient who arouses from the coma will be left with a hemiplegia and homonymous hemianopsia.

Hence, the patient will present with unilateral tone-strength abnormalities and visual neglect.

Oculomotor, Trochlear, Abducent

Cranial nerves III, IV, and VI are often tested together. The oculomotor, trochlear, and abducent nerves control the movements of the eyeball itself. Damage to various areas of the tracts or nuclei of these nerves in the midbrain lead to different difficulties with visual tracking (Table 6-2).

Table 6-2 Oculomotor, Trochlear and Abducens Nerves

Nerve	Paralysis
Oculomotor	Cannot look up, down, or medially Ptosis of lid and pupil dilation
Trochlear	Cannot look down and laterally
Abducens	Cannot look laterally

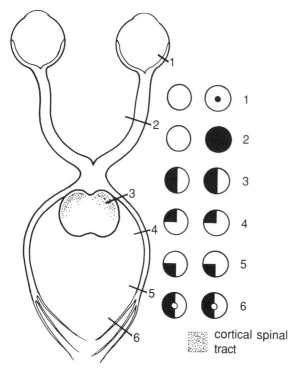

Fig. 6-1 Lesion sites along the optic pathway with corresponding visual field deficits.

the masseter and temporal muscles; and maxillary reflex (jaw jerk). Lack of response or evidence of damage in the pons and medulla directly affects a choice of treatment approach. Damage to this large tract precludes the effectiveness of tactile input to the face for arousal or oral motor control.

Facial

Cranial nerve VII is the facial nerve. Damage to this nerve can produce a variety of symptoms including disturbance in salivation and crying, hyperresponsivity to noises (hyperacusis), paralysis of the muscles of facial expression, and a loss of taste sensation. Damage to this nerve will result in the appearance of a flat affect because the patient is unable to express nonverbal communication with the paralyzed facial muscles. It is important to differentiate between the patient with paralysis of facial muscles and the receptive aphasic patient. The first may understand verbal cues but not be able to give nonverbal responses, whereas the second cannot understand verbal stimuli. Should the patient have difficulty with the hyperacusis, any loud noise, such as talking too close to that ear, can produce an excessive aversion response including increased tone or startle reaction.

Vestibular

Cranial nerve VIII is the vestibular auditory nerve. It is practically impossible clinically to identify accurately a lesion of the vestibular nuclei or nerve. Several clinical behaviors have been used to infer damage in this area: nystagmus, balance reactions, and audition. Clinically, the appearance of nystagmus is often used to determine presence or absence of an intact vestibular occular reflex. It is important to note that on clinical testing (i.e., spinning the patient) a lack of nystagmus may be due to damage of the vestibular nerve, damage to the vestibular nuclei, or damage to the occular motor nuclei. A clinical assessment of hyperresponsivity or hyporesponsivity to vestibular input based on increased or decreased saccadic movement during nystagmus is difficult because norms do not exist for a normal amount of nystagmus that should be present in the adult (see also Ch. 7).

A lack of equilibrium reactions may be due to vestibular nerve-nuclei damage, interruption of

This test requires that the patient be able to track an object vertically and horizontally. If the patient does not track, the test is deferred. As the patient regains consciousness, difficulties with the control of these nerves may lead to double vision. This double vision may interfere with the patient's regaining motor skills such as balance, steering of the wheel chair, or ambulation.

Trigeminal

The fifth cranial nerve is the trigeminal nerve. It carries information from the face. Damage to a branch of the trigeminal nerve will produce isolated sensory loss to that are of the face. Damage to the whole trigeminal nerve or to the small autonomic fibers that run near it results in a loss of sensation to the face with possible absence of autonomic response in the ciliary nerves to the eyes, a lack of proprioception within the face, and a lack of pain and temperature sensation within the face. This nerve is tested by touch, pinprick, and temperature stimuli to the face; strength of

tracts from nuclei to the muscles, muscle weakness, or decreased range of motion. Because the vestibular role cannot be clinically assessed, the other problems must be assessed and corrected, if necessary, before conclusions can be drawn regarding the lack of response to vestibular input.

Damage to the auditory portion of cranial nerve VIII on one side will lead to same side hearing loss. More central damage (i.e., from the nuclei centrally) leads to decreased hearing bilaterally. This is due to the bilaterality of the auditory pathway connections within the brain stem itself. Almost all of the nuclei that mediate auditory reflexes receive input from both sides. Consequently, isolated damage to unilateral hearing loss may cause asymmetrical posturing in the patient. Since the patient will tend to turn the intact nerve toward the speaker, it is critical to differentiate the asymmetry due to hearing loss from asymmetry seen in an asymmetrical tonic neck reflex (ATNR). For example, a patient who faces right in the supine position and left in the prone position may not have an alternating ATNR; rather he simply may not be able to hear out of the right ear and has turned the left one in response to the therapist's verbal cuing. Postural symmetry might be obtained when verbal input ceases.

Glossopharyngeal

Cranial nerves IX and X are the glossopharyngeal and vagus nerve respectively. They innervate muscles of the larynx and pharynx. These nerves are tested by assessing the gag reflex, swallowing, movements of the palate (as in "Ah"), and clarity of speech (no hoarseness).

Spinal Accessory

Cranial nerve XI is the spinal accessory nerve. This nerve innervates the sternocleidomastoid and the trapezius muscles. Assessment of its function is determined by resistance to contraction of those muscles and is graded according to manual muscle testing guidelines.

Hypoglossal

Cranial nerve XII is the hypoglossal. It plays a critical role in coordinating swallowing. It is as-

sessed by noting any lateral deviation, atrophy, or tremor of the tongue. Dysphagia may be a result of damage to the hypoglossal nerve.

As the patient regains consciousness, more specific information regarding the cranial nerves previously deferred and the proprioceptive reflexes can be obtained. Refer to previous discussion to assess the deferred cranial nerves.

Proprioceptive reflexes include an awareness of kinesthesia, position in space, and response to vestibular input.[1]

To test kinesthesia hold the proximal interphalangeal joint by a bony prominence so that no pressure is applied on the joint in the direction of movement. For example, hold the medial and lateral borders of this joint then raise the finger up or down while asking the patient to tell in which direction the joint is moved without looking at it. The more distal the joint, the more sensitive the patient to smaller amounts of movement.

To test for position in space a similar maneuver is used. Place the joint on one side of the body in a position, then ask the patient to mimic the position on the other side, again without looking.

The integrity of the vestibular responses can be estimated by testing the balance reactions in sitting and standing (as with CN VIII). These include slight shifts of the patient on a stable surface or slight shifts of the base of support. The patient should be able to maintain an upright position of the head and alignment of the body over the new base of support. Balance requires slight postural adjustments as in sit to stand, or sit on moving surface. It does not necessarily require large ranges of movement. It should be noted that the absence of any of these responses does not necessarily indicate that the vestibular nuclei are damaged but that the reflexes may not be able to be expressed due to tone, joint limitations, or weakness. To assist the patient in expressing his balance reactions the therapist should determine if the limitation to balance is due to tone, joint limitations, or weakness. To accomplish this a musculoskeletal evaluation must be integrated with the neurological examination.

An assessment of higher functioning would indicate the ability to perform more integrated activities, such as stereognosis, two-point discrimination, praxis, etc. These activities usually cannot be performed at the initial examination. However, as the patient becomes more aware, these functions should be assessed. Because they are not critical to the assessment of the early comatose patient, the appropriate tests are listed in Table 6-1, but are not discussed in this chapter. Cerebellar function can also be assessed but only in the patient who has made marked progress in recovery from the coma (Table 6-3). Consequently, those tests have also been listed within the examination table but are not pertinent to the treatment of the initial comatose patient and will not be discussed within this text.

Musculoskeletal Evaluation

The neurological examination must be interpreted in conjunction with the musculoskeletal examination. The musculoskeletal evaluation assesses the patient's ability to respond to stimuli. This information is necessary to differentiate between the patient's ability to perceive and process (neurological) a stimulus and the inability to respond (musculoskeletal) to a stimulus (Table 6-4).

Skeletal Assessment

The patient must have an intact and appropriately aligned skeletal system to be able to move. Because one of the primary causes of head trauma is motor vehicle accidents, the integrity of any fractures must be assessed before allowing the patient to move.

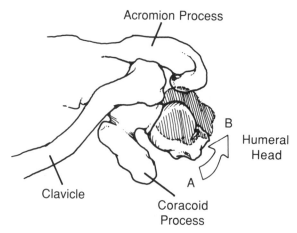

Fig. 6-2 Possible anatomic effects of prolonged supine positioning: humeral head (shaded area) drops backward into a position of reduced mobility.

Resting skeletal alignment can be assessed with the patient in bed or on the mat table. Alignment of the shoulder girdle can give clues to the potentially subluxed shoulder. Normally the clavicle is relatively horizontal and the humerus points into the glenoid fossa.

This alignment may be altered in the bedridden patient in a variety of ways. The humerus may pull away from the scapula (Fig. 6-2) and the clavicle may be elevated or protracted.

Alignment of the spine is critical if the patient is to maintain balance in sitting or standing. Normally, the spine is S-shaped, with a posteriorly

Table 6-3 Assessment of Cerebellar and Cortical Functioning

	Cerebellar Assessment	
Stimuli	Response	Interpretation
Finger to nose	Smooth movement of hand no past pointing	Weakness and poor endurance must be ruled out as a source of error in these activities
Rapid alternating movements	Smooth alternating movements	
Heel toe walking	Accurate, smooth movements	
Standing with feet together, eyes open/eyes closed	Ability to balance	
	Cortical Assessment	

Areas to include: level of consciousness, intellectual performance, emotional status, thought content, sensory interpretation, language, and praxis.
Watch for behavioral responses, affect, language and motor skill. Note changes over time.

Table 6-4 Musculoskeletal Assessment

Skeletal		
A. Alignment	Normal Alignment	Pathological Alignment
1. Shoulder Girdle	Head of humerus in line with glenoid fossa, clavicle relatively horizontal	Subluxed shoulder or elevated/protracted clavicle will limit reach; may be painful
2. Spine	Posterior concavity of cervical and lumbar spine, extension of thoracic spine	Bedrest tends to flatten the lumbar spine and flex the thoracic spine
3. Hip	Full hyperextension available for gait	Bedrest tends to maintain the hip in flexion.
4. Foot	Talocrural dorsiflexion with subtalar inversion, eversion needed for weight shift and gait.	Bedrest tends to place the talocrural joint in plantarflexion, subtalar joint is variable.
B. Joint Assessment	Movements of Particular Importance to the Neurological Patient	Rationale
1. Shoulder Girdle: a. Sternoclavicular joint	Protraction, retraction, elevation, depression	Mobility needed for midrange shoulder flexion and abduction.
b. Glenohumeral	Inferior glide	Inferior glide necessary for abduction/flexion often is overstretched.
2. Spine	Posterior, anterior flexibility for extension	Full extension flexibility is critical for rolling, sitting, and standing balance.
3. Hip	Inferior capsule and anterior capsule mobility	Full inferior capsule flexibility is needed for sitting on the ischium; anterior capsule flexibility is needed for standing balance and weight shift in gait
4. Foot	Posterior capsule of talocrural joint, lateral aspect of subtalar and transverse tarsal joints	Full flexibility of the talocrural capsule is needed to shift weight forward to come to stand and balance in standing. Subtalar and midtarsal mobility is needed to lock the foot into a rigid lever for push off

Muscular

A. Flexibility

1. Stimuli: Place muscle on maximum stretch.
2. Interpretation: Muscle tightness may be imitated by capsular limitations. Joint capsular flexibility must be normal before testing muscle length to rule out the joint's role.

B. Strength

concave lumbar spine. In the comatose patient who has been in bed for any length of time, the spine may go into a relatively straight (flat) position, which, for the lumbar spine, is flexion.

Alignment of the hip joint will influence sitting and standing balance. The ability of the hip to come into more than 90° of flexion with abduction and external rotation is critical for sitting balance. The ability of the hip to come into hyperextension is critical if the patient is to be able to achieve control of the center of gravity during standing and walking. The patient on bedrest spends time in a position of slight flexion and adduction.

The effects of immobilization of a joint in a

given alignment on the available range of motion must be assessed. Because difficulties in alignment due to fractures are treated by the orthopaedist, they will not be discussed further here. Difficulties in alignment seen by the physical therapy clinician include limited range or subluxation due to increased tone, joint limitations, or weakness.

The true role of increased tone in movement dysfunction is still difficult to ascertain. Increased tone is a result of the neurological damage, but much of that tone may be due to spasm to prevent excessive range in a tight joint. This can only be differentiated clinically. Consequently, a joint play assessment of the shoulder girdle, including sternoclavicular and acromioclavicular joints, the spine, hip, and foot, are critical to assess the true role of tone. If any of these joints are limited because of capsular tightness, secondary to the immobility seen from bed rest or the weakness and inability to move against gravity, that tightness must be treated before tone is assessed. As long as the joint is tight, any tendency to push it into full range (i.e., passive range of motion) will tend to overstretch some parts of the joint or compress other parts of the joint, possibly producing a protective spasm.

Joint play is assessed by stabilizing one bone that participates in the joint and moving the other in an anteroposterior cephalocaudal or lateral direction as appropriate to the angle of that joint surface. For example, to assess the mobility of the sternoclavicular joint, the sternum must be stabilized. The only way to stabilize the sternum is to make sure that the ribs and sternum cannot move on the spine. Grasping the distal end of the clavicle, and moving the clavicle on the sternum in a forward-backward direction will determine the amount of the anteroposterior play available at that joint (Fig. 6-3). Grasping the inferior portion of the glenoid fossa of the scapula in the patient's axilla will allow you to move the clavicle in a cephalocaudal direction to assess the superior-inferior mobility of the sternoclavicular joint. These motions are critical for normal scapulohumeral rhythm during all upper extremity activities. Tightness felt within the joint will reflect in an inability to raise the arm past midrange in flexion or abduction. Other joint play assessments are listed within the evaluation (see Table 6-4).

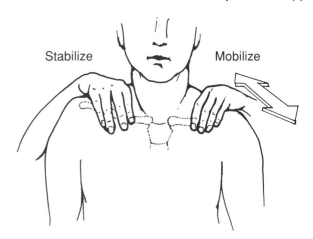

Fig. 6-3 Anterioposterior joint mobility of the sternoclavicular joint.

Muscular Assessment

Once the skeletal system is assessed, the flexibility and strength of the muscles need to be determined.

Muscle Flexibility

After the full joint flexibility is obtained, the flexibility of the muscles (i.e., the length of the muscles) can be evaluated. The joint flexibility must be achieved first because any tightness in the

Table 6-5 Functional Activity Assessment

Rolling
  Abnormalities in rolling may be due to reflexes (ATNR, STNR, TLR*), weakness (back extensors, pectorals, etc.), limited range (back and hip extensors) or tone.
Coming to Sit and Sitting
  Abnormalities in sitting may be due to reflexes (ATNR, STNR, TLR, lack of equilibrium), weakness, limited range (especially lumbar extension, full hip flexion) or tone
Coming to Stand and Standing
  Abnormalities may be due to reflexes (ATNR, STNR, TLR, lack of equilibrium), weakness, limited range (especially lumbar extension, hip extension, talocrural dorsiflexion, subtalar/midtarsal inversion) or tone
Walking
  Abnormalities may be due to reflexes (ATNR, STNR, TLR, lack of equilibrium), weakness, limited range (lumbar spine, hip hyperextension, ankle dorsiflexion) or tone

* ATNR = assymmetrical tonic neck reflex, STNR = symmetrical tonic neck reflex, TLR = tonic labyrinthine reflex.

joint will result in an apparent shortening of the muscle because of limited range at the joint. For example, during pectoralis major flexibility testing in which the patient is supine, the shoulder is flexed and abducted to approximately 120°. The pectoralis major is put on stretch. Should there be any tightness in the sternoclavicular joint, it will be impossible for the shoulder to get true flexion and abduction of that range. The patient will appear to have a tight pectoralis major when in fact it is the sternoclavicular joint that is tight. Specific flexibility testing can be found in the assessment (see Table 6-4).

Muscle Strength

After the joint is free to move and the muscles are flexible enough to cross the full joint range, an assessment of the muscular strength must be obtained. All of the muscles require minimal strength in isometric, eccentric, and concentric contractions for functional activities. If the patient shows an ability to perform isolated muscle contractions, a manual muscle test can be performed. However, since many of the recovering comatose patients are so weak that they must recruit other muscles to assist them in performing an activity, manual muscle tests are often replaced by functional activities (Table 6-5). By looking at the type of contraction that the muscle can perform, some idea of the patient's strength can be obtained. For example, the "plopping" that is often seen (i.e., the falling backward into the chair) in a patient with an extended knee who is asked to go from stand to sit, may be due to the patient's inability to perform an eccentric contraction of the quadriceps. Instead he maintains the knee extension and falls into the chair. If eccentric weakness of the quadriceps limits the patient's function, the therapeutic program needs to work on eccentric contraction of these muscles.

Functional Activities Evaluation

Depending on the degree of mobility and awareness available to the recovering patient, active mobility can be assessed grossly. This assessment usually progresses from gross motor movements, as in the developmental sequence, to fine motor control, such as isolated movements of specific joints. During the functional mobility portion of the assessment, it is important to note the following:

1. Can the patient do the activity voluntarily or does the patient need manual assistance or verbal cuing?
2. What is the active range available to the patient in a given position?
3. Can the patient maintain the position with and without disturbing influences; that is, can he balance there?
4. Does the patient have the strength to obtain and maintain a given position? To which muscles can the strength be attributed?

For example, as the patient rolls from a prone to supine position, does he have enough active mobility to perform the activity himself or does he need verbal or manual cues? Does the patient have enough thoracic and lumbar extension to get his head up or his arm free during the roll? Does he have enough concentric strength of the back extensors and/or the pectorals to roll with control? Specific assessment of tone, range of motion, and strength during the developmental activities and common substitutions and their causes are reviewed in the assessment chart.

Treatment is designed to correct the causes of the limitation in the ability to move. For example, if the difficulty in rolling is a lack of lumbar and thoracic extension to allow the head to come up, then spinal range of motion must be increased. If the problem is due to lack of strength, then strengthening activities are designed. If, on the other hand, the problem is due to the neurological damage itself, the cause may not be amenable to therapeutic treatment.

Often it is noted that the difficulty with the individual movements is due to interference of reflexes, such as the ATNR, symmetrical tonic neck reflex (STNR), or tonic labrynthine reflex, which were released because of the neurological damage. In the intact human, these reflexes are normally present and are often called on to assist in performance of an activity (i.e., the fencer uses the ATNR as does the basketball player when making a shot). The recovering comatose patient also calls on these reflexes to aid him in performing functional activities. For example, the patient may have difficulty rolling prone to supine because of an inability to overcome the tonic labrynthine reflex. It must be determined whether it is the reflex that is limiting the ability to roll or if the patient has resorted to the reflex because he does not have the range or the strength to roll in any other way. This can only be assessed by

1. Determining strength and range
2. Treating any limitations
3. Reassessing the patient's ability to roll to determine if he still requires the tonic labyrinthine reflex.

Often when the strength and range limitations are removed, the use of the reflex disappears.

PRINCIPLES OF TREATMENT

Before applying treatment strategies to the comatose patient, a thorough understanding of recovery of function and mechanisms of disability is required to guide the intervention strategies. After damage is inflicted on the nervous system, it attempts to repair itself. During this neural recovery of function, the patient is often confined to bed to allow stabilization of the repairing organism.

This neural recovery of function may occur through several mechanisms, including diaschisis, equal potentiality, vicarious function, behavioral substitution, functional reorganization, denervation supersensitivity, or collateral sprouting[2] (Table 6-6).

As can be seen from Table 6-6, much of the improvement noted in neurologically impaired patients can be attributed to natural improvements occurring within the brain itself, regardless of any therapeutic intervention.

While the nervous system is attempting to repair itself, the prolonged bed rest may lead to musculoskeletal complications because of the immobility and weakness from the inactivity. These musculoskeletal complications may include

1. Connective tissue tightening within the joint capsule itself
2. Muscle atrophy
3. Weakness resulting from disuse and stretch due to unusual positioning

During the acute phase of therapy, these musculoskeletal complications must be minimized. Later, as the patient is ready for more intensive

Table 6-6 Mechanisms of Recovery of Function

Mechanism	Neural/Anatomical Basis of Mechanism	Influence of Therapy
Diaschisis	Injury to one part of the nervous system may cause alteration of functioning in other parts (neural shock)	As the nervous system repairs itself the function of noninjured parts may return. Therapy will not necessarily affect this.
Equal potentiality	Undamaged areas of the brain may have the capacity to acquire functions of the damaged area	May or may not affect this area
Vicarious function	Undamaged areas of the brain may be able to "learn" the lost function but subtle deficits in its primary role may be apparent	May or may not affect this area
Behavioral substitution	The ability to perform an activity without the neural substrate i.e. elbow extension in C5 quad is accomplished by joint locking.	May assist this area
Collateral sprouting	Anomalous nervous connections can be established as nondamaged neurons attempt to innervate an area	May or may not affect this area
Denervation supersensitivity	Postsynaptic membrane can become more sensitive to smaller amounts of transmitter such that minimal transmitter can produce a response	An anatomical/physiological response; may or may not affect this area

Table 6-7. Principles of Treatment During the Acute Phase

Treatment Modality	Rationale for Modality
Positioning in bed	1. Variety of positions for each joint to prevent the joint capsule from excessively tightening and muscles from excessively shortening 2. Support joints so that excessive stretch is not placed on them (i.e. glenohumeral joint) 3. Minimize vascular stasis and pressure sores
Passive range of motion	1. Maintain muscle flexibility (cardinal plane range of motion) 2. Maintain capsular flexibility (joint play)
Maintenance of clear respiratory tract	Clear secretions to allow efficient oxygen transport
Sensory stimulation	Sensory stimulation may influence the reticular activating system (RAS). Activation of this system is required before the patient can arouse from the coma

exercise, the program must include exercise principles that will minimize the effects of immobility on the musculoskeletal and cardiovascular system so that endurance can be regained. Principles of motor learning that may influence the nervous system can be incorporated to assist the patient in coping with the damaged part of the nervous system.

Physical therapy intervention can be categorized into an acute phase and a later rehabilitation phase.

Physical Therapy in the Acute Phase

Positioning

The deleterious effects of immobility during the acute phase can be minimized by

1. Accurate positioning in bed.
2. Performance of appropriate passive range of motion.
3. Maintenance of a clear respiratory tract (if indicated).
4. Sensory stimulation to produce appropriate responses (Table 6-7)

Variations in positioning of all joints are critical in the immobile patient in order to

1. Maintain the flexibility of the ligaments around and within the joint capsule
2. Maintain the flexibility of the connective tissue within the muscle
3. Prevent the occurrence of decubitus ulcers.

Three positions used are supine and sidelying on either side.

It should be noted that good positioning will help maintain the skeletal alignment and joint integrity of the body. Each joint has specific characteristics that must be considered in positioning. The patient needs to be positioned so that the humerus is supported within the glenoid fossa to prevent gravity from pulling it away from the glenoid fossa. For example, in the supine position, the humerus is pulled toward the bed by gravity, but the glenoid fossa points approximately 40° above the horizontal. This position can put an abnormal stress on the anterior capsule and could contribute to overstretching as seen in subluxation. To prevent this from happening, the humerus must be supported in line with the joint (see Fig. 6-2).

Principles of good positioning require that a change of position be incorporated throughout the day. This change will help to move the joints and to decrease pressure over isolated areas of the skin. The positioning itself will not maintain the flexibility of the connective tissue surrounding the joints in these ranges.

Passive Range of Motion

Passive range of motion assists in maintaining the flexibility of the connective tissues, including muscles, ligaments, and joint capsules, and may possibly provide neural input to the recovering nervous system.[3] During passive range of motion, the goal is to maintain joint alignment throughout the range. This becomes particularly important at joints, such as the shoulder, where overstretching of parts of the capsule can lead to subluxation. For example, at the shoulder, the glenoid fossa normally faces approximately 40° above the horizontal in the supine patient. Consequently, when providing passive range of motion to the supine patient, abduction with the humerus lying along the bed or supporting surface is actually performed with some horizontal extension, which allows the potential for overstretching of the anterior capsule and structures including the coracohumeral ligament. This ligament maintains the scapulohumeral integrity in an upright position,[4] and overstretching it may lead to instability or predispose to a subluxation of the glenohumeral joint. The rationales to remember while doing passive range of motion at each joint are identified in Table 6-7.

Sensory Stimulation

Sensory stimulation is given to the comatose patient to (1) activate the nervous system, and to (2) elicit reflex responses. Changing the stimuli prevents habituation to constant input regardless of the modality. Various forms of sensory stimulation have been advocated. (Table 6-8)

Treatment During the Rehabilitation Phase

As the patient begins to show evidence of gaining motor control, three key problems underlying his motor deficits emerge.

1. Weakness

2. Limitation of range
3. Increased tone

The weakness is a result of (1) neural damage, (2) immobility, and/or (3) excessive stretching or shortening. The weakness caused by neural damage may be a result of damage to descending motor tracts. Input from these tracts go to the alpha motor neurons in the spinal cord and influences the amount of force a given muscle can produce. The imposed immobility can produce weakness from disuse. Excessive stretching or shortening will produce weakness because of the decreased numbers of crossbridges available within the muscle to create tension.

Limitation of range is usually not a function of the neurological damage per se, but rather a function of the imposed immobility. This immobility then produces tightness in the joint capsules, ligaments, and muscular tissues.

Increased tone is thought to result from the neural damage itself. This concept is supported by the observation that the tone only occurs after neural damage. It is thought to be caused by a release of inhibitory mechanisms from higher neural centers.[1] Another source for the increased tone seen in some orthopaedic patients seems to be related to a protective spasm mechanism. The mechanism requires the muscle to contract to maintain tension as a joint is placed near the end of its range. In the joint where the capsule and ligamentous structures are prematurely signaling the end of range, the muscles respond by spasming

Table 6-8 Sensory Stimulation

Modality	Method	Expected Response to Modality
Olfaction	Hold vials of vinegar, ammonia etc. under patient's nose	Turns head away, facial grimacing
Audition	Radio or television, talking to the patient	Turns head toward sound, response to conversation (i.e., squeeze fingers, raise arm)
Vision	Television or other visual stimuli	Orienting to stimulus
Proprioception	Deep pressure or traction through a joint, change position (i.e., sit from supine, quick stretch)	Occasional muscle contractions, attempted balance reactions, muscle contractions
Vestibular input	Changing positions, weight shift in sitting	Righting/equilibrium responses, muscle contractions
Tactile input	Rubbing/stroking skin in dermatome matching muscle innervated	Contraction of muscle

to keep the joint from becoming overstretched. The appearance of this spasm may be interpreted as increased tone. This spasm must be reduced before the assessment of the tone problem. The same mechanism may be at work in neurological patients, including the comatose patient.

An Exercise Approach

Because it is difficult to assess any one of these problems (weakness, limitation in range, tone) due to the overlying effects of the other two, treatment needs to be directed to all three. This can be done in a number of ways. The following progression illustrates the integration of techniques that will strengthen a given set of muscles, stretch ligaments and capsules of the appropriate joints to the appropriate amount of range for an activity, and decrease tone. These combinations allow a progression of functional activities.

One approach to solving both muscular and structural problems secondary to bed rest is to combine techniques that affect both problems into one exercise. Neurological techniques produce exercises that can strengthen muscles, while mobilization techniques stretch the tightened structural elements (capsules, ligaments, muscles, etc.)

Mobilization techniques use specific hand placement and pressure to stretch joint capsules and ligaments. These techniques provide the joint supportive structures enough flexibility to allow normal arthrokinematic (roll and slide) movements for (1) normal peripheral input from the joints to the CNS, (2) smooth joint movement with a minimum of muscle force, and (3) normal wear of the joint surfaces.[4] Neurological techniques can incorporate principles of mobilization to pinpoint hand placement, pressure, and joint play for adequate range of motion.

Mobilization techniques can incorporate principles of neurology to use joint receptors to influence muscle tone and coordinate sensory input from joints, muscles, and skin as a base to relearn normal movement. The following treatment program uses principles of neural treatment techniques and mobilization treatment techniques to

1. Strengthen muscles
2. Increase range
3. Influence tone

4. Improve the functional abilities of the neurological patient

The following sections are organized by joint problem. Each problem includes an assessment and techniques that incorporate neurological and orthopaedic principles to obtain full range while strengthening areas around the joint to produce normal functional activity. Because a common sequence followed in the rehabilitation of the comatose patient involves the developmental sequence, techniques for each joint will be illustrated that can be incorporated at any stage during the developmental sequence.

Hip

One of the most common limitations that prevents normal movement throughout the developmental sequence is limitations in range of motion at the hip. This is particularly true for abduction and extension range. The presence of these limitations require that the entire hip capsule be assessed, especially the anterior and inferior portions. Tightness in the anterior capsule limits extension and external rotation. Tightness in the inferior portion limits extension and abduction.

Before treating the patient, it must be determined if the limitation is due to (1) weakness, (2) muscle or (3) capsular tightness, or (3) increased tone. Before assessing muscle flexibility or tone, the joint capsule flexibility must be assessed. To assess hip joint play, stabilize the pelvis and move the femur sequentially laterally, anteriorly, posteriorly, and inferiorly. If appropriate play is not available, the capsule is tight and must be stretched (mobilized) before continuing the assessment.

After capsular flexibility has been obtained, muscle flexibility can be assessed. Stabilize the pelvis by flexing one hip as far as it will go and letting the other leg fall to the table. If the leg does not go all the way to the table, the iliopsoas, rectus femoris, or tensor fasciae latae could be tight, in which case they must be stretched before determining the deleterious effects of tone and weakness on movement.

The next phase of the assessment is muscle strength. Allowing the patient to move in functional activities can give an indication of strength. While observing a patient's movements note the type of contractions that the patient uses with each

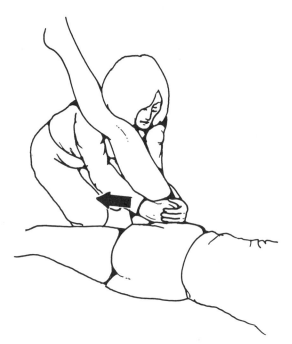

Fig. 6-4 Caudal glide of the hip: supine.

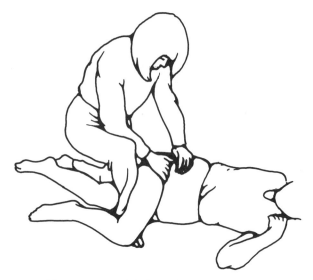

Fig. 6-5 Caudal glide of the hip: sidelying.

muscle group. Activities can be designed to increase isometric, eccentric, or concentric strength.

Finally, the influence of tone on the patient's motor performance may be estimated. Since it is difficult to define tone it is also difficult to treat it.

Treatment of the Hip. The joint capsule may be stretched either directly through mobilization techniques or indirectly through careful hand placement and pressure, as in the neurophysiological techniques used in neurodevelopmental treatment (NDT)[5], proprioceptive neuromuscular facilitation (PNF)[6], Rood [7], etc. To stretch the anterior and inferior capsule directly you may use specific mobilization techniques. To incorporate the mobilization with neurological techniques

1. Begin with the patient supine and with the hip in as much flexion as possible.
2. Stabilize the pelvis.

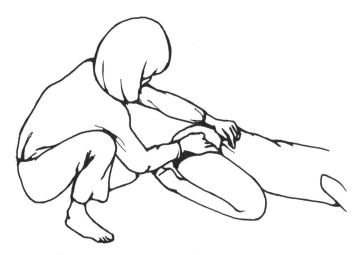

Fig. 6-6 Caudal glide of the hip: forward crouch.

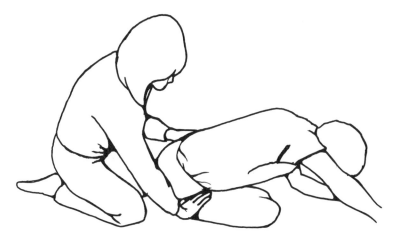

Fig. 6-7 Caudal glide of the hip: side sitting.

3. Grasp the anterior surface of the thigh as close to the inguinal ligament as possible.
4. Your pressure will then be to pull the femur inferiorly and laterally. As you gain abduction range begin to incorporate the rolling techniques from the neurophysiological principles (Fig. 6-4). Maintain the leg in as much abduction and flexion as possible as the patient rolls. By using the hip as a "key point" and maintaining the pressure in an inferior and lateral direction, you may see changes in the patient's tone as he begins to participate in rolling. If you allow the leg to go into extension, the patient will roll from supine to prone. (Fig. 6-5) If you maintain the hip in flexion and abduction you can then continue to put your pressure from your hand placement inferiorly and laterally and have the patient go from supine to sitting on a mat.

Independent sitting requires that the pelvis come forward on the hips so that the lumbar spine can extend (align itself) and sitting balance can be maintained on the ischia. The stretch you have just placed on the inferior capsule of the hip as you assisted the patient to roll will help the patient to sit better (i.e., with the pelvis lying over the femurs (Figs. 6-6 and 6-7). Inferior capsule mobility can be further enhanced by allowing the pelvis to shift forward and backward several times as the patient practices weight shift in preparation for standing (Fig. 6-8).

To continue the developmental sequence in allowing the patient to go from sit to stand, the anterior hip capsule must also be flexible enough to allow the patient to come into full hip hyperextension. If the patient cannot come into this full hip hyperextension, he will require too much muscle to maintain his balance in standing. Ante-

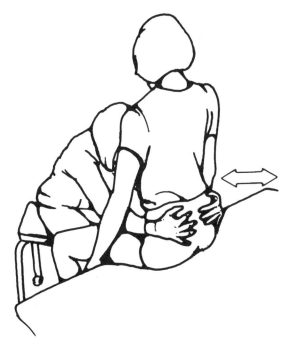

Fig. 6-8 Pelvic shift forward and backward to enhance inferior capsule mobility.

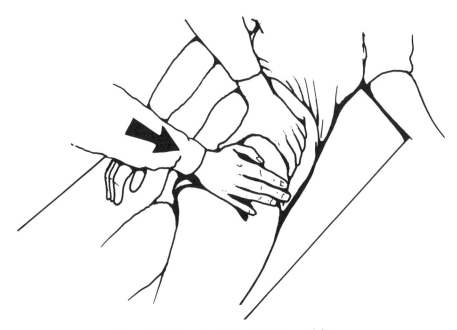

Fig. 6-9 Anterior glide of the hip: sidelying.

rior hip capsule mobility can be achieved also in rolling by stabilizing the pelvis and placing your hand over the neck of the femur approximately along the gluteal fold. With the pelvis stable, anterior pressure of the femur into the capsule will stretch the anterior capsule, allowing full extension of the hip (Figs. 6-9, 6-10). After this capsule flexibility has been obtained and the patient has achieved sitting, exercises that emphasize sit to stand will strengthen the necessary muscles to get into standing. Full range at the hip will decrease the need for muscles to maintain standing.

Achievement of these developmental skills may require range of motion in motor control at joints other than the hip. Using the same sequence, hand placements can be described and illustrated that will use mobilization and neurological techniques and principles to gain range and control at joints other than the hip. The joints illustrated include the spine and shoulder girdle, as these are primary problem areas. Other joints may also benefit from the combination of mobilization and neurological techniques, but assessment of other joints is difficult until the hip, spine, and shoulder are mobile. Consequently, emphasis will be placed on proximal mobility.

Spine Sequence

Patients who have been on prolonged bed rest, such as those in a coma, lose extension mobility in the lumbar and thoracic spine. This loss of mobility contributes to the difficulty in (1) rolling, (2) maintaining prone on elbows, (3) sitting balance, and (4) standing balance.

If the difficulty in performing the intended activity (such as rolling, coming to sit, or coming to stand) is caused by a limitation in spinal mobility, joint play of the spine needs to be checked. Usually the lumbar and thoracic spines are tight in flexed

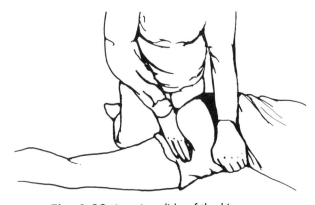

Fig. 6-10 Anterior glide of the hip: prone.

positions (compared to normal, alignment) due to positioning in bed. Therefore, extension techniques are often helpful to achieve improved sitting and standing balance, as well as rolling.

Initial assessment of the spine can be performed by observing the patient in prone or sitting. If the patient is unable to achieve normal lumbar and thoracic extension in either of these positions, it is possible that the joints themselves are tight. To assess the tightness of the spinal joints

1. Place your pisiform on the spinous process of each vertebra.
2. Press down (posterior to anterior) to assess the amount of spring in the ligaments.
3. Assess each joint progressing up or down the spine, avoiding the cervical spine.
4. Compare the flexibility that you feel with what should normally exist (i.e., there should be less extension available in the thoracic spine than in the upper or midlumbar spine, but all parts of the spine should have some give to them.)
5. If you find decreased flexibility you can use standard mobilization techniques, repeat the assessment movements, or incorporate the techniques into the neurophysiological approaches.

Spine Treatment. Hand placement over each vertebra with anteriorly directed pressure starting with the patient in prone should increase the flexibility of the spine, allowing improved rolling or the ability of the patient to come prone on elbows (Fig. 6-11). Resisting the patient's attempts to come to prone on elbows will increase the strength necessary to achieve the position, as well as allow the patient to gain mobility to the joints themselves.

The same principle can be incorporated into weight shifting forward with the patient in the sitting position. Place your fingers along the transverse process of the lumbar spine and pull anteriorly as the patient shifts weight forward from the hips, maintaining the head position. Continue pressure until a normal lumbar alignment is achieved.

If the weight shifting is continued forward the activity progresses from sitting balance to a coming-to-stand exercise. Spinal alignment is critical in standing to place the center of gravity over the

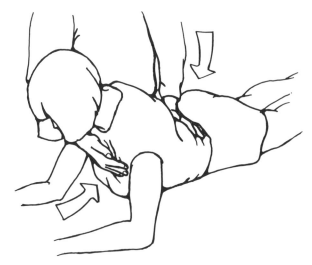

Fig. 6-11 Anterioposterior glide of the spine: prone.

base of support, thus allowing maintenance of balance with minimal muscle contraction. This alignment structurally decreases the muscular effort needed to maintain the position and improve efficiency in standing.

Shoulder Sequence

The third area of proximal tightness in patients who have been immobile for prolonged periods of time is the shoulder girdle. This is particularly the case at the sternoclavicular joint, which allows (1) protraction, (2) retraction, (3) elevation, (4) depression, and (5) rotation of the clavicle. These movements are critical to position the scapula as the humerus is elevated in abduction or flexion. Limitation in mobility produces

1. A reach in abduction or flexion of less than 90°
2. Inability to weight shift in prone on elbows (which requires sternoclavicular protraction and retraction)
3. An inability to crawl or creep backwards and forwards (which requires sternoclavicular elevation and depression).

Immobility at this joint can be assessed by observation during elevation of the arm and by assessing the joint play. If limitation is found, specific mobilization techniques can be used or the techniques can be incorporated in the neurophysiological treatment approach.

Shoulder Treatment. Using the sample treatment outlined for the other joints, pressure can be exerted through the sternocclavicular joint by grasping the clavicle (Fig. 6-12) and protracting/retracting it as the patient shifts weight anteriorly and posteriorly (as pushing up prone on elbows) or elevating and depressing the clavicle (as the patient weight shifts by pushing backwards in a prone on elbows position).

The same principles can be incorporated into techniques used to improve reach in sitting. "Shaking," a technique used to decrease tone, can be used to increase the shoulder range by shaking (protraction or retraction) the clavicle enough to produce a movement in the sternoclavicular joint (see Fig. 6-12). This can allow the clavicle scapula complex enough range to provide more normal reach. While doing this it should be noted that the spine must be stabilized to allow the motion to occur at the sternoclavicular joint alone (Fig. 6-13). The stability of the spine helps to stabilize the ribs and thereby stabilizes the sternum. After mobility and strength have been achieved, the patient can practice the developmental sequence or perform other exercises to improve activities.

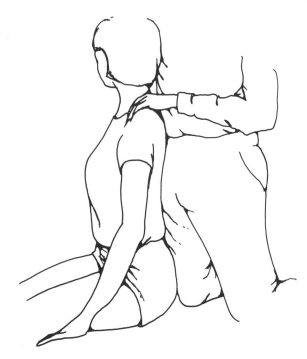

Fig. 6-13 Shoulder retraction isolating motion to the sternoclavicular joint.

Providing motion and strength at the shoulder girdle, spine, and pelvis may improve functional activities considerably. It is feasible that tightness at other joints may limit function. This is particularly true of the sacroiliac joint for weight shifting, ankle for standing, and wrist for grasping. The same principles for treating these joints can be applied during the developmental sequence.

Sacroiliac Joint

The sacroiliac joint provides minimal measurable mobility when normal range exists but marked dysfunction when limited range is found. This joint absorbs forces coming up from the floor and down from the trunk. It also appears to be critical to allow full dissociation of the lower extremities. That is, movement in this joint is necessary to allow one hip to flex while the other extends in activities such as

1. Rolling
2. Coming to sit from prone
3. Sit to half kneel
4. Half kneel to stand
5. Stride length in gait (clinical observations)

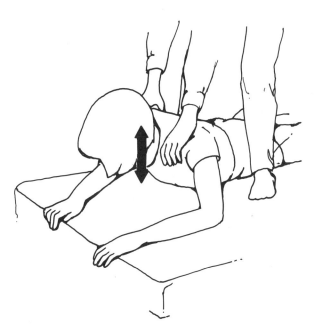

Fig. 6-12 Sternoclavicular retraction and protraction (shaking): prone.

Orthopaedic assessment of this joint requires movement on the part of the patient usually not available to the neurologically involved patient. Instead, immobility in this pair of joints can be inferred by observing the patient's movements. Can the client (1) roll with one hip fully flexed and the other extended, (2) obtain runner's stretch position, (3) come to half kneel or (4) show normal stride length? Inability to be placed in these positions suggests immobility in the sacroiliac joints.

Treatment of the Sacroiliac Joint. Modification of therapist's hand placement while working from prone to sit can achieve increased mobility in the sacroiliac joints. As depicted in Figure 6-14, the therapist's right hand and patient's right leg stabilize the patient's right ilium. The therapist oscillates the patient's left ilium forward. This can be followed by a functional activity requiring this range (i.e., coming to sit over the right hip). Rolling

and getting into half kneel are other activities that can use sacroiliac mobility while gaining functional strength. Oscillating movements at the appropriate joint or repetition of exercises stressing mobility at the appropriate joint will assist the patient in achieving active strength and control of his mobility.

The Ankle/Foot Complex

The ankle and foot quickly lose their normal alignments with prolonged bed rest. Three separate joints must work together correctly for normal weight-bearing, weight shifting, and push off in gait. The three joints necessary for these activities are the (1) talocrural joint, (2) subtalar joint, and (3) transverse tarsal (midtarsal) joint.

The talocrural joint produces dorsiflexion and plantarflexion. The posterior aspect of the joint capsule can become tight preventing dorsiflexion. Figures 6-15 and 6-16 show test and treatment techniques to assess and gain range at the talocrural joint. These techniques should be performed before assessing the gastrocsoleus tightness.

The joint principles can be incorporated into neurological techniques. For example begin with the patient sitting in a wheelchair. As the patient pulls forward as if to come to stand, the therapist

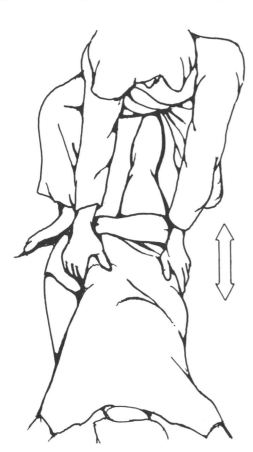

Fig. 6-14 Sacroiliac mobility.

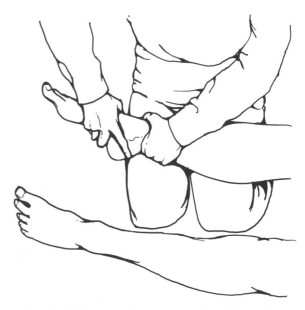

Fig. 6-15 Talocrural anterioposterior glide: supine.

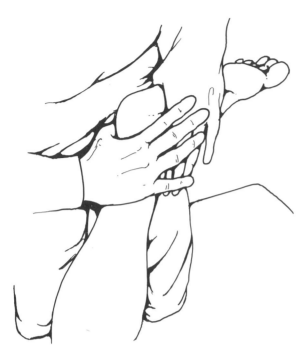

Fig. 6-16 Ankle dystraction for stretching the posterior aspect of the joint capsule.

stabilizes the talus and moves the articular surface of the tibia forward. This forward motion can be achieved by oscillation from the therapist's hand or active weight-shifting by the patient over the stabilized talus.

The subtalar joint produces inversion and eversion, a motion necessary to (1) shift weight through the hind foot, (2) absorb rotary stresses from the superimposed leg, and (3) in inversion, lock the foot into a rigid lever for push off.

Figure 6-17 demonstrates the technique to assess and treat this joint using mobilization principles (medial-lateral slides). Medial and lateral weight shifting over the fixed talus is an exercise from neurological techniques that incorporates the same principle to gain range while increasing muscle strength and active control of this joint.

The transverse tarsal (midtarsal) joint contributes to the total inversion-eversion range available in the foot. This joint is responsible for (1) abduction-adduction, (2) dorsiflexion-plantarflexion range, and (3) supination-pronation range, which makes up inversion and eversion. Because this is the only joint in the foot that can contribute to dorsiflexion if range is limited at the talocrural joint, it is not uncommon for this joint to be hypermobile in dorsiflexion and hypomobile in adduction and inversion. Consequently, it is critical that dorsiflexion occur only at the talocrural joint and not by overstretching the transverse tarsal joint.

Figure 6-18 illustrates hand position to assess this joint. The therapist's left hand stabilizes the patient's calcaneus bone, while the right hand moves the navicular and cuboid bone on the talus

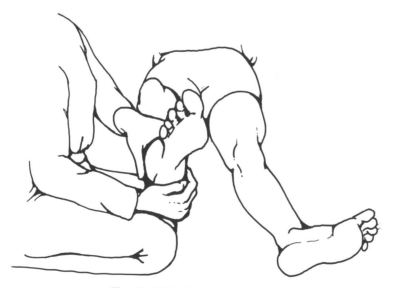

Fig. 6-17 Subtalar joint inversion.

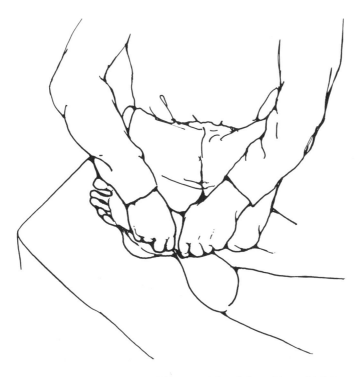

Fig. 6-18 Abduction-adduction glide of the midtarsal joint.

and calcaneus. To incorporate this technique into an exercise requires control of the subtalar joint. For example to assist the patient in gaining the range and strength necessary for push off, the subtalar and transverse tarsal joint must lock into inversion. This can be accomplished by assuring that the joints invert on lateral weight shifting through the foot. Combining this activity with gastrocsoleus strengthening occurs when the patient practices push off.

Wrist
Through a series of movements, the wrist adjusts the length tension relationship of the multiarticular hand muscles. Table 6-9 shows the sequence of joints and the range they contribute to dorsiflexion.

Functional grasp and weight-bearing on the hand both require dorsiflexion. Any limit in dorsiflexion range will limit grasp strength and weight shifting over the hand. This is often seen as an inability to shift forward in quadruped or the tendency to bear weight on the fingers instead of the palm.

Figure 6-19 demonstrates hand placement to assess the movement of the capitate bone on the scaphoid bone. To attain full range, each joint in the wrist must have full mobility. Once the joint mobility is obtained, active control of the joint must follow. This can be accomplished in weight-bearing over the hand, being careful to note that each joint contributes its range in the correct sequence to total dorsiflexion.

Table 6-9 Relationship Between Movements of the Wrist and the Joints Producing the Movement

Range	Movement
Palmar flexion to zero degrees dorsiflexion	Between capitate (with the distal carpals) and the scaphoid
Initial dorsiflexion (exact range variable)	Between scaphoid (with capitate and distal carpals) and the lunate
Terminal dorsiflexion (exact range variable)	Between scaphoid (with lunate and distal carpals) and the radius

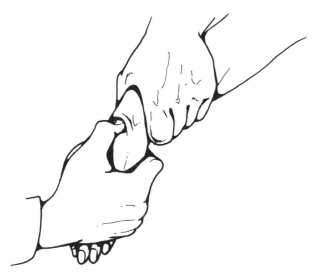

Fig. 6-19 Anterioposterior glide of the wrist.

Regaining control after neurological insult and its concomitant immobility depends on an accurate assessment and treatment program to influence the problems identified in the assessment. These problems are an interaction between neurological damage and the secondary effects of immobility, including increased tendency for (1) respiratory infiltrates, (2) decreased cardiac endurance, (3) muscular weakness and (4) ligamentous tightness. To achieve maximal functional return, the treatment program must incorporate activities to ameliorate problems in each of these areas. The previous sample treatment program stressed one approach: mobilization and strengthening as part of the developmental sequence commonly integrated into neurological techniques. The following section is a brief review of other aids advocated in the rehabilitation of the comatose patient.

Other Aids in the Rehabilitation of the Comatose Patient

Various authors have advocated the use of modalities to aid the rehabilitation of the neurologically involved patient. These include the use of

1. Ice
2. Brushing
3. Vibration[7]
4. Balance reaction[5]
5. Electrical stimulation
6. EMG biofeedback
7. The kinetron[2]
8. Casting[6]

Ice has been advocated by Rood[12] to assist in gaining motor control and by Knott and Voss[8] to influence spasticity. Few studies have documented the effects of this approach.

Small-amplitude, high-frequency vibration produces a state of contraction in the muscle. This has been used clinically on the antagonist to a spastic muscle to produce a reflex inhibition of the muscle. For example, vibration can be applied to the muscle belly of the triceps, to attempt inhibition of the biceps in the upper extremity. Some clinicians have suggested positive effects when using the vibratory reflex, whereas Bishop[9] suggests that the tonic vibratory reflex be used with care and that the patient be carefully selected because motor control may be worsened in cerebellar disorders.

Biofeedback
Biofeedback has been used by many workers to enhance the learning of new skills. The literature shows conflicting results, with some researchers noting significant functional gains[10] and others[11] reporting no significant gains.

Tone-Reducing Casts, Inhibitive Casting, Total Contact Casting
This technique involves applying plaster or resin cast to an appropriately prepositioned joint to maintain its position during functional activities. Reports of effectiveness vary with the researchers, some finding them very effective in decreasing tone and thereby increasing motor ability.[7] In contrast, unrealistic goals for the casting, as well as side effects resulting from inaccurate application of the technique, may account for some apparent ineffectiveness. These techniques must be used cautiously, as improper casting can lead to problems, such as nerve palsies, decubitus ulcers, and overstretching of joint support structures.

Isokinetic Devices
Nelson[2] reports that hemiparetic patients be treated with bilateral reciprocal isokinetic exercise via kinetron. After treatment his patients showed significantly increased unilateral stance, velocity,

and ambulation and ability to rapidly shift weight and step from one foot to the other.

SUMMARY

Coma is a state of altered consciousness that has many causes. It could be as a result of direct injury to the brain stem, injury to other parts of the brain putting pressure on the brain stem, or severe and massive injury throughout the neural axis. Its presence is generally noted as an unresponsiveness to any stimuli, no active movement, and no communication. Because these patients are often put on bed rest, subsequent problems develop including

1. Shortening of connective tissue structures, such as joint ligaments, capsules, muscles, and tendons
2. Unusual joint alignment as seen in the flexed posture of the lumbar spine and the plantar flexion of the ankles
3. Compromise to the cardiovascular system
4. Muscle weakness and hypertonicity

Given this list of problems, treatment and assessment needs to be aimed at each of the different systems. Cardiorespiratory function must be stabilized and the airways maintained for appropriate respiratory function. Some have suggested that the use of reflexive responses to sensory input helps alert and orient the comatose patient. These stimuli may include sight, sound, smell, proprioception, and touch. Flexibility of the connective tissue structures needs to be maintained should any motor control return. This is accomplished using range of motion and maintaining joint play in all of the joints. This flexibility may decrease the amount of spasm becaue the joint is protected upon movement, which occurs as initial return of motor control becomes evident. Finally, active exercise, either through the use of the developmental sequence or specific exercises for specific groups of muscles, needs to be incorporated into the program so that the muscle strength can be redeveloped. As the patient improves these exercises, along with maintenance of the joint flexibility, need to be incorporated into a training program that will stress the cardiovascular system enough to build up functional endurance to allow the patient to participate in normal activities of daily living without becoming excessively fatigued.

REFERENCES

1. Kandel E, Schwartz J: Principles of Neural Science. Elsevier, New York, 1981
2. Nelson A: Strategies for improving motor control. In Rosenthal M, Griffith E, Bond M, Miller J (eds): Rehabilitation of the Head Injured Adult. p. 241 FA Davis, Philadelphia, 1983
3. Lundberg A, Malmgren K, Schomburg E: Role of joint afferents in motor control exemplified by effects on reflex pathways from 1b afferents. J Physiol (London) 284:327, 1978
4. Norkin C, Levangie P: Joint Structure and Function; A Comprehensive Analysis. F. A. Davis, Philadelphia, 1983
5. Bobath B: Adult Hemiplegia: Evaluation and Treatment. Heinemann, London, 1978
6. Cusick B, Sussman M: Short leg casts: their role in the management of cerebral palsy. Physical and Occupational Therapy in Pediatrics. 2:93, 1982
7. Stockmeyer S: A sensorimotor approach to treatment. p. 186 In Pearson P, Williams C (eds): Physical Therapy Services in the Developmental Disabilities. Charles C Thomas, Springfield, IL, 1972
8. Knott M, Voss DE: Proprioceptive Neuromuscular Facilitation. Harper & Row, New York, 1968
9. Bishop B: Vibratory stimulation, Part 3. Phys Ther 55:139, 1975
10. Brundy J, Grynbaum B, Korein J: Spasmodic torticalles: treatment by feedback display of EMG. Arch Phys Med Rehabil 55:403, 1974
11. Lee K, Hill E, Johnston R, Smichorowski T: Myofeedback for muscle re-training in hemiplegic patients. Arch Phys Med Rehabil 57:588, 1976
12. Stockmeyer S: An interpretation of the approach of Rood to the treatment of neuromuscular dysfunction. In Proceedings: An Exploratory and Analytical Survey of Therapeutic Exercise. Arch Phys Med Rehabil 46:900, 1967

7 Vestibular Stimulation in the Treatment of Postural and Related Deficits

Anne G. Fisher and Anita C. Bundy

OVERVIEW

There has been a recent trend toward an increased emphasis on the use of vestibular stimulation as a therapeutic modality. This trend is reflected not only in recent reviews of research on the use of vestibular stimulation,[1-5] but also in the number of physical and occupational therapy textbooks that discuss the use of vestibular stimulation in treatment.[6-11]

The objective of this chapter is to describe and discuss vestibular stimulation as it may be used to treat postural and associated disorders in patients with (1) vestibular deficits arising from hypothesized central nervous system (CNS) dysfunction at the level of the brain stem vestibular nuclei, and (2) higher level CNS damage. Because all static positions and/or movement patterns facilitate the vestibular system, *vestibular stimulation is a component of all therapeutic activity.* However, the emphasis in this chapter is on techniques to enhance stimulation of the vestibular mechanism to remediate deficits believed to respond to *augmented vestibular stimulation.* After a brief review of the anatomical, neurophysiological, and functional principles that underlie treatment planning, evaluation procedures and the use of vestibular stimulation to treat (1) abnormalities of muscle tone (including postural-ocular movement disorder), (2) gravitational insecurity, and (3) intolerance to movement and provoked vertigo are presented. Indications for the use of linear versus rotary vestibular stimula-tion are included. The final section discusses precautions in the use of vestibular stimulation.

BASIC NEUROANATOMICAL, NEUROPHYSIOLOGICAL, AND FUNCTIONAL PRINCIPLES FOR TREATMENT PLANNING

The vestibular receptors include the semicircular canals and the otolith organs (utricle and saccule). Both are able to detect movement in the three orthogonal planes of three-dimensional space; hence, they respond to movement of the head in any direction[12,13] (Table 7-1).

The semicircular canals are angular accelerom-eters, which detect changes in the rate of angular or rotational movements of the head in space.[12,13] They respond most efficiently to high frequency stimuli (i.e., head movements greater than 0.01 to 0.10 Hz).[13-15] This response is primarily short-term or transient (i.e., phasic).[12,13,15]

The otolith organs are linear accelerometers, which detect both changes in rate of linear move-ment of the head and static position of the head in space.[12,13] They respond to low-frequency stim-uli (i.e., head movements less than 0.01 to 0.10 Hz).[13-15] The response of the otolith organs is primarily long-term or sustained (i.e., tonic).[12,13,15]

Semicircular canal spinal afferents project to the medial, descending, and lateral (Deiters') vestibu-lar nuclei which, in turn, primarily project bilat-erally, via the medial vestibulospinal pathway, to

Table 7-1   Summary of Semicircular Canal and Otolith Organ Response Characteristics

	Semicircular Canals	Otolith Organs
Effective stimuli (Head movement)	Angular Transient High frequency	Linear Sustained Low frequency/position
Response	Phasic extension of downhill limbs and flexion of uphill limbs Phasic righting of the head and upper trunk	Tonic extension of downhill limbs and flexion of uphill limbs Maintained (tonic) righting of the head and upper trunk

axial muscle alpha and gamma motoneurons of the neck and upper trunk. To a lesser extent, semicircular canal afferents also project ipsilaterally, via the lateral vestibulospinal pathway, to limb and axial alpha and gamma motoneurons.[12,13]

Otolith organ spinal afferents project primarily to the lateral vestibular nucleus, which, in turn, projects ipsilaterally, via the lateral vestibulospinal pathway, to primarily limb, but also axial, alpha and gamma motoneurons of the neck and upper trunk. To a lesser extent, otolith organ spinal afferents also descend to neck and upper trunk alpha and gamma motoneurons via the medial vestibulospinal pathway.[12,13]

Medial and lateral vestibulospinal responses act on antigravity extensor muscles so as to elicit *compensatory* head, trunk, and limb movements, which serve to oppose head perturbations, postural sway, or tilt. Transient tilt or rotational head movements stimulate the semicircular canals such that the neck muscles, which oppose the motion, phasically contract to stabilize the head in space. Transient head movements, which stimulate the semicircular canals, also result in phasic extension of the limbs on the side of rotation or tilt (downhill limbs) and phasic flexion of the contralateral uphill limbs. Sustained tilt or movement of the head stimulates primarily the otolith organs such that there is maintained downhill limb extension, maintained contralateral uphill limb flexion, and maintained head righting.[12,13]

Transient semicircular canal mediated responses contribute to phasic equilibrium reactions, whereas, otolith organ mediated responses contribute to tonic postural extension and support reactions.[12,13]

Although the beneficial effects of vestibular stimulation as a therapeutic modality have not been proven, behavioral and neurophysiological experimental research suggests the following trends:

1. Vestibular stimulation has the greatest effect on motor/reflex function and visual/auditory ability.[3]
2. Vestibular stimulation has more impact on the development of cerebral palsied or mentally retarded children than on normal, at risk, or premature infants.[3]
3. Vestibular stimulation has a more pronounced effect in younger children and those children with CNS damage who do not demonstrate spasticity.[3,16,17]
4. Linear vestibular stimulation results in relaxation and soothing (inhibition of distress) in infants. Stimulation of greater amplitude and higher frequency results in more pronounced effects.[18-20]
5. The tonic labyrinthine inverted position is more likely to increase extensor tone in normal adults than in adults with spasticity.[21-23]
6. Rotary vestibular stimulation has been shown to have a greater therapeutic effect than linear vestibular stimulation; however, this effect may reflect a confound because a much higher percentage of research studies have used rotary stimulation to influence motor/reflex function.[3] We hypothesize that certain deficits are better treated using linear vestibular stimulation; further research is clearly indicated.

SIGNS AND SYMPTOMS INDICATING VESTIBULAR STIMULATION

Disorders of Sensory Integration[6,24–27]

Postural-Ocular Movement Disorder

It is hypothesized that postural-ocular movement disorder is caused by inefficient processing of vestibular inputs at the level of the brain stem vestibular nuclei and is characterized by the *presence of a meaningful cluster of the following symptoms*:

1. Shortened duration of postrotary nystagmus[27]
2. Inability to assume and/or to maintain the pivot prone (prone extension) position
3. Hypotonicity of extensor muscles
4. Poor equilibrium and support reactions
5. Poor joint stability (co-contraction)
6. Deficient postural background movements

Gravitational Insecurity

Gravitational insecurity is thought to result from hyperresponsiveness to, or poor modulation of, otolith organ input. It is characterized by (1) excessive emotional reactions to vestibular stimuli that are out of proportion to the real threat or danger; and (2) excessive fear of new positions or postures, especially those in which the feet are no longer in contact with the floor.

Intolerance (Adverse Response) to Movement

The cause of intolerance to movement is hypothesized to be hyperresponsiveness, primarily to semicircular canal input. It is characterized by (1) feelings of discomfort, (2) nausea, (3) vomiting, and (4) dizziness or vertigo.

Abnormalities of Muscle Tone Caused by Higher Level CNS Lesions

Abnormalities of muscle tone caused by higher level CNS lesions are characterized by general hypotonicity or hypotonicity of the proximal extensor muscles (especially neck and trunk) with spasticity, athetosis, or ataxia of limb muscles.

Provoked or Positional Vertigo

Provoked or positional vertigo is associated with traumatic head injury and is defined as sensation of apparent self-motion relative to the surround, or sensation of apparent background motion relative to the self.

EVALUATION

Disorders of Sensory Integration

Postural-Ocular Movement Disorder

Duration of Postrotary Nystagmus

1. The use of the Postrotary Nystagmus Test (PRN) is recommended when evaluating children between the ages of 4 and 9 years without frank CNS damage.[27]
2. Shortened duration of postrotary nystagmus is interpreted as indicating hyporesponsiveness or inefficient processing of vestibular inputs at brain stem levels.
3. Prolonged duration of postrotary nystagmus is interpreted as indicating lack of inhibition of the vestibular system by higher CNS structures; prolonged duration of postrotary nystagmus *is not suggestive of a vestibular system disorder.*
4. Although emphasis in the diagnosis of postural-ocular movement disorder is often placed on the results of the PRN, the validity of this emphasis is questionable. Further, a valid diagnosis can be made without the results of this test.[28]
5. Normative data for the PRN are lacking for other age groups or for populations with CNS deficits. Although numerous studies have found depressed scores on the PRN in populations with a variety of diagnoses,[29–34] the interpretation that depressed durations of postrotary nystagmus are indicative of vestibular dysfunction is not recommended until the validity of such an interpretation is demonstrated.

Pivot Prone Position (Fig. 7-1)

1. The pivot prone position is demonstrated to the patient.

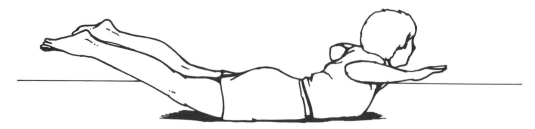

Fig. 7-1 Normal pivot prone (prone extension) position.

2. The patient is requested to assume the pivot prone position. Assistance is given as necessary until it is determined that the patient understands what is being requested.
3. After a brief rest period, the patient is asked to independently assume and maintain the pivot prone position.
4. The length of time the patient can maintain the position is timed with a stopwatch.
5. The quality of response is graded using the form in Table 7-2 (Fig. 7-2).
6. Adults and children 6 years of age and older should obtain quality scores of 6 and be able to maintain the position for 30 seconds.
7. Patients with tight hip flexors and older adults will have difficulty assuming a full pivot prone position.

Hypotonicity of Extensor Muscles
Look for a meaningful cluster of the following signs:

1. Hyperextensibility of distal joints
2. Hypotonic posture in standing, including lordosis or hyperextended and/or locked knees
3. "Mushiness" of muscles upon palpation

Before concluding the patient is hypotonic, rule out the following:

1. Joint laxity
2. Lordosis compensatory to tight hip flexors
3. Normal joint mobility and lordosis seen in toddlers

Equilibrium
Assessment should be made using a variety of tests and in a variety of positions. Objective tests include

1. Standing balance: eyes open and standing balance: eyes closed[26]
2. Bruininks-Oseretsky balance subtest[35]
3. Floor ataxia test battery[36]
4. Standing and walking balance[27]

Table 7-2 Pivot Prone (Prone Extension) Administration and Quality Scoring Criteria[a]

_____	Assumes position smoothly, quickly, and nonsegmentally
_____	Head position held steady and within 45° of vertical
_____	Upper trunk (shoulders, chest, and arms) raised off of floor, arms abducted and externally rotated approximately 90°, elbows flexed approximately 90°
_____	Distal one-third of thigh raised far enough off floor to allow examiner to place fingers between distal thigh and floor; knees can be flexed
_____	Knees flexed 30° or less; thighs do not have to be off floor, but feet cannot touch floor
_____	Able to talk out loud (patient counts time in seconds with stopwatch)

[a] After demonstration and practice (patient is manually assisted into position if necessary), the patient is asked to assume the position independently. Verbal and tactile cues can be given if patient does not initially assume the correct position. Timing begins from when the correct or "best" posture is assumed. Timing stops when (1) the patient's head, upper trunk, or distal thigh touch the floor; (2) the knees flex more than 30°; (3) the patient can no longer talk out loud; or (4) the patient has held the posture for 30 seconds. If the patient's "best" posture does not include all of these components, timing ceases when the patient can no longer maintain any one of the components (not including assumes smoothly, etc.) that the patient could initially perform. Each category, if checked, equals 1. A total score of 6 is possible and indicates a high quality position.

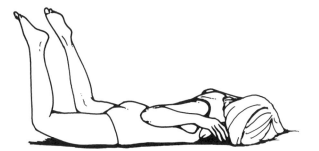

Fig. 7-2 Abnormal pivot prone (prone extension) position. Head position not held within 45° of vertical and knees flexed more than 30°.

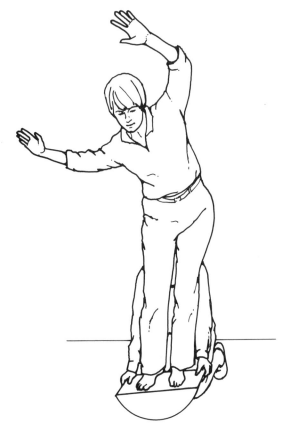

Fig. 7-4 Abnormal adult tilt reaction in standing with arms in "high guard" position and lack of hip and knee flexion of uphill leg.

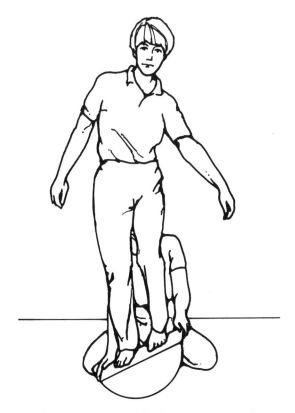

Fig. 7-3 Normal adult tilt reaction in standing.

Subjective tests include tilt reactions (Fig. 7-3) and lateral reach. Vestibular dysfunction in tilt reactions may be indicated by[37–44]

1. Loss of balance at speeds and inclinations readily tolerated by normal subjects of similar age, even when the response behaviorally appears normal

2. Impaired protective or support reactions of the downhill limbs (lack of or failure to maintain downhill extension)
3. Exaggerated abduction or "high guard" position of non-weight-bearing upper extremities (Fig. 7-4)
4. In standing, excessive external rotation of the uphill hip, or lack of uphill hip and knee flexion (normal in 2-, 3-, and 4-year-olds) (Fig. 7-4)

Vestibular dysfunction during lateral reach while standing on a stable and an unstable surface (Fig. 7-5) may be indicated by[37]

1. Failure to lift the uphill foot from the support surface (normal in 2-, 3-, and 4-year-olds) (Fig. 7-6)
2. Knee flexion of the uphill leg (Fig. 7-7)

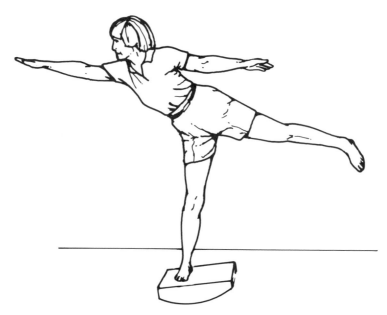

Fig. 7-5 Normal adult equilibrium response during lateral reach while standing on an unstable surface.

3. Elbow flexion and/or failure to abduct the uphill arm (Fig. 7-7)

Poor Joint Stability (Co-contraction)

Joint stability is best tested by asking the patient to assume the quadruped position. An attempt should be made to correct the patient's posture by using verbal and tactile cues. The normal position includes

1. Head neutral
2. Hips, shoulders, and knees flexed 90°
3. Fingers pointing forward
4. Elbows *slightly* flexed
5. Back straight

The patient should be evaluated for persistent

1. Lordosis
2. Hyperextension and/or locking of the elbows
3. Raising of the entire medial border of the scapula
4. Excessive lifting of the inferior angle of the scapula
5. Excessive scapular abduction

Hypotonicity may be ruled out if lordosis is seen in the standing but not in the quadruped position.

Poor Postural Background Movements

Poor postural background movements are characterized by excessive or lack of appropriate postural adjustments during movement or functional use of the extremities. The patient is evaluated by

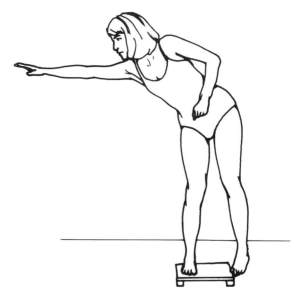

Fig. 7-6 Abnormal adult equilibrium response during lateral reach while standing on a stable surface. Uphill foot remains in contact with support surface and elbow of uphill arm is flexed.

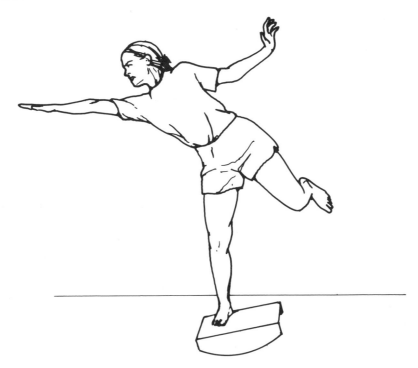

Fig. 7-7 Abnormal adult equilibrium response during lateral reach while standing on an unstable surface. Uphill knee and arm are flexed.

observation during functional activity. The condition is frequently associated with and/or due to poor tonic postural stabilization.

Gravitational Insecurity and Intolerance to Movement

Evaluation for these problems are based on patient interview and clinical observation of relevant signs and symptoms.

Abnormalities of Muscle Tone Caused by Higher Level CNS Lesions

Generalized Muscle Hypotonia

The evaluation for generalized muscle hypotonia is identical to that for postural-ocular movement disorder, but symptoms are frequently more pronounced.

Hypotonicity of Proximal Extensor Muscles With Spasticity, Athetosis, or Ataxia of Limb Muscles

Unlike the patient with generalized hypotonia or postural-ocular movement disorder, the patient with hypotonicity of the proximal extensor muscles frequently (1) fixates the trunk or (2) demonstrates an intermittent overlay of trunk hypertonicity. When inhibitory techniques are used to mobilize the trunk or reduce hypertonicity, the trunk becomes hypotonic. Evaluation is as described for postural-ocular movement disorder but is preceded by appropriate inhibitory techniques. The evaluation is modified according to the functional capabilities of the patient; positions that elicit stereotyped abnormal patterns of movement are avoided (Fig. 7-8).

A meaningful cluster of postural-ocular movement disorder signs and symptoms is interpreted as an indication for the use of vestibular stimulation in treatment, *but not necessarily as indicative of vestibular dysfunction, per se*.

Provoked or Positional Vertigo

Evaluation and treatment of vertigo has not typically been the responsibility of physical or occupational therapists. However, patients with traumatic head injury or other CNS disorders, and

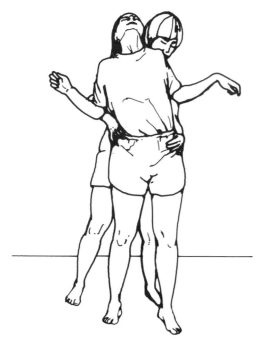

Fig. 7-8 Abnormal posture elicited when evaluating equilibrium in standing by lateral push.

who are treated using vestibular stimulation, may be asked to assume positions or move in a manner that elicits vertigo. Because vertigo can interfere with ongoing therapy, as well as function, evaluation and treatment is indicated. Since the evaluation is an integral part of treatment, evaluation methods are discussed in detail below (see Case J.).

PRINCIPLES OF TREATMENT

Postural-Ocular/Tone Disorders
Normalization of Extensor Muscle Tone

Objective

The objective of treatment is to normalize tone of the tonic postural extensor muscles to provide a basis for (1) trunk, neck, and proximal limb stability; (2) improved reflex and motor performance; and (3) enhanced functional abilities.

Method

Vestibular stimulation is designed to emphasize input to the otolith organs. Activities should in-

volve linear movement in all planes of three-dimensional space.

Rationale

The most efficient receptors for linear stimulation are the otolith organs. Otolith organ stimulation results in the facilitation of tonic postural extensor muscles. Linear acceleration and deceleration in all planes and in all positions result in stimulation of all hair cells of the otolith organs. However, *the prone position is emphasized* because it facilitates maintained contraction of the tonic extensor muscles of the neck and upper trunk (i.e., maintained tilt results in maintained righting of the head and upper trunk).

Treatment

Jumping and Bouncing Activities
Standing/Kneel Standing
1. Jumping up and down on a large inflated inner tube lying on its side on the floor

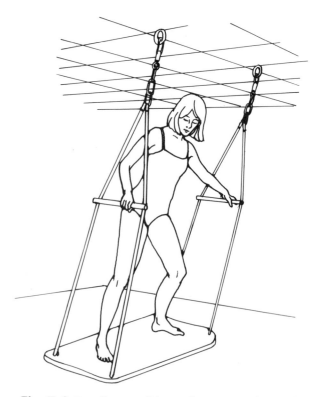

Fig. 7-9 Standing on glider and swinging side to side.

2. Jumping up and down on a trampoline
3. Upper trunk stability and control increase if the patient holds onto ropes suspended from the ceiling; shoulder retraction should be avoided.

Sitting

1. Bouncing on an inflated inner tube lying on its side on the floor
2. Bouncing on a trampoline
3. Sitting inside a large inner tube suspended from the ceiling and bouncing up and down
4. Bouncing up and down on a partially deflated therapy ball or hippity-hop
5. Sitting on equipment suspended by springs or shock cord from the ceiling
6. Upper trunk stability and control increase if the patient holds onto ropes suspended from the ceiling; shoulder retraction should be avoided.

Swinging (Linear)
Standing/Kneel Standing
1. Glider (Fig. 7-9)
2. Platform swing

Sitting
1. Net hammock
2. T-swing (Fig. 7-10)
3. Bolster swing
4. Platform swing

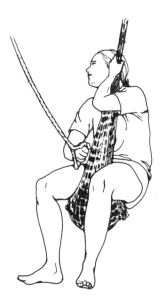

Fig. 7-11 Sitting on top of ball placed inside of net hammock. Direction and speed of swinging is controlled by the patient.

5. Glider
6. On top of a ball placed inside of a suspended net hammock (Fig. 7-11)
7. Adapted and standard swings

Quadruped
1. Platform swing
2. Glider

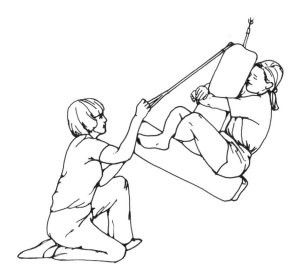

Fig. 7-10 Sitting on T-swing. Direction and speed of swinging is controlled by the therapist.

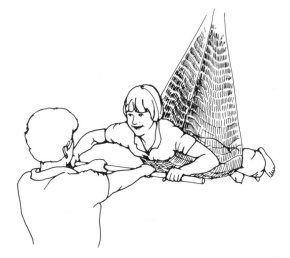

Fig. 7-12 Prone in the net hammock, the patient pulls into the pivot prone position and then releases to initiate swinging.

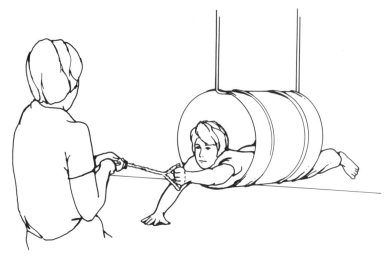

Fig. 7-13 Prone in a barrel suspended from two points in the ceiling to prevent angular rotation.

Prone/Supine
1. Net hammock (Fig. 7-12)
2. Barrel (Fig. 7-13)
3. Glider
4. Platform swing
5. Bolster swing (Fig. 7-14)

Other Linear Activities
Sitting and Prone/Supine
1. On a scooter board: (1) self-propelled by pulling on a rope attached to the wall; (2) holding onto a hoop held by the therapist who pulls the patient across the room (Fig. 7-15); or (3) self-propelled down a ramp

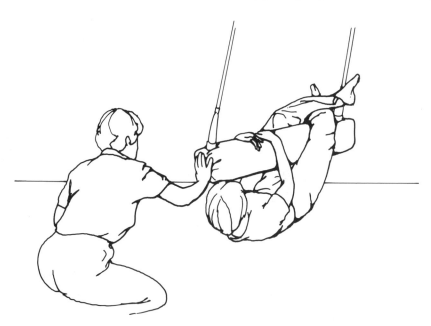

Fig. 7-14 Patient hangs in a supine position from a bolster swing as the swing is accelerated by the therapist.

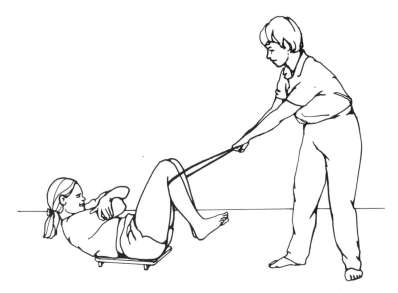

Fig. 7-15 In supine, the patient holds hoop with flexed knees as therapist pulls patient across the room.

2. Slide
3. Wheelchair and gurney

Jumping or Falling onto Pillows or Mattress (Fig. 7-16)

Considerations for Spastic Patients
Patients who exhibit the tonic labyrinthine reflex should avoid the supine position if it increases extensor spasticity. Jumping or bouncing activities that would cause the patient to land on the balls of the feet should be avoided if it elicits a positive

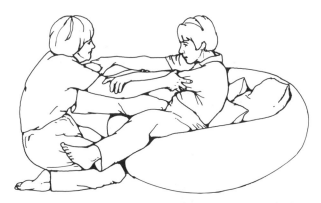

Fig. 7-16 With the patient's leg position controlled by the therapist, the patient is bounced up and down on an inner tube. After falling back onto the pillows, the patient is assisted back into the sitting position.

support reaction and an increase in extensor spasticity. In general, positioning techniques should be used to prevent excessive internal rotation and adduction of the hips and retraction of the shoulders. The application of linear vestibular stimulation to the treatment of a patient with cerebral palsy is demonstrated in the following case study.

Case Study. B. was a 6-year-old girl, of normal intelligence, with a diagnosis of spastic cerebral palsy. She had fair head control and poor trunk control. Her left extremities were more involved than her right. Although the muscle tone in her extremities was predominantly hypertonic, the muscle tone in her trunk fluctuated between hypertonicity and extreme hypotonicity. B.'s gross motor skills were at the 5- to 6-month level. She could sit unsupported momentarily; she moved around by rolling or commando crawling. B.'s fine motor skills were at a slightly higher developmental level than were her gross motor skills. She reached for objects with either hand, using an ulnar grasp; however, bilateral manipulation was impossible. B. did not demonstrate equilibrium reactions in any position. Protective extension sideways was present on the right but was not reliable; righting reactions were present, but delayed and labored.

B.'s therapists felt that many of her skills were compromised by the lack of stability in her trunk and neck. Controlling (by positioning) for B.'s tendency to assume stereotyped, abnormal positions, the therapists incorporated several types of primarily linear vestibular stimulation into B.'s ongoing therapy. B. was treated four times weekly for 1 hour each session. At least one session each week included augmented vestibular stimulation. The other three sessions were based on a neurodevelopmental approach, and included the development of daily living skills. Augmented vestibular stimulation included activities such as the following:

1. B. was placed in a long sitting position, facing the therapist, on top of a large inflated inner tube, her arms extended for support. Grasping just above B.'s knees, the therapist bounced B. up and down 10 to 15 times and then allowed her to fall backward onto a large pile of pillows placed inside the inner tube. B. was then assisted to right herself back into the sitting position (see Fig. 7-16).

2. B. straddled a bolster swing suspended by two points from the ceiling. B. held onto the rope in front of her. The therapist also straddled the bolster swing behind B. and stabilized B. at her hips. B. and the therapist swung back and forth several times, playing games that required various postural adjustments.

3. B. was seated, fully supported, in an adapted swing suspended from two overhead points. As B. was swung back and forth, she was asked to fixate visually on specified objects and to perform tasks such as breaking bubbles.

The most dramatic immediate effects of augmented vestibular stimulation included the normalization of muscle tone in B.'s trunk and extremities. After a few minutes of vestibular stimulation, her sitting posture became more erect. She could more easily support herself with her arms; hypertonicity of lower extremity extensors and adductors was reduced. Although no controlled experimental design was employed, long-term (6 months to 1 year) functional gains were also noted, which were assumed to be, at least in part, a result of the augmented vestibular stimulation. B.'s head control improved from fair to good; her trunk control increased from poor to fair. B.'s sitting balance improved so that she could sit independently for more than 1 minute. Perhaps the most dramatic change was in B.'s ability to use her upper extremity. Protective extension became more reliable on the right and began to emerge on the left. She developed a pincer grasp with the right hand and began to consistently manipulate objects bilaterally.

Postural-Ocular/Tone Disorders Development of Equilibrium Reactions

Objective

The objective of treatment is to increase functional equilibrium.

Method

Vestibular stimulation is provided, which results in transient perturbations of the head and body.

Rationale

The rationale of treatment is based on the belief that semicircular canal mediated responses contribute to equilibrium reactions. In patients with deficient processing of vestibular inputs, vestibular stimulation is hypothesized to normalize the response. In patients with absent vestibular responses, transient perturbations are hypothesized to enhance compensation by visual and somatosensory (muscle and joint proprioceptors and cutaneous inputs from the support surface) inputs.[45]

Treatment

An efficient equilibrium response requires a background of tonic postural extension. Therefore, patients with instability of neck, trunk, and limbs, secondary to extensor hypotonicity or weakness, should first be treated according to the principles for normalization of extensor muscle tone.

Treatment is comprised of transient perturbations that challenge the center of gravity and result in phasic head movements. Perturbations should be provided in all directions with the patient in a variety of positions. Initially, they should be of small amplitude, and progress according to the tolerance of the patient. However, they should be of sufficient magnitude to challenge the patient.

As the patient progresses, activities are introduced that maximize the potential for visual-somatosensory conflict. Visual-somatosensory conflict increases when on unstable, unpredictable surfaces.[45]

Activities providing transient perturbations include displacement of the patient's center of gravity by push or pull, and active or passive displacement of the patient's center of gravity by movement of the support surface. This may be accomplished by means of a

1. Tilt board (see Fig. 9-3)
2. Therapy ball
3. Barrel lying on its side
4. Bolsters placed on the floor

Activities that maximize visual-somatosensory conflict include

1. Active maintenance of balance on a tilt board, therapy ball, barrel, or bolster
2. Active maintenance of balance on uneven surfaces (e.g., stairs, ramps)
3. Active maintenance of balance during locomotion on foam or other unpredictable surfaces

Gravitational Insecurity

Objective

The objective of treatment is to reduce disproportionate fear of movement or positional change.

Method

The method used is self-initiated linear vestibular stimulation in nonthreatening positions, with speeds and durations tolerable to the patient.

Rationale

Because gravitational insecurity is hypothesized to be the result of poor modulation of otolithic input, linear vestibular stimulation is used to facilitate adaptation and normalization of the response.

Treatment

The use of linear vestibular stimulation activities previously described is emphasized. The following precautions should be considered.

1. It is important that the patient be in control of the movement and that he not become overaroused.
2. Generally, positions used in the early stages of treatment of gravitational insecurity are those where the patient's feet are in contact with the floor.
3. Initially, activities are slow and of small amplitude; speed and amplitude increase as the patient's tolerance increases.
4. When gravitational insecurity occurs in conjunction with conditions of frank CNS pathology, care should be taken to avoid eliciting stereotyped, abnormal patterns of movement.

The use of linear vestibular stimulation in the treatment of gravitational insecurity is illustrated in the following case study.

Case Study

M. was a 9-year-old child diagnosed as having spastic cerebral palsy, with a triplegic distribution. M. had a normal IQ and age appropriate verbal and visual perceptual skills. She had excellent head control, fair to good trunk control, near normal use of her right arm and hand, and very little functional use of her left arm or hand. She could stand with assistance but was extremely fearful when upright.

M. had been receiving physical and occupational therapy since she was an infant. Her therapy had been primarily based on a neurodevelopmental framework; as a result, a great deal of movement, including frequent use of the therapy ball, was incorporated into her treatment. Although she had never fallen or been dropped, M. was terrified unless a large proportion of her body was in contact with a stable supporting surface, preferably the floor. For example, when M. was held in standing, or in any position on the therapy ball, she demonstrated pallor and sweating, verbalized fear disproportionate to the risk involved, and clutched the therapist. In addition, her muscle tone became so hypertonic as to minimize any gains that might otherwise have resulted from treatment. In an attempt to reduce her gravitational insecurity, M. was given a 3 week, 45 minute, daily trial of linear vestibular stimulation in lieu of her more traditional physical and occupational therapy.

The following criteria were used in the selection of activities:

1. The activities were performed low to the ground and in positions where M. had as much control over starting and stopping the movement as possible.
2. The activities were adapted to control, as much as possible, for undesirable movement into stereotyped positions (i.e., adduction and internal rotation of the lower extremities and excessive flexion of the left upper extremity).

M. participated in the following activities.

1. M. was placed prone on a scooter board, which supported her body from her shoulders to her knees. A triangular-shaped block was fastened to the board between her knees to prevent excessive adduction. For safety, and to maintain her hips in extension, a wide (webbing strap) seat belt was fastened across her hips. With her left elbow extended and her arm flexed over her head, M. grasped a hula hoop in her left hand while she was pulled back and forth across a gymnasium floor.
2. M. was positioned prone in a net hammock suspended from a single point on the ceiling (see Fig. 7-12). Her hips were positioned in abduction and external rotation. M. held onto a towel with her left hand as she was pulled forward and then allowed to swing back and forth in a straight line.
3. M. was placed prone inside a carpeted barrel (see Fig. 7-13), suspended horizontally about 6 inches off the floor from two points on the ceiling. M.'s hips were held in abduction and external rotation as she was linearly propelled forward and backward while holding onto a towel with her left hand.

Although M. was not informed of the reason for her change in program, she obviously enjoyed it. She became eager to go to therapy, and her affect during the session was characterized by laughing and joking and willing participation. Sweating and pallor were eliminated. At the end of 3 weeks, the therapist brought M. into the therapy room and stood her up. It was M. who immediately remarked "I'm not afraid! I'm not grabbing for you."

M.'s therapy program continued to include some augmented linear vestibular stimulation during each treatment session, but she also resumed participation in activities that had been a part of her prior program. Her gravitational insecurity had not returned after 8 weeks.

Three months after the initiation of linear vestibular stimulation, M.'s therapist left the state and M.'s program changed once again. Linear vestibular stimulation was eliminated from her treatment program. When M.'s original therapist returned for a visit 4 months later, all of M.'s original symptoms of gravitational insecurity had returned.

Provoked Vertigo and Intolerance to Movement

Objective

The objective of treatment is to decrease provoked or positional vertigo and/or increase tolerance to movement.

Methods and Rationale

Two related approaches for the treatment of persistent provoked or positional vertigo using exercise programs have been reported in the literature.[46–51] Both approaches appear to enhance vestibular habituation of hyperresponsive vestibular end organ responses and/or central vestibular compensation by visual and somatosensory substitution[45,52–54] and, therefore, may be applicable to the treatment of intolerance to movement or other adverse vestibular responses seen in patients with sensory integrative disorders. The first approach, Cawthorne-Cooksey exercises, is comprised of a series of graduated exercises that encourage head and eye movements designed to improve balance and train the visual and somatosensory systems to compensate for permanent vestibular dysfunction.[46,47] The exercises are nonspecific to the patient's symptoms. The second approach, vestibular habituation training, involves the use of exercises specifically prescribed based on those movements or positions that elicit vertigo.[48–51]

Treatment

Cawthorne-Cooksey Exercises

The exercise program is graduated so that the patient progresses from easily tolerated movements to movements more likely to elicit an adverse response or vertigo. Because adverse symptoms are more likely to increase in the dark (or with eyes closed), ascending and descending stairs, or walking on inclined planes or unstable surfaces, these conditions are only introduced later in the treatment program when they are more readily tolerated by the patient. Each exercise is repeated 10 to 20 times a day and progresses from slow to fast movement, and toward potentially more stressful exercises. The following exercise progression is based on this approach.

1. Eye movements
   a. Looking up and down, head stationary
   b. Looking side to side, head stationary
2. Head movements with eye fixation
   a. Alternating neck flexion and extension with the arm flexed 90°, the elbow and thumb extended, and visual fixation on the thumb (Fig. 7-17)
   b. Neck rotation with visual fixation on the extended thumb
   c. Alternating neck flexion and extension with visual fixation on a target placed on the wall
   d. Neck rotation with visual fixation on a target placed on the wall
3. Head movements with eyes closed
   a. Alternating neck flexion and extension
   b. Neck rotation
4. Speed up head and eye movements; mix fast movements with slow ones
5. Assume a standing position from sitting (eyes open, eyes closed)
6. Ascending and descending stairs and ramps (eyes open, eyes closed)
7. Ambulation on an unstable surface (eyes open, eyes closed)
8. Games involving bending, stooping, and turning
   a. Throwing a bean bag from hand to hand overhead or between the legs
   b. Playing ball, catching overhead, and throwing between the knees
   c. Bending to pick up balls or bean bags from the floor, and then standing and rotating to throw them into a container placed on the contralateral side
   d. Other games and activities involving bending and turning

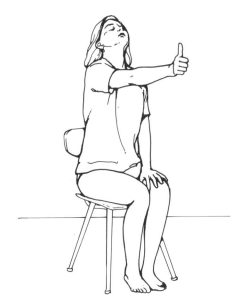

Fig. 7-17 Alternating neck flexion and extension with visual fixation on stable thumb.

Vestibular Habituation Training

This approach is based on the hypothesis that a response decline occurs as a result of repeated stimulation (versus prolonged stimulation resulting in adaptation). Therefore, effectiveness is dependent on the repeated stimulation of those receptors, which, when stimulated, elicit vertigo. Treatment, then, is based on a thorough evaluation of the patient to determine what positions or movements elicit vertigo, and notation of the type, intensity, and duration of the vertigo. Specific exercises, which include the exact positions or movements that elicited the adversive response, are then prescribed. The exercises selected must elicit vertigo as intensely as possible. Five repetitions of each exercise are performed twice each day. After each repetition, the patient is instructed to stay in the position eliciting the vertigo for as long as the vertigo persists. Marked improvement should be seen within the first 2 weeks; adverse symptoms should resolve within 2 months.

Evidence that vestibular habituation training also may be effective in reducing or eliminating other types of adverse vestibular responses is demonstrated in the following case study.

Case Study. J. was a 28-year-old woman with vestibular dysfunction associated with sensory integrative dysfunction and learning disability. Clinical assessment of posture revealed poor co-contraction; low extensor muscle tone; inability to assume or maintain the pivot prone position; impaired protective extension and equilibrium; and, when posture was challenged, a tendency to assume a "high guard" position with neck and trunk extended, arms abducted 90° and externally rotated, and elbows flexed 90°. Electronystagmography and electro-oculography of visual-vestibular control of eye movements confirmed dysfunction of tonic vestibular system processing.[28] During treatment, especially rolling activities, J. complained of "dizziness" and a feeling of "sloshing" within her head. Because these latter symptoms were interfering with her ongoing therapy program, an attempt to reduce their adverse effects through modified vestibular habituation training was initiated. The training proceeded as follows.

At initial evaluation, J. was asked to assume a variety of positions and to carry out a number of head and body movements to establish what head positions and/or movements elicited the adverse sensations of "dizziness" and "sloshing." Positions that the patient assumed were

1. Prone
2. Side lying (right, left)
3. Supine, head neutral
4. Supine, neck hyperextended
5. Supine, neck hyperextended and rotated (right, left)
6. Sitting, neck flexed
7. Sitting, neck extended

The patient's head movements were (1) rapid, alternating neck flexion and extension, and (2) rapid head rotation.

Body movements included (1) rolling, (2) somersaults, and (3) rapid inversion over therapy ball (prone, supine).

In establishing baselines, rolling and somersaults were found to be the only positions or movements that elicited adverse sensations. One somersault or four complete rolls were the maximum number J. could tolerate. "Dizziness," described as light headedness or a "floating" feeling, persisted more than 20 minutes.

To initiate vestibular habituation training, rolling was selected as the activity of choice. Somer-

saults were difficult for J. to perform independently, a prerequisite for a home program. Furthermore, because J. was susceptible to "sensory overload" (see section on sensory overload), a conservative, strictly designed, modified vestibular habituation training program was developed. J. was instructed to perform four rolling cycles, each comprised of four complete rolls, with a rest period between cycles. This four-cycle sequence was performed one time each day, a minimum of 5 days a week.

J. reported her progress in a daily journal.

1. *Day 1.* "I felt dizzy after the first complete roll. During the third cycle I wondered if I could go on. After the fourth cycle, I was unable to get up into quadruped. Twenty minutes later, I continued to have a floating feeling in my head. I felt as if I was not totally in contact with the ground."
2. *Day 8.* "I still began to feel dizzy with the first roll. Immediately after the fourth cycle I felt disoriented; 20 minutes later I felt only slight light headedness."
3. *Day 15.* "I felt only slight discomfort until the third roll, then I felt dizzy. When I was all done, I was light headed but not disoriented. While I was rolling, I kept waiting for the feeling to get worse, but it never did. I could have rolled more."
4. *Day 60.* "I only felt slight dizziness as I slowed down at the end of each cycle. The dizziness stopped immediately when I stopped rolling." When asked to perform her first somersault in 2 months, no adverse sensation was elicited. This was in contrast to expectations of vestibular habituation training.
5. *8-month follow-up.* J. continued not to experience "dizziness" or "sloshing" during rolling or somersaults. Although rigid experimental control was lacking, the reduction in adverse sensations was felt to be attributable to her modified vestibular habituation training program because (1) no other changes in her ongoing therapy were made, and (2) J. had been receiving therapy, based on sensory integration theory[6,24–27] for slightly more than 2 years before modified vestibular habituation training was initiated.

Precautions

Sensory Overload

Sensory overload is a very serious consequence of apparent overstimulation and should not be confused with gravitational insecurity, intolerance to movement, or provoked vertigo. Sensory overload is a poorly understood reaction that can result from a variety of sensory stimuli, including vestibular, and appears to result in disorganization of the CNS. Stimuli observed to cause sensory overload have sometimes been comprised of stimuli that would have a minimal effect on the normal nervous system. Further, sensory overload can occur even with cautious use of sensory stimuli. The following guidelines are suggested.

1. Avoid overstimulation.
2. Monitor patient for signs of overarousal or underarousal before, during, and after vestibular stimulation.
3. Allow the patient to set his own pace.

The following case study reflects the seriousness of a patient's reaction to sensory overload.

Case Study

R. was a 26-year-old graduate student, diagnosed as having sensory integrative (including tactile and vestibular) dysfunction. R.'s sensory overload occurred after a 45-minute testing period involving rotary vestibular, full-field optokinetic, and combined visual-vestibular stimulation in a motor driven rotary chair.[28] Immediately after testing, R. experienced vertigo and nausea; these initial symptoms subsided after a 1-hour rest period. Approximately 3 hours later, R.'s symptoms of sensory overload began to appear and became progressively worse over the next several hours. She complained of extreme hypersensitivity to sound ("noise hurt"), feeling as if she was floating in space, and of being *extremely disoriented* (she no longer knew where up or down was or where she was in relation to the ground). R.'s most alarming symptom was that she felt as though her arms, legs, and head were not attached to her body. For 2 days, "I felt as if I was somewhere else. I was all disconnected and my parts were floating around. I didn't want to move because when I moved everything came apart and left, and then I had to go find it and reattach it and make it stay."

Although nothing totally alleviated R.'s symptoms, deep pressure and proprioceptive input reduced her discomfort. She was most comfortable when lying down and covered by a sleeping bag and approximately 100 pounds of weight evenly distributed over her body.

It was 4 days before R. felt well enough to return to her classes and 10 days before she "felt like a human being again." Approximately 1 month later, the somatosensory tests of the Southern California Sensory Integration Tests[26] were administered to R. She had a milder recurrence of her symptoms suggesting that tactile, as well as visual and/or vestibular stimuli, are capable of eliciting sensory overload.

Because R. was an adult, she was able to vividly describe her experience, a description that reminds one of what a "bad drug trip" or a psychotic episode might be like. But R. was not unique. While sensory overload is rare, we treated four other such patients within a 2-year period. The symptoms each experienced were lessened by the application of neutral warmth and firm, deep touch-pressure (i.e., wrapping up in comforters with heavy objects on top of the patient). There was no other identifiable commonality.

Overinhibition of the Brain Stem

According to Ayres,[6]

Perhaps the greatest potential harm arising from [sensory stimulation] is overinhibition of the brain stem. Reports of this occurrence are rare but deserving of every clinician's awareness. In one case a child appeared to become unconscious and in another case a child became cyanotic. Both cases appear to represent depression of vital functions through inhibitory vestibular stimuli. (p. 132)

Seizures

Vestibular and other types of sensory stimuli have the potential to induce seizures.[55–57] However, seizures activated by peripheral sensory inputs are extremely rare, accounting for less than 1 percent of all seizures.[58] Furthermore, nonvestibular sensory inputs (e.g., auditory, visual), as well as fatigue or excitement, are more likely to induce seizures than are vestibular stimuli.[55–57] Rotation (i.e., spinning in a suspended net hammock) in the light with eyes open, in addition to providing vestibular stimulation, also provides optokinetic stimulation.[27,28,30] The resultant rhythmic stimulation of the visual system is a potential trigger for seizures.[56,57]

Investigations of the effect of vestibular stimulation on seizure activity have failed to find an increase in seizure activity following vestibular stimulation.[58–60] Because the results of these investigations do not suggest that rotary vestibular stimulation could not trigger seizures in some patients, the following guidelines are suggested.

1. Patients with a history of seizure activity should be monitored carefully before, during, and after vestibular stimulation. If fatigue, hyperexcitability, or hyperventilation are observed, sensory stimulation should be discontinued.[6,56,58]
2. Rotary vestibular stimulation, especially when applied in a lighted room to patients with eyes open, should be avoided in patients with active seizure disorders.
3. The use of a particular type of stimulation (rotary versus linear) in treatment should be discontinued if it is observed to trigger seizures.

Muscle Tone

Although poorly documented in well-controlled research studies, there are a number of indications in the literature that vestibular stimulation may have an adverse effect on muscle tone. Increasing tone in patients with hypertonicity is a common concern;[6,7,11] decreasing tone in the hypotonic patient may be another. In general, fast vestibular stimulation has been thought to result in increases in muscle tone, and slow vestibular stimulation has been associated with relaxation and reduction in muscle tone.[6–11] However, *each patient will have his own individual response to sensory stimulation.* Therapists should monitor each patient carefully and avoid overgeneralizations about the effects of any given stimulus. Experimental evidence suggests that fast vestibular stimulation has a soothing effect.[18–20] Increases in muscle tone noted during treatment may be less due to the direct effects of vestibular stimulation than to fear (see Case M.), environmental factors, level of arousal, or initial state of the CNS. Further, some hypertonic pa-

tients may show increases in muscle tone after slow vestibular stimulation and a reduction or normalization of tone as a result of fast vestibular stimulation (see Case B.). These observations may suggest that certain patients who lack stability may fixate their trunks and/or extremities, to allow themselves to perform functional tasks. When slow vestibular stimulation is administered, these patients must fixate more strongly to counteract the effects of the inhibition.

Safety

The following safety measures are advised.

1. When using suspended equipment, use high quality carabiners and be sure that eye bolts are firmly secured into the support beams of the ceiling. Expert installation is indicated; shearing forces during swinging readily break or loosen an improperly installed eye bolt.
2. To protect the patient from potential falls, always cover the floor with mats; guard the unstable patient.
3. Remember that vestibular stimuli can have a powerful effect on the nervous system. In general, *vestibular stimulation should only be provided by professionals with a thorough understanding of the nervous system, and knowledge of signs of autonomic nervous system distress.*
4. Be responsive to the patient. Respect his desire to discontinue stimulation. Conversely, discontinue stimulation if, in the therapist's judgment, continued stimulation might result in adverse responses, even when the patient expresses a desire to continue. Patients with deficits in vestibular processing are not always aware of their limitations.

ACKNOWLEDGMENTS

The authors express appreciation to Lee A. Quintana, Lucia G. Littlefield, Deirdre E. Curran, Jacquelyn Ott, and Ruth M. Atwood for their assistance in the preparation of this chapter.

REFERENCES

1. Montgomery PC (ed): The Vestibular System: An Annotated Bibliography. Center for the Study of

Sensory Integrative Dysfunction, Pasadena, CA (now Sensory Integration International, Torrance, CA), 1981

2. Ottenbacher K: Developmental implications of clinically applied vestibular stimulation: A review. Phys Ther 63:338, 1983

3. Ottenbacher KJ, Petersen P: The efficacy of vestibular stimulation as a form of specific sensory enrichment: Quantitative review of the literature. Clin Pediatr 23:428, 1983

4. Weeks ZR: Effects of the vestibular system on human development. I. Overview of functions and effects of stimulation. Am J Occup Ther 33:376, 1979

5. Weeks ZR: Effects of the vestibular system on human development. II. Effects of vestibular stimulation on mentally retarded, emotionally disturbed, and learning-disabled individuals. Am J Occup Ther 33:450, 1979

6. Ayres AJ: Sensory Integration and Learning Disorders. Western Psychological Services, Los Angeles, 1972

7. Farber S: Neurorehabilitation: A Multisensory Approach. WB Saunders, Philadelphia, 1982

8. Heiniger MC, Randolph SL: Neurophysiological Concepts in Human Behavior: The Tree of Learning. CV Mosby, St. Louis, 1981

9. Powell NJ: Children with cerebral palsy. p. 312. In Clark PN, Allen AS (eds): Occupational Therapy for Children. CV Mosby, St. Louis, 1985

10. Trombly CA: Motor control therapy. p. 59. In Trombly CA (ed): Occupational Therapy for Physical Dysfunction. 2nd Ed. Williams & Wilkins, Baltimore, 1983

11. Umphred DA, McCormack GL: Classification of common facilitory and inhibitory treatment techniques. p. 72. In Umphred DA (ed): Neurological Rehabilitation. CV Mosby, St. Louis, 1985

12. Roberts TDM: Neurophysiology of Postural Mechanisms. 2nd Ed. Butterworths, Boston, 1978

13. Wilson VJ, Melvill Jones G: Mammalian Vestibular Physiology. Plenum Press, New York, 1979

14. Booth JB, Stockwell CW: A method for evaluating vestibular control of posture. Trans Am Acad Ophthalmol Otolaryngol 86:ORL-93, 1978

15. Nashner LM: Sensory Feedback in Human Posture Control. MIT Rep MVT-70-3. Man-Vehicle Laboratory, MIT, Cambridge MA, 1970

16. Chee FKW, Kreutzberg JR, Clark DL: Semicircular canal stimulation in cerebral palsied children. Phys Ther 58:1071, 1978

17. Ottenbacher K, Short MA, Watson PJ: The effects of a clinically applied program of vestibular stimulation on the neuromotor performance of children with severe developmental delay. Phys Occup Ther Pediatr 1:1, 1981

18. Freedman D, Boverman H: The effects of kinesthetic stimulation on certain aspects of development in premature infants. Am J Orthopsychiatry 36:223, 1966

19. Pederson DR, TerVrugt D: The influence of ampli-

tude and frequency of vestibular stimulation on the activity of two-month-old infants. Child Dev 44:122, 1973

20. Van den Daele LD: Modification of infant state by treatment in a rockerbox. J Psychol 74:161, 1970

21. Fisher AG: An electromyographic investigation of the effect of the tonic labyrinthine inverted position on the tonic activity of normal muscle. Unpublished masters thesis. Boston University, 1977

22. Stejskal L: Postural reflexes in man. Am J Phys Med 58:1, 1979

23. Tokizane T, Murao M, Ogata T, Kondo T: Electromyographic studies of tonic neck, lumbar and labyrinthine reflexes in normal persons. Jpn J Physiol 2:130, 1951

24. Ayres AJ: Learning disabilities and the vestibular system. J Learn Disabil 11:18, 1978

25. Ayres AJ: Sensory Integration and the Child. Western Psychological Services, Los Angeles, 1979

26. Ayres AJ: Southern California Sensory Integration Tests Manual: Revised 1980. Western Psychological Services, Los Angeles, 1980

27. Ayres AJ: Sensory Intergration and Praxis Tests. Western Psychological Services, Los Angeles, 1988

28. Fisher AG, Mixon J, Herman R: The validity of the clinical diagnosis of vestibular dysfunction. Occup Ther J Res 6:3, 1986

29. Jensen GM, Wilson KB: Horizontal postrotary nystagmus response in female subjects with adolescent idiopathic scoliosis. Phys Ther 59:1226, 1979

30. Ornitz EM: Normal and pathological maturation of vestibular function in the human child. p. 479. In Romand R (ed): Development of Auditory and Vestibular Systems. Academic Press, New York, 1983

31. Ritvo ER, Ornitz EM, Eviatar A, et al: Decreased postrotary nystagmus in early infantile autism. Neurology 19:653, 1969

32. Shuer J, Clark F, Azen SP: Vestibular function in mildly mentally retarded adults. Am J Occup Ther 34:664, 1980

33. Torok N, Perlstein MA: Vestibular findings in cerebral palsy. Ann Otol Rhinol Laryngol 71:51, 1962

34. Zee-Chen EL-F, Hardman ML: Postrotary nystagmus response in children with Down's syndrome. Am J Occup Ther 37:260, 1983

35. Bruininks RH: Bruininks-Oseretsky Test of Motor Proficiency Examiner's Manual. American Guidance Service, Circle Pines, MN, 1978

36. Fregly AR, Graybiel A: an ataxia test battery not requiring rails. Aerospace Medicine 39:277, 1968

37. Fisher AG: Equilibrium: Development and Clinical Assessment. Unpublished doctoral dissertation, Boston University, 1984

38. Fisher AG, Bundy AC: Equilibrium reactions in normal children and boys with sensory integrative dysfunction. Occup Ther J Res 2:171, 1982

39. Martin JP: The Basal Ganglia and Posture. Pittman Medical Publishing, London, 1967

40. Rademaker GGJ, Garcin R: Note sur quelques réac-

tions labyrinthiques des extrémités chez l'animal et chez l'homme: Étude physiologique et clinique. Rev Neurol (Paris) 1:637, 1932

41. Rademaker GGJ, Garcin R: L'épreuve d'adaptation statique: Suite a l'étude de quelques réactions des extrémités d'origine labyrinthique. Rev Neurol (Paris) 2:566, 1933

42. Radmark K: Tipping reaction in cases of vertigo after head injury. Acta Otolaryngol [Suppl] (Stockh) 52:1, 1944

43. Weisz S: Studies in equilibrium reaction. J Nerv Ment Dis 88:150, 1938

44. Zador J: Less réactions d'équilibre chez l'homme: Étude physiologique et clinique des réactions d'équilibre sur la table basculante. Masson, Paris, 1938

45. Nashner LM, Black FO, Wall C: Adaptation to altered support and visual conditions during stance: Patients with vestibular deficits. J Neurosci 2:536, 1982

46. Cawthorne T: Vestibular injuries. Proc R Soc Med 39:270, 1946

47. Cooksey FS: Rehabilitation in vestibular injuries. Proc R Soc Med 39:273, 1946

48. Guidetti G: La rieducazione vestibolare: Considerazioni sui risultati ottenuti in 46 casi. Acta Otorhinolaryngol Ital 3:125, 1983

49. Norré ME, De Weerdt W: Treatment of vertigo based on habituation. I. Physio-pathological basis. J Laryngol Otol 94:689, 1980

50. Norré ME, De Weerdt W: Treatment of vertigo based on habituation. II. Techniques and results of habituation training. J Laryngol Otol 94:971, 1980

51. Norré ME, De Weerdt W: Positional (provoked) vertigo treated by postural training: Vestibular habituation training. Aggressologie 22B:37, 1981

52. Bles W, de Jong JMBV, de Wit G: Compensation for labyrinthine deficits examined by use of a tilting room. Acta Otolaryngol 95:576, 1983

53. Bles W, de Jong JMBV, de Wit G: Somatosensory compensation for loss of labyrinthine function. Acta Otolaryngol 97:213, 1984

54. Pfaltz CR: Vestibular compensation: Physiological and clinical aspects. Acta Otolaryngol 95:402, 1983

55. Behrman S, Wyke BD: Vestibulogenic seizures. Brain 81:529, 1958

56. Gastaut H, Tassinari CA: Triggering mechanisms in epilepsy: The electroclinical point of view. Epilepsia 7:85, 1966

57. Green JB: Reflex epilepsy. Epilepsia 12:225, 1971

58. Kantner RM, Clark DL, Atkinson J, Paulson G: Effects of vestibular stimulation in seizure-prone children. Phys Ther 62:16, 1982

59. Barac B: Vestibular influences upon the EEG of epileptics. Electroencephalogr Clin Neurophysiol 22:245, 1967

60. Ottenbacher K: The effect of a controlled program of vestibular stimulation on the incidence of seizures in children with severe developmental delay. Phys Occup Ther Pediatr 2:25, 1982

8 Parkinson's Syndrome and Other Disorders of the Basal Ganglia

Barbara S. Oremland

EXTRAPYRAMIDAL DISORDERS

The extrapyramidal system works with the cerebellum and the cortex to produce normal movement.[1] Located within the diencephalon of the brain, it is responsible for inhibiting unwanted movement and controlling posture and tone.[1,2] The main components of the extrapyramidal system are the basal ganglia, consisting of the caudate, putamen and the globus pallidus; and related subcortical nuclei, known as the substania nigra, subthalamic nucleus, and the red nucleus.

The most common disorder of the extrapyramidal system is Parkinson's Disease, which will be discussed later and is predominantly characterized by hypokinesia. Other extrapyramidal or basal ganglia disorders, as they are sometimes called, are characterized by excessive involuntary movements known as hyperkinesias; they are athetosis, chorea, ballismus, Wilson's Disease, and spasmodic torticollis. Common to all these disorders is the fact that the hyperkinetic movements cease during sleep[3] and symptoms increase with stress.

Athetosis

Pathology

Athetosis is characterized by slow, involuntary, wormlike movements, mainly of the distal extremities. Patients exhibit uncoordinated, purposeless movements and postural instability with abnormal postural tone.[3,5]

The main lesion is usually in the putamen. Athetosis is usually associated with cerebral palsy. Thirty percent of cerebral palsy lesions involve extrapyramidal tract damages, usually with a lack of oxygen to the basal ganglia, resulting in athetosis and other hyperkinetic disorder.[11]

Clinical Manifestations

The clinical picture of athetosis involves problems with involuntary movements and in initiating willed movement. The patient exhibits

1. Tremendous fluctuations in body tone
2. Alteration of posture
3. Asymmetry and poor body alignment
4. Poor eye-hand coordination due to lack of head control and visual fixation
5. Dysarthria and hearing deficiencies[3,5]

These patients may be of normal intelligence but because of the facial grimacing, dysarthria, awkward movement, and associated hearing loss, the mental capabilities are easily camouflaged.[2] Athetoid movements can vary in speed, be unpatterned or patterned, and intended or purposeless.[2]

Treatment

Because patients vary so dramatically, treatment is individually designed. Instability is caused by fluctuations in tone and uncontrolled movements, as well as poor body alignment. Compression force through the weight-bearing joints, such as the use of weighted caps for athetotic children, is suggested by Atkinson.[2]

Poor body image is caused by proprioception deficits.[3,5] Improved body image and sensory feedback, which allows the patient to experience normal activity and to enhance more functional movement, should be an essential part of the physical therapy program.[2,5] Inhibiting involuntary movements should also be one part of the program (e.g., allowing the patient to lie prone).[12] The goal is to inhibit activity by allowing the patient to experience normal purposeful movements.[2] Additional areas of concentration should be on activities to stimulate and improve (1) hand-eye coordination, (2) orofacial function, and (3) relaxation.

Effort should be concentrated on regaining control on one body part at a time. Excitation of the patient will exaggerate symptoms; nevertheless, activities to maintain an active recreational program are recommended.[5]

Chorea

Pathology

Chorea is a movement disorder characterized by sudden involuntary purposeless and quick movements or jerks of the extremities and head, as well as facial grimaces.[3]

The lesion is usually in the caudate and can result from disease or hereditary defects. The basic principles for treatment for athetosis apply to chorea, especially in the early stages.[2,5,13] There are two major types of chorea.

Sydenham's Chorea or Acute Chorea

Sydenham's chorea is a movement disorder, which usually occurs between the ages of 5 and 15. It is characterized by wild flinging movements and can result from streptococcal throat infections or rheumatic fever. The disease is self-limiting, disappearing in a few months to a year. The lesion is believed to be in the caudate.[3,11]

The only recommended treatment in most cases is penicillin for the infection and sedation for the patient because of the exhausting nature of wild movements. The patient is usually on bedrest, and padding is suggested on the bedside if the movements become too violent.[14]

Huntington's Chorea

Usually diagnosed between the ages of 30 and 50, Huntington's chorea is a familial, chronic, progressive disorder. The disease is fatal, usually 10 to 15 years from time of onset. The corpus striatum is involved, as well as parts of the cortex.

Signs and symptoms include the following:[11,13]

1. Severe grimacing
2. Incoordination
3. Explosive speech
4. Major involuntary movements involving sudden lightening-like contraction, as well as slow sinuous movement
5. Memory loss and mental deficits
6. Difficulty in gait and self-care

No specific treatment is available. Warfel and Schlagenhauf (11) state that "Huntington's chorea . . . has the highest suicide rate of all neurological entities" (p. 79).[11] They attribute this to the patients knowledge of their disease.

Ballismus

Ballismus is an involuntary movement disorder characterized by wild flinging movements involving the arms and legs. The disease usually affects the elderly.[2,3,11]

The lesion is in the subthalamic nucleus and is most often caused from arteriosclerotic-thrombotic damage. Usually, only one side of the body is involved.[3,11] The disease could be threatening if both sides are involved because so much energy is expended in continuous movement. The patient is eventually unable to walk or care for himself. Sedation is the only form of recommended treatment in more advanced stages.[11]

Wilson's Disease (Hepatocerebral Degeneration)

Wilson's disease is a genetic defect in copper metabolism resulting in bilateral degeneration in the putamen and sometimes the caudate. It occurs in patients between the ages of 1 and 20 years. The disease shortens life expectancy by 10 to 15 years.[11–13]

Spasmodic Torticollis

Patients present with head jerking to one side. The disease results in a hypertrophic sternocleidomastoid muscle contralaterally and is usually a result of psychogenic causes; however, the basal ganglia, mainly the putamen, may be involved in about 10 percent of patients following encephalitis.[2,11]

Treatment consists of (1) psychotherapy, (2) neck collars, (3) tranquillizers, and (4) touching the face with one finger to prevent jerky movements of the head.[11]

PARKINSONISM

Parkinson's disease is a disorder of movement that is part of a larger syndrome known as Parkinsonism. The Parkinson's syndrome presents clinically with four basic symptoms.[4,5,15]

1. Tremor
2. Rigidity
3. Bradykinesia
4. Poor postural reflexes

The types of Parkinsonism are defined by causes according to the following classification:

1. *Idiopathic.* Idiopathic Parkinsonism is characterized by deterioration mainly in the substantia nigra and the basal ganglia. This form of the disease occurs for no apparent reason. Known as Parkinson's disease, it is the most common form of Parkinsonism.[4,5]
2. *Toxic exposure.* Toxic exposure Parkinsonism results from carbon monoxide, manganese, or methyl bromide exposure.[5,6] Another recently investigated potential toxin, MPTP (1-methyl-4-phenyl1-1,2,3,6-tetrahydropyridine), was found to cause an irreversible, rapidly progressive form of Parkinsonism.[7] It was found to be a contaminant in illegally prepared street drugs, such as synthetic opiates. Many young drug addicts ingested MPTP, which itself is not harmful. Once inside the body, however, it turns into a destructive toxin known as MPP+, which is specific in destruction in the substantia nigra. Most of the young addicts developed rapidly progressive Parkinsonism, with severe irreversible disability.[7] MPTP is also speculated to be toxic if inhaled or absorbed through the skin and is thought to be an environmental toxin.[7]
3. *Arteriosclerotic.* Arteriosclerotic Parkinsonism is characterized by little strokes in areas of the basal ganglia; a full-scale Parkinson's

appearance is not present, but the patient may have dementia. Often anti-Parkinson's medication is not effective. Tremor is rarely present. Primitive sucking and palmarmental reflexes appear.[5]

4. *Shy-Drager syndrome.* This type of Parkinsonism is associated with hypotension. Some patients exhibit urinary incontinency and frequent fainting.[5,8]
5. *Postencephalitic.* Postencephalitic Parkinsonism occurs after episodes of encephalitis lethargica, sometimes many years later. Usually, widespread damage occurs in the basal ganglia.[4,5]
6. *Steele-Richardson-Olszewski syndrome.* This form is a fairly common degenerative disease of the brain stem. The patient exhibits blurred or double vision, with a tendency for falling backwards.[8]
7. *Drug induced.* Many of the major tranquilizers in the phenothiazine group, such as chlorpromazine (Thorazine), can induce Parkinson's syndrome, as well as many drugs for high blood pressure. If the patient has not been on the medication for too long, in many cases the Parkinson's can be reversed if the medication is removed.[5,6]
8. *Trauma.* Any severe injury to the head or a series of continuous blows to the head, such as those experienced by boxers, can also precipitate the condition. In this case, most anti-Parkinson's medication are ineffective, and intellectual impairment often occurs.[6]

PARKINSON'S DISEASE

The most common form of Parkinsonism, Parkinson's disease is progressive and degenerative. Although onset of the disease is usually between 50 and 60 years of age, it can occur as early as age 20 to 40; juvenile cases are rare. Parkinson's disease affects 1 percent of the population over 50.[4]

Sources disagree as to the sexual prevalence of the disease. Some say men and women are affected equally;[4] others maintain that men are slightly more predisposed. The disease is not contagious, fatal, or hereditary. It is important to note that there is no apparent time table for Parkinson's involvement. No two patients parallel each other regarding duration of the disease or level of disability.[5]

There is no diagnostic test for Parkinson's disease.[4] The diagnosis is usually arrived at through the clinical picture and elimination of other possible diagnostically confirmable etiologies.

Physiology and Pathology of Parkinson's Disease

There is still much to be understood about the causative factors of Parkinson's disease. However, the main symptoms of bradykinesia, tremor, and rigidity are caused by extrapyramidal deterioration. The main lesion in Parkinson's disease is in the substantia nigra, with the globus pallidus showing the next level of severe involvement.[3,5] The degeneration results in a deficiency of an important neurotransmitter in the brain known as dopamine.[15]

Godwin-Austen[6] explained that the substantia nigra and the basal ganglia contain practically all the dopamine in the human brain. Afifi[3] described two main fiber systems connecting the substantia nigra and the striatum as an inhibitory dopaminergic system and an excitatory cholinergic system. Dopamine and acetylcholine are antagonistic toward each other in the striatum. Perlik et al.[15] described Parkinson's disease as a deficiency of dopamine and an overactivity of striatal acetylcholine.

For normal movement to occur, the cortex, cerebellum, and the basal ganglia all interact through important feedback loops or circuits.[16] Understanding that dopamine is an inhibitory substance,[17] Perlik[15] explains that the loss of dopamine transmission disrupts the equilibrium with acetylcholine, allowing the cholinergic or excitatory pathway to dominate.

The ensuing loss of inhibitory function of the extrapyramidal system, secondary to the loss of dopamine, results in abnormal motor behavior or involuntary movements called release phenomena. Without the inhibitory effect of the extrapyramidal system supplied by the dopamine, there is unwanted movement and a lack of control in willed movements. Without the normal influence of the extrapyramidal system, automatic movements are disrupted, and tone and posture are altered.

Histologically, Parkinson's appears with depigmentation in the substantia nigra and shows the formation of Lewy bodies in the substantia nigra. Lewy bodies are a special type of nerve cell degeneration and are prevalent in 90 percent of idiopathic forms of Parkinsonism.[18] They appear as an unusual cytoplasmic inclusion in the cells and can be observed only on autopsy. In the postencephalitic form of Parkinsonism, neurofibrillary tangles are the main form of degeneration noted.[18]

There is also a loss of neurons and an increase of glial cells in the pallidus and substantia nigra in Parkinson's. Chemically, there is a decrease or absence of dopamine.[18]

For normal movement, there must be stimulation of the desired muscles and inhibition of unwanted movement.[2] Initiation of many movements is attributed to the pyramidal system, and the extrapyramidal system allows required movement to occur without involving unwanted activity.[2]

The basal ganglia, in addition to modifying movement, also may play a role in its initiation. The globus pallidus and the putamen have shown discharge patterns before the actual beginning of movement.[2]

Some of the major effects of extrapyramidal system are on posture; righting responses; muscle tone; and control of automatic movements, such as arm swing in gait and spontaneity of facial expression. In a decorticate primate, almost normal posture and movements can be maintained, except for very precise movements, such as those of the hand.[3]

The Parkinsonian gait is often described as resembling an immature walking pattern.[19] Primitive gait in small children may be transformed to an adult pattern of gait by the descending influences involving dopaminergic pathways.[19] The Parkinson's gait is unique, with its shuffling steps and forward propulsion, once initiated. When a bilateral lesion ablates an animal caudate and putamen, the result is forced progression, where the animal has an irresistible tendency to move forward.[3] This is not unlike the Parkinson's gait, which is also described as repetitive forward falls, halted by successively placing the feet further ahead; the patient looks as if he is trying to catch up with his center of gravity.[19] When forward motion does occur, it appears as a festinating gait because of the bent over posture and the stiffness, which prevents the patient from straightening up.[17] The lack of dopamine in severe Parkinson's disease may be responsible for the more primitive locomotion patterns. This gait pattern would include a wide course, difficulty in initiating movement, and apparent lack of smooth gradual transitions in the gait cycle.

The extrapyramidal system also plays a major role in maintaining a certain amount of muscle tone. Disruption of this tone appears in Parkinson's disease as rigidity, the most commonly occurring symptom.[17] Rigidity is a result of the stretch reflex, which involves the intrafusal fibers of the muscle spindle. These fibers are linked partially to the extrapyramidal pathways.[2,17] Subcortical nuclei help produce postural fixation by affecting the stretch reflex mechanism. Damage in the area linking the cortex and the basal ganglia, such as in Parkinson's disease, can lead to excessive postural fixation so that voluntary movement is disturbed.[2]

The diffuse endings of the muscle spindle are enlarged in Parkinson's patients. This may be related to rigidity, which has been defined as physiological hyperactivity of the static gamma system.[20] The diffuse endings are thought to be innervated by the static gamma nerve fibers, and considerable control from the reticular system and the basal ganglia is exercised on the gamma neurons.[16,20]

Rigidity is a co-contraction of agonist and antagonist and, unlike spasticity, favors no particular set of muscles. It sometimes is released spontaneously by L-dopa medication and is very exhausting to the patient. It will increase with stress, such as occurs from resistive exercises.

Another major symptom associated with Parkinson's disease is the slowness in movement described as bradykinesia. The inability to initiate willed movement, such as when the patient freezes in the middle of gait, is referred to as akinesia and is caused by massive cell deterioration in the globus pallidus.[5] If the caudate and putamen are stimulated in an animal, it leads to a slowing of limb movement, such as that in bradykinesia.[3] Bilateral ablation of the globus pallidus in animals results in a hypoactive, sleepy animal, which seldom moves around or even changes position.[3] These are also characteristics in the Parkinson's patient associated with bradykinesia. The actual mechanisms involved in bradykinesia is suggested as an abnormal recruitment and abnormal firing of motor units.[21] A long reaction time, which refers to the time from the initiation of a stimulus until a movement is performed, is found in Parkinson's patients.[21] An example is normal elbow flexion, which normally takes about 240 ms but in Parkinson's patients take 660 ms.[22] Physiologically, bradykinesia is independent of rigidity. However, when both are present, the gait becomes shuffling and the patient is often unable to lift his feet high enough to allow a normal swing-through gait pattern.

One of the earliest symptoms of Parkinson's disease is tremor. Most often it is a resting tremor, usually appearing first in the hand muscles presenting at a frequency of 3 to 6 cycles/sec with the fingers and thumbs moving opposite each other. The wrist can also alternate in flexion and extension in tremor. Tremor may also appear in the neck, face, and sometimes the foot.[19] Occasionally, an action tremor is present; when it occurs with rigidity, it produces a cogwheeling effect.[5] The tremor may appear on only one side and increases with stress. Prolonged stimulation of the globus pallidus results in contralateral tremor.[3]

Clinical Picture of Parkinson's Disease

Signs and Symptoms

1. *Tremor.* Usually a resting tremor involving the thumb and index finger, alternating in flexion and extension known as "pill rolling." Tremor may occur on just one side and appears at a rate of 3 to 6 cycles/sec. It may also be present in the anterior neck muscles, as well as the foot. About 20 percent of patients show no tremor.[15] However, in those that do, it is usually the earliest occurring symptoms.[15,19]

2. *Rigidity.* Range of motion is limited due to rigidity. Target areas for involvement are neck, shoulders, hips, knees, and sometimes the trunk and ankle. Attention should be given to the rotatory components of movement. When an action tremor is present with rigidity, it appears as a series of jerky movements during passive range of motion and is known as cogwheel rigidity.[5]

3. *Strength* is usually not a problem with Parkinson's patients, but one area that may need attention is the abdominals. Because of the continuous flexed posture, these muscles never reach their full length and lose some of their control.

4. *Posture*. Simian posture with head and shoulders forward. While sitting, patient often slumps to one side. Usually, most joints are in slight flexion and postural reflexes may also be slowed.[15]

5. *Balance* is often unstable; protective and righting reflexes are diminished or gone. There is a lack of upper trunk rotation. Usually when the patient is pushed forward or back, he either propulses or retropulses.[15] There is a history of frequent falls.

6. *Gait* is slow, with shuffling steps. There is low height of steps and poor or no arm swing during gait. Gait may progress to a pattern of quick, short steps (festination gait). There is difficulty with initiating or stopping gait, changing direction, or turning. This is especially a problem in narrow or confined spaces. There is limited upper trunk rotation. Glue foot or freezing is described as a patient coming to a complete stop and remaining there momentarily. He says he cannot move and feels like his foot is frozen. This also may occur before walking starts and may be triggered by obstacles or crowded areas or stress.

7. *Facial mobility*. Decreased facial expression; patient can perform but lacks spontaneity; decreased blinking. The patient sometimes complains of blurred or double vision and difficulty in reading, as eyes do not scan a line easily.[4] Eyelids may close inappropriately and have to be reopened manually. Lack of eye blinking results in decreased lubrication in the eyes.

8. *Orofacial and speech*. The patient has difficulty in chewing and swallowing. Speech is slowed, low toned, and unclear, usually due to poor lung capacity from stooped posture.[4] Often the patient cannot move his jaw freely to both sides when the mouth is open, (usually only to one), but when practiced or given a visual cue, such as a finger to follow, movement improves.

9. *Hand dexterity*. Movement of small muscles of the hand are greatly affected; there is a loss of dexterity and coordination.[19] Handwriting becomes smaller and illegible. Use of eating utensils is awkward, and cutting food is difficult. Grooming, such as cleaning after toileting and brushing teeth, is a problem; buttoning and zippering are also difficult, as are handling change and using keys. Grasp and release of grasp is slowed, and dropping objects may be a problem.

10. *Reciprocal motion*. In normal gait, there is foward movement of the right arm with the left leg and vice versa. This automatic pattern is usually greatly decreased or nonexistent. When drilling on this pattern sitting or standing, the patient may have difficulty using both sets of extremities and can only point the left arm and then the right arm, without correlating leg movements.

11. *Activities of daily living (ADL)*. The patient has difficulty in getting in and out of a chair, positioning himself on a couch or chair, getting in and out of a car, turning in bed, carrying something while walking doing two things at once, grooming, and dressing. The patient also has a tendency to overestimate weights and may complain of sheets or clothing feeling too heavy.

12. *Mental*. Depression is present in many patients and is often not just a reaction to the illness but to a neurological manifestation of the disease process. Some dementia and hallucinations also are reported, as well as problems with recent memory and a lack of interest in activities.[15,19] Slowing of the thought processes and loss in concentration and lack of attention can occur.[23]

13. *On-off phenomena*. The patient experiences extreme fluctuation from very mobile to complete inability to move, or with much slowness. This can be a phenomenon of the disease or of medication and may also fluctuate with the time of day.[23]

14. *Autonomic*. There is increased sweating, constipation, swelling in the lower extremities, and loss of appetite.[4,23]

15. *General*. There is a general slowing of movement (bradykinesia) in all activities; a decreased tendency to change positions is

prevalent; fatigue may occur easily and is to be avoided. Slowness in initiating movement is very common.

Interview and History

One of the most important parts of the evaluation is the history. There is much to be learned from the responses to relevant and appropriate questions. The following questions should be asked of all patients.

1. When did you first notice the signs of Parkinson's disease and what were they?

2. When did you first seek the help of a physician? Note the time period between questions 1 and 2. It is usually much longer than expected; this may give some insight on how long they have been in poor movement patterns. There is a theory that trauma or a major crisis may trigger the onset in one who is prone to Parkinson's.[8] If the patient indicates he is a widower, ask for how long, and see if the date parallels the onset of the illness. If there is not tactful way to approach this question, avoid it.

3. What is your occupation? (Get an answer, even if the patient is retired.) This is important because of the many environmental factors influencing the onset of Parkinson's disease. For example, many miners and steel workers have unusually high exposure to manganese, which can be a cause of Parkinsonism.

4. Do you smoke? Did you ever smoke? How often do you smoke? Recent articles indicate those who smoke have a lesser chance of getting Parkinson's or may get a less severe form of the disease.[7,8] These are important patterns to observe.

5. Do any of your relatives have Parkinson's disease? If so, when did they contract it? Because of many ongoing studies to further investigate the possibility of heredity, these answers may present a pattern. Also, if two relatives are different ages but contracted the disease at the same time, it may point to environmental factors.

6. What are the dates of your two most recent falls? This is important in establishing a frequency or a pattern to the falls. What were the conditions under which you fell? If the

conditions were similar, a goal of therapy might be to learn how to avoid these situations.

7. What medication are you taking? At what time today did you take the medication containing L-dopa? (actually ask the name of the medication such as "Sinemet." First, some medications can cause Parkinsonism. Many patients see several doctors and do not always communicate a complete history to each one. It is important to note familiar drugs they might be taking, that are contraindicated for Parkinson's and inform the physician. In addition, many Parkinson medications have an on-off effect on the patient, which means that after a certain amount of time, the patient "shuts down" or cannot perform well. In addition, the disease itself, often goes through unpredictable fluctuations. Most often, though, a patient will know these periods, or at what point into their medication, or even into the day, that they are less functional. If so, then seeing the patient at his "on" time may be more beneficial during therapy. However, seeing the patient once or twice during the "off" periods may also be of help to work on goals for the patient to get through those difficult periods.

8. Do you have or have you ever had any episode of low back pain? In some articles, low back pain has been documented as one of the earliest symptoms of the disease.[24] Often this pain will not respond to analgesics or heat. It results from the early let down in postural reflexes causing too much demand on the low back. The one treatment that often will eliminate the pain is the anti-Parkinson's medication containing L-dopa.

9. Do you live alone? This is important to determine the goals of the program in ADL.

In addition to these questions, ask the patient exactly what problems he is having. This is often easier for him to describe when presented with a problem list as shown in Table 8-1.

Ask the traditional history questions (i.e., a history of major surgery, high blood pressure, or a heart condition, that could affect performance in therapy). After concluding the history, a focus of the patient's goals can be obtained by asking what three things have changed most since he has had

Table 8-1 Problem List for Patient

Please check if you have ever had any difficulty with the following:
1. Getting out of a chair _____
2. Sitting down in a chair _____
3. Getting out of bed _____
4. Turning in bed _____
5. Carrying things while walking _____
6. Brushing teeth _____
7. Chewing _____
9. Drooling _____
9. Handwriting _____
10. Getting stuck _____
    If so, check below when it occurs:
    In a crowd _____
    In a narrow space _____
    When changing directions _____
    When asked to rush _____
    Other _____
11. Getting dressed _____
    If so, check below for which items are difficult:
    Tops _____
    Slacks _____
    Underwear _____
    Shoes _____
    Other _____
11. Losing balance _____
    If so, check below for when it happens:
    Getting up to walk _____
    Changing directions _____
    After bending down to get something _____
    For no reason at all _____
    Other _____
12. What has changed most since you found you had Parkinson's?

13. Would you like to have more information about Parkinson's?

Parkinson's disease. This will usually present a good focus of what goals are most important to the patient.

At this time, it is also effective to offer the patient more information about Parkinson's disease. (See Educating the Patient, this chapter).

Principles of Treatment

Because of the use of L-dopa, which became available in 1970, the picture of a Parkinson's patient has changed greatly, from a rapidly deteriorating individual to one who is slowly losing control of his movements and coordination. Carr and Shepherd explain that in addition to L-dopa, physical therapy is necessary to help the patient "adjust to his new situation (created from the use of L-dopa) and to enable him to make full use of his new capabilities."[5]

The main principles involved in the physical therapy treatment for Parkinson's patients receiving L-dopa are as follows:

1. "Prior to the use of L-dopa, the course of Parkinson's disease was completely downhill"[10] (p. 39) and physical therapy could offer only maintenance care.
2. The patient has often been using poor movement patterns for longer than is documented, and what is abnormal often seems normal to them. Imprinting of poor movement patterns often occurs with the Parkinson's patient, even one who may be on L-dopa but receives no physical therapy, and is allowed to continue to practice in error, movements that he perceives as normal.[5]
3. The goal of therapy is to help the patients relearn normal movements. Often this is done through intense, repetitive drilling of simple movements to create a proper movement pattern and establish it as a habit. Be sure to emphasize upper trunk rotation. Inhibiting and avoiding abnormal patterns previously established is essential.
4. The Parkinson's patient seems to have lost an innate goal or direction of movement but responds well to visual and audio cues to aid movements. Improvements in movements, decreases in reaction time, and improved coordination have been demonstrated through the use of audio and visual cues in the treatment of Parkinson's patients.[25–27]
5. The patient often has to relearn movements on a conscious level, as opposed to automatic or subconscious, and requires much effort.
6. Lack of motivation, associated with depression, is the one symptom that is not helped by L-dopa.
7. Fatigue occurs easily, is slow to disappear, and should be avoided. Stress, which may include resistive exercises, increases all symptoms. Just as the Parkinson's patient shows slowing of all major movements, as well as some autonomic

functions, such as bowel and bladder, he is also slow to recover from stress. The rigidity that grips his muscles so much of the time is an unpleasant and exhausting experience. Resistive exercises only enhance this feeling in the rigid patient and should be discouraged or used minimally.

Assessment and Individual Treatment Techniques

In assessing the Parkinson's patient, one can create numerical scales on which to rate involvement, or involvement can be rated as mild, moderate, or severe. Timing and distance are the most objective assessments, such as walking 10 feet, sitting down, getting up, and walking back in 2 minutes.

Preliminary assessment of the patient is made during the history taking and includes observation of (1) gait, (2) facial expression, (3) spouse interactions, (4) recent memory, and (5) apparent mental status. The main areas of concern in the treatment of the Parkinsons' patient in physical therapy are (1) extension, to work against the Parkinson's posture of flexed trunk and extremities; (2) upper trunk rotation; (3) reciprocal motion, which is no longer automatic (e.g., arm swing during gait); (4) weight shifting, which is a problem from slowed postural and balance reflexes; (5) facial mobility; (6) hand dexterity; and (7) activities of daily living (ADL).

For the ease and tolerance of the patient, position changes should be minimized. The assessment and treatment sequence described will follow a typical session, with specific techniques at each different position level. The levels considered are lying supine on a plinth, lying prone on a plinth, sitting on a plinth, sitting on a chair, standing, and working on the floor.

Lying Supine on the Plinth

Assessment is made of range of motion of

1. Shoulders (flexion and external rotation)
2. Hips (flexion and extension)
3. Knee (extension)
4. Ankle (dorsiflexion, plantarflexion, inversion/ eversion)
5. Forearm supination and pronation are sometimes affected, but supination is usually more involved.

Strength can be tested generally; however, weakness is not a major problem with the Parkinson's patient. One area of concern, however, is the abdominals. Asking the patient to do a sit-up while lying supine on the plinth is a good opportunity to assess the strength of the abdominals. Working toward independence in coming to sitting should be a goal of therapy. This is important for carry over to control while sitting down in a chair and to avoid the usual plopping back that is characteristic of a Parkinson's patient. Also emphasized in this position is upper trunk rotation. Exercises include

1. Upper extremity. Active, active-assistive exercise to tolerance, shoulder flexion, and rotation are usually uncomfortable due to rigidity in approximately the last 80°. Supination is usually limited in second half of range.
2. Ankle range of motion is sometimes slow and limited; active or active-assistive for ankle circles and dorsiflexion and plantarflexion.
3. For low back and hip flexion, have patient bend knees so that feet are flat on mat in hooklying position. Bring both knees to chest. After returning feet to mat, patient should then bridge, raising hips toward the ceiling. Alternately bring knees to chest, and finally bring both knees to chest and make a circle with the knees, while the feet are off the mat.
4. Sit-ups (for abdominals and upper trunk rotation). While patient is lying down, have him hold a cane above his head, but parallel to the floor as in Figure 8-1A. Then swiftly have the patient come to sitting, bringing the cane toward his ankles (Fig. 8-1B). The therapist may hold the patient's feet, as needed, or he may even pull slightly on the cane to assist as the patient is coming up. Also, the cane provides the patient with a visual reference. When the patient is sitting upright, ask him to rotate with cane at shoulder level, all the way to the right and then to the left for upper trunk rotation. When the patient is returning to the lying position, have him begin with the cane at shoulder height and go back slowly "with control," maintaining the cane at approximately 90° shoulder flexion, as the patient returns to mat (Fig. 8-1C). Tell the

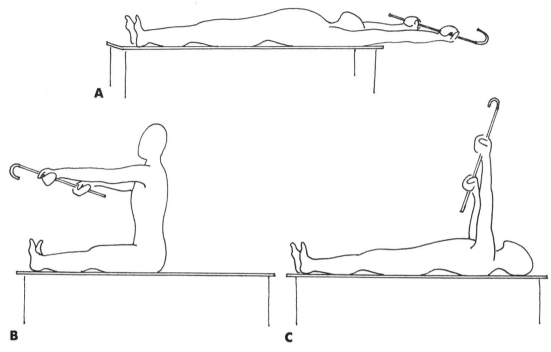

Fig. 8-1 Sit-ups.

patient to tighten the abdominal muscles and to focus his eyes on the cane and not to plop back down. Because of the stooped over posture, the abdominals often never have a chance to reach their normal length, and these muscles are important for control in sitting down in a chair and in coming to standing.

Lying Prone on the Plinth

Range of motion for knee flexion and hip extension is best assessed with the patient in this position. Knee flexion range is consistently limited in the last 90°, especially caused by rigidity in the quadriceps femoris. If the patient has been inactive or sits a great deal, just getting to a prone position will be painful due to the tightness in hip extension, which is also characteristic. Prone is also a good position to check and work through scapular ranges of motion, which are not usually limited.

To help reduce the rigidity temporarily, use rapid assisted reciprocal flexion-extension in both knees as demonstrated in Figure 8-2. In addition slow, gradual stretching to tolerance is necessary for the patient to eventually gain range. Sitting

for long periods during the day, with much inactivity, should be discouraged.

Hip flexors are often a target area for rigidity due to the classical position of the Parkinson's posture. Lying prone will help stretch the hips into a more neutral position. With proper pillow placement under the patient to allow support for the spine, lying prone for a few minutes should be a daily requirement for the patient.

Sitting over the Edge of the Plinth

Many Parkinson's patients are unable to right themselves after they have leaned to one side because weight transfer is difficult. From supine, ask the patient to come to sitting over the edge of the plinth. Here with legs hanging down, the patient rocks from side to side, shifting weight from one hip to another. Check for sitting balance.

The patient should use whole body motion to allow the shift in weight from right hip to the left, getting one hip in the air and then the other (Fig. 8-3). Raising the knee with the hip will allow more leverage.

For weight shifting forward to back, and also

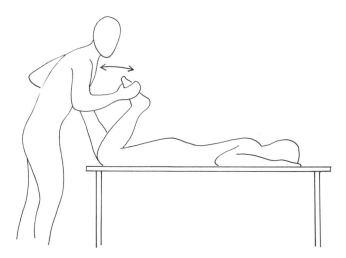

Fig. 8-2 Rapid reciprocal movements to enhance knee flexion and release rigidity.

for bringing in the abdominals, the patient rocks front to back. The patient sits over the plinth, with feet hanging down, and leans back and brings the knees slightly up from the mat (Fig. 8-4). Stand behind the patient, and ask him to try to maintain his balance without putting his hands on the mat. Have the patient then rock forward, lowering knees to the mat and leaning forward over them. Repeat rocking motion again for five to seven repetitions.

Sitting in a Chair

To assess reciprocal motion, ask the patient to sit in a chair opposite the therapist. Ask the patient to point his left arm and right leg, and then to reverse the pattern. If the patient is having difficulty, then ask him to work with just one set of extremities. Patients with more involvement of the disease usually cannot work with both arms and legs together. This previously automatic pattern

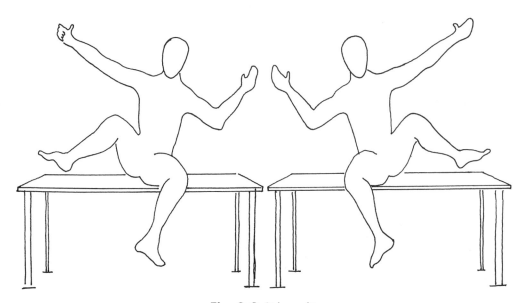

Fig. 8-3 Side rocking.

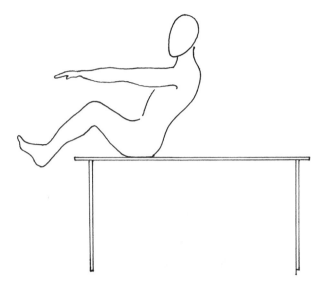

Fig. 8-4 Rocking forward and back.

now can be performed only on a conscious level. This is an important pattern that carries over into gait because it allows for more stability.

For these exercises the therapist sits opposite the patient and presents a mirror image of what the patient is to do.

Point Opposites

The therapist points the left arm and right foot, and asks the patient to point his right arm and left foot (Fig. 8-5). If the patient gets confused or frustrated at not being able to coordinate his movements, go on to reciprocal movements of one set of extremities. For example, ask the patient to point the right arm and then the left, as you mirror the motions. Then work with the legs separately. As this action progresses and the patient can perform it well, attempt to combine arms and legs. The mirror image gives the patient the needed visual guides for movement, and the verbal cues

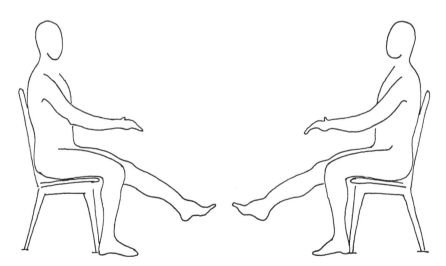

Fig. 8-5 Reciprocal motion—point opposites—using a mirror image.

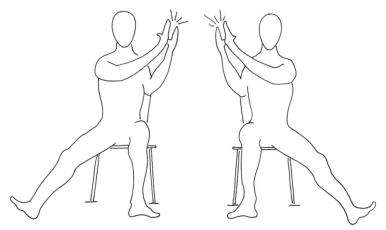

Fig. 8-6 Sit and clap.

helps the patient to "think opposites," reminding him that you should never have an arm and a leg pointing from the same side.

Sit and Clap

In addition to reciprocal motion, sit and clap develops the ability of performing two activities at the same time. Ask the patient to point his right foot forward and clap hands to the left. When he switches to point the left foot forward, turn and clap to the right at the same time the foot touches the floor (Fig. 8-6). This exercise also brings in upper trunk rotation as the patient claps to the side.

Shift Opposites

Shift opposites is used to develop reciprocal motion, as well as weight shifting (Fig. 8-7). Ask the patient to shift both arms to the left and both feet to the right, and then to switch.

Supination—Pronation

Have the patient bend forearms at 90° elbow flexion. Have one palm facing the ceiling and one facing the floor. Switch them simultaneously. This is an important motion and is usually greatly limited in supination. This dysfunction carries over into the problems with grooming, such as brushing teeth, holding and manipulating silverware. The

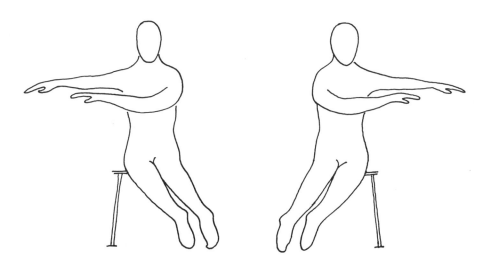

Fig. 8-7 Shift opposites.

patient usually needs much daily stretching (active or active-assistive), to increase the supination range.

Scapular Muscle Stretching

For scapular muscle stretching, have the patient hold the cane with the left hand under and the right hand over (Fig. 8-8). Rotate the cane so that the patient's left hand moves the cane upward and then rolls over toward the floor, with the two elbows extended, until the arms are crossed with the left arm over the right. Then return to the starting position as shown in the figure, and repeat a few times. Switch hand positions and reverse movement of the cane and repeat. Coach the patient to keep the elbows straight, and push the cane away from the body. This is mainly to stretch the rhomboids and other scapular muscles, which often are not stimulated to their full range.

Neck Range of Motion

While the patient is in the chair, neck range of motion can be assessed. Usually, there is limitation due to rigidity and poor posture in neck extension. The sitting patient provides a good opportunity to perform active or active-assistive neck flexion-extension, neck rotation, and lateral movements, all of which are usually limited in the last 25 percent of movement.

Trunk Flexion–Extension, Eye Muscles

For trunk flexion-extension, eye muscle stimulation, and coordination, the patient is asked to hold a cane, with hands about 14 inches apart. Begin with the cane lowered to the ankles. Then raise it up toward the ceiling. The patient is asked to follow the cane with his eyes, as it moves, to stimulate the eye and neck muscles. Then, the patient is to lower the cane down again and repeat. Following with the eyes also gives a goal of direction to the movement and serves as a visual cue. To assess eye movement only, the patient is asked to move his eyes up and down, and then side to side, and told *not* to move his head. This is often a problem, and proper feedback from the therapist or a family member is important, so they know they are isolating the movements.

Grasp and Release

To assess grasp and release, ask the patient to toss a cane into the air and catch it or to throw a ball. The cane toss is intended to develop better control of grasp and release. The patient is asked to hold the can upright in one hand and toss the cane fully away from his hand into the air and then to catch it. Repeat with each hand. often, the difficulty arises in letting go of the cane. If so, let the patient drop the cane toward the floor, so as to experience the feeling of releasing the cane. Then slowly work toward tossing it into the air.

Fine Motor Control of the Hand

Fine motor control of the hand is usually greatly impaired, as reflected by handwriting, which becomes smaller and illegible; use of silverware; and dressing. To assess fine motor control, have the patient write his name; check the signature. Usu-

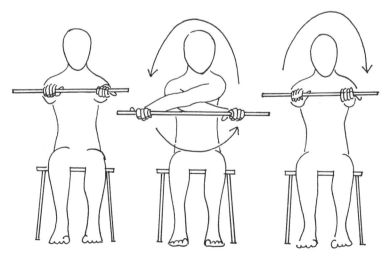

Fig. 8-8 Cane rowing.

ally, the handwriting gets smaller and cramped. Check regularly the date samples. Dressing, including buttoning and zippering, involves hand dexterity problems and must also be assessed, especially for the patient who is alone. To improve hand coordination, typing is recommended, even if there is no knowledge of how to type. Just to have the exercise of using the fingers individually on each key as they press down can be beneficial. For handwriting, since visual cues are important, the use of a children's script book aids in relearning normal writing, through tracing or copying the large figures illustrated in the book.

Activities of Daily Living

Often the following problems are associated with Parkinson's and should be assessed:

1. Getting in and out of a car
2. Getting in and out of a bathtub
3. Getting in and out of a shower
4. Getting up from the floor
5. Getting out of a chair at a table
6. Walking and carrying things
7. Dressing

Suggested ADL devices include card holders and an adapter to enlarge the buttons on push button phones. Also, placing a fluorescent sticker with an arrow pointing over the key hole is a visual cue for placing keys in locks properly.

Check forearm supination and pronation while the patient is sitting, as limitations in supination carry over to difficulty with eating utensils and personal grooming, such as shaving and teeth cleaning. Ask the patient to hold silverware and simulate eating to judge for problems. For eating aids, built up handles on utensils and scoop plates for ease in getting the food on the utensils are suggested. When the patient is eating out, cutting food is often difficult and sometimes cause for embarrassment. It is wise and a lot less conspicuous to ask the waiter to cut the patient's food before he brings it to the table.

Facial Mobility

Facial mobility, which is an automatic motion, including spontaneous expressions and natural unpremeditated movements of the face, is usually decreased or nonexistent in patients with Parkinson's disease. To assess orofacial and facial mobility, constantly talk to the patient and look for

appropriate responses. Ask the patient to make the following expressions: (1) smile-whistle, (2) wrinkle nose, (3) relax, and (4) open and close eyes. The ability to move the muscles is present, but the spontaneity is lost, and often the decreased resulting movement leads to muscle tightness. The muscles involving all expressions need to be stimulated and worked daily. The therapist should do these exercises with the patient during therapy, but for visual guidance at home and for feedback on how well he is doing, the patient should exercise in front of a mirror.

Have the patient go through the following movements:

1. Smile (all teeth showing) in front. Then move lips to a whistling position.
2. Wrinkle the muscles around the nose and upper lip and then relax.
3. Close eyes tightly, and then open wide, raising the brow.
4. Open the mouth and move the lower jaw side to side (Fig. 8-9). This is often difficult for the patient; many patients demonstrate an ability to move the jaw with ease to only one side or not at all.

In addition to facial movements, speaking, swallowing, and chewing are all movements that are slowed in Parkinson's. Any activity that will help define and increase mobility in these actions is helpful. Many patients have difficulty with choking; large pieces of meat, pasta, and any difficult food to swallow should be avoided. If at all possible, the patient should *not eat alone*. Teach the Heimlich maneuver to family members.

Mental Assessment

To assess mental acuity, note if the patient is able to follow directions, and check his memory when

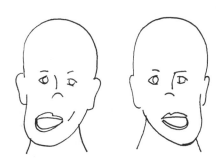

Fig. 8-9 Jaw movements—facial mobility.

asking questions. Be alert to the possibility of depression.

Standing Position

Evaluate for gait, balance, posture, and the ability to come to standing. Be sure to assess rotatory components of movement. Determine if the patient needs help to stand from a chair or if he maintains his balance once up, an area that usually requires much work for the Parkinson's patient. Independence is the goal for gait assessment. Look for height of steps; arm swing during gait; and posture, keeping head upright and shoulders back; and the ability to maintain gait as he turns or changes direction.

Glue foot, which affects many patients, involves getting stuck before or during walking. It is important to observe if the patient can get started on his own from the glue foot or if work needs to be concentrated on this activity.

Observe if patients can maintain an upright position if pushed sideways, forward, or back, and even during gait. The ability to keep an upright posture standing and sitting should be assessed, as well as the position of the head during gait and while sitting at a table.

Frequent falls in the Parkinson's patient are a result of the slowed or absent righting and protective reflexes. Assess for balance and watch the patient in the clinic where frequent episodes of poor balance can occur. It is important to attempt to reduce the number of falls and/or at least to teach how to fall with more control or protection.

The following exercise plan is recommended.

Getting In and Out of a Chair

If at all possible, the patient should not use the arms of the chair, if he can do without them. First, the patient should move to the edge of the chair and bend forward so that his arms are reaching out and down, and his shoulders are over his knees as in Fig. 8-10. At that point, the patient should begin to raise up, with the weight of his body shifting on to the balls and toes of his feet. After standing, he will then straighten his posture and level out his feet so that both heels also touch the floor. If the patient uses the handrests (as suggested in many patient guides) when the patient gets to standing, often he is still holding onto the

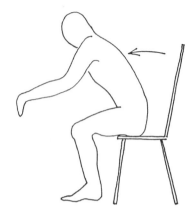

Fig. 8-10 Getting up from a chair.

handrests, which are slightly behind him. After he lets go, the weight of his body usually shifts to his heels, and the toes are raised, resulting in the patient often falling back into the chair. For this reason, coach the patient to lean forward in an attempt to raise up, and always shift the weight onto the front part of the feet.

Often the greatest error in sitting down in a chair is the tendency to lead with the head and the upper body. This usually results in the patient plopping back into the chair, often landing in an awkward position, which he is unable to correct because he is so far back in the chair. The objective is to maintain control, which is achieved through proper posture in lowering the body to the chair. This is accomplished by telling the patient to lower his hands down his thighs toward his knees, causing him to lean forward slightly and bend at the hips (Fig. 8-11). As his hands are running down his legs toward his knees, ask the patient to lower his buttocks toward the chair. By maintaining this posture when he reaches the chair, the patient has his head forward and is in a position of control. After sitting in the chair, the patient is often able to slip himself back into a position of choice.

Gait

Most Parkinson's patients have poor posture, leaning forward slightly or a great deal. There is poor arm swing, usually with the wrong pattern. They usually have low, shuffling steps. To help the patient relearn the normal pattern of gait first list the elements needed, demonstrate them for him, and then do them with him, usually right beside him. Show and tell the patient to stand erect, look

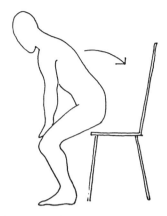

Fig. 8-11 Sitting down in a chair.

ahead, and move the left arm forward with the right leg simultaneously. Explain that the shoulders rotate opposite to the hips. Next, move the right arm forward with the left leg. When working with the patient, tell him to think of the parts he will start with and to say them aloud. Coach the patient to think "opposites" and to check visually the parts he has moved forward. Move slowly for the first few steps, saying the parts for him to move, such as "right arm, left leg." If this progresses well, as you are moving beside him, say "switch" for the next step. If the correct parts are

moved, then move to a cadence such as "1, 2, 3, 4," or "left, right." If there is a problem, slow the patient down, and work very slowly again. Working beside the patient for training in gait patterns gives the visual cues helpful to re-establish the pattern.

Mirrors help the patient see the pattern correctly. Allow the patient to walk in the correct pattern while you stay behind and count. Always remind the patient to stop walking when he observes the pattern to be incorrect. If he tries to miss a step or move arms swiftly to correct the pattern while in gait, this usually sets the patient up for a fall. It is better to create a habit of stopping to correct the pattern when the patient himself or an observer indicates that the pattern is incorrect.

Often, the Parkinson's patient has difficulty doing two things at once. That is, it is difficult for the patient to walk in a pattern that involves direction changes and to also keep the proper walking pattern of moving the opposite arm and leg forward. All these activities often have to be performed on a conscious level. These types of movements are important in ADL. To simulate frequent problem situations, have the patient walk a figure 8 pattern between two chairs placed about 6 feet apart (Fig. 8-12). It is important to remind

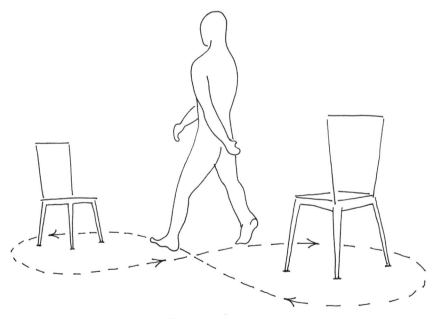

Fig. 8-12 Figure 8.

the patient to maintain the proper walking pattern of right arm and left leg and then reverse as he continues in the figure 8 pattern. Usually, he will lose the pattern as he rounds the back of each chair. Have him check the pattern visually and continue to coach "lift and swing" in a rhythmic voice or count a cadence so that he can maintain an even pattern and not slow down around the chairs.

Any change of direction poses a problem; however, turning around poses an especially hazardous one. These situations often cause the patient to get his feet tangled under him, lose his balance, and fall or nearly fall. He may also go into small shuffling steps or even get stuck. Even maneuvering in the kitchen may require many 180° turns. Therefore, try to have the patient establish turning as a very consistent and controlled pattern. The newly learned pattern is always in one direction and always with the same footwork pattern. Even if a patient wants to turn in the other direction to save steps, I usually insist that he turn in the same direction at all times to be consistent, as they are creating a new habit, which may become more automatic with repetition.

The pattern recommended is shown in Figure 8-13. Beginning with the standing position, ask the patient to move his right foot slightly behind him, and point the toes to the right to create an "L" with the shape of his two feet. Then, the patient steps around toward his right, bringing his left foot to the right, as in the third sequence. Begin the L-pattern again, until the patient is turned in the direction he wants.

To stimulate looser arm swing and mobility of the upper trunk, before the patient walks, have him swing his shoulders around, with the arms swaying one in front and one in back, and then reverse (Fig. 8-14).

Walk and Clap. When the patient is standing, have him point the right foot forward and clap his hands to the left (Fig. 8-15). When he takes his next step and moves his left foot forward, he should also clap his hands to the right at the same time his left foot touches down, to practice doing two things at once. The exercise also stimulates reciprocal motion and upper trunk rotation.

Balance and righting reflexes are slowed or even

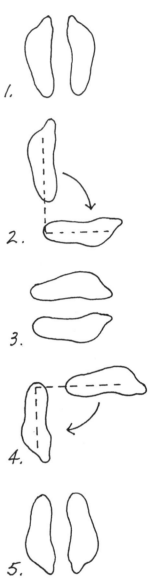

Fig. 8-13 Turning pattern.

nonexistent with many Parkinson's patients. The ability to shift weight properly from one foot to the other rapidly, or even in a walking situation, is difficult. It is important in relearning how to stop a fall, but also just to enhance the fluidity or normal gait.

Forward Shifting. Initially, in retraining weight shifting, visual cues are usually helpful but should not be used continually. Place an envelope or some other small piece of paper on the floor in front of

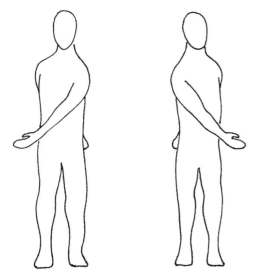

Fig. 8-14 Swing shoulders.

the patient's dominant foot and ask the patient to step over it with his dominant foot. At the same time, have him put both arms forward with the wrists extended as though to push something away. Ask him to shift his weight completely onto the dominant foot. Then ask the patient to return to the upright position, returning his hands to his side.

Lean and Rock. Have the patient place his dominant foot forward, and lean onto it shifting both hands forward (Fig. 8-16). When leaning forward make sure the foot behind him lifts up as the weight is shifted onto the dominant foot ahead. As the patient shifts back onto the nondominant foot make sure the arms pull in and the dominant foot still stays ahead but lifts up.

Glue-foot Release. To help the patient learn to get out of a glue foot have him rock from side to side, shifting his weight from one foot to the other. If the patient has a cane, it is helpful to turn the cane sideways (Fig. 8-17) and sway it from side to side. It is also helpful for the patient to set up a cadence to establish a rhythmic background, such as left-right-left. Instead of struggling to go on and getting more unstable, the patient should be encouraged to stop, relax, and take deep breaths to regain control before continuing.

Backstroke. The backstroke emphasizes upper extremity extension, upper trunk rotation, and weight shifting and encourages fluidity of movement. Demonstrate the maneuver while standing opposite the patient. Encourage the patient to keep his left elbow straight as it comes up across the hips and toward the ceiling (Fig. 8-18). Note the shift in weight to the right foot and the upper trunk rotation as shown. When the arm reaches 180° flexion with the wrist in a neutral position, the body shifts back toward both feet to share the weight and the trunk faces forward. As the arm

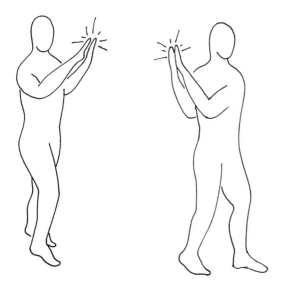

Fig. 8-15 Walk and clap.

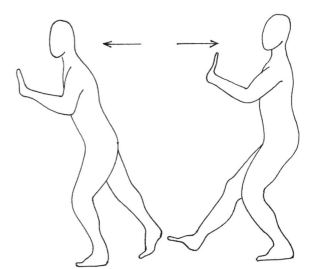

Fig. 8-16 Shift forward. Lean and rock.

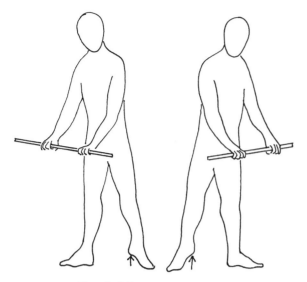

Fig. 8-17 Glue foot release.

begins to lower behind the patient, the contralateral arm begins to cross the hips and go toward the ceiling. The weight shift to the left foot begins and upper trunk rotation also occurs.

Speed Drill. Many patients indicate difficulty in getting up from a chair or walking when they have to get somewhere fast. The highest risk for possible falls occurs during these times. Work through this problem situation by simulating it with three chairs arranged in a circle. Have the patient begin by sitting in one chair, and then getting up quickly and going to the next chair and sitting down. Then have him get up quickly from chair two and go to chair three and sit down. If the patient can tolerate this, go through a few chair changes. Work with this each session to observe the problems that occur when the patient is hurried and to help him become aware of them and how to eliminate them.

Floor Exercises

Floor exercises are usually for the patient who is in a very early stage of the disease. These exercises are more demanding and require more balance and coordination efforts. Be careful to note the tolerance level of the patient.

Weight shifting-siderocking is done in the long sitting position on the floor with arms at 90° abduction. Have the patient rock side to side (Fig. 8-19), lift one hip completely in the air, then rock to the other. Hip walk is done for weight shifting and upper trunk rotation.

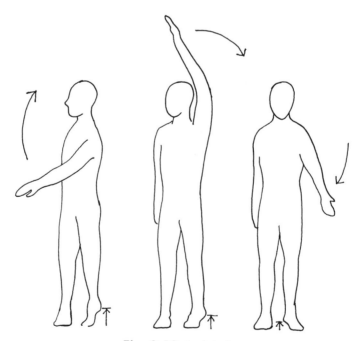

Fig. 8-18 Backstroke.

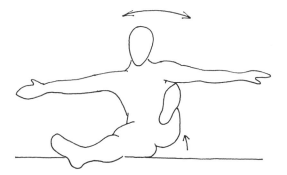

Fig. 8-19 Floor exercises—side rocking.

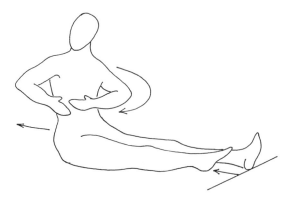

Fig. 8-21 Hip walk backwards.

Forward Hip Walk

Begin in long sitting position, with shoulders at 90° flexion, and hands extended forward over the feet. Begin by thrusting the left arm and leg forward so that the left hip comes off the floor, and move forward on the left leg. Then thrust the right arm and leg forward, pulling the body and leg forward, so that the patient is actually moving forward on his buttocks across the floor (Fig. 8-20).

Backward Hip Walk

Begin with long sitting position, and move upper body quickly to the right with elbows bent (Fig. 8-21) while pulling right hip and leg backwards. Then turn upper body rapidly to the left with elbows bent, and pull left hip and leg backwards, so that the body is moving backwards on the floor. This is very good for upper trunk rotation. If the movements are performed rapidly, the patient may develop better coordination and movement; the exercise also helps with performing movements quickly.

Knee Flexion and Balance

Have the patient stand on his knees (Fig. 8-22), arms out to the side at 90° abduction, and no flexion at the hips. The therapist stands behind the patient with knee behind his back and hands in a protective position behind the patient's scapular areas. Instruct the patient to lean back as a unit, not bending at the hips, and then to come upright again to the starting position. The patient will feel the quadriceps stretching out as he goes into more knee flexion. The ability to hold the knee standing position and to regain it after leaning back requires good balance and also taps the abdominals.

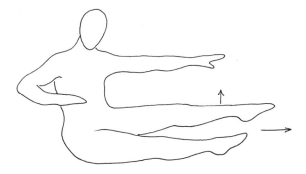

Fig. 8-20 Hip walk—forward.

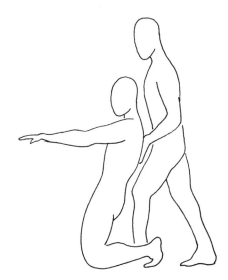

Fig. 8-22 Knee standing.

Treatment Techniques for Group Exercise Sessions

The goals of the group exercise session for Parkinson's patients are manifold. If you consider that most of the week's activities of the Parkinson's patient are spent in competition with non-Parkinson individuals. For the Parkinson's patient, the group exercise session offers the patient a chance at peer competition. In addition, it is a coming together, a sharing of abilities and pleasures, and empathy to understand limitations.

In Parkinson's patients, the basic natural rhythm of gait and fluidity of movement is greatly decreased or even nonexistent. In the group session, the exercises are performed to music, which provides a controlled, rhythmical background. All types of music have been successful in the group setting. Varying the types within one session is often more interesting to the patients. Anything with a marching beat is extremely helpful, whereas any basa nova beat is very difficult. Extremes in tempo, either too fast or too slow, are awkward. Many ballads, modern rock, classical, and country tunes can be successful. Alternatively, a metronome can be used, which provides a good controlled metered background for exercise and is somewhat less conspicuous than a tape deck in a physical therapy clinic.

The basic exercise group for Parkinson's patients consists of six to eight patients. One therapist and, if possible, an aid or assistant should be present to help with spotting and for general safety precautions. The session lasts 45 minutes and is often held once a month. Many of the patients find it helpful to come for individual sessions and then work with the group monthly.

It is usually less threatening if all the patients in a group are of the same level of involvement. This reduces self-consciousness. All the exercises can be modified to fit the patient. Goals should be realistic and relevant, and fatigue should be avoided whenever possible. Remember that facial mobility can be worked throughout all the exercises, by continually reminding the patient to "smile." Considering the many problems facing a patient with a chronic, deteriorating illness, and remembering that physical therapy can be fun, the program is often more beneficial when this philosophy prevails.

Because of the controlled, metered background provided by the music, a basic goal of the group session is to improve the flow and spontaneity of motion by correlating movements with the music and triggering a more fluid response to movement.

Some patients do not prefer working in a group. Many of the group exercises can be done with just the patient and the therapist to a music background. Nevertheless, I have noted that a majority of patients benefit the most from group activity and have also enjoyed it.

The routine begins with warmup, and general stretching without music, then progresses through the following musical tempos: slow, moderate, fast, then back to moderate and ends with a cool down or slow rhythm. Activities can be performed on the floor, sitting, and standing. Chairs are placed in a semicircle, the therapist stands or sits front and center. The four basic areas of concentration for the group exercises are extension, reciprocal motion, upper trunk rotation, and weight shifting. Also, the combining of two activities at once taps and aids coordination.

Initially, the therapist demonstrates the motions they are going to cover in the group session. After demonstrating a movement, the name of the movement is given, and then the group is asked to do the activity along with the therapist before the music begins. Note that the therapist is facing the group for both the standing and sitting exercises and, therefore, is presenting a mirror image of movement. Name the next movement you are going to perform a few seconds before you perform it so that patients can get ready for the position change.

During the music, one exercise follows another in time to the music. A great deal of thought should be developed to selecting the appropriate music and in choreographing appropriate movements. It is also helpful, once you are familiar with the group, to survey the participants' musical preferences.

Reciprocal Motion

1. *Reach opposites, sitting.* The patient points his right arm into full shoulder flexion, and slightly to the right and extends his left knee. Then reverse.

2. *Clap opposites, sitting.* The patient claps and then hits his right palm to the left knee. Claps again and then hits the left palm to the right knee.
3. *Point opposites.* Can be done sitting or standing. Patient points left arm and right foot then reverses.
4. *Side opposites, standing.* Patient points the right leg to the right and left arm to the left. Then brings both arms to the side and both feet together (Fig. 8-23). He then points the left leg to the left, and the right arm to the right.

Upper Trunk Rotation

1. *Sweep the floor.* This exercise can be done sitting or standing. Put arms into 90° shoulder flexion and move them parallel, first all the way to the right slightly flexing right elbow, and then all the way to the left, slightly flexing left elbow, using a very fluid movement. As you sway arms from side to side, turn the upper trunk.
2. *Hit hips, standing.* Place both hands on the left hip, slightly posteriorly and turn head to look at the hands (Fig. 8-24). Then swing arms to place hands on right hip, also slightly to the posterior, and turn head to look at hands. In addition to upper trunk mobility, this is good for the eye and neck muscles.

Weight Shifting

1. *Sideways lean and rock, standing, feet and arms apart.* Lean to the left so that right foot comes up and then lean to the right, so the left foot comes up.
2. *Touch step, standing.* Beginning with feet apart and hands out to the side, touch right foot to the left foot and then return to starting position. Then touch the left foot to the right foot.

Extension

1. *Arms overhead.* Have the patient stand, with the arms at 90° abduction. Bend left arm laterally into extreme abduction, at which point the patient bends the elbow over the head pointing to the right (Fig. 8-25). Return left arm to start position and proceed with right arm. The shoulders often do not get into full shoulder flexion or abduction, and the elbows are often flexed. This exercise allows good elbow extension and movement of the arms away from the body.

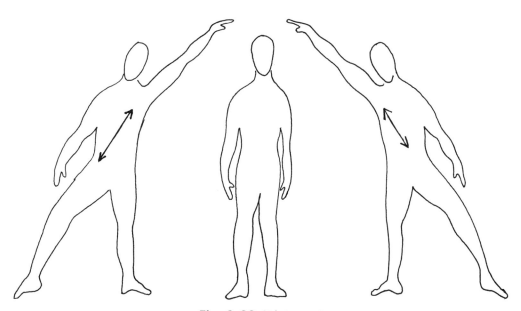

Fig. 8-23 Side opposites.

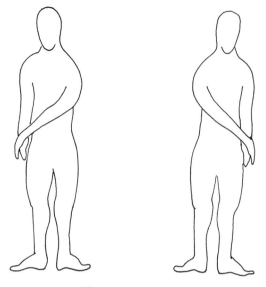

Fig. 8-24 Hit hips.

wrists can aid fluidity of movement in gait. This exercise works the wrists into full extension and flexion. Standing or sitting, begin with arms at 90° abduction, and wrists extended. Then as arms move slowly toward 90° horizontal adduction, keeping them parallel to the floor, simultaneously flex and extend wrists (Fig. 8-27). Then move arms into horizontal abduction, away from each other, maintaining wrist flexion-extension movement throughout as you reach starting position. the whole pattern can be repeated.

Combination of Movements

1. *Sway arms and turn.* For coordination in gait and arm activity simultaneously, and for balance. Raise arms above head. As you sway them from side to side, turn in a circle.
2. *Sway arms and step.* Two activities at once are worked on involving arm motion and stepping sideways. Begin in standing position, and bend elbows. After the elbows are bent in front of the patient, with palms facing away, have the forearms move side to side, in a "window wiper" fashion. When that motion is established, as the arms sway to the left, have the patient step sideways to the left. When the arms sway back to the right, then the patient

2. *Arms across.* Standing or sitting, begin with arms at 90° abduction, and bring both arms across each other into horizontal adduction (Fig. 8-26). Then, open arms again, into horizontal abduction, back to starting position. This activity is good for stretching elbows and pectorals.
3. *Wave wrists.* Often during gait the wrists are locked into flexion and are very right. Floppy

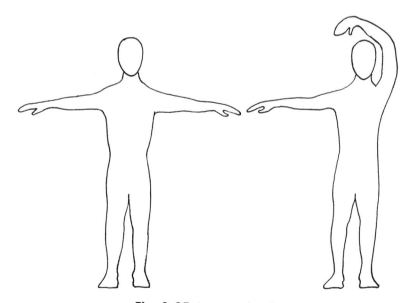

Fig. 8-25 Arms overhead.

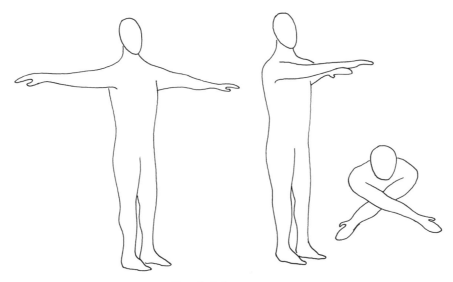

Fig. 8-26 Arms across.

brings his right foot toward his left foot. Continue pattern for a few steps in each direction.

3. *Side step, standing*. Patient has hands together in a clapping position and feet together. Patient steps to the left and opens arms wide (Fig. 8-28). As the patient brings his right foot toward his left foot, he closes his hands to a clapping position simultaneously.

Many props such as canes and balls can be

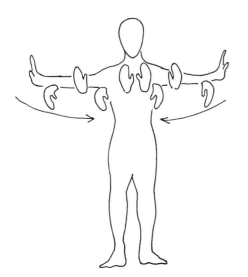

Fig. 8-27 Wave wrists.

used during the group sessions. The canes offer a visual cue and help as a goal in the direction of movement. Many patients find it easier to use them when working to music. They are held sideways, parallel to the floor, with both hands holding them. *Sway arms and step* is a marvelous exercise for use with the canes, and really helps with the focus on the swaying motion of the arms. The concept of simulating the patient's problem situations and establishing a working model in the clinic is important, so that what goes wrong in these situations can be observed and corrected. Allowing the patient to rely on himself when recovering from a difficult situation, such as glue foot and getting off pattern in gait, is a major step toward the patient's independence. I refer to these activities as independent recovery techniques, and they are a source of pride for the patient and family when they do occur.

Families should be instructed and a home exercise program should be established after about eight to ten weekly treatments. As the disease progresses, patients may want to check in accordingly. The exercise group is a very good way for the early Parkinson's patient to keep in shape and it often meets on a monthly basis. Many patients, however, prefer to have their workout once a week with their therapist; for many who live alone it is their only motivation for exercising.

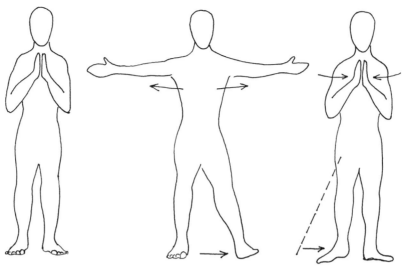

Fig. 8-28 Side step.

Psychosocial Aspects of Parkinson's Disease

Understanding the patient's psychosocial status and needs is essential in planning an appropriate physical therapy program.[28] His feelings and attitudes have a profound influence on his motivation and the possible success of a therapy program. The most important part of the physical therapy program in Parkinson's disease should not be exercises, but motivation.[10]

Parkinson's patients often have a low self-opinion regarding their abilities, and progress needs to be documented in meaningful ways.[5] Realistic goals are paramount in making the treatment relevant to the patient's goals.

Depression

Depression is a common symptom among Parkinson's patients[29,30] and is significantly more severe than in other major disabilities, even paraplegia.[29]

That depression is more than just a reaction to illness is supported by the pathological findings indicating decreases of dopamine, noradrenaline, and serotonin in the patient's brains; functional deficiencies of these compounds can result in depression.[31] Mesolimbic and mesocortical dopamine projections degenerate in Parkinson's disease, and this might indicate reduced capacity to experience reward or pleasure.[31]

Many patients, when given a diagnosis of a chronic disease, go though the same stages of grieving as one mourning the loss of a loved one. Whether the patient is in the denial, anger, bargaining, depression, or acceptance stage will make a major difference in their receptiveness to therapy and their motivation. Family members also go through these stages when the patient is diagnosed and may not always be in the same stage as the patient. This may be a factor in carry over of the therapy to a home exercise program. The drug L-dopa is not effective against the depression resulting from Parkinson's disease.

Parkinson's Personality Profile

The basic personality traits of a Parkinson's patient include the following:[32]

1. Self-reliant
2. Over-control of emotionality
3. Goes his own way
4. Moral rigidity[8]

It is also suggested that there might be a pre-morbid personality showing a state of perpetual emotional tension and constant worrying.[8]

Basic Social Interferences from Parkinson's

Many Parkinson's patients suffer embarrassments socially from physical effects of the disease, such as

1. Difficulty with eating (food slips out of mouth due to poor chewing coordination; inability to

cut food at table due to poor fine motor hand coordination and tremor)
2. Tremor (embarrassing shaking, cause for self-consciousness)
3. Difficulty with toileting activities (inability to clean, or zip or button, often requiring assistance)
4. Lack of facial expression (usually triggers poor social relationships)
5. Depression and self-consciousness (often causes patient to withdraw from social activities)
6. Role reversal with spouse (often a source of friction and difficulty in relationships)
7. Many people at the Parkinson's age are in second marriages. The impact of taking care of another spouse with a long-term illness is a great source of stress to the Parkinson's spouse.

Educating the Patient

Fear of the unknown appears to be a great source of stress to the Parkinson's patient. Local support groups are important media for the patient and family members to air their feelings and get important information about the disease. Many national organizations offer much information, usually at no cost and through toll free numbers. Political action on drug research and benefits for the disabled can be a source of strength and pride for these patient groups. National Parkinson's organizations have been engaged in this activity in the past. A list of these patient organizations is contained in the Appendix. These groups can offer lists of local support groups to the patient. The physical therapist may be the first one in the health care system to offer the patient this information.

The Parkinson's patient is experiencing a great deal of change in his life. The therapist should try to understand these changes and to help the patient understand the relevance of the treatment goals. This can help the patient regain some control and responsibility over his life.

Medications Used in the Treatment of Parkinson's Disease

To understand the treatment of Parkinson's disease, the effect and principles of medication cannot be overlooked. Understanding the side effects, as well as the effects of the medication the Parkinson's patient is using, is important in understanding what the patient is experiencing. The medications can have a profound effect on performance and attitude in therapy, and a solid knowledge of this aspect of their management is important in planning a relevant treatment program.

L-DOPA

L-dopa, a medication to replace the dopamine depleted in the Parkinson's patient, is the main hope for slowing the symptoms of tremor, bradykinesia, and rigidity, although it does not stop the progression of the degeneration in the Parkinson's disease process. It is only useful for a limited time. It is during this time, however, that physical therapy plays a major role in helping the patient relearn normal patterns of movement and improve his quality of life. Because L-dopa loses its effectiveness with time, the physician usually has to individualize doses for the Parkinson's patient. The physical therapist, who usually has more contact time with the patient than many other health professionals, can be an important source of information to the physician regarding the effectiveness of the medication.

With the use of L-dopa, the rapid functional decline of the Parkinson's patient is slowed, and a whole new approach to treatment can be established. L-dopa is the precursor of dopamine, which will not pass through the blood-brain barrier when given to humans. When L-dopa is administered, it crosses the blood-brain barrier and enters the brain where it is converted to the needed dopamine.[17] The major side effects of L-dopa are[33]

1. Decreased effectiveness with increased use. Therefore, gradually increased doses are necessary for the patient to benefit from the drug.[15]
2. Dyskinesia, or uncontrolled undirected movements
3. On-off phenomena, which is an abrupt transition from profound dyskinesia, or even a highly mobile state, to marked akinesia[15]
4. Hallucinations and dementia
5. Nausea, vomiting, and loss of appetite

The goal in medicating the Parkinson's patient

is to allow the minimal dose of L-dopa to be as effective as possible, for as long as possible.[15] A study of Parkinson's patient conducted at Northwestern University revealed that a combination of L-dopa medication and physical therapy results in an earlier greater level of functioning than when L-dopa is administered without physical therapy.[10]

Sinemet

For patients who cannot tolerate the dramatic nausea usually associated with L-dopa, a compound was created adding a decarboxylase inhibitor known as carbidopa, to the L-dopa.[15] This prevents most of the L-dopa from being used up before it reaches the brain and allows a lesser amount of L-dopa to be effective. Commercially, this compound of L-dopa and carbidopa is known as Sinemet, one of the most frequently used medications in Parkinson's treatment.[34] Most of the side effects for L-dopa compound, including high dose dyskinesia, are also associated with Sinemet, except that the nausea is greatly reduced.

Acetylcholine Inhibitors

Another approach to treatment, although not as effective as L-dopa, is to manipulate the level of acetylcholine, which exists in a seesaw arrangement with dopamine. Whichever one of these neurotransmitters is depleted, the other will predominate. With the depletion of dopamine, acetylcholine predominates in Parkinson's disease.

Anticholinergic medication eliminates some of the acetylcholine, allowing the dopamine that does exist to be more effective. One commercial anticholinergic is known as Artane. Some side effects associated with anticholinergics are (1) dry mouth, (2) blurred vision, and (3) constipation.[33]

The use of both anticholinergics and L-dopa to prolong the effectiveness of the L-dopa compounds is not unusual, but in general the anticholinergics are not as effective as L-dopa.[15]

Dopamine Agonists

Another type of medication that is used, particularly for those who do not respond well to L-dopa, are the dopamine agonists, such as bromocriptine (commercial name—Parlodel). These medications imitate the action of dopamine in the brain.[4] It is not as effective as dopamine but has some of the same side effects. Of particular concern are the hallucinations that patients sometimes experience while on the medication.[4,34]

Antihistamines

Antihistamines are also used for patients with mild complaints of sleep disorders. It serves as a mild sedative and also helps reduce tremor. A common antihistamine used is Benadryl. The antihistamines can cause drowsiness, which can be a problem for the patient who has a tendency to fall.

Table 8-2 summarizes the main medications used in the treatment of Parkinson's disease. Some commercial names and their side effects are listed.

Other Medications

Amantadine (Symmetrel) was initially used as an antiviral medication. When given to a flu victim who was also suffering from Parkinson's the Parkinson's symptoms markedly improved. The drug decreases rigidity, bradykinesia, and tremor. Mild swelling of the feet is another side effect.[33]

Drug Holiday

Because L-dopa loses its effectiveness with time, it is useful to put the patient on what is known as a "drug holiday." This is a period of time when the patient is taken off all medication to increase the sensitivity to L-dopa. A very traumatic experience for the patient, the drug holiday usually takes place in a hospital setting, under strict medical supervision. It often allows the patient to start with lower doses of medication after the few days he has been taken off all medication, and less amount of L-dopa seem to be effective. Hence, it alleviates the serious side effects associated with high doses of the medication.[19]

Medications Contraindicated for Parkinson's Disease

Phenothiazines are contraindicated for Parkinson's disease. They are known to have extrapyramidal side effects, one of which is tardive dyskinesia.

Another medication of concern to the therapist working with Parkinson's patients is Haldol. This

Table 8-2 Medications in Parkinson's Disease

Type	Examples	Comments	Side Effects
L-DOPA (levodopa)	Larodopa, Bendopa, Dopar	Decreases bradykinesia, rigidity, and tremor; Counteracted by vitamin B_6	Nausea and vomiting, dyskinesia, confusion, on-off effect
L-DOPA with decarboxylase inhibitor (L-DOPA/Carbidopa)	Sinemet	Same as above No effect from vitamin B_6	Less nausea, dyskinesias, confusion, on-off effect
Anticholinergics	Kemadrin, Artane, Pagitane, Cogentin	Decreases shaking and rigidity	Dry mouth, blurred vision, constipation, confusion, mottling of the skin
Dopamine Agonists (bromocriptine)	Parlodel	Not as effective as L-DOPA; Mild reduction in bradykinesia, rigidity, & tremor	Hallucinations, nausea, visual disturbances
Antihistamines	Benadryl, Disipal	Mild sedative decreases tremor	Drowsiness
Other Amantadine	Symmetrel	Not as effective as L-DOPA; Mild reduction of bradykinesia, tremor, and rigidity	Mild swelling of the feet

(Data from Afifi et al.[3], Sweet et al.[33], and Angel.[34])

medication is often prescribed for Parkinson's patients who show psychotic disturbances, such as hallucinations. The medication is basically contraindicated for Parkinson's disease is that it too can cause dyskinesias. However, in patients with severe mental complications it is sometimes prescribed.

Parkinson's patients often see many doctors simultaneously—a neurologist, a general practitioner, and sometimes a psychiatrist. One physician may not know what medications the other has given, or even the other ailments for which the patient is undergoing treatment. It may be necessary for the physical therapist to discuss with the physician the patient's disease and the effect of the prescribed medication.

REFERENCES

1. Gatz AJ: Manter's Essentials of Clinical Neuroanatomy and Neurophysiology. FA Davis, Philadelphia, 1972
2. Atkinson HW: Principles of Treatment—2. p 117. In Downie PA (ed): Cash's Textbook of Neurology for Physiotherapists. JB Lippincott, Philadelphia, 1982
3. Afifi AK, Bergman RA: Basic Neuroscience. Urban & Schwarzenberg, Baltimore, 1980
4. DuVoisin RC: Parkinson's Disease, A Guide for Patient and Family. Raven Press, New York, 1978
5. Carr J, Shepherd R: Physiotherapy in Disorders of the Brain. Aspen Systems, Rockville, MD, 1980
6. Godwin-Austen RB: Parkinsonism—Clinical. p. 292. In Downie PA (ed): Cash's Textbook of Neurology for Physiotherapists. JB Lippincott, Philadelphia, PA, 1982
7. Snyder SH: Clues to aetiology from a toxin. Nature 311:514, 1984
8. Lees AJ: Early diagnosis of Parkinson's disease. Br J Hosp Med 81:511, 1981
9. Sine RD, Holcomb JD, Roush RE, et al: Basic Rehabilitation Techniques, A Self-Instructional Guide. Aspen Publication, Rockville, MD, 1981
10. Blonsky ER, Minnigh EC: The changing picture of Parkinsonism, Part I & II. Rehab Lit 32:34, 1971
11. Warfel JH, Schlagenhauff RE: Understanding Neurologic Disease, A Textbook for Therapists. Urban & Schwarzenberg, Baltimore, 1980
12. Levitt S: Cerebral Palsy. p. 378. In Downie PA (ed): Cash's Textbook of Neurology for Physiotherapists. JB Lippincott, Philadelphia, 1982
13. Anderson WA, Scotti TM: Synopsis of Pathology. CV Mosby, St Louis, 1972
14. Lyght CE (ed): The Merck Manual of Diagnosis and Therapy. Merck Sharp & Dohme Res Lab, Rahway, NJ, 1966
15. Perlik SJ, Kollner WC, Weiner WJ, et al: Parkinsonism: is your treatment appropriate? Geriatrics 1980:65
16. Clark RG: Manter and Gatz's Essentials of Clinical

Neuroanatomy and Physiology. FA Davis, Philadelphia, 1975

17. Gordon VC, Oster C: Rehabilitation of the patient with Parkinson's disease. Journal AOA 74:308, 1974
18. Davis JC: Team management of Parkinson's disease. Am J Occup Ther 31:301, 1977
19. Forssberg H, Johnels B, Steg G: Is Parkinsonisan gait caused by a regression to an immature walking pattern? Adv Neurol 40:375, 1974
20. Saito M, Tomonaga M, Narabayashi H: Histochemical study of the muscle spindles in Parkinsonism, motor neuron disease, and mysasthenia. J Neurol 219:261, 1978
21. Milner-Brown HS, Fisher MA, Weiner WJ: Electrical properties of motor units in Parkinsonism and a possible relationship with bradykinesia. J Neurol Neurosurg Psychiatry 42:35, 1979
22. Sandyk R: The role of cortical and subcortical mechanisms in voluntary movement in Parkinson's disease. S Afr Med J 20:283, 1982
23. Birkmayer W, Danielczyk W, Reiderer P: Symptoms and side effects in the course of Parkinson's disease, J Neural Transm [Suppl] 19:185, 1983
24. Sandyk R: Back pain as an eary symptom in Parkinson's disease. S Afr Med J 2:3, 1982
25. Cooke JD, Brown JD, Brooks VB: Increased dependence on visual information for movement control in patients with Parkinson's disease. Can J Neurol Sci 5:413, 1978
26. Stefaniwsky L, Bilowit DS: Parkinsonism: facilitation of motion by sensory stimulation. Arch Phys Med Rehabil 54:75, 1973
27. Yanigasawa N, Fukimoto S, Tanaka R: Visuomotor control of leg tracking in patients with Parkinson's disease or chorea. Adv Neurol 39:883, 1983
28. Doneson IR: The role of the physical therapist in emotional rehabilitation. p. 201. In Kreuger DW (ed): Rehabilitation Psychology. Aspen Publications, Rockville, MD, 1984
29. Mayeux R, Williams JB, Stern Y, Coté L: Depression and Parkinson's disease. Adv Neurol 40:241, 1984
30. Robins AD: Depression in patients with Parkinsonism. Br J Psychiatry 128:141, 1976
31. Fibiger HC: The neurobiological substrates of depression in Parkinson's disease: a hypothesis. Can J Neurol Sci 11 (Suppl):105, 1984
32. Ogawa T: Personality characteristics of Parkinson's disease. Percept Mot Skills 52:375, 1981
33. Sweet R, McDowell F: A Manual for Patients with Parkinson's Disease (booklet), American Parkinson's Disease Association, New York, (no date given)
34. Angel JE (ed): Physicians' Desk Reference. 38th Ed. Medical Economics Company, Oradell, NJ, 1984

Appendix:
National Parkinson's Organizations

American Parkinson's Disease Association
116 John Street
New York, NY 10038
800-223-2732 (toll free)

National Parkinson Foundation
1051 N. W. 9th Ave.
Miami, FL 33136
800-327-4545 (toll free)

Parkinson's Disease Foundation
William Black Research Building
640 West 168th Street
New York, NY 10032
800-457-6676 (toll-free)

Parkinson Foundation of Canada
Suite 232 ManuLife Centre
55 Bloor Street West
Toronto, Ontario M4W 1A6 Canada
416-064-1155

PEP of Newport Beach, CA (national
patient's organization)
Parkinson's Educational Program
1800 Park Newport, Suite 302
Newport Beach, CA 92660
714-640-0218 or 800-344-7872

United Parkinson's Foundation
360 West Superior Street
Chicago, IL 60610
312-664-2344

9 Stroke

Pamela W. Duncan and Mary Beth Badke

INCIDENCE

Cerebral vascular disease affects approximately 2 percent of the civilian population in the United States.[1] The rate of stroke incidence nearly doubles in every 10 year age group from 45 to 85[2] and costs American society over $7 billion per year in health care expenses, institutionalization, and loss of manpower due to disability.[3] The prevalence of acute stroke has been estimated at 794 per 100,000 population,[4] and stroke victims use more days in short-stay hospitals than any other major diagnostic grouping.[5] It is particularly relevant to note that when a patient survives a stroke, all but a small percentage of them suffer from limitations in functional activities and subsequently do not become self-sufficient. The most commonly recognized risk factors for stroke are (1) hypertension, (2) heart disease, (3) diabetes, and (4) previous transient ischemic attacks.

DEFINITION AND PATHOLOGY

Stroke or cerebral vascular accidents (CVA) may be defined as a sudden onset of focal neurological deficits caused by a vascular lesion to the brain. In general, vascular lesions may be divided into hemorrhagic strokes, cerebral infarcts caused by thrombosis, and cerebral embolism.

The three most frequent causes of hemorrhagic strokes are (1) hypertensive intracerebral hemorrhage, (2) ruptured saccular aneurysm and vascular malformation, and (3) hemorrhage associated with bleeding disorders.[6] Hypertensive hemorrhage forms a roughly circular or oval mass, which displaces and compresses adjacent brain tissue. After a period of 2 to 6 months, the volume of blood gradually decreases in size. Saccular aneurysms are small protrusions from the arteries of the circle of Willis or its branches and are thought to be caused by deficits in the media and the elastica, which vary in size (8 to 10 mm) and are located most often at bifurcations; the site of the rupture is usually at their dome.[6] An arteriovenous malformation has been described as a mass of dilated vessels that form an arteriovenous fistula; it is a developmental abnormality that varies in size from a few millimeters in diameter to a huge tangle of dilated vessels located in the posterior half of the cerebral hemispheres. Although the lesion is present at birth, most malformations are clinically silent for a long time. The onset of symptoms most often occurs between the ages of 10 and 30.[6] Bleeding disorders that commonly give rise to intracranial hemorrhage are leukemia, aplastic anemia, and thrombopenic purpura.

Atherosclerotic lesions are the primary cause of cerebral infarcts associated with thrombosis. Atheromatous lesions tend to form at branchings and bifurcations of the cerebral arteries. The three most frequent sites are the internal carotid arteries at the carotid sinus in the neck, at the point where the vertebral arteries join to form the basilar artery, and at the main bifurcation of the middle cerebral arteries. The atheromatous plaques are clinically silent as they grow over a period of 20 to 30 years. Intermittent blockage of the circulation eventually leads to permanent impairment of function in the ischemic area of the brain. Sudden thrombus overlying a plaque results in acute signs of infarction. The early stages in the thrombic process may

291

explain the clinical symptoms of transient ischemic attacks (TIA).[6]

A cerebral embolus most often is a fragment of material that has broken away from a thrombosis within the heart. Ischemic infarction occurs after the embolus becomes arrested at a site of narrowing of the lumen. The area most frequently involved is the upper division of the middle cerebral artery. Because of the speed with which the lesion develops, chances of establishing collateral circulation are diminished; thus the chances of sparing brain tissue distal to the area of embolic infarct is less than in thrombosis.[6]

The clinical manifestations of stroke are variable and are determined by the size and location of the lesions. The clinical syndromes and incidences of neurological deficits are summarized in Tables 9-1 and 9-2.

RECOVERY OF FUNCTION

Many studies of the natural history of stroke indicate that most recovery from stroke occurs during the first 6 months after infarct. There are, however, reports in the clinical literature of patients who continue to recover several years after stroke.[7-9] Factors that influence rate of recovery are (1) age, (2) sensation, (3) cognitive function, (4) severe weakness, and (5) delaying therapy.

The fact that the CNS is able to recover and the recent reports of the success of pharmacological

Table 9-1 Clinical Syndromes of Cerebral Vascular Accidents

Vessel	Clinical Symptoms
Internal carotid	Unconsciousness at the time of occlusion Contralateral hemiplegia cortical sensory loss Aphasia when the dominant hemisphere is infarcted
Anterior cerebral artery	Contralateral hemiplegia (lower extremity more involved than upper extremity) Cortical sensory loss Aphasia and mental confusion when the dominant hemisphere is infarcted
Middle cerebral artery	Contralateral hemiplegia (face and upper extremity more involved than lower extremity) Contralateral hemianesthesia Homonymous hemianopia Aphasia when the dominant hemisphere is infarcted Apraxia Alexia Agnosia
Posterior cerebral artery	Homonymous hemianopia Fleeting hemiplegia Thalamic syndrome Choreoathetoid movement Ataxia Tremor
Basilar artery	Loss of consciousness Pupillary abnormalities Disorders of eye movements Facial paralysis Contralateral hemiplegia or quadraplegia Dysarthria Dysphagia Horner's syndrome

(Adapted from Merritt HH: A Textbook of Neurology. Philadelphia, Lea & Febiger, 1970, with permission.)

Table 9-2 Primary Clinical Manifestations of Stroke

	Frequency
Sensorimotor Loss on Contralateral Side of Body	
Motor weakness	50–80%
Sensory function	25%
Difficulty swallowing	30%
Cognitive Dysfunction	
Level of consciousness	30–40%
Mental confusion	45%
Communicative Disorders	
Dysphasia/aphasia	30%
Slurred speech	30%
Visual Disturbances	
Visual field defects	7%
Diplopia	
Perceptual-Motor Problems	
Visual-spatial neglect	Not known

(Adapted from Wade DT, Langton R, Hewer CE, et al: Stroke. © Chapman and Hall Ltd, London, 1985.)

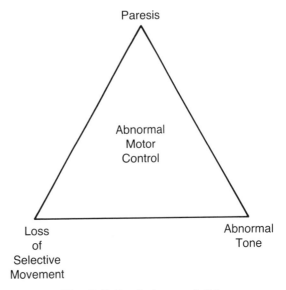

Fig. 9-1 Triad of motor deficits.

agents in facilitating recovery[10] should encourage the perception of stroke as a disease in which the patient has a reasonable chance for recovery and return to a high degree of function.

MOTOR SYMPTOMS OF STROKE

Stroke patients usually present with three primary motor deficits: (1) paresis, (2) loss of selective motor control, and (3) abnormal tone (Fig. 9-1). Paresis (the inability to produce an appropriate voluntary muscle contraction) is the most common characteristic of stroke. Many clinicians have previously assumed that paresis is not a primary motor deficit but rather secondary to an overactive antagonist muscle.[11,12] Recent research, however, has demonstrated that paresis is a primary motor problem caused by abnormal recruitment of motor units and inappropriate frequency of firing of the motor neuron pool.[13–15]

Loss of selective motor control interferes with the capacity to use a variety of movement and postural synergies for functional activities. In stroke, movement is limited to a few stereotypical synergies characterized by poor organization and timing. Brunnstrom[12] has previously described in detail the stereotypical synergies of stroke (Table 9-3).

Table 9-3 Stereotypical Movement Synergies of Stroke as Described by Brunnstrom

	Flexor Synergy	Extensor Synergy
Upper Extremity	Elbow flexion	Elbow extension
	Forearm supination	Forearm pronation
	External rotation of shoulder	Internal rotation of shoulder
	Abduction of shoulder	Adduction of shoulder
	Retraction/elevation of shoulder girdle	Protraction of shoulder girdle
Lower Extremity	Toe dorsiflexion	Toe plantarflexion
	Dorsiflexion and inversion of ankle	Ankle plantarflexion and inversion
	Knee flexion	Knee extension
	Hip flexion	Hip extension
	Hip abduction and external rotation	Hip adduction and internal rotation

Abnormal tone is the most salient feature of stroke. Initially the patient may be flaccid, with decreased resistance to passive movement. As recovery occurs, there is a gradual increase in deep tendon reflexes and increased resistance to passive movement. The distribution of abnormal tone is variable, but the typical patterns involve the flexors of the upper extremity and the extensors of the lower extremity. Clinical observation reveals a relationship between abnormal tone and the ability to move and develop selective control (i.e., flaccid, no voluntary motor control; increase in tone, semivoluntary control of the stereotypical synergies; and decline in hypertonicity, increase in selective control of movement). The assumption has been that paresis, abnormal tone, and loss of selective control have cause and effect relationships. More recently, clinicians have re-examined this assumption and suggest that the three motor deficits are independent symptoms of central nervous system damage, which may correlate with but do not necessarily cause the other. Unless the independence of these symptoms is recognized, therapeutic programs become wishful rather than rational.

SENSORY DISTURBANCES

Stroke patients may experience disturbances in exteroception, proprioception, and vision. With any of these disturbances, the patient may quickly develop a nonuse syndrome with an inability to perform efficient and coordinated movements. In addition, sensory loss deprives the patient of feedback about motor performance. This severely impairs the patient's ability to relearn motor skills.

PERCEPTUAL DEFICITS

Perceptual impairment is intimately related to the sensorimotor deficits of stroke. The degree and type of perceptual deficit in stroke is determined by the side and site of hemispheric lesions. Commonly observed perceptual deficits include problems with left-right discrimination, unilateral neglect, altered spacial relationships, visual inattention, abnormal vertical perception, and poor figure-ground discrimination.

Apraxia is the inability to program a movement sequence when motor and sensory functions are apparently preserved. The apraxic patient is unable to integrate available sensory information with his motor systems to produce purposeful movements. The general apraxias are ideomotor (the patient is able to perform a movement automatically but not volitionally) and ideation (the patient is unable to perform a sequence of motor tasks but can do the different parts of the movement). In addition to the general apraxias there are several specific types of apraxias: dressing apraxias, constructional apraxias, and apraxias of gait and speech.

MEASUREMENT AND EVALUATION PROCEDURES

The assessment of sensorimotor functions after stroke is complex. Many aspects of the disability need to be measured: specific motor and sensory functions, tone, balance, activities of daily living, and gait. Unfortunately, many of the evaluation methods are qualitative rather than quantitative. In addition, the validity and reliability of the assessments have not been established. More recently, however, several separate valid and reliable tests have been developed that quantitatively measure specific functions.

Fugl-Meyer[16] designed an assessment of physical performance that evaluates 50 different movements, and performance is graded on a 3-point ordinal scale (0, unable to perform; 1, performs partially; 2, performs faultlessly). The test evaluates range of motion, pain, sensation, movement, and balance. The reliability and validity of this test have been independently established.[9,17–19] The reader is referred to Fugl-Meyer's original article for specific instructions and guidelines for performing this assessment.[16]

Many activities of daily living (ADL) assessments have been devised, but the Barthel Index, which measures 10 different activities and has a maximum score of 100 points, is the most widely known and used. The advantages of the Barthel Index is its simplicity and well-documented usefulness in evaluation of patients. The reader is referred to the original description of the Barthel Index for specific details and scoring.[20]

In addition to the quantitative measurements of recovery of function after stroke, clinicians need to assess specific sensorimotor deficits (cognition, perception, range of motion, strength, tone, sensation, selective motor control, balance, and adaptability). Guidelines for this assessment are presented in Table 9-4. After all components of abnormal motor performance are assessed, the therapist must evaluate which sensorimotor deficits are contributing to the observed moment dysfunction and select appropriate intervention strategies. (See Table 9-5 for an *example*.)

PRINCIPLES OF TREATMENT

1. The successful rehabilitation of stroke patients uses a problem solving approach. The therapist must assess the patient, define the specific cause of the movement disorders, and select appropriate treatment strategies based on this process.

2. Motor relearning is an active process. In order for there to be a carryover of learned behaviors to activities of daily living the patient must be able to participate actively in all exercises and activities.

3. The ultimate goal of therapy is to improve functional performance. Muscles should not be continually exercised in isolation; rather (as soon as possible) muscle groups should be facilitated in patterns of movement and in goal-directed activities.

4. Relearning of a motor skill requires a lot of practice. Just as in sports, many repetitions of therapeutic exercise and activities are required for skill acquisition.

Table 9-4 Assessment of Motor Control Poststroke

1. Cognition—Perception
   a. Is patient motivated?
   b. Does patient understand instructions and goals of therapy?
   c. Does patient have good long- and short-term memory?
   d. Does patient have perceptual deficits?
   e. Does patient have apraxia?

2. Range of Motion—Pain
   a. Are there range of motion and pain limitations during passive movement?

3. Sensation
   a. Does patient have somatosensory, visual, vestibular, or auditory deficits?

4. Weakness
   a. Does patient have ability to produce muscle force?
   b. Can patient produce force repetitively (endurance)?
   c. Can the patient generate force at faster speeds of movement?

5. Muscle Tone
   a. What resistance to passive movement is present? Increased? Decreased?
   b. What is the distribution pattern of the resistance?
   c. Does resistance change with position?

6. Synergies
   a. Observe movements. Are they stereotyped or varied?
   b. Observe selectivity in movement as patient makes effort, changes position or environment, moves faster.
   c. Are movements coordinated? Are there tremors, dysmetria, slowness, and inability to reciprocate?
   d. Postural Synergies
      1. Does patient have corrective and protective balance responses in upper extremities, trunk, lower extremities during:
         a. Perturbations
         b. Self-initiated movements (observe in come-to-sit, sit, sit-to-stand, stand)
      2. Does patient have balance and weight shift in sitting, standing, walking?

7. Adaptability
   a. Does patient use available movement patterns in functional activities? (rolling, sitting, standing, walking)
   b. What are influences of environmental changes and speed on movement patterns?

Table 9-5 Analysis of All the Factors that Could Contribute to a Motor Deficit

I. Observe motor deficit	Inability to weight shift on involved extremity
II. Assess factors that could cause the motor deficit	1. Perception—The patient's perception of vertical is distorted.
	2. Range of Motion—The patient lacks sufficient hip, knee, or ankle ROM to provide adequate biomechanical alignment for weight shift.
	3. Tone—The patient has excessive and prolonged muscle activity in certain muscle groups.
	4. Weakness—The patient cannot generate appropriate muscle force to maintain body weight or adjust to postural displacements.
	5. Sensory—The patient has inadequate sensory integration to provide feedback about foot placement and weight shift.
	6. Synergistic organization—The patient's movement is restricted to the stereotypical flexion and extension synergies of stroke that do not provide selective and efficient use of flexor and extensor muscle groups for postural adaptations and movements.
	7. Coordination—The patient has deficits in timing and reciprocation of muscle activity.
	8. Adaptability—As the speed and force requirements vary, environmental conditions change and the volitional control of the movement is reduced, the patient cannot respond quickly and efficiently to postural displacements.
III. Evaluate	Decide which of these factors are contributing to the patient's motor deficits.
IV. Select intervention strategies	
V. Treat	

SUGGESTIONS FOR TREATMENT

Individual stroke patients exhibit variable mixtures and intensities of the eight sensorimotor deficits that contribute to movement dysfunction. Therapeutic strategies for stroke rehabilitation must be individualized and based on the patient's primary motor deficits, age, degree of involvement, cognition, related medical problems, and family support.

Many other clinicians have described in detail therapeutic strategies to restore functional movement in stroke. The purpose of this section is not to give a detailed description of each treatment technique but rather to outline and give examples of treatment alternatives for specific motor deficits.

Sensory Deficits

The patient who is experiencing specific sensory deficits should be taught to use alternative methods of feedback. For example, if the patient has diminished proprioception, the patient is encouraged to orient visually to his extremities (Fig. 9-2). Sensory stimulation (stroking, stretching, tapping, vibration, and compression) may also be used to reinforce feedback. Electromyography (EMG) biofeedback is an external mode of feedback that may minimize sensory deficits and augment motor performance.

Range of Motion

When the patient has little voluntary motor control, passive and active assistive exercises must be performed to maintain range of motion (ROM) and flexibility. During upper extremity range of motion, shoulder range of motion must be accompanied by scapula motion (upward rotation and abduction) and depression of the head of the humerus so that the humeral head is not jammed

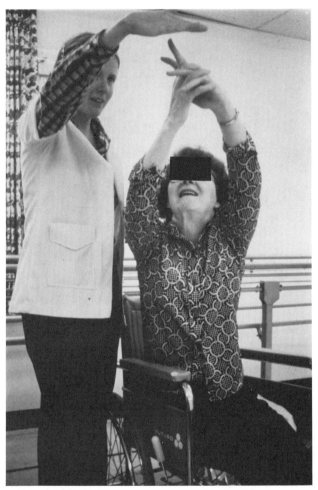

Fig. 9-2 Bilateral activities help integrate both sides of the body.

against the acromial process, causing soft tissue impingement and pain (Fig. 9-3).

Proper bed positioning and splinting will minimize the range of motion limitations. The following positions should be emphasized

1. Shoulder protraction
2. Slight abduction and external rotation of the shoulder
3. Elbow extension
4. Wrist extension and radial deviation
5. Finger extension and abduction
6. Slight hip and knee flexion
7. Ankle dorsiflexion
8. Elongation of the trunk on the involved side.

Proper positioning can be maintained by changes in bed position, pillows, conventional splints, and air inflated splints advocated by Johnstone.[21]

Inhibitive casting, a relatively new technique in stroke rehabilitation, is reported to increase range of motion and decrease muscle tone.[22] Inhibitive casting maintains biomechanical alignment of the ankle that minimizes the risk for developing contracture and enhances weight-bearing on the involved extremity (Fig. 9-4).

Weakness

Paresis is a common problem in stroke. Physical therapy procedures available for facilitation of muscle contraction include tapping, quick stretch, touch, vibration, brushing, resistance, electrical stimulation and biofeedback. When a stroke patient has difficulty in developing an appropriate muscle force, the following sequence of activities is recommended:

1. Use the facilitatory techniques as you passively move the joints.
2. Ask the patient to attempt voluntary movement as you provide necessary assistance.
3. After the patient has developed some volitional control during active assistive exercise, ask him to hold the body part against gravity (isometric muscle contraction) and lower the body part against gravity (eccentric muscle contraction).
4. Ask the patient to move actively against gravity (concentric muscle contraction).
5. Withdraw all facilitatory techniques and assistance.
6. Ask the patient to generate force against resistance repetitively and at different rates of movement. The therapist's role is to help the patient recognize the optimal conditions for development of muscle forces and to minimize excessive effort. This muscle re-education sequence must not be continually performed in isolated movements but rather incorporated immediately into patterns of movements and functionally goal-directed activities.

Abnormal Tone

Restraint to passive movement is a major problem in stroke. It is generally accepted that the hyperactive stretch reflex causes hypertonicity. If ig-

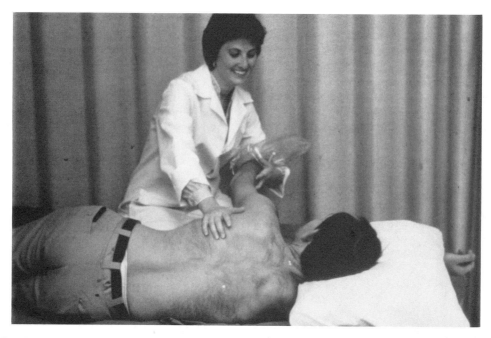

Fig. 9-3 Forward flexion must be accompanied by scapula protraction and upward rotation and external rotation of the humerus.

nored, the hypertonicity causes decreased ROM, contractures, pain, poor biomechanical alignment, and impaired motor control. Many techniques are available to counter hyperactivity; some are based on practical experience, but in others the mode of action is well known. The therapeutic modalities to reduce hypertonicity include cold, slow stroking of the extremity, slow elongation of the spastic muscle groups, rhythmical rotation of the body part, air splints, inversion of the head, and vibration of the antagonist muscles. Several pharmacological agents (diazepam, dantrolene, and baclofen) and surgical procedures (tenotomy and neurotomy) are considered when physical treatment is not effective. The reduction of hypertonicity by any of these techniques is usually temporary and does not necessarily carry over to active movements.

Researchers have suggested that restraint to movement during active volitional contractions is due to an abnormal regulation of the motor neuron pool rather than increased or hyperactive stretch reflex.[23] When the patient volitionally contracts a typically spastic muscle, excessive and prolonged motor unit activity occurs which impairs reciprocal

movement. Suggestions for intervention in this situation include the following:

1. Do not reinforce contraction of the typically spastic muscle before an active contraction of the less active muscle (i.e., if there is restraint to elbow extension do not reinforce active elbow flexion before active elbow extension).
2. Reduce the effort of movement. Excessive effort increases the prolonged motor activity of "spastic" muscles.
3. Use active assistive exercises to encourage slow smooth reciprocal movements. Gradually withdraw your assistance as the patient's volitional and reciprocal control increases.
4. Feedback therapy may be also used to help the patient minimize the excessive motor unit activity.

Selectivity

The movements of most stroke patients are characterized by stereotypical synergies. The flexor synergy predominately prevails in the upper extremity and the extension synergy predominately prevails in the lower extremity. The purpose of

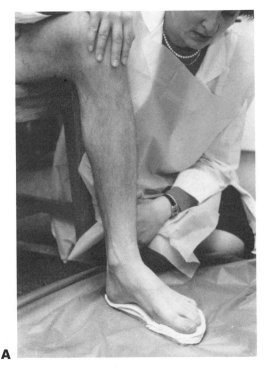

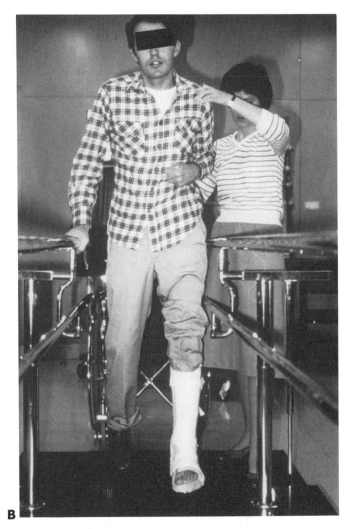

Fig. 9-4 (A) Inhibitive casting used to maintain biomechanical alignment of ankle and prevent development of plantarflexion contracture. **(B)** Enhanced weight-bearing on the involved extremity.

physical therapy is to increase the number of available movement patterns. This is accomplished by

1. Eliciting gross patterns of flexion and extension
2. Combining the components of the flexion and extension patterns
3. Reconstructing new movements
4. Increasing the coordination of the movements
5. Incorporating the new movement patterns in the functional task.

Examples of suggested activities to increase the

variety of movements of the upper arm are as follows:

1. Sidelying—The therapist assists the patient to flex the arm and slowly reverse into extension. This forward flexion must be accompanied by upward rotation and abduction of the scapula.
2. Supine—Encourage the patient to flex his shoulder with elbow extension. Initially the therapist should position the arm and ask the patient to hold the position (isometric muscle contraction) then lower the extremity against gravity (eccentric muscle contraction).

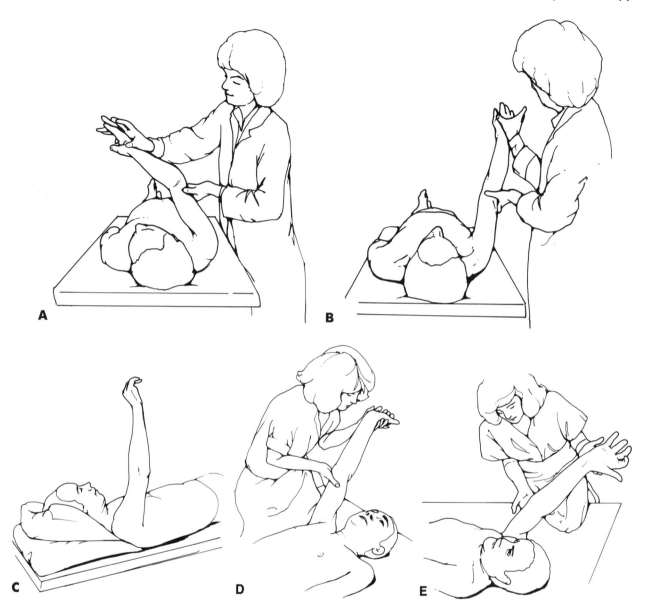

Fig. 9-5 (A) Therapist assists the patient to flex the arm and **(B)** slowly reverse into extension. **(C)** Patient holds the arm in flexion with elbow extension (isometric muscle contraction). **(D)** and **(E)** Patient practices D2 flexion PNF patterns. (*Figure continues.*)

3. Practice D2 flexion proprioceptive neuromuscular facilitation (PNF) patterns.
4. Supine—The patient actively holds his shoulder in flexion as he attempts to alternately flex and extend the elbow.
5. Sitting—The patient practices hand-to-mouth patterns.

6. Sitting—The patient holds the arm in forward flexion with elbow extension.
7. Sitting—Practice raising and lowering the arm with elbow extension.
8. Reinforce the use of the upper extremity in rolling activities, reaching, and in postural displacements (Fig. 9-5).

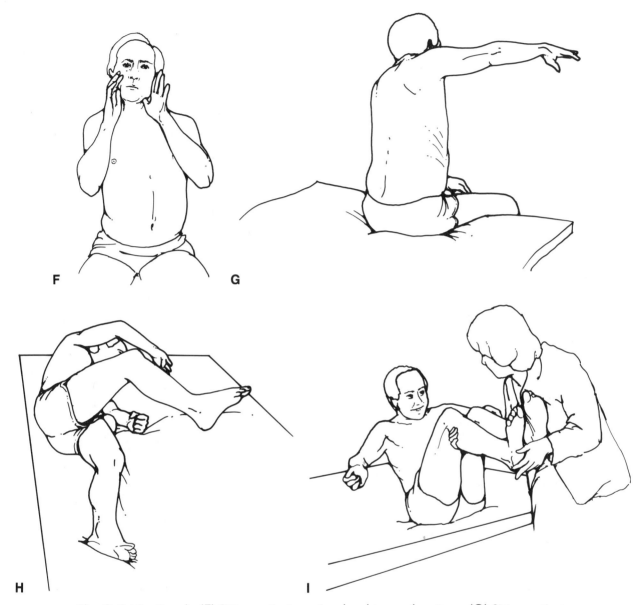

Fig. 9-5 (*Continued*). **(F)** Sitting, patient practices hand-to-mouth patterns. **(G)** Sitting, patient practices raising and lowering the arm with elbow extension. **(H)** Use of the upper extremity is reinforced in rolling and **(I)** in postural displacements.

Balance

The ability to adjust to gravity is a prerequisite for any movement. There are two types of balance responses: corrective and protective. Corrective responses maintain equilibrium in any upright position. This type of response involves specific and discrete sequences of muscle contractions in the ankle, knee, and hip. Protective responses occur when balance is lost and attempt to minimize the effect of an inevitable fall. Protective extension of the upper extremity is an example of a protective response that serves to absorb the impact of landing.[24]

Balance responses are elicited via feedback and feedforward mechanisms. Under the conditions of feedback, the subject is alerted by sensory systems that his balance is threatened. During feedforward the balance responses are programmed with self-initiated movements. Researchers have shown that postural adjustments actually precede the voluntary movement.[25-26] The central nervous system, therefore, is capable of predicting the balance requirements of any movement.[26]

The essential components of balance responses are intact sensory systems that reference the upright position; a peripheral motor apparatus that produces appropriate muscle contractions; functional range of motion and appropriate biomechanical alignment; and finally an intact central nervous system that programs the correct sequence, force, and timing of muscular contractions.

Vision, proprioception, and vestibular functions are the primary sensory systems that alert or trigger a balance response. There is some evidence that as individuals age, the visual system becomes less important for balance responses and the proprioceptive system becomes more important.[27] The chance for falling increases dramatically when two sensory systems are compromised. In stroke, vision and proprioception are often compromised, leading to increased risk of falling and a subsequent fear of falling. In these cases, therapeutic intervention should include (1) sensory stimulation in the weight-bearing position (i.e., stretch, joint compression, resistance, etc.) to enhance feedback and (2) increasing the patient's awareness of subtle displacements in his center of gravity.

A normal biomechanical alignment allows the stroke patient to make efficient and subtle movements for balance responses and minimizes the excessive effort or "stiffness" often observed in the upright postures. For example, a frequent problem in the stroke patient is lack of proximal stability. This leads the stroke patient to fix the pelvis in a posterior tilt.[28] The patient uses positional stability to stabilize his spine, pelvis, and the center of gravity. The feet are usually widely abducted to add more postural stability. If the patient has lateral trunk shortening, the problems in compensations are exaggerated and his posterior tilt becomes tighter. This interferes with the patient's ability to develop a normal process for forward/backward and lateral weight shift. When the stroke patient attempts to weight shift in

standing, he may laterally flex on the weight-bearing side instead of elongating. An abnormal kinematic chain is set up, which increases the posterior tilt of the pelvis, retraction of the pelvis, and hip flexion. With this fixed position, normal mobility and control cannot develop and, therefore, interferes with normal automatic postural adjustments. Furthermore, stroke patients with limited mobility at the joints of the hip and lumbar spine have difficulty controlling the center of gravity over the base of support. In an attempt to prevent falling, the patient will increase his effort in order to compensate for postural instability. This results in a synchronous co-contraction of many muscles rather than a dynamic response of synergistic muscles working together. In addition to the poor proximal alignment, the stroke patient often has improper foot placement. If the base is not in proper alignment, the rest of the lower extremity kinematic chain will be affected.[29] The feet must be aligned correctly and ankle joint motion must occur. With the feet placed in the appropriate position, control of ankle movement, weight shifts, and weight-bearing on the affected extremity will be more easily facilitated.

Forceful and quick muscle contractions are necessary to make rapid adjustments of the center of gravity in order to prevent falls. Stroke patients have profoundly diminished muscle strength and speed of contraction. In addition, they often lack the ability to synergistically organize muscle contractions for postural adjustments. Therapeutic interventions should

1. Facilitate muscular contractions (i.e., biofeedback, neuromuscular electrical stimulation, stretch, resistance, vibration, etc.) volitionally and automatically
2. Increase speed of muscle contraction
3. Reinforce the muscular contractions in a variety of movement patterns and in a variety of positions (i.e., ankle dorsiflexion should be reinforced with the knee and hip flexed, with the hip and knee extended)
4. In standing, ankle dorsiflexion should be elicited in response to a subtle displacement of the center of gravity.

Specific training for correct balance responses should include (1) subtle external perturbations by the therapist in the sitting and standing posi-

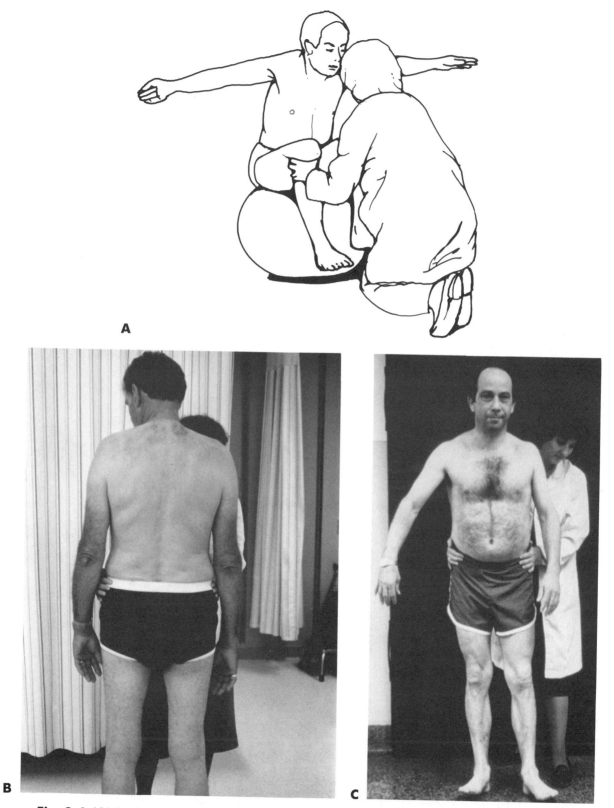

Fig. 9-6 (A) Subtle external perturbations in sitting. **(B)** Lateral displacements of center of gravity in standing. **(C)** Subtle backward displacements in standing.

tions, (2) subtle volitional forward/backward and lateral sways in sitting and standing, and (3) self-initiating movements that require postural responses (i.e., standing, lifting the arm over the head or sitting the patient reaches diagonally backwards for an object). The therapist must avoid using excessive resistance and threatening the patient beyond the limits of his stability. These methods will force the patient to become rigid and prevent the desired subtle corrective balance responses (Fig. 9-6).

If the purpose of therapy is to improve protective responses, the patient must reach the limits of his stability, or he must believe that a fall is inevitable. The protective responses are very different from the corrective responses previously described. Protective responses include quick extension and abduction of the extremities or stepping to prevent falling. It is important to facilitate protective responses in stroke patients, but if they are elicited prematurely, the patient will experience increased muscular effort, increased tone, and lose selective control of available movement patterns.

Adaptability

To adapt the relearned motor skills to a variety of force, speed, movement, and sensory conditions, the patient must develop the basic components of motor control: range of motion, strength, tone, and selective motor control. Many patients do not develop these necessary prerequisites and subsequently do not attain adaptability; yet other patients should be trained for increasing adaptability. Changing the speed and force requirements for movement and altering the environment contexts are methods of adaptability training. Isokinetic training on the Cybex II dynamometer is an appropriate strategy to increase adaptability in movement responses. Isokinetic training should emphasize fast reciprocation of movement at a variety of exercise velocities (i.e., 60°/sec, 90°/sec, 180°/sec, 240°/sec).

FUNCTIONAL ACTIVITIES

The ultimate purpose of any therapeutic intervention is to improve function. In stroke rehabilitation, activities must focus on integrating the two sides of the body immediately and reinforcing the avail-

able and developing motor control of the hemiparetic side. The key functional activities that should be practiced in stroke rehabilitation are rolling, supine-to-sit, sitting, sit-to-stand, standing, and walking.

Rolling

Rolling from supine to sidelying should be practiced to both sides; however, the patient will be more reluctant to roll toward the good side. Reaching forward with the involved upper extremity, trunk rotation, and flexion of the lower extremity should be facilitated while rolling toward the good side (Fig. 9-7).

Supine-to-Sit

Sitting up from a sidelying position requires lateral flexion of the head and trunk, a weight shift on to the abducted "down" upper extremity, and a

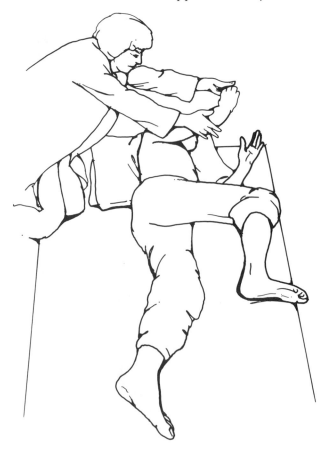

Fig. 9-7 Reaching forward with the involved upper extremity and flexion of the lower extremity is facilitated while rolling toward the good side.

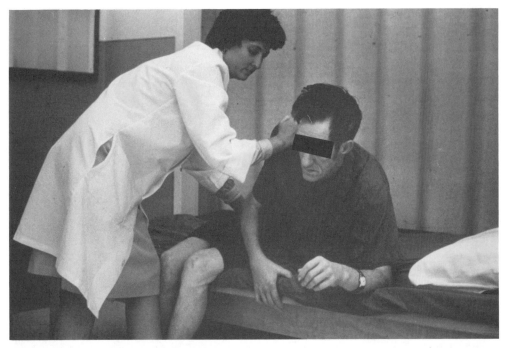

Fig. 9-8 Patient shifts weight onto abducted upper extremity as he moves from supine to sit.

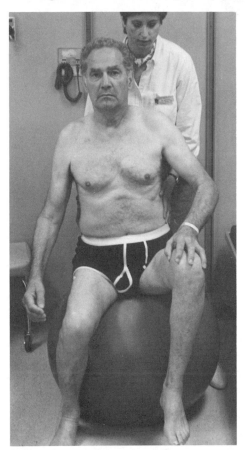

Fig. 9-9 Self-initiating movements that require postural responses.

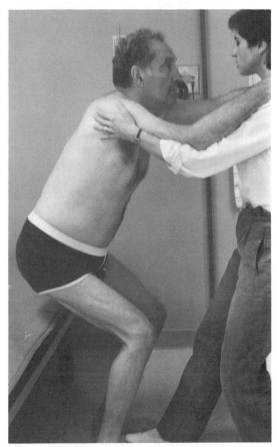

Fig. 9-10 Alignment of both feet and forward inclination of trunk are two key components during sit to stand.

reach across midline and push off with the leading upper extremity. The lower extremities must flex and be moved over the edge of the bed. Moving from supine to sit with the involved side leading willl reinforce lateral head and lateral trunk flexion, whereas leading with the uninvolved side will encourage weight shift over the involved upper extremity and elongation of the trunk (Fig. 9-8). If weight-bearing is forced on the involved upper extremity, the therapist must assist the patient in developing scapula and shoulder control until adequate stability is developed.

Sitting

In sitting, the appropriate alignment of the head and trunk should be emphasized, corrective responses to displacement of the center of gravity should be practiced, and trunk rotation should be encouraged. In addition, during sitting subtle weight shift to the contralateral hip should be facilitated before asking the patient to lift his extremities (Fig. 9-9).

Sit-to-Stand

The alignment of both feet under the patient provides a more normal kinematic chain for shifting the weight forward and standing up. To bring the center of gravity over the feet, forward inclination of the trunk should be facilitated (Fig. 9-10). Finally, hip and knee extension must be reinforced to allow weight-bearing through the lower extremity.

Standing

During standing, symmetrical weight shift is encouraged over properly positioned and aligned feet. Self-initiated, subtle weight shifts forward, backward, and laterally should be encouraged (Fig. 9-11). If the upper extremity tone increases and stereotypical synergies are reinforced as the patient moves to standing, the patient may simultaneously practice some weight-bearing through his upper extremities with the therapist's assistance or independently as he stands next to a plinth.

Walking

Walking is a complex movement that requires reciprocal movements of the lower extremity, exquisite control of displacements of the center of gravity, and unilateral weight shift. The specific

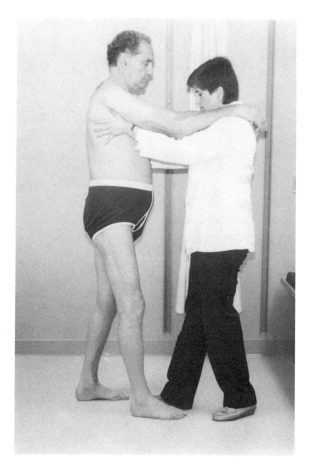

Fig. 9-11 Patient practices self-initiated subtle weight shifts diagonally and backward.

activities for improving gait should be selected by carefully analyzing the missing components of the swing and stance phase of gait. Once a particular gait deviation is recognized and the cause of the disorder is established, specific therapeutic intervention can be selected and reinforced in the context of walking. For example, if lack of heel strike is identified as a gait deficit and insufficient ankle dorsiflexion is recognized as the cause, contraction of the ankle dorsiflexors must be reinforced with knee extension and the patient must practice ankle dorsiflexion with knee extension in the context of gait.

SUMMARY

Rehabilitation of the stroke patient is a complex clinical problem. Although we have discussed strategies to improve motor function, we realize that some patients have such devastating lesions that their movements will never be completely normal. At this time the ability to predict who will benefit from rehabilitation is at best empirical. Successful therapists, however, consider the many factors that facilitate recovery and rehabilitation and attempt to document objectively the value of their intervention. Continued physical therapy that does not produce measurable improvement in functional outcomes is frustrating for the patient and costly for the current health care programs.

REFERENCES

1. Baum HM: Stroke prevalence: An analysis of data from the 1977 National Health Interview Survey. Public Health Rep 97:24, 1982
2. Robins M, Baum HM: The National Survey of Stroke, Chapter 4—Incidence Stroke Part II, 12:I-45, 1981
3. Adelman SM: The National Survey of Stroke, Chapter 6—Economic Impact Stroke Part II, Vol 12(2):I-69-I-78, 1981
4. Baum HM, Robins M: The National Survey of Stroke, Chapter 5—Survival and Prevalence Stroke, Part II Vol 12(2):I-59-I-68, 1981
5. Vital Health Statistics—Series 13 No. 41 Utilization of short stay hospitals. U.S. Dept. Health, Educ., Welfare, National Center for Health Statistics, March 1979
6. Adams RD, Victor M: Principles of Neurology. McGraw-Hill, Inc, New York, 1981
7. Bach-y-Rita P (ed): Recovery of function: Theoretical considerations for brain injury rehabilitation. University Park Press, Baltimore, 1980
8. Bach-y-Rita P: The process of recovery from stroke. In Brandstater ME (ed): Stroke Rehabilitation. Williams & Wilkins, Baltimore, 1988
9. Fugl-Meyer AR, Jaasko L: Post-stroke hemiplegia and ADL performance. Scand J Rehabil Med [Suppl] 7:140, 1980
10. Feeney DN, Gonzales A, Law WA: Amphetamine, haloperidol and experience interact to affect rate of recovery after motor cortex injury. Science 217:855, 1982
11. Bobath B: Adult Hemiplegia: Evaluation and Treatment. William Heinneman, London, 1978
12. Brunnstrom S: Movement Therapy in Hemiplegia. Harper & Row, New York, 1970
13. Edstrom L, Grimby L, Hannerz J: Correlation between recruitment order of motor units and muscle atrophy patterns of upper motor neuron lesions:

significance of spasticity. Experimenta 29:560, 1973
14. Rosenfalck AM, Andreassen S: Impaired regulation of force and firing pattern of single motor units in patients with spasticity. J Neurol Neurosurg Psychiatry 43:907, 1980
15. Tang A, Rymer WZ: Abnormal force—EMG relations in paretic limbs of hemiparetic human subjects. J Neurol Neurosurg Psychiatry 44:690, 1981
16. Fugl-Meyer AR, Jaasko L, Leyman T, et al: The post-stroke hemiplegic patient. 1. A method for evaluation of physical performance. Scand J Rehabil Med 7:13, 1975
17. Duncan, PW, Propst M, Nelson SG: Reliability of the Fugl-Meyer assessment of sensorimotor recovery following cerebrovascular accident. Phys Ther 63:1606, 1983
18. Kusoffsky A, Wadell I, Nilssen BY: The relationship between sensory impairment and motor recovery in patients with hemiplegia. Scand J Rehabil Med 14:27, 1982
19. Badke MB, Duncan PW: Patterns of rapid motor responses in normal and hemiplegic subjects during postural adjustments in standing. Phys Ther 63:13, 1983
20. Mahoney FI, Barthel PW: Functional evaluation: the Barthel index. Maryland State Med J 14:61, 1965
21. Johnstone M: Restoration of Motor Function in the Stroke Patient. Churchill Livingstone, Edinburgh, 1978
22. Winstein CJ: Short leg casting and gait training in adult hemiplegic patients. Unpublished Master's Thesis, Downey, CA, University of Southern California, 1984
23. Sahrmann SA, Norton BS: The relationship of voluntary movement to spasticity in the upper moto-neuron syndrome. Ann Neurol 2:460, 1977
24. Stelmach G, Worringham CJ: Sensorimotor deficits related to postural stability: implications for falling in the elderly. Clin Geriatr Med 1:679, 1985
25. Belen'kii V Ye, Gurfinkel VS, Pal'tsev Ye I: Elements of control of voluntary movements. Biofizika 12:154, 1967
26. Cordo PJ, Nashner LM: Properties of postural adjustments associated with rapid arm movements. J Neurophysiol 47:287, 1982
27. Woollacott M, Shumway-Cook A, Nashner L: Postural reflexes and aging. p. 99. In Mortimer JA, Pironyzolo FJ, Maletta GJ (eds): The Aging Motor System. Praeger Publishers, New York, 1982
28. Ryerson SD: Hemiplegia resulting from vascular insult or disease. p. 474. In Umphred DA (ed): Neurological Rehabilitation. CV Mosby Co., St. Louis, 1985
29. Carr JH, Shepherd RB: Motor Relearning Programme for Stroke. Aspen Systems Corporation, Rockville, MD, 1983

10 Muscular Dystrophy, Spinal Muscle Atrophy, and Related Disorders

Kent Allsop

A myopathy is a disease in which there are morphological, neurophysiological, or biochemical changes in muscles that are not secondary to abnormalities of the central nervous system, anterior horn cell, peripheral nerve, or neuromuscular junction. The muscular dystrophies are a group of myopathies characterized by progressive degeneration, which appear to have a hereditary basis and which, for historical purposes and clinical convenience, have been grouped together.

Duchenne muscular dystrophy (pseudohypertrophic) is the most common dystrophy affecting children and will be emphasized in this chapter. Other dystrophies presented are Becker's dystrophy, limb-girdle dystrophy, myotonic dystrophy, and facioscapulohumeral dystrophy. These myopathies will be discussed in a subsequent section with Charcot-Marie-Tooth disease and three common anterior horn cell diseases, Werdnig-Hoffman, Kugelberg-Welander, and amyotrophic lateral sclerosis. Two collagen vascular disorders, dermatomyositis and polymyositis, will also be presented.

DUCHENNE MUSCULAR DYSTROPHY

Pathology

Duchenne Muscular Dystrophy (DMD) is the most frequently occurring and most disabling of the childhood neuromuscular disorders. It is characterized by progressive weakness, typically leading to death from respiratory insufficiency in the late teens. Estimates of incidence vary from 13 to 33/100,000 live male births.[1]

Another name for DMD, pseudohypertrophic muscular dystrophy, is derived from the abnormally large calves, resulting from an excessive amount of adipose tissue surrounding the muscle tissue of the gastrocnemius and soleus muscles (Fig. 10-1). DMD shows X-linked inheritance: passed to boys from unaffected mothers (passed from mother to son in 50% of cases).

Muscle enzyme serum creatine phosphokinase (CK) is elevated, resulting in a significant diagnostic blood test, not available for the other diseases discussed in this chapter. Carrier detection with the same test is reasonably accurate.

Signs and Symptoms

There is a marked tendency to develop contractures; plantar flexion contractures occur occasionally within the first 3 years of onset. A tendency toward toe walking is an early sign.

Loss of ambulation usually occurs because of the development of hip, knee, plantar flexion and inversion contractures. These contractures are frequently precipitated by bed confinement.[2]

The classical pattern and sequence of weakness exhibited by boys with DMD results in their inability to rise from the floor in the usual fashion. The sequence of movements of rolling to the all-fours position and "climbing up the legs" is de-

remaining on the floor, he places the other hand on the knee to assist in locking the knee in extension. The other hand is placed on the other knee. Both hands alternate as they "walk" up the thighs until the body has achieved the upright position. The maneuver substitutes for both the weakened quadriceps muscles, which lack the strength to lock the knees into extension, and the weakened gluteus maximus muscle, which is unable to bring the trunk to the upright position against gravity.

Other signs are progressive scoliosis, which is difficult to control. Frequent respiratory infections and dystrophic cardiomyopathy[3] are common.

DMD can exhibit nonprogressive intellectual deficit[1,4,5] Misdiagnosis in early years is common.[6] The young boy with DMD frequently begins walking later than siblings and may exhibit difficulty in rising from the floor or climbing stairs.

The progression of weakness is proximal to

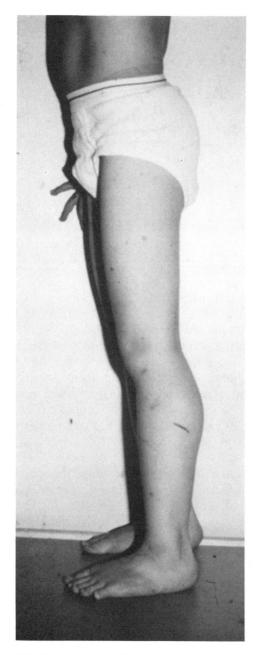

Fig. 10-1 Large calves characteristic of pseudohypertrophic muscular dystrophy.

scribed as Gowers' maneuver (Fig. 10-2). The young boy rolls to the prone position and maneuvers to the all-four position. He then plants both feet on the floor while both palms remain flat on the floor. He walks his hands on the floor closer to his feet while flexing at the hips. With one hand

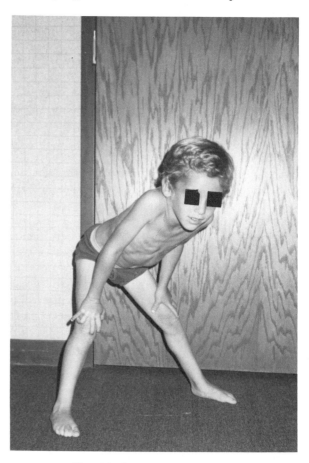

Fig. 10-2 Gower's maneuver.

distal. Early involvement of the gluteus maximus and the quadriceps results in an exaggerated lordotic curve in order to get the center of gravity behind the fulcrum of the hip joint and anterior to the fulcrum of the knee joint. Standing stability at the hip is provided by the structures anterior to the hip joint, primarily the Y ligament of Bigelow.

The boy can no longer climb stairs with the use of a rail when the quadriceps are weakened and the latissimus dorsi muscles lose the strength to pull the trunk up to and over the weight bearing lower extremities. When the boy is in this weakened stage, even minimal knee flexion contracture would make ambulation impossible.

The youngster can no longer rise from the floor when the combined strength of the gluteus maximus and triceps muscles cannot elevate the trunk over the hip joints against gravity. The arms are pulled posteriorly with the elbows, seldom moving anterior to the line of gravity during gait to keep maximum weight behind the fulcrum of the hip joint.

A waddling gait occurs secondary to the weakened gluteus medius and to the broadened base of support. The child weakens and gait alters to provide improved stability.

Contractures of the iliotibial (IT) band result from the wide stance, not vice versa. The IT band accommodates to the shortened position. A boy with noncontracted IT band will ambulate with a stance as wide as a boy with those contractures (Figs. 10-3 and 10-4).

Isolated muscle testing of the pelvic and shoulder girdle reveals weakness. The latissimus dorsi muscle is the first to exhibit marked weakness clinically.

Over time, functional ability can appear to plateau, whereas actual strength continues an insidious decline.[7,8] For a patient on therapeutic drug trials, this period of uniform task completion and essentially normal performance will not indicate the progressive decline; had the stable patients been given drug therapy, one might have concluded that there had been therapeutic benefit.

Physical Therapy Evaluation

The evaluation, based on the functional significance of the therapist's findings, will determine the plan of care.

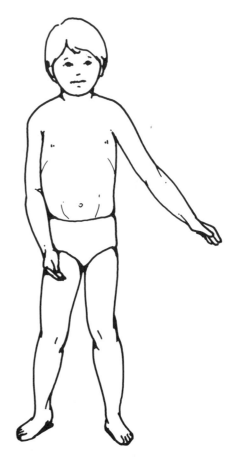

Fig. 10-3 Patient with DMD with wide-based gait.

Functional Ability

Timing common functional activities (i.e., stair climbing, standing from supine) assists in determining the patient's current functional status.

Serial recording of standard functional tasks demonstrates that the DMD youngster passes through one of two phases. The first phase is the stable period where there is no indication of actual progressive decline and can appear to last several years. The second phase is the declining period. Strength exhibits insidious progressive decline, and functional tasks are failed.

There is marked variability in age at the time that functional tasks are failed. For instance, in a report by Ziter and Allsop[9] on functional decline in six functional tasks, one functional task, loss of walking, occurred within the narrowest age range, yet it spanned 5.2 years.

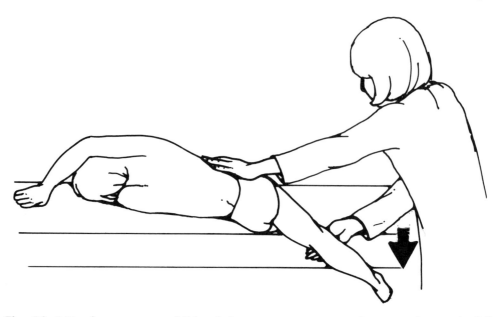

Fig. 10-4 Test for contracture of IT band. Contracture not present when upper leg can be fully abducted as shown.

Age is only a crude indicator of muscle strength and functional impairment. Muscle strength closely parallels loss of function late in the disease. The functional task that reflects muscle strength most accurately is the standing from supine position.[9] Strength loss at failure of this task is 50 percent of normal strength, plus or minus 7 percent, at the time the youngster can no longer achieve a standing position from the floor, irrespective of the youngster's age.

Muscle Testing

Manual muscle testing techniques are the most valid methods of determining strength in DMD. This testing assists in differentiating and determining the diagnosis. It outlines the natural history of the disease. It is also critical to the evaluation of therapeutic drug trials. Serial muscle testing will determine if there is linearity in strength decline and the severity of the disease. If there are plateau or acceleration of the disease process,[7,9] use of braces does not slow the rate of deterioration.[10] Use of wheelchair does not increase the rate of deterioration.[10] By approximately 7 years of age or with 1 year's collection of muscle strength

score, the tempo of the disease can be established for any particular child. The tempo may be rapid (greater than 10 percent deterioration per year), average (5 to 10 percent deterioration per year), or slow (below 5 percent deterioration per year). DMD, as shown by muscle strength linear scores, is not a homogeneous disease (Fig. 10-5). Manual muscle testing assists in prognosticating and determining when bracing or wheelchairs may be indicated.

The following muscles have been routinely graded.

1. Upper trapezius
2. Deltoid
3. Serratus anterior
4. Pectorals
5. Latissimus dorsi
6. Triceps
7. Middle trapezius
8. Lower trapezius
9. Abdominals
10. Gluteus maximus
11. Gluteus medius
12. Iliopsoas
13. Anterior tibialis

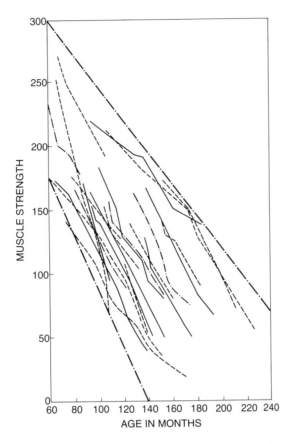

Fig. 10-5 Plotted composite strength scores over time. Each line indicates the progressive measurements of one patient.

These muscles were chosen because they deteriorate at different rates. The composite manual muscle test score of these muscles as they deteriorate approximates the overall decline in total body muscle strength.

In grading the pectoral muscles, no attempt is made to differentiate the strength of the diminished or nonexistent sternal portion from the clavicular portion. Abdominal muscle strength in the fair and less range is difficult to differentiate. Neck flexors are weak, the head does not completely flex forward on the thorax, and the abdominal muscles contract against the resultant longer lever arm. The iliopsoas muscle is tested from the routine position; however, in the weakened stage of hip flexion, the attempted motion is performed by the long head of the rectus femoris and the sartorius muscles.

The sequence of muscle deterioration of eight muscles in a sample of boys with DMD at the time ambulation ceases, from strongest to weakest was (1) deltoid, (2) upper trapezius, (3) triceps, (4) gluteus medius, (5) quadriceps, (6) iliopsoas, (7) gluteus maximus, and (8) latissimus dorsi. These subjects were followed from 20 to 105 months.[9]

The percentage of muscle strength lost in those subjects from the time of the first test to the time ambulation ceased was (1) iliopsoas, 74 percent; (2) gluteus maximus, 74 percent; (3) latissimus dorsi, 60 percent; (4) quadriceps, 56 percent; (5) triceps, 51 percent; (6) deltoid, 47 percent; (7) upper trapezius, 47 percent; and (8) gluteus medius, 44 percent.[9]

Joint Range of Motion (ROM)

Early loss of ambulation occurs from a decrease in joint ROM more frequently than from weakness.[10] Decreased ROM of foot dorsiflexion, knee extension, and hip extension is the cause of early bracing.[10]

Management

No known pharmacological or physical agent can retard the insidious linear decline in strength caused by this myopathy. Proper management can prolong maximum functional ability.[2]

Functional Ability

After the diagnosis has been confirmed, management begins with counseling of the parents who may suffer from guilt, hostility, depression, helplessness, and a myriad of other emotions.

The clinician, faced with this situation can propose a positive approach based on the following: (1) some of the complications which magnify the functional disability of DMD are predictable and preventable; (2) an active program of physical therapy and the timely application of braces can prolong ambulation and more closely approximate the normal independent of later childhood; and (3) if a specific treatment ever becomes available, those in optimal physical condition are most apt to benefit.[2]

Problems in Management

The problems in DMD are

1. Weakness
2. Decreased active and passive ROM
3. Loss of ambulation
4. Family and patient emotional trauma
5. Decreased functional ability
6. Decreased pulmonary function

Home Program

Home program is the *most* important aspect of management. Sustaining enthusiasm for compliance with the home program is a challenge. Success is dependent on keeping the instructions simple, requiring only one or two different stretches to be performed once a day (in repetitions of 10), and providing extensive feedback to the family or support system.

There appears to be improved compliance and rapport when the anxiety of repercussion or guilt for noncompliance is minimized. Immediate, as well as long-term, goals should be outlined to the parents. In the single-parent home, additional support with the home program from older siblings, clergy, social groups, neighbors, school, etc. may be sought.

The purchase of elaborate rehabilitation equipment is unnecessary. Physical therapy once or twice a week is neither warranted nor cost-effective, but monthly or quarterly training and motivation sessions for parents are mandatory. The therapist's examination will identify the current problems. Knowledge of the disease process allows the prediction of the major difficulties that will next occur.

Goals

Once the specific concerns are identified, there are four major goals.

Prevent Deformity

The earliest problem will be the tendency for the development of plantar flexion contractures. Passive stretch of the heelcords performed five or six times a week, one time per day for 10 repetitions of 10 seconds each, will maintain reasonable ROM into dorsi flexion and will prevent necessity for heelcord tenotomies before bracing. Night foot splints are not effective and are not a substitute for the stretching program. When the therapist's evaluation reveals less than normal hip abduction, stretch for tight iliotibial band should begin.

Assist Gait and Mobility
Orthoses
Bilateral long leg orthoses are indicated for the majority of patients with DMD. In addition to the benefits of an upright position, the use of long leg braces enhances the transfer of the patient by an assistant. Long leg braces with no pelvic band, gravity knee locks, and double adjustable ankle stops similar to those proposed by Vignos are used.[11]

Surgery
Early aggressive management and home program compliance can eliminate the need for the orthopaedic surgery so commonly advocated.[1,12] The only surgery deemed necessary (in less than 20

percent of patients) is the heelcord percutaneous tenotomy.[10] Hospitalization has not been used. The orthopaedic surgery is performed on an outpatient basis. Ambulation in walking casts is begun the next day. Surgical procedures and hospitalization performed in association with bracing appears to have little effect on the duration of walking ability.[13] The most useful factor in predicting the duration of walking ability is the percentage of residual muscle strength at the time of bracing. Although more extensive operations may improve mobility in orthoses, data substantiating such claims are not convincing.

The youngster has poor to zero latissimus dorsi strength and triceps strength in the poor range in this stage, thus, upper extremity ambulation aids are of questionable value. An aggressive walking program should be stressed. Only minimal support or standby assistance should be given. The boy must learn to transfer from sitting with unlocked braces to locked braces to the standing position without assistance.

Initially, the patient should be on his feet a minimum of 4 hours a day; the eventual goal is for the boy to spend as much as 12 hours a day in the standing position. (The boy is actually in a modified sitting position on the top cuff of the braces.) The first week after bracing determines whether the braced candidate will be a successful ambulator.

Postpone the Nonambulatory Phase

Discourage wheelchair purchase until extended ambulation becomes impractical. Youngsters enjoy the newfound independence, peer attention, increased comfort, and decreased fatigue that a wheelchair allows and will seldom become braced ambulators if a wheelchair is convenient to them. Secondary problems of hip, knee, and ankle flexion contracturs, as well as scoliosis, accelerate rapidly once ambulation ceases. By maintaining the upright position, in a standing table if ambulation is no longer feasible, those secondary problems will be postponed, as well the concomitant pulmonary complications of scoliosis. If allowed to increase, plantar flexion contractures, with resultant secondary knee and hip flexion contractures, will force the child to the late ambulation stage much sooner than necessary.

Wheelchair

Once wheelchair bound, the long leg braces are cut down to short leg braces and worn throughout the day to prevent the common plantar flexion and inversion foot deformity (Fig. 10-6). Wheelchair is *home* for the youngster so he must be the one to choose the color. Other critical aspects of a wheelchair prescription are

1. Wraparound removable desk arms (wraparound saves almost 2 inches of overall width and desk arms allow access to tables and desks more functionally
2. Swing-away, elevating, detachable leg rests with heel loops (the leg rests can be elevated periodically to stretch knees into extension; the swing away allows easier toileting)
3. Solid seat (the eyes will maintain a horizontal position to the floor; both ischial tuberosities must also be maintained on a horizontal plane to the floor or a scoliosis is imminent. The top end of the spine will align to the eye level, and the bottom end of the spine will align to one ischial tuberosity being higher than the other (Fig. 10-7)

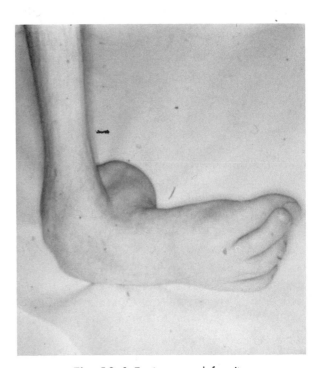

Fig. 10-6 Equinovarus deformity.

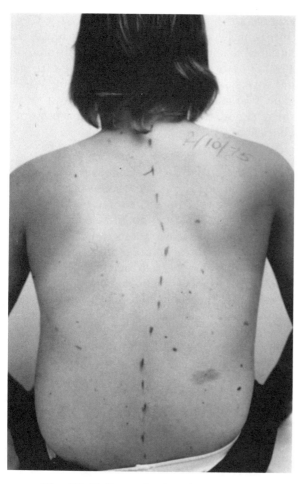

Fig. 10-7 Elevated right ischial tuberosity.

4. Lateral trunk supports (before the development of scoliosis)
5. Narrow width to place as much lateral support to the upright position of the spine as possible
6. Reclining back (facilitates comfort in later stages and, if the back is zippered can be used to help in toileting)
7. Seat cushion for comfort and decubiti prevention.

In addition to ordering the wheelchair, we have frequently ordered a polypropylene body jacket but tend to share Johnson's doubt about the corrective ability credited to spinal braces in DMD.[14]

Late Wheelchair Phases
Order an electric wheelchair if it is financially feasible. Also order a proportional drive for ease and safety of the driver to manipulate the wheel-

chair. Some scoliosis is inevitable, and the convexity will be toward the dominant extremity (see Fig. 10-7).[15] If the youngster is ambidextrous enough to operate the wheelchair with either hand, the drive may be switched from the right to the left side approximately every 6 months to attempt to make scoliosis functional rather than structural and to minimize the curvature.

Obesity will eliminate a boy's ambulation much too early. Even after he is in the wheelchair stage it remains a critical problem. The use of calories as a reward system must be forbidden. Education of the family regarding the complications of obesity must be stressed. Excessive weight transfers become difficult. Less transferring curtails socialization drastically.

It is the therapist's responsibility to train family members or guardians in appropriate transfer techniques and body mechanics. In the wheelchair stage, a hydraulic lift may be indicated. A family member must be appropriately trained in its use. The family or guardians need training in the techniques of postural drainage and the indications of its use at home also.

A few clients with DMD have been taught the technique of glossopharyngeal breathing to facilitate a cough and maintain chest excursion. A hormonica is encouraged and compliance at playing with it appears to be much higher than the use of the three ball inhalator that used to be stressed during the wheelchair stage of this disease.

Active resistance exercises are not encouraged. The youngster is encouraged to participate in all regular activities. Concern about overfatigue should occur only if after a full night's sleep the child is not rested. Routine examination of major activities of daily living, i.e., patient's ability to feed himself, turn pages, take care of some hygiene tasks, etc. must be assessed.

If occupational therapy has not been a major contributor to the child's plan of care throughout, the physical therapist should initiate that involvement no later than the early wheelchair stage.

The therapist's success as counselor, motivator, trainer, etc. of the patient and the family is dependent on getting involved very early in the plan for future management. Assessing the social situation at each visit and stimulating adherence to the home program are major factors to the therapist's success.

Mild to moderate intellectual impairment in these boys may impose educational and emotional handicaps. The child eventually learns that this disease will continually erode the quality and quantity of his existence, and his resultant reliance on others frequently gives rise to intrafamily strain. A healthly emotional environment is at least as important to a child as the prevention of contractures. The therapist must be aware of the emotional factors and should be prepared to assist in providing strong emotional support, reinforcing goals and preventing conflicts.

Pain management should not be a problem if previous goals are met. Pain occurs at the end of the range of motion. Contractures reduce that range resulting in the increased opportunity for pain. Routine physical therapy pain modalities and appropriate positioning techniques should minimize pain if it does occur.

A successfully managed patient will have fewer orthopaedic surgeries than are commonly proposed;[16] will have several years of independent walking, greater self-sufficiency, and substantial postponement of the restrictions imposed by a wheelchair; and will maintain the maximum functional independence that his strength will allow.

Despite ignorance of the cause and the cure of many muscle diseases, it is not helpful for one to take on a defeatist attitude. Many disorders of the musculoskeletal system have common problems and can be managed by applying similar principles.[12] Treatment should be directed at preventing complications during the span of each disease. None of the rehabilitative approaches we have available can alter the underlying disease process. Our best approach to these potential problems is preventive. The basic tenets of such treatment are to assure that the home program is executed and to appropriately monitor and supervise the patient and his support system.

OTHER NEUROMUSCULAR DISORDERS

Other muscular dystrophies include Becker's, limb-girdle, myotonic, and facioscapulohumeral muscular dystrophy. Charcot-Marie Tooth disease, a peripheral neuropathy, and three anterior horn cell diseases—Werdnig-Hoffman types I and II and Kugelberg-Welander. Dermatomyositis and polymyositis collagen vascular disorders are also discussed. Finally, amytrophic lateral sclerosis is presented. The prognosis of all of these diseases worsens after the initial diagnosis is made. Treatment is based on maintaining functional capabilities for as long as possible and slowing or stopping deterioration if possible.

Becker's Dystrophy

Becker's dystrophy is the same disease as Duchenne with precisely the same inheritance pattern and pattern of muscle involvement. The only difference between the two dystrophies is that Becker's dystrophy progresses more slowly. Misdiagnosis of slower progressing youngsters with DMD or more rapid progressing youngsters classifed as having Becker's dystrophy is common. Use of the diagnosis of DMD may be more traumatic to parents.

The major difference in management is that the youngster with Becker's dystrophy will survive much longer, many past the age of 40.[17] Joint pain, especially in the back from hyperextension during gait and in the knees from abnormal joint pressure, is common. Bilateral long leg braces reduce knee joint pain, compensate for quadriceps muscle weakness, maintain ambulation longer, and actually decrease the lordotic curve to relieve back pain with many.[10]

Precautions in the late ambulatory and nonambulatory phases are identical to DMD.

Limb-Girdle Muscular Dystrophy
Pathology

Limb-girdle dystrophy is an autosomal recessive disease affecting both sexes. It is possible that this disease could in fact be several disease entities that exhibit initial weakness in the pelvic and shoulder girdles. Cause of the disease is unknown.

Signs and Symptoms

The primary clinical difference between limb-girdle muscular dystrophy and Duchenne muscular dystrophy is that the pattern of weakness appears to be more generalized, althouth still a proximal to distal weakness. Moreover, the pattern is not as precise and predictable as is the DMD or Becker's form of dystrophy.

Age of onset of limb-girdle muscular dystrophy varies greatly but usually begins in the second decade. In many patients, the progression of the disease is slow, with long periods of apparent plateauing. In others, there is an insidious progression over a 10 to 15 year period, leading eventually to severe disability.[18] A general rule is that the earlier the onset of limb-girdle disease, the more rapidly the progression. Many individuals with this disease are severely disabled within 20 years of onset. Death earlier than normal is not uncommon.

Evaluation

The hallmark of limb-girdle dystrophy is proximal weakness of most major muscle groups. Eventually, distal musculature may also become weakened. Serial muscle testing of key muscles over time will trace the tempo of the disease.

Management

The home program will be the primary emphasis of therapy. Weakness around any joint can lead to a tendency toward joint contractures. Evaluation of ROM of most major joints of the body should be performed routinely. Stretching joints that may eventually exhibit contractures must be stressed. Pain may result from secondary complications of the contractures and may be treated as any other joint contracture pain. Moderate active exercise is encouraged by overexertion is discouraged. If the patient is not fully rested after a full night's sleep, the activity of the previous day must be considered too strenuous.

The nonambulatory phase of limb-girdle muscular dystrophy should be treated similarly to that previously described for Duchenne muscular dystrophy.

Goals

The most important goal is compliance with the therapist's individually designed and periodically reviewed home program. The primary goal is to maintain ambulation until it is no longer functional.

Standing tables can be beneficial for many years after functional ambulation has ceased. Their use can minimize contractures. Periodic interviewing and counseling are required to ascertain motivational level of maintaining the home program.

Myotonic Muscular Dystrophy

Pathology

Individuals with myotonic dystrophy exhibit sustained contractions and abnormally slow relaxation after voluntary contraction, percussion, or electrical stimulation. The genetic transmission of myotonic dystrophy is autosomal dominant, with variable penetrance and expressivity.[19]

If myotonic dystrophy is seen in a child, one must check for myotonic dystrophy in one of the parents. The incidence is 3 to 5/100,000.[20] Frequently, the female will pass on a more severe expressivity than the male.

Signs and Symptoms

Generally, the younger the onset of symptoms, the more severe the disease. In the adult form, the age of onset of symptoms is commonly between ages 20 and 50, but detectable disease is usually present in the second decade.

The course of the disease is frequently a very slow but insidious deterioration. Functional decline may be greater than actual decline in strength from factors such as weight gain, reduction in motivational level, inability to follow a home program, etc.

Intellect is usually affected, creating major problems with compliance in the home program. Unlike DMD, there can be marked variation in severity of the disease in members of the same family.

Evaluation and Management

The myotonia will not interfere with the determination of muscle strength through muscle testing. Serial muscle testing over years assesses the tempo of the disease effectively.

In the lower extremities, the anterior tibialis and peroneals exhibit initial weakness. Prefabricated bilateral ankle-foot orthoses (AFO) have worked well.

Absence or weakness of sternocleidomastoid muscle is a hallmark of myotonic dystrophy. Occasionally, a soft cervical collar is used to support the anterior compartment of the neck. A cane may be of some benefit in assisting with gait; however, the handles usually need to be built up in circumference to facilitate grip. Intrinsic hand musculature is usually markedly weakened. Obesity is particularly problematic with this type of dystrophy. Caloric intake must be closely monitored. Abdominal musculature is severely weakened in the disease process, and abdominal support for cosmetic reasons might be considered.

Facioscapulohumeral (FSH) Muscular Dystrophy

Pathology

Both sexes are affected, and it is a dominantly inherited disease. Onset can be at any age from childhood until adult life. It is not uncommon for this disease to appear in the third or fourth decade of life. A youngster at risk cannot be pronounced free of the risk of future disease simply because no signs of weakness are present.

There is initial involvement of the face and shoulder girdle muscles, with subsequent spread to the pelvic girdle. The progress of the disease is insidious, with prolonged periods of apparent arrest. In some cases, primarily males who received the transmission of the disease from a female, the disease progresses unusually rapidly.[21] Females who receive the transmission of the disease from males are the least affected. The majority of patients remain active to a normal age.[18] Serum enzymes remain within normal limits.

Signs and Symptoms

Although the weakness in FSH dystrophy proceeds from proximal to distal, the particular muscles involved differ from those involved in Duchenne muscular dystrophy. The latissimus dorsi muscle remains intact, but the lower trapezius and face musculature are the first muscles to exhibit weakness.

Evaluation and Management

Manual muscle testing is the preferred method of diagnostic testing. The easiest test for orbicularis oris weakness is to have the patient attempt to blow air into both cheeks with the lips tight so air cannot escape. The patient should be able to resist external pressure applied to the cheeks without losing air from the mouth. Attempting to blow up

a balloon can also provide a rough estimate of strength loss.

The orbicularis oculi muscles also weaken and are tested by attempting to open the tightly closed eye with the thumb of one hand and the index finger of the other. Surprisingly, strong resistance should be felt during active contraction. The therapist's major concern is to be familiar with what normal facial musculature feels like.

The brachioradialis is characteristically very weak or absent in FSH; palpation and visible observation are the only valid tests for examining its strength because a strong biceps muscle makes the test of the brachioradialis invalid.

Hand dynamometer grip strength tests on approximately 150 patients with FSH and on 50 physical therapy students showed the students to have strength in their dominant hand equal to or, in the majority of cases, superior to the nondominant extremity. However, in testing the FSH group, the nondominant hand was strongest in the vast majority of patients.[21]

These findings, along with additional dominant lower extremity weakness data, tend to make the author question the advisability of strenuous active exercise for the weakened muscles in this particular type of dystrophy. The therapist working with a youngster whose disease was transmitted from the mother needs to provide early counseling toward a physically nonstrenuous life style and occupation. If the youngster wishes, he should be encouraged to participate in athletics, but with realistic expectations.

The initial major problem may be pain in the upper thoracic region resulting from the lack of stability from the scapular girdle musculature, specifically the trapezius and rhomboid muscles. The only orthotic device that I have found effective in the most severe cases has been a modified Taylor brace. It supports the midthoracic region and retracts the scapulae when applied properly. It must be well stabilized at the pelvis with straps.

Charcot-Marie Tooth Disease

Pathology

Charcot-Marie Tooth disease is one of the infrequent distal to proximal neuromuscular diseases. There are several different classifications with similar patterns of involvement.[22] The usual pattern of inheritance is autosomal dominant, although autosomal recessive patterns may occur occasionally. Another name for this disease is peroneal muscular atrophy.

Signs and Symptoms

The peroneal muscles bilaterally weaken, allowing the near normal posterior tibialis muscles to pull the foot into a pes cavus deformity early in the disease. Pes equinovarus and some gait disturbances appear by the second decade due to progressive atrophy of the anterior tibial and peroneal muscles. Progressive foot drop develops with a steppage gait. Hand dexterity decreases as the intrinsic muscle of hands atrophy. Sensory impairment appears later and is less severe than motor involement.[23] The condition is very slowly progressive and many are still walking with aids 30 years after the onset.

Management

The anterior tibial muscles weaken early, along with the peroneal atrophy. This creates not only a tendency toward foot drop but also ankles that invert toward the strong posterior tibials upon weight-bearing. An ankle-foot orthosis (AFO) as described in the myotonic dystrophy section is appropriate in the early stages. The individually fabricated AFO is necessary in the later stage to control the instability at the ankle. The toes frequently exhibit a tendency to contract into dorsiflexion at the metatarsophalangeal joint and plantar flexion at the proximal interphalangeal joint (hammer toes). Simple stretching and splinting of the most affected toes can initially relieve the symptoms. Shoes with extra toe depth facilitate comfort and decrease calluses; however, surgery is occasionally warranted.

Periodical serial muscle testing of frequently involved muscles will determine the tempo of the disease process and assist in prognosticating when orthopaedic devices will become necessary.

Spinal Muscular Atrophy

Infantile spinal muscular atrophy (Werdnig-Hoffman) types I and II, along with juvenile spinal muscular atrophy (Kugelberg-Welander) Type III, will be discussed (Fig. 10-8). These are diseases of the anterior horn cells. Upper neuron signs are absent, but fasciculations and flaccidity are frequently present. The diseases are fairly static. In general, the earlier the onset of the disease the more severe and the poorer the prognosis.

All three are inherited as autosomal recessive diseases, with one defective gene coming from each parent. Both sexes can exhibit the symptoms. Any one particular type tends to exhibit a particular kindred although there are cases of some families having types I, II, and III in the same sibship. This, along with other similarities in disease pattern, suggests that they are all variations of the same disorder.

Infantile Spinal Muscular Atrophy (SMA) (Werdnig-Hoffman) Type I

The highest percentage of SMA patients have type I disease and usually die within the first 2 years of life.[20] The pattern of weakness of type I is identical to types II and III; only the severity differs.

The legs frequently assume a froglike posture in supine position. Smiling and alert recognition are appropriate for the age, although normal neuromuscular development is delayed.

Type I usually begins in utero and results in the most serious prognosis. Breathing and feeding difficulties followed by respiratory failure are the most common causes of death. Weak or absent

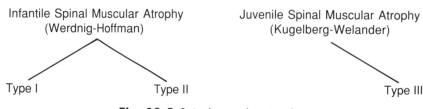

Fig. 10-8 Spinal muscular atrophy.

neck flexors result in complete head lag when the infant is pulled to a sitting position (Fig. 10-9). This is the most common cause of the "floppy baby syndrome" in disorders of neuromuscular origin.

Infantile Spinal Muscular Atrophy, (Werdnig-Hoffman), Type II

Signs and Symptoms
If the infant lives beyond 2 years of life, the potential for living a moderate life span is high. The majority of these youngsters are very bright and should be encouraged to participate in intellectual endeavors in school. If desired, long-term employment should be a major goal.

Most joints are hypermobile. However, contractures of the hip, knee, and plantar flexors are not uncommon, with unilateral severity being the rule rather than the exception. In the upper extremities, contractures of the supinators are frequently overlooked. Elbow and wrist flexion contractures occur with less frequency.

Management
It is necessary to begin the home stretching program on the first visit. The key to long-term success in the functional arena will be compliance with the home program. The goal is to begin very early to maintain the range of motion in all joints to allow the patient to take advantage of the musculature that has been salvaged and is still effective. The home program should be carried out daily and re-evaluation should take place at 1 to 3 month intervals, depending on the severity of the disease and the compliance with the home program.

Type II disease is characterized by a district pattern that makes it subject to unproven health practices. The weak infant will appear to gain strength as neurological maturation takes place.

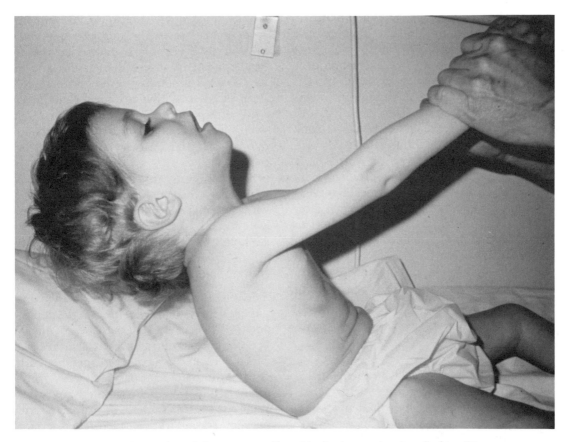

Fig. 10-9 Weak neck flexors cause "head lay" when patient is pulled to sitting.

The child will continue in functional improvement until the increase in the skeleton size creates an apparent plateau in strength. As the skeleton continues to increase in size with the additional body tissues that accompany growth, there will be an apparent decrease in functional ability (i.e., sitting to standing and independent braced ambulation to loss of ambulation at 6 to 9 years). The unwary therapist who intervenes with a particular pediatric approach during the phase when normal neurological development is taking place may believe that they are responsible for the improvement in the child's functional ability.[7]

The activity level should be maintained at the maximum level; controlling the weight down of these youngsters must become a way of life. Calories as a reward system should not be allowed.

One of the strollers that provides appropriate positioning should be purchased from a reputable supply house. Before the attaining complete skeletal maturation, the child may benefit from long leg braces, a standing table, or a standing platform of the type described by Motlach.[24] When it is apparent that walking will not occur or will cease, an appropriately measured wheelchair should be ordered. It is not uncommon to order electric wheelchairs for these intelligent youngsters at earlier ages than previously considered (i.e., 3 to 4 years). Very narrow wheelchairs with lateral trunk supports are sometimes helpful, as are polypropylene trunk supports.

Scoliosis is the major secondary problem associated with type II disease. Early surgical intervention is becoming common. I routinely teach glossopharyngeal breathing to these patients to facilitate a cough and maintain lung capacity. Switching the drive on the electric wheelchair from right to left and back approximately every 6 months appears to postpone the scoliosis or to minimize it.

Juvenile Spinal Musculature Atrophy, (Kugelberg-Welander), Type III

If the disease first expresses itself in the 5- to 15-year-old age group, it is termed Kugelberg-Welander disease. Each milestone that the patient attains, such as sitting, standing, or walking, increases the chances for increased longevity and increased functional ability.

It is my belief based on serial muscle testing experience over many years, that once the disease is expressed, deterioration in muscle strength is minor and occurs over decades rather than months.

The role of the therapist as motivator, counselor, facilitator, and provider of emotional support is more important than the role of the therapeutic exercise instructor. A defeatist attitude is inappropriate in this disease. These bright youngsters need an emphasis on career goals.

Dermatomyositis, Polymyositis

Pathology

The primary difference between these two diseases is that dermatomyositis manifests itself in the skin, as well as the underlying tissues, whereas polymyositis exhibits only in the underlying tissue.[25] Both are inflammatory myopathies of presumed autoimmune etiology often resulting in muscle lesions. The course is extremely variable, ranging from mild cases with complete spontaneous remission to a chronic progressive type with the development of severe deformities and disability to a severe fulminating disease with rapid death.[1] Both diseases exhibit proximal limb-girdle weakness, affecting the pelvic girdle first and most seriously. Neck and abdominal musculature is frequently affected. Muscle pain and tenderness is common.

Systemic signs with general malaise, fever, and weight loss occur. Movement restrictions occur with systemic symptoms and although the joints are normally unaffected, they may occasionally swell and become red and tender.[26]

Management

The therapist's primary goal is to maintain the patient's functional capacity (i.e., the ability to walk and carry on the usual activities of daily living). Prevention of contractures is critical because reversal of established contractures is very difficult.[27] During the acute exacerbation stage, exercise programs are neither well tolerated nor appropriate. When bed rest is suggested, proper positioning to prevent secondary contractures is critical. Pain management can be accomplished through routine applications of heat. Stretching of the major joints should be carried out but not to the point of pain. Weight-bearing and ambulation are the preferred methods of maintaining strength and range of motion in the lower extremities.

Serial muscle testing is important in assisting the physician in monitoring the medication dose, especially when steroids are used. The dose should be high enough to obtain desired results, but low enough to minimize side effects. The primary role of the therapist is that of counselor to motivate the family to perform the home program.

Motor Neuron Disease

Four noninherited motor neuron diseases are frequently classified under the rubric amyotrophic lateral sclerosis (ALS) (Table 10-1). These diseases usually affect adults in the 40 to 70 year age range; men are affected more than women.[5]

Progressive Bulbar Palsy

Progressive bulbar palsy is a very severe disease that exhibits primarily upper motor neuron signs with occasional lower motor neuron signs. Many patients die within 6 months to 1 year after diagnosis.

Progressive Muscular Atrophy

Progressive muscular atrophy is a relatively mild motor neuron disease that primarily shows lower motor neuron signs. The patient frequently sur-

vives for 15 years or longer from age of initial diagnosis.

Primary Lateral Sclerosis

Primary lateral sclerosis is an upper motor neuron disease frequently misdiagonsed as multiple sclerosis. Characterized primarily by upper motor neuron signs, the patient is usually spared from death for 5 to 10 years from initial diagnosis.

Amyotrophic Lateral Sclerosis

The most common form and the most diffuse form of motor neuron disease is amyotrophic lateral sclerosis disease (ALS), more informally known as Lou Gehrig's disease. ALS involves both upper and lower motor neurons and is characterized by four classical signs: (1) hyperreflexia and/or spasticity, (2) fasciculations, (3) weakness, and (4) wasting or atrophy.

Progression is relentless, with death frequently occurring within 3 years of onset. ALS can sometimes appear to plateau, which accounts for the apparent success of various experimental treatments or therapeutic interventions.

Spinal musculature is often weak, making standing in the complete upright position very difficult for some patients. Proximal, as well as distal, muscles weaken, resulting in an expressionless face in many patients.

Management

Medical attempts, such as plasmapheresis, have been unsuccessful in slowing or stopping the progression of the disease. No cure has been found yet. Various therapeutic drug trials (i.e., administration of thyrotropin release hormone) have been attempted with only minimal success. Any new treatment in ALS emphasizes the importance of having therapists involved in evaluating the drug efficacy through serial manual muscle testing.

The physician has little to offer once a diagnosis is made, but the therapist can play a vital role in the management of these patients. The primary goals are to (1) prevent deformity, (2) prolong functional capacity, and (3) facilitate the existing family support system or attempt to create one. Intervention focuses on treating the symptoms and maintaining the patient's function at the maximum level feasible.

Table 10-1 Motor Neuron Disease

Disease	Signs	Prognosis
Progressive bulbar palsy	Upper and lower motor neuron signs	Death may occur within 6 months of diagnosis
Progressive macular atrophy	Lower motor neuron signs	Death may occur within 15 years of diagnosis
Primary lateral sclerosis	Upper motor neuron signs	Death may occur within 5–10 years of diagnosis
Amyotrophic lateral sclerosis	Upper and lower motor neuron signs	Death may occur within 1–3 years of diagnosis

Shoulder pain is common in over half of ALS patients seen in our clinic. Maintaining normal range of motion appears to decrease or minimize but not prevent that pain.

The sequence of events is predictable based on a thorough evaluation of weakness. As the disease progresses, the base of support widens to enhance stability during ambulation. A cane helps improve stability, not only by bearing weight on the upper extremity but also through the additional proprioceptive input a cane offers when neurological deficit occurs. Hand involvement with atrophy of the intrinsic muscle occurs early, making use of a cane no longer feasible. Polypropylene posterior shell AFOs are helpful when the anterior tibials weaken. Occasionally, bilateral long leg braces effectively maintain ambulation in the slower form of the disease. When a wheelchair becomes necessary, a powered chair should be ordered if it is financially feasible.

Even when there is rapid progression in ALS, it is not uncommon for a plateauing or period of stabilization to take place, resulting in extensive time in a wheelchair. As with all wheelchairs, they must be narrow enough to postpone scoliosis. A solid seat insert is important (see wheelchair information under DMD, this chapter). Pulmonary hygiene during the wheelchair phase must be taught to family members.

Patient care and patient satisfaction with their situation may be enhanced with occupational therapy intervention. Many assistive devices make the patient's world much more tolerable. Because of the bulbar involvement, dysphagia, drooling, and speech impairment are present. As verbalization ceases, communication devices need to be considered. Unfortunately, costs of the majority of the electronic devices are prohibitive.

A major task is to maintain the range of motion within normal limits in all major joints. Decreasing spasticity through appropriate positioning techniques is an important task. Maintaining independence in activities of daily living through adaptive equippment, modifying the daily routine, and training family or support group in appropriate methods of assisting are major goals. It is important to assist and adapt feeding with oral facilitation techniques, altering the food size and texture, and using adaptive equipment.

It is critical to establish coping mechanisms. Too often we become preoccupied with exercises and devices and pay little attention to the emotional conflicts. The therapist plays a crucial role in the support, motivation, and training of the patient and family members. Success is dependent on being involved early in the management of the patient and facilitating adherence to the program you outline and revise at each visit.

A successful patient will have fewer surgeries and will have the maximal functional independence his strength will allow for as long as possible.

REFERENCES

1. Dubowitz V: The muscular dystrophies. p. 19. In Muscle Disorders in Childhood. WB Saunders, Philadelphia, 1978
2. Ziter FA, Allsop KG: The diagnosis and management of childhood muscular dystrophy. Clin Pediatr (Phila) 15:540, 1976
3. Perloff JK: Cardiomyopathy associated with heredofamilial neuromyopathic disease. Mod Conc Cardiov Dis 40:23, 1971
4. Prosser EJ, Murphy EG, Thomson MW: Intelligence and the gene for Duchenne muscular dystrophy. Arch Dis Child 44:221, 1969
5. Siegel, IM: Muscle and Its Diseases. Year Book Medical Publishers, Chicago, 1986
6. Crisp, DE, Ziter FA, Bray PF: Diagnostic delay in Duchenne's muscular dystrophy. JAMA 247:478, 1982
7. Allsop K: ISMA, DMD, a comparison of two childhood neuromuscular disorders and their implication for therapists. Clinical Management in Physical Therapy 5:46, 1985
8. Ziter FA, Allsop KG, Tyler FH: Assessment of muscle strength in Duchenne muscular dystrophy. Neurology 271:981, 1977
9. Allsop KG, Ziter FA: Loss of strength and functional decline in Duchenne's dystrophy. Arch Neurol 38:410, 1981
10. Ziter FA, Allsop KG: The value of orthoses for patients with Duchenne muscular dystrophy. Phys Ther 59:1361, 1979
11. Vignos PJ: Rehabilitation in progressive muscular dystrophy. p. 584. In Licht S (ed): Rehabilitation and Medicine. E. Lich, New London, CT, 1968
12. Kentenjian AY: Muscular dystrophy: diagnosis and treatment, symposium on pediatric orthopedics. Orthop Clin North Am 9:25, 1978
13. Vignos PJ, Wagner MB, Sakaplan J, Spencer GE: Predicting the success of reambulation in patients with Duchenne muscular dystrophy. J Bone Joint Surgery (Am) 65A:719, 1983

14. Johnson EW: Letter to the editor. Dev Med Child Neurol 22:401, 1980

15. Johnson EW, Yarnell SK: Hand dominance and scoliosis in Duchenne muscular dystrophy. Arch Phys Med Rehabil 57:462, 1976

16. Siegel IM: The Clinical Management of Muscle Disease. JB Lippincott, Philadelphia, 1977

17. Gilroy J, Holliday P: Basic Neurology. Macmillan, New York, 1982

18. Walton JN, Gardner-Medwin D: Progressive muscular dystrophy and the myotonic disorders. p. 561. In Walton JN (ed): Disorders of Voluntary Muscle. 3rd Ed. Churchill Livingstone, Edinburgh, London, 1974

19. Downey JA, Low NA: The Child with Disabling Illness. WB Saunders, London, 1974

20. Brooke MH: A Clinician's View of Neuromuscular Diseases. Williams & Wilkins, Baltimore, 1978

21. Allsop K: Evaluation of facioscapulohumeral muscular dystrophy. Paper presented at the American Physical Therapy Association Convention, Phoenix, AZ, July, 1980 (produced and sold on tape)

22. Dyck PJ: Neuronal atrophy and degeneration predominantly affecting peripheral sensory and motor neurons. p. 1557. In Dyck P, Thomas P, Lambert E, Bunge R, (eds): Peripheral Neuropathy. 2nd Ed. WB Saunders, Philadelphia, 1984

23. Bradley WG: The neuropathies. p. 804. In Walton JN (ed): Diseases of voluntary muscle. 3rd Ed. Churchill Livingstone.

24. Motlach W: The parapodium: an orthotic device for neuromuscular disorders. Artificial Limb 15:36, 1971

25. Bohan A, Peter JB: Polymyositis and dermatomyositis. New Engl J Med 292:244, 1975

26. Huskisson EC, Hart FD: Joint Disease: All the Arthropathies. 3rd Ed. John Wright & Sons, Ltd. Birstol, England, 1978

27. Rose A, Walton J: Polymyositis: a survey of 89 cases with particular reference to treatment and prognosis. Brain 89:768, 1966

Section II

Orthopaedic Dysfunction

Edited by
Stanley V. Paris

11 Principles of Management

Stanley V. Paris

The authors of the orthopaedic section realize that the reader's experience of orthopaedic physical therapy can range from an entry level knowledge to significant experience. We have therefore sought to provide a nearly complete reference on the basic treatment of most common and not-so-common spinal and extremity dysfunctions. Since each of the spinal and extremity syndromes are presented in a concise, uniform format, we strongly urge the reader to take the necessary time to become fully acquainted with this first chapter, which sets forth our philosophy of practice, before reading the following discussions.

In this chapter, we present our operative definitions and principles and practice of patient management, which may be somewhat different from the reader's experience. We illustrate a selected number of techniques, which, while they cannot be fully learned from a text such as this, can be aptly introduced and reviewed within this reference. We select techniques that may be familiar to the reader or, if not, are easily acquired at continuing education courses conducted by various organizations. The material presented here has been selected from the courses instructed at the precertification level of the Institute of Graduate Health Sciences. We omit those techniques of treatment that require advanced skill and instruction beyond the level of basic postgraduate courses.

OPERATING PRINCIPLES

Within the orthopaedic section, we use the term *dysfunction* to represent abnormalities in physical functioning that are treated by physical therapists. By contrast, our physicians are schooled in the diagnosis and treatment of *disease*. We believe quite strongly that the role of the physical therapist is in differential evaluation and treatment of dysfunction, while the physician is concerned with the differential diagnosis and treatment of disease. Therapists do not directly treat disease, but we should treat the dysfunctions that result from or may even contribute to disease.

The *medical diagnosis of orthopaedic dysfunction* has a very poor inter-rater reliability; for example, a painful shoulder may be diagnosed as a strain, capsulitis, or supraspinatus tendinitis by different physicians seeing the same patient. Therefore, physical therapists must treat the dysfunction, or the objective signs of altered function. When the therapist has successfully achieved this end, the patient's "diagnosis," whatever it may be labeled, will be relieved.

Our emphasize in patient management is *not on the patient's pain but rather on the cause of that pain*. Both physicians and physical therapists have a variety of means for relieving pain. But only when the cause of the pain has been addressed will a continuing relief of pain and a return to optimal function follow. When the pain prevents treatment, it must be attended to. However, for the most part, pain can be ignored.

The term *professional physical therapist* denotes the responsibility of the physical therapist for the evaluation and treatment of the patient. Inevitably, therefore, as physical therapists may disagree among each other, they will frequently disagree with the referring physicians should they choose to dictate or prescribe treatment. Physical therapists therefore, as a rule, cannot accept prescriptions for treatment.

The patient has a primary role with regard to his own rehabilitation, both mentally and physically. Programs such as back schools are therefore an integral and understood part of the patient management processes.

The term *joint manipulation* is used here to mean "skillful passive movement applied to a joint." It is used in conformity with arthrokinematic principles, that is, the intimate mechanics of joints, as opposed to the term *range of motion,* which is an unskilled movement, related more to osteokinematics, that is, the movement of bones with little regard to the joint. The use of the terms *manipulation* and *mobilization* are synonymous.

PRINCIPLES OF PRACTICE

There are at least four concepts in treatment that should be applied to the management of spinal and extremity syndromes. The first of these is the perceived level of acuteness or stage of the condition, and the second is perceived response or reactivity of the tissues to treatment. Physical therapists must have a reasonable idea of these two states if they are to effectively manage the syndrome and to avoid aggravating it. The third concept is to recognize that the perception gained must be tested with a trial treatment. And finally, it is helpful to consider whether the primary effect of the treatments is palliative, preparatory, corrective, or supportive.

Stages of the Condition

Traditionally, the terms *acute, subacute,* and *chronic* have been the principal labels for denoting the stage of the condition. However, these are inadequate for our present purposes, and so the following is offered.

Immediate

The immediate stage may exist from a few moments to a number of minutes after injury. Doing the "right thing" during this stage can be of significance in the later course of the condition. Of course, the therapist is rarely present at the time of injury. However, since most conditions that patients suffer are in fact recurrences of previous conditions, the opportunity for giving the patient advice as to what he should do in this immediate stage should it occur again is often available. Such advice should be part of the patient's discharge summary.

It is at this stage that restoring a locked knee or shoulder dislocation is easiest. The same is true for an acute attack of cervical or low back pain from facet capsular impingement. The immediate application of ice to joint sprains will lessen tissue reaction.

Treatment is therefore directed at immediate correction or efforts to lessen the spread of the problem, either geographically or by degree.

Acute

The acute stage is characterized by increasing symptoms (patient complaints) and signs (that which the therapist can observe). The concern here is to judge correctly the nature and intensity of the syndrome and to give treatment only if it will aid the reparative process. It may be that rest is the only treatment indicated in the case of a ligamentous injury of, say, the cervical spine or knee, or maintaining movement in the case of a synovitis.

Subacute

The subacute stage is characterized by a plateauing of signs and symptoms. Great care must be taken not to interfere with the healing process and thus recreate the acute state. It is at this stage that physical treatment, although making the patient feel better, may actually delay the healing process—such as in giving cervical traction to a "whiplash" (ligamentous) injury. The intermittent traction and gentle movements may gate the discomfort while aggravating interstitial bleeding.

At this stage, it may still be difficult to conduct a full and competent evaluation to determine the true nature of the syndrome, and thus great care must still be exercised in administering treatment.

Settled

In the settled stage, the syndrome has stabilized and shows a good tolerance to moderate stress or insult, thus permitting a full evaluation, which may now include provocation techniques. The effect of manipulative and exercise treatments can be easily measured as muscle guarding is now minimal.

Chronic

By convention, this term *chronic* is applied to static conditions that are at least 3 months old. The use of the term is valid as by this time primary healing has already taken place and the patient has no doubt made or failed to make adjustments in lifestyle.

Rate of Healing

Part of the basis for the above scheme is in the perceived rate of healing of soft tissues after injury:

50 percent of healing occurs in the first 2 weeks.
80 percent of healing occurs in the first 6 weeks.
100 percent of healing has occurred by the 12th week.

Certainly any healing that occurs after 6 months is by remodeling rather than by primary intention. Furthermore, at 6 months, if not sooner, there may be considerable behavioral changes that add to the chronicity of the condition.

Joint Reactivity

The concept of *joint reactivity* (or severity) is related to the degree of injury, the sensitivity of the tissues, and the tolerance of the patient. It can form a useful guide to the management of the condition. It is different from the stage of the condition; for instance, a patient with a minor acute strain to the knee should be encouraged to keep walking; but a major acute strain may require ice, elevation, and compression. Both are clearly acute conditions, but their reactivity, or severity, is different.

High Reactivity

A painful response is evoked before the end of joint range. For treatment, rest and limited range of motion are prescribed. Oscillations may help, as may ice, transcutaneous electrical stimulation (TENS), and acupressure.

Moderate Reactivity

A painful response is evoked at the end of joint range. The prescribed treatment is progressive oscillations and gentle stretching of the capsule. Heat is used as opposed to ice.

Minimal Reactivity

There is no pain at the end of range of motion. For treatment; mechanical stretch or thrust manipulations may now be commenced.

Trial Treatment

Even the most experienced clinician cannot be certain about the amount of treatment the patient can receive without experiencing an adverse reaction. Therefore, it is important that the first treatment be briefer in intensity and duration than what the patient might be expected to tolerate.

Modalities—Palliative, Preparatory, Corrective, and Supportive

In treating orthopaedic conditions, it is essential at each succeeding session to be able to assess the objective and subjective effect of the previous treatment session. If too many treatments were administered, it will be impossible to determine which modality or procedure either benefitted or hindered the patient. By arbitrarily placing modalities and procedures into distinct groups (palliative, preparatory, corrective, and supportive), we gain an advantage in reassessing outcomes of treatment (See Table 11-1). As a rule, I tend to use palliative modalities in acute and painful conditions and preparatory modalities in subacute and later stages, followed by *one* corrective procedure to *one* joint at that session. Finally, I may conclude with a supportive treatment to help maintain the benefits of treatment.

For example, for a subacute low back condition, I may use the palliative treatments of rest and heat, the preparatory treatments of massage and oscillations, and then finally a corrective treatment of manipulation supported by postural advice and perhaps taping. Should the patient have an adverse reaction, it is probable that the cause was the manipulation. Had I also added muscle stretching or distraction, I would be at a loss to know the cause of the adverse reaction, and valuable time in patient rehabilitation would have been lost.

I acknowledge that the classification of modalities in this manner is somewhat arbitrary. It is

Table 11-1 Classification of Modalities for Orthopaedic Dysfunction

Palliative
  Rest
  Heat
  Ice
Preparatory
  Massage
  Oscillations
  TENS
  Acupressure
Corrective treatment
  Manipulation
  Distraction
  Exercises
  Transverse frictions
  Ultrasound
Supportive
  Back school
  Posture
  Exercises
  Home program

understood that heat, for instance, could be palliative on one occasion and preparatory to a corrective treatment on another (Table 11-1).

FIRST VISIT

Closely related to the concept of the "trial treatment" is the advisability of resisting the temptation to treat a patient by attempting corrective measures during the first visit. In an acute-stage condition, it is of course appropriate to offer treatment even though a full evaluation cannot be performed. However, in the subacute or settled condition, the conducting of a full evaluation combined with supportive treatments of, for example, back school, is certainly enough for one session. If on top of this complete evaluation a trial treatment is added, there is a very high risk of doing far too much. As a result, the patient impressed by the therapist's skills and thoroughness of evaluation, and with justifiably high expectations for relief, may be plunged into despair when awakening with increased discomfort the next day.

In the acute case, palliative treatment is sufficient. In the subacute or later stages, the evaluation alone with supportive patient education is enough for the first session. The next session commences

with the trial treatment, and during the third session, the therapist offers the best and most appropriate treatment.

COMMON DYSFUNCTION ENTITIES AND PRINCIPLES OF TREATMENT

There are a number of orthopaedic terms and conditions common to both the spine and extremities. They are presented in this chapter to avoid redundancy within the discussions that follow, since the treatment principles may be applied, in general, to the specific body regions.

Stress, Strain, and Sprain

Stress is a force. It will cause a change in the tissues. In a compressive stress, the structure will shorten; in a distractive stress, it will lengthen (strain). Moderate and frequent stress is good for tissues as the stimulus it provides is a stimulus for cellular activity that maintains the strength and viability of all tissues. Too much stress may accumulate in the tissues at a rate faster than the structures can biologically adapt, and failure or fracture may ensue.

Strain is the increase in length caused by a stress. Pulling on a spring or tight joint capsule will in both cases create a change in length or strain. Strains are not unhealthy when defined in this biomechanical sense. Indeed, in biological structures a stress or strain results in increased cellular activity and thus has a beneficial effect. Strains performed within the elastic range of the tissue will cause it to toughen within that range (e.g., stretching a hamstring). Strains performed beyond the elastic range and into the plastic range will lengthen the strained structures (e.g., manipulating a tight joint capsule).

Sprain is what occurs when fibers or elements within the tissues lose their normal integrity by tearing, rupturing, etc. It is a harmful incident that requires the sprained tissues to be immobilized for a period to reduce bleeding and aid healing, particularly in the first 2 weeks after the sprain.

In a *rupture*, the sprain is of such magnitude that the entire structure is disrupted. It will require immobilization and perhaps surgical reduction, realignment, suturing, or other forms of fixation.

Dysfunction by Structure

Ligamentous Sprain

A ligamentous sprain is a serious condition in any region of the spine or extremities, for weak ligaments may lead to or be associated with joint instability or joint degeneration, including disc degeneration. The intervertebral disc is to all intents and purposes a ligament with a enclosed fluid nucleus.

Causes

Postural misuse and abuse, for example, sustained stooping or falling asleep on the sofa with the knees hyperextended on a stool or the neck hanging unsupported

Trauma, such as jumping from a height

Acceleration injuries (motor vehicle and whiplash)

Symptoms

Dull ache, at first local and later diffuse pain

Inability to sit or stand still for a period

In extreme cases, difficulty in finding any position which provides for comfort

Treatment

Postural re-education

Support, such as corset, brace, or tape

Correct neighboring restrictions of movement that may be contributing to the joints needed to compensate

Management

Patient must recognize his key role in postural correction

Back school education is very necessary

Progress

Unless the patient takes the condition seriously, and accepts a role in treatment, ligamentous injuries invariably lead to joint degeneration, including, in the case of the spine, disc degeneration. Even with excellent patient cooperation and initial rapid progress, once the ligaments become desensitized by appropriate postural behavior, the ligaments may never regain their original and full strength, particularly in the spine.

Synovitis and Haemarthrosis

The closely related conditions of synovitis and hemarthrosis occur when a joint is either forced beyond its normal restraints or when the capsule of the joint is pinched. Since synovial fluid is natural to a joint its presence is considered harmless, but if blood, that is, serofibrinous exedate, is present (haemarthrosis), then this is a very different and serious matter. Blood is rich in fibrinogen, which may not only form adhesions between the capsule and bone ends but may actually damage the surface of the cartilage. It is therefore important to distinguish between synovitis and hemarthrosis since the latter may require medical aspiration (Table 11-2).

Muscle Spasm and Holding/Guarding

The terms *muscle spasm* and *holding/guarding* are used very loosely and usually at variance with their dictionary definition. As a result, there is much misunderstanding when the term muscle spasm or muscle holding is used.

Table 11-2 Distinguishing Between Synovitis and Hemarthrosis

	Synovitis	Hemarthrosis
Signs and symptoms	Gradual onset of swelling	Swelling within minutes
	Passive range limited but joint moves freely	Passive movement sluggish
	Uncomfortable	Painful
	Warm joint	Hot joint
Treatment	Rest from further activity while maintaining function	Rest, support, aspiration
	Ice, elevation, and compression if desired	Ice, elevation, and compression
	Manipulation after 10 days	Manipulation after 10 days

Spasm

Spasm is an uncontrolled involuntary jerking of the muscle. It is occasionally observed in orthopaedics when attempting to move a painful joint in the direction of its dysfunction. It is a term more commonly applied in neurological disorders.

For a better understanding of the changes that do occur in muscles, and for the format that will be used throughout this section, the following is presented.

Myofascial Restrictions

Causes
Poor posture
Joint injury, such as a painful low back being maintained in lordosis for a prolonged period owing to voluntary, or chemical muscle holding
Obesity or inactivity

Symptoms
Minimal symptoms at first, but later the loss of function will lead to muscular and joint discomfort

Signs
Restricted active range of motion and altered function
All passive movements free but with limited range

Treatment
Heat, massage, and connective tissue techniques
Proprioceptive neuromuscular facilitation (PNF)
Sustained stretch

Muscle Spasm of Orthopaedic Origin

As stated above, muscle spasm is a commonly misused term. It is used here to denote the sudden twitching of muscle when a joint is moved in such a manner or direction that it triggers the spasm response.

Cause
Painful movement "pinching" sensitive tissues such as facet capsule or nerve root
Reflex response from a facillitated segment
Neurological conditions not of orthopaedic origin

Symptoms
Pain (possibly quite severe)
Tugging sensation

Signs
May be triggered by provocation of affected segment
Observed flicking of muscle

Treatment
Correction of underlying cause
Posture correction to avoid triggering the spasms

Muscle Holding—Involuntary

Involuntary muscle holding is a state of muscle tone that may be palpated or observed and that signifies an underlying clinical or subclinical lesion.

Causes
Joint or ligamentous dysfunction
Disc lesion or instability

Symptoms
None

Signs
In an extremity, the limb may feel "heavy" when the therapist is moving it passively. This feeling of heaviness results from the muscles surrounding the joint being in a state other than complete relaxation. They are in effect "involuntarily" holding, guarding, or protecting the joint, creating a heightened resting tone and desire to guard against passive movements. It is the first and most subtle of all clinical signs of joint dysfunction.

Treatment
Correct the cause (see conditions within this section)

Muscle Holding—Chemical

Chemical muscle holding is a state in which the muscles of the patient appear pudgy and dense and somewhat nonelastic to palpation.

Causes
Sustained involuntary or voluntary muscle holding
Diminution of blood flow with accumulation of waste products of metabolism within the muscle belly

Symptoms
Discomfort and fatigue
Restricted and cramped movements

Signs
Muscle tightness and doughiness-pudginess to palpation
Is not relieved by altering posture

Treatment
Hot packs and massage to remove waste products
Treatment of the cause
Have the patient perform activities that use the muscles in a healthy manner
Muscle stretching

Muscle Guarding—Voluntary

With voluntary muscle guarding, the patient, aware of pain from a joint of other tissue, chooses to voluntarily restrict motion in the belief that it will reduce pain and suffering.

Causes
Pain on movement
Fear and anxiety
Mistaken impression that no movement is good

Symptom
Pain

Sign
Patient unable, unwilling, or refuses to move the part

Treatment
Determine whether the muscle guarding should be continued, as in fracture, disease, etc. Be aware that its presence could signify a serious condition
Otherwise, get the part moving by such activities as pendular movements
Oscillations of grade I or II intensity. For the extremities, the best movements are pendular (Codman for the shoulder) or oscillations of grades I or II intensity.

Fibrositis

The term *fibrositis* is one of the most confusing in orthopaedics. Since fibrositic nodules exist only in the living and can be provoked in all individuals by an appropriate stimulus, such as rolling the finger over and into scapular muscle, they must be considered as physiological and not pathological entities. They occur in response to stimuli: pal-patory, mechanical, or perhaps from a joint dysfunction. They are not present in cadavers and disappear at death. They are thus a response to stimuli or a pathologic condition and do not represent a pathologic condition in themselves. Any beneficial effect from treating them is indirect and would have more to do with mechanisms akin to acupressure, gating, and similar procedures.

Trigger Points

Somewhat related to fibrositic nodules are (so-called) trigger points. These anatomical locations are sites that, when a segmentally related condition exists, are capable of provoking both symptoms and signs of that condition such as pain, increased reflexes, muscle tone, muscle twitch, etc. Injections into or frictions of these locations may, as in fibrositis, be of assistance, but again the effect is reflexive for the trigger point is not a clinical entity.

Osteoarthritis or Osteoarthrosis

The terms *osteoarthritis* and *osteoarthrosis* are synonymous and reflect the argument as to whether or not there is indeed any inflammation. Since inflammation is generally considered not to be present the term osteoarthrosis is preferred.

The degenerative process affects both the joint capsule and the cartilaginous joint surfaces. Since stiff joints are not usually painful, these conditions frequently go unnoticed until the stage of degeneration has been reached at which there is destruction of the insensitive cartilage down to the level of the sensitive raw bone.

To treat osteoarthritis, the therapist should restore function (notably range of motion), establish good muscle support, and correct patterns of use.

Arthritis

The term *arthritis* needs to be qualified. The word arthritis means joint inflammation, of which there are many types ranging from rheumatoid to osteoarthritis. Or the term may refer to a problem in some part of the joint, such as synovitis.

Osteoarthritis has been referred to above and rheumatoid arthritis will not be considered in this contribution for it is not a condition commonly treated in orthopaedic physical therapy. Ankylosing spondylitis will, however, be listed as a syndrome.

Joint Lock or Block

On occasion, a joint may be locked. The condition is common, and may affect half of the population, occurring mostly in joints with menisci such as the knee, wrist, elbow, and spinal facet joints.

Causes
Forced full range or awkward motion producing a catch

Symptoms
Unable to move the joint, with some discomfort that is often acute

Signs
The joint cannot return to the neutral or rest position

Treatment
Manipulation

Hypermobility

Hypermobility is a term applied to a range of motion believed to be excessive to the joint in question.

Causes
Genetic
Response to repeated stress, such as standing on one leg, may produce sacroiliac hypermobility
Compensation for loss of motion in a neighboring joint

Symptoms
Ligamentous type of pain, that is a dull ache on assuming a fixed position

Signs
An excessive range of motion

Treatment
Manipulation of neighboring stiffness
Postural instruction
Stabilization exercises

Dislocation

In dislocations, joint surfaces have lost their normal relationship and cannot easily of their own accord be restored to their neutral or rest position.

Subluxation

Subluxed joint surfaces, owing to either hypermobility or loss of normal muscle tone, have assumed a rest position beyond that which is normal for the joint.

A patient with flaccid hemiparesis may display a subluxed shoulder, the position of which, on an individual with normal muscle tone, would be described as dislocated.

Tenosynovitis

The synovial sheath around a tendon may become inflamed. The inflammation may deposit synovial crystals that appear to lead to recurrences of the condition.

Causes
Unaccustomed overuse
Faulty use

Symptoms
Pain
Crepitus

Signs
Palpable crepitus

Treatment
Transverse friction
Ultrasound

Tenovaginitis

Tenovaginitis is similar to tenosynovitis but is related to the common extensor of the thumb.

Nerve Entrapment Syndromes

Receiving increasing attention in orthopaedics are those incidences in which pain may be caused by entrapment of the nerve over, against, or in between structures. The nerve does not have a nerve supply as such, but the sympathetics to the veins that accompany the nerve may give rise to the vascular pain so often experienced.

Causes
Degenerative conditions, for example, disc disease, stenosis
Posture
Myofascial restrictions

Symptoms
Pain reference is vague and intermittent
Altering posture may increase or decrease pain
Increasing activity may increase the pain
Pain type is pins and needles

Signs
The signs will depend greatly on the location and severity of neurological involvement. The classic neurological signs are: loss of skin sensation; weakness of muscle (beware of reluctance and disuse atrophy, neither of which is neurological); altered reflexes (unreliable); transient neurological deficits typical of lumbar spine stenosis.

Treatment
Posture
Myofascial stretches, for example, the thoracic outlet
Positional distraction, for example, disc protrusion

Overuse Syndromes

With the current emphasis on endurance sports such as aerobic running and triathalons, there is an increase in syndromes that appear to develop when the stress to tissues is greater than the tissues' ability to respond either by repair or by increasing their strength. Common examples are the stress fractures to tibia, femur, and posterior arches of the lumbar vertebra, that is, spondylosis leading to spondylolisthesis.

First Level
Discomfort comes on some hours after use. This is normal whenever we exceed our accustomed activity level. It is due no doubt to the inefficiency of the vascular system in carrying away the waste products of activity.

Treatment. Do not increase level of activity
Rest one or more days between efforts
Consider taking aspirin before the activity
Heat, massage, or hot tub after exercise
Stretch the muscles after the activity

Second Level
Pain comes on during or immediately after use. This is not normal and could be due to overuse or faulty technique. In this case, there is a definite need for professional coaching advice on technique.

Treatment. As for the first level
Check for dysfunction that may influence technique
Advise on exercise that may lessen the effects of overuse; for example, strengthen rotator cuff in the case of swimmer's shoulder, which is a friction syndrome occurring under the acromial arch

Third Level
Pain or discomfort is present even at rest. Damage has no doubt been done, and the athlete must stop the performance to avoid worsening the injury. In addition, it must be recognized that the athlete who has gone through the above two stages and has now reached this stage is one who does not listen to his body and thus has a common athletic behavioral problem, namely, denial.

The "no pain-no gain" philosophy is totally without merit in any athlete who has a serious interest in continued sports participation. Although it is perfectly acceptable to exercise through muscular discomfort of fatigue, it is never acceptable to continue any activity to the point of or beyond pain. Discomfort and pain need to be differentiated.

Postural Syndromes

Increasingly, the positions in which we sit, stand, and even sleep are being recognized as contributing factors in cases of back pain, craniomandibular dysfunction, and, of course, scoliosis.

Causes
Poor postural sense
Injury, age, pain

Symptoms
Few primary symptoms, but other conditions may develop as a result of postural change, for example, thoracic outlet syndrome, temperomandibular occlusal dysfunction

Signs
Poor postural appearance, slouching
Tight myofascia on attempting correction

Treatment
Education
Release of tight myofascia

Lesion Complex

Lesion complex is a useful term to draw attention to the fact that rarely do single entities such as those listed above exist without the involvement of adjacent structures as well. Hence, any attempt to create a diagnosis that nominates one structure to be at fault, for example, disc protrusion, will inevitably fail to state the entire story. Physicians and surgeons are required to determine a diagnosis. Physical therapists are free from that requirement. When an evaluation is completed the therapist should be able to construct a list of objective findings that can be treated. It is to these findings and not the diagnosis to which the therapist's attention is addressed.

A disease can be diagnosed, but dysfunctions are best served by a complete listing or description rather than by a catchall term. A surgeon may diagnose the patient with disc disease. Table 11-3 lists the findings of the therapist on completing the evaluation of this patient.

PRINCIPLES OF EVALUATION

Although this text does not fully address the subject of evaluation, we feel that it is important to stress the need for a full and comprehensive evaluation of patients and to recognize the need for continual reassessment. Much of the advice presented in the following chapters, although correct in principle, may not apply in a specific case because of what may be observed during a complete and competent evaluation.

The ten steps of the evaluation are listed below, along with a brief presentation on the manner in which physical therapists use "end feels" in both evaluation and treatment. This material, particu-

larly with regard to end feel, will be essential to the section on extremity dysfunction (see below).

Steps in Patient Evaluation

1. Pain drawing and assessment
2. Initial observation
3. History and interview
4. Structural assessment
5. Active movements
6. Palpation
   a. Condition
   b. Position
   c. Mobility
7. Neurological findings
8. Radiological findings
9. Correlation and treatment planning
10. Prognosis

End Feel

The above ten steps can be applied to examination of the spine and extremities. However, in the extremities and in advanced spinal evaluations, the therapists greatly rely on the condition of the articular tissues, which defines the end of joint range (e.g., cartilage, bone, and muscle). Since every joint is eventually limited in its motion, the therapist must decide whether that range is normal (i.e., normal end feels) or abnormal (as in the case of abnormal end feels). Abnormal end feels can occur from a variety of structures, and each requires a separate approach for optimal results of treatment.

SUGGESTED READINGS

1. Akeson W: An experimental study of joint stiffness. J Bone Joint Surg
2. Bourdillon JF: Spinal Manipulation. 3rd Ed. Appleton-Century-Crofts, East Norwalk, CT 1982
3. Cyriac J: Textbook of Orthopaedic Medicine Vol. 1. Diagnosis of Soft Tissue Lesions. 6th Ed. Williams & Wilkins, Baltimore, 1975
4. Daube JR: Nerve conduction studies in the TOS. Neurology 25:347, 1975
5. DePalma A, Rothman R: The Intervertebral Disc. WB Saunders, Philadelphia, 1970
6. Williams PL, Warkwick R (ed): Grays Anatomy. 36th Ed. WB Saunders, Philadelphia, 1980

Table 11-3 Findings after Evaluation by Therapist of Patient with Disc Disease

Findings	Treatment
Tight myofascia	Stretches
Hypermobility of L4-L5 segment	Stabilization
Restriction L5-S1 segment	Manipulation
Short right leg	Heel lift
Restricted capsule in the right hip	Manipulation

7. Gregersen G, Lucas D: An in vivo study of the axial rotation of the human thoracolumbar spine. J Bone Joint Surg 49A:247, 1967

8. Grieve G: Common Vertebral Joint Problems. Churchill Livingstone, Edenburgh, 1981

9. Hoppenfeld S: Physical Examination of the Spine and Extremities. Appleton-Century-Crofts, East Norwalk, CT, 1976

10. Janda V: In Koss I (ed): Muscles, Central Nervous Motor Regulation, and Back Problems: The Neurobiologic Mechanisms in Manipulative Therapy. Plenum, New York, 1978

11. Kapandji IA: The Physiology of the Joints. Vol. 3. The Trunk and the Vertebral Column. 2nd Ed. Churchill Livingstone, Edinburgh, 1974

12. Kendall H, Kendall F, Wadsworth G: Muscle Testing and Function. 2nd Ed. Williams & Wilkins, Baltimore, 1971

13. Kendall H, Kendall F, Boynton D: Posture and Pain. Robert E. Krieger Publishing, Malaba, FL, 1952

14. Kopell H, Thompson W: Peripheral Entrapment Neuropathies. Robert E. Krieger Publishing, Huntington, NY, 1976

15. Mennel J: The Science and Art of Joint Manipulation. Vol. 2. The Spinal Column. J. and A. Churchill, London, 1952

16. Panjabi M, White A: Clinical Biomechanics of the Spine. JB Lippincott, Philadelphia, 1978

17. Panjabi M et al. Thoracic spine centers of rotation in the sagittal plane. J Orthop Res 1:387, 1984

18. Roos DB: Congenital anomalies associated with TOS. Am J Surg 132:771, 1976

19. Spence E: The slipping rib syndrome. Arch Surg 118:1330, 1983

20. Stallworth JM, Quinn GJ, Aiken AF: Is rib resection necessary for relief of TOS? Ann Surg 185:581, 1977

21. Stoddard A: Manual of Osteopathic Practice. Hutchison, London, 1969

22. Steindler A: Kinesiology of the Human Body under Normal and Pathological Conditions. Charles C Thomas, Springfield, IL, 1973

23. Vo N: TOS: ten years later. Conn Med 48:143, 1984

24. Zohn D, Mennell J: Diagnosis and Physical Treatment: musculoskeletal pain. Little, Brown, Boston, 1976

12 Lumbar Spine

Stanley V. Paris

COCCYDYNIA

Coccydynia is an uncommon condition at the bottom of the spine that can be very painful. There is also a reluctance on the part of clinicians to examine this area. It is good policy to be accompanied by a member of the patient's sex during both examination and treatment and to use an appropriate glove and lubricant.

Causes

Direct trauma by a fall onto the coccyx, for instance, sitting on a hard object

During childbirth the sacrococcygeal joint may be strained or the coccyx itself fractured

Indirect trauma in which a hypermobile sacroiliac joint causes a pull on the coccyx via the sacrococcygeal ligament

Symptoms

Pain at the base of the spine aggravated by sitting on a medium-soft surface

Pain on exertion during either passing a stool or climbing stairs

Signs

Difficulty in sitting still

Tender to palpation

Tender to passive movement testing

Possible positional fault

Treatment

This is one of the rare occasions in manual therapy when a "routine" may be most suitable. The point of the treatment is to stretch out the sacrococcygeal joint to free the capsule or joint adhesions. Additional positional faults may be corrected by the following routine (Fig. 12-1).

First Treatment Session

With the patient prone and two pillows under the pelvis, the legs are abducted and internally rotated (prevents gluteal contractions). A gloved index finger is inserted into the anus while the thumb of the second gloved hand supports the coccyx from the posterior aspect. The coccyx is then given traction along the long axis in the position in which it is observed to rest. This is repeated about three times to the point of increasing discomfort.

Second Treatment Sesstion

The above routine is repeated and in addition some attempt is made to change the position of the coccyx to a more normal alignment while it is held under traction. The traction is not released until the coccyx is returned to its original position.

Third Treatment Session

The third treatment session proceeds as described above, but now the traction may be released at various points.

These three treatments should be sufficient to free the coccyx for normal function. If not, repeat aspects of the last two treatments. In addition, ultrasound may be given after each treatment.

Management

Sitting to be avoided when possible

Coccygeal pillow (not a ring) is best (Fig. 12-2)

Dietary advice to reduce firmness of stools

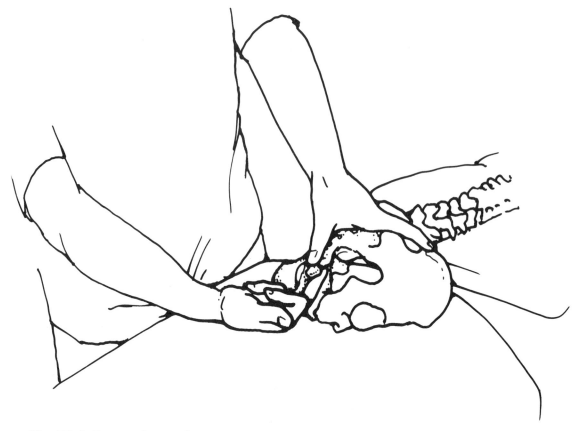

Fig. 12-1 Coccygeal manipulation. *Patient*: Prone lying over one or more pillows with the legs abducted and internally rotated. *Therapist*: Accompanied by a member of the patient's sex, inserts the gloved and lubricated index finger of the right hand into the anal passage so that it comes to rest against the anterior surface of the coccyx. The thumb of the other hand, also gloved but not lubricated, is placed on the dorsum of the coccyx to effect a good grasp between the two fingers. *Technique*: The coccyx is distracted along its long axis. *Use*: Release of coccygeal adhesions that presumably trigger the capsular discomfort and synovitis.

Prognosis

It usually takes 2 weeks for 90 percent relief. Two months may need to pass without further stress for the area to quiet down.

LUMBAR FACET CONDITIONS

1. Facet synovitis/haemarthrosis.
2. Facet stiffness.
3. Painful entrapment of facet.
4. Mechanical block of facet.

Facet Synovitis-Hemarthrosis

Facet synovitis-hemarthrosis is a painful low back injury usually caused by twisting or lifting.

Cause
Lifting or twisting against a heavy load
Could be a "sudden" catch, where perhaps capsule is momentarily nipped, resulting in synovitis or haemarthrosis
Stiff facet more liable to this kind of injury owing to lack of tolerance to insult

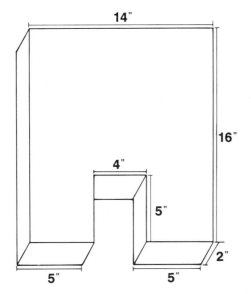

Fig. 12-2 Coccygeal pillow. This item can be easily cut from 1½ to 2 inch thick foam rubber and measures 16 by 14 inches. The patient sits on the pillow, with the coccyx over the 4 by 5 inch opening.

Symptoms
Painful low back
Difficulty in moving freely secondary to associated strong involuntary muscle holding

Signs
Demonstrated reluctance to move
Difficulty arising from or getting down into a chair and preferring to rest on the side of the table or against a wall. Patient can take all the weight on the spine, but must move carefully

Treatment
Rest for 10 days from activity, but not function. If muscle guarding restricts function and fear produces immobility with consequent retiring to the bed then this must be corrected.
Passive assisted motion on a manipulator (Fig. 12-3)

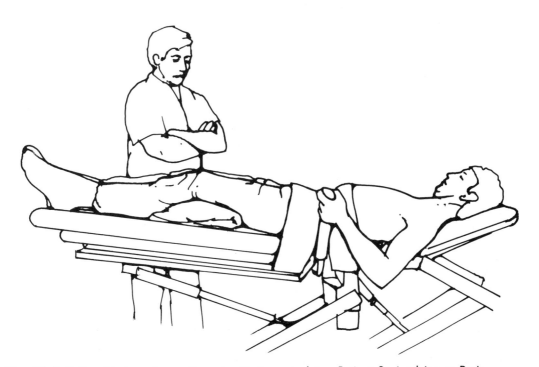

Fig. 12-3 Self-assisted passive motion using Paris manipulator. *Patient*: Supine lying on Paris manipulator and position in maximal comfort. *Therapist*: Once having set up the patient, the therapist may help begin the initial motion while the patient grabs the horns of the table. *Technique*: Patient moves his own spine within his own comfort range. May also let go of the horns and use the low back muscles when able to do so. *Use*: Acute facet traction. Postoperative remobilization.

Heat, massage, transcutaneous electrical nerve stimulation (TENS), oscillation. Patient must be made to ambulate.

TENS or other palliative treatment may be of assistance or could be tried.

Management

Other than providing for pain relief, there is little that can be done during the first 10 days. Movement should be encouraged, but it must not be to the limits of discomfort. The joint has been injured and, as with other extremity joints, must be allowed to rest and heal. Bed rest is permitted for short periods, but too much bed rest will lead to excessive muscle guarding, particularly of the chemical type, and could result in further stresses to the back. Heat, ice, or massage may help. Grade one and two oscillations may also be used as may a mobilization table for movement within the range.

After 10 days, provided the joint has not been aggravated by any of the preceding activities, the therapist may begin to mobilize the joint, restoring it gradually to full range.

Facet Stiffness

Facet stiffness is surely the most common condition affecting the spine, causing segmental loss of movement. Stiff joints do not of themselves cause pain, but they are more liable to reinjury and hence strain and thus to repeated attacks of synovitis.

Within their own segment, stiff facets may result in reduction of nutrition to the disc. In neighboring segments, they may produce ligamentous and joint instability (hypermobility).

The decision as to whether or not stiff facets require treatment will depend on the following factors:

1. Being subject to repeated acute attacks of synovitis.
2. The facets appear to be causing hypermobility at an adjacent level.
3. In the athlete, treatment may help achieve optimal range.

Causes
Previous strain
Disuse

Symptoms
None

Signs

Restriction of active and passive movements showing a capsular pattern. For example, in the lumbar spine, a stiff facet on the left side would cause the spine to deviate to the left side on forward bending while limiting side bending to the right side and rotation to the left side. All other movements would be free.

Treatment

Manipulation to restore full range motion to lessen degenerative changes within that segment and the need for compensatory changes at segments above (Figs. 12-4 to 12-7).

Painful Entrapment of the Facet

In entrapment, the sensitive facet joint capsule is caught between the articular surfaces. Unstable joints are those that are most likely to have their capsules entrapped.

Causes

An awkward movement usually involving rotation and backward bending to the involved side. This appears to open up and "suck in" the capsule, causing it to get nipped.

Symptoms

Acute pain on trying to straighten up.

Signs
Fixed posture with voluntary muscle holding.
Secondary lateral shift. Here because of pain which increases with any attempt to resume the fully erect position, the intervertebral discs will adapt to the new position by a fluid shift.

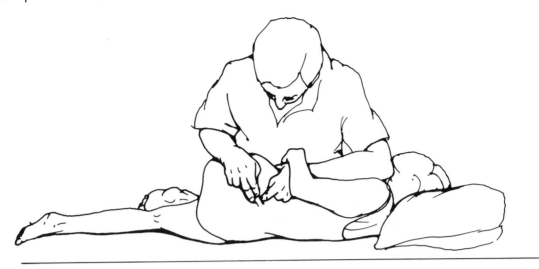

Fig. 12-4 Midlumbar manipulation-distraction. *Patient*: Side lying facing therapist. *Therapist*: Flexes up to and rotates down to the involved level. Contacts cephalid vertebra of the segment on the left side and caudal vertebra on the right side of their respective spinous processes with the middle finger of each hand. *Technique*: In time with breathing exerts a rotational motion through finger contacts plus those on the shoulder and pelvis and illustrated. *Use*: Distraction of the lumbar facet on the left side primarily to assist rotation left.

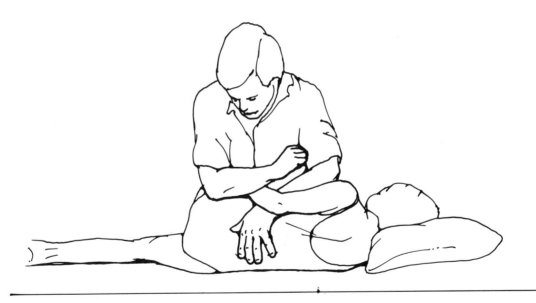

Fig. 12-5 Lumbosacral manipulation-distraction. *Patient*: Side lying facing therapist. *Therapist*: Places patient's top leg over side of table to flex to level and rotates the spine from above to the same level. The left thumb is now placed on the left side of the spinous process of L5 and the right elbow is placed on the posterior iliac crest. *Technique*: The left thumb fixes while the right elbow delivers a small but sharp impulse to the pelvis. *Use*: Distracts the left lumbosacral facet to assist rotation at that level.

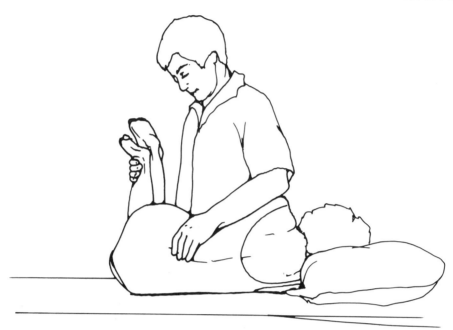

Fig. 12-6 Side bending manipulation of the midlumbar spine. *Patient*: Side lying flexed to the level with hip and knees at a right angle. *Therapist*: Blocks the spinous process on the left side with the middle fingers and then after supporting patient's thighs on therapist's thighs. *Technique*: Therapist raises legs to effect a stretch at the level just below the blocking fingers. *Use*: Causes a sliding motion in the facet that is a component of side bending and will thus assist side bending to the opposite side.

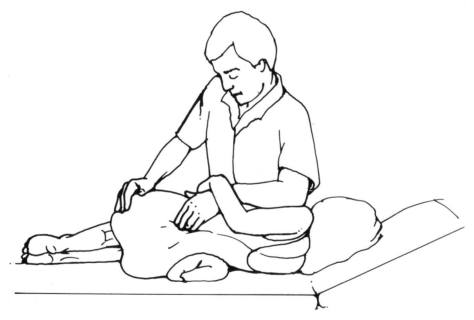

Fig. 12-7 Side bending manipulation of the midlumbar spine. *Patient*: Side lying over pillow to begin the side bending. *Therapist*: Blocks the vertebra above the level by contacting the spinous process with the middle fingers of the left hand. *Technique*: By pushing on the pelvis while blocking with the fingers a side bending technique is effected. *Use*: As in Fig. 12-6.

Treatment

Midlumbar manipulation—distraction technique (Fig. 12-4)

Isometric manipulation using the patient's own muscles to pull the capsule out from between the joint surfaces (Fig. 12-8)

Correction of the lateral shift (see Fig. 12-16)

Management

Once the joint capsule has been freed and the patient can move about more easily, the condition should be treated as an acute facet synovitis (see above).

If, once the condition has settled, it is observed that the segment is unstable, then stabilizing exercises directed at the multifidus will need be taught.

Mechanical Block of a Facet

When a facet is mechanically blocked, patients suddenly find themselves locked over and unable to move. The exact pathophysiology is unknown, but is is speculated that roughness between the joint surfaces or an entrapped synovial meniscus is the cause. Many researchers think that this is due to a fragment displacement of the disc, but I do not share this belief because, surgically, such fragments are not observed and mechanical blocks are easily treated by manipulation, whereas manipulation is of little or no assistance to disc conditions.

Causes

Entrapped meniscus or degenerative facet joint surface, brought on by a full-range awkward or twisting movement

Symptoms

Minimal pain and some shock

Signs

Patient is bent over in a manner that would be expected if the facet were to ride up on the one below and get stuck there

Secondary fluid shift (see Lateral Shift, below)

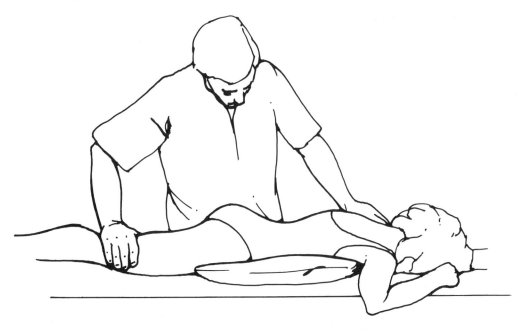

Fig. 12-8 Isometric manipulation of multifidii on the facet capsules. *Patient*: Prone lying over one or more pillows to attain a position of comfort and to avoid backward bending. *Therapist*: One hand on the patient's left shoulder and the other on the right thigh. *Technique*: Patient is asked to raise the right leg, which the therapist resists. *Use*: As isometric stretch to the facet capsules via the attachment of multifidus. This will stretch the capsules and thereby assist range of motion and in addition may be successful in releasing capsular impingement.

Treatment

Manipulate facet by rotating to side away from side to which the patient is bent (see Fig. 12-4). The effect may be enhanced by increasing the degree of side bending with a rolled-up pillow under the waist.

Management

Pay attention to any lateral shift (see Fig. 12-15) or loss of lordosis once the facet has been freed.

The prognosis is excellent.

MUSCLE GUARDING—CHEMICAL

Chemical muscle guarding is discussed in Chapter 11. It commonly accompanies low back dysfunction.

Treatment

Heat and massage

MYOFACIAL RESTRICTIONS

Cause

Secondary to chemical muscle guarding, which in turn is secondary to lumbar spine dysfunctions

Symptoms

Stiffness
Fatigue

Signs

Limited forward bending
Free side bending

Treatment

Sustained stretch. For a stretch to be effective other than in the short term, it must exceed the elastic range of the muscles' connective tissue elements, which can only be done when the muscle has been either tricked into relaxing (contract-relax-stretch) or when it has been inhibited (pressure over origin-insertion) or fatigued.

Knees to chest (Fig. 12-9).
Prone kneel squat (Fig. 12-10).
Assisted prone kneel squat (Fig. 12-11).
Sustained stretch on Paris manipulator (Fig. 12-12).

LIGAMENTOUS DEFICIENCY

The ligaments of the lumbar spine include not only those described in anatomy texts, but in addition must include for all practical purposes the fibrous outer anulus of the intervertebral disc.

Causes

Poor posture, sitting slouched
Obesity
Repeated trauma, twisting

Symptoms

Constant dull back pain on sitting
Need to keep moving
May awaken stiff and then be pain free but pain worsens as day goes on
May obtain relief by "cracking" back (reflex muscle relaxation and perhaps endorphin release)

Signs

Difficulty in sitting still

Treatment

Posture correction by the back school method
Stabilizing exercises

Management

These patients must be made to appreciate the seriousness of their condition. Ligamentous insufficiency leads to segmental instability and intervertebral disc rupture.

ILIOLUMBAR LIGAMENT STRAIN-SPRAIN

Iliolumbar ligament strain-sprain is an unusual condition often mistaken for sacroiliac problems.

Causes

Traumatic twist or jerking of the low back

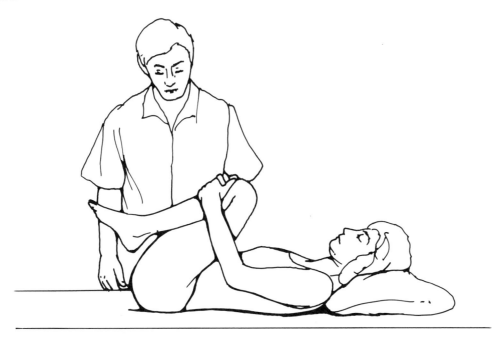

Fig. 12-9 Self stretch of lumbar myofascia with knees to chest. *Patient*: Supine lying. *Technique*: Knees are pulled gently yet firmly to the chest. Pull is maintained to fatigue. *Use*: Stretch lumbar myofascia.

Symptoms

Pain on the side of the low back, overlying the sacroiliac and lumbosacral region

Signs

Pain on forward bending, backward bending, side bending away, and rotation to the affected side. Each of these movements places stress on the iliolumbar ligament, whereas rotation and side bending to the affected side is unlikely to produce discomfort.

Treatment

Rest and perhaps support with an abdominal corset

Management

The patient needs to know that a period of some 6 weeks of avoiding stress to this ligament will be necessary for it to repair. There is

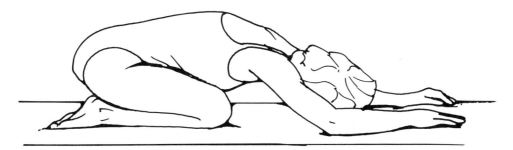

Fig. 12-10 Myofascia stretch to the posterior lumbar muscles. *Patient*: Kneels on the table and then squats back on the heels. Once this position is relaxed into, the patient pushes back with the hands while relaxing his lower back to affect the stretch. *Use*: To stretch out myofascial restriction.

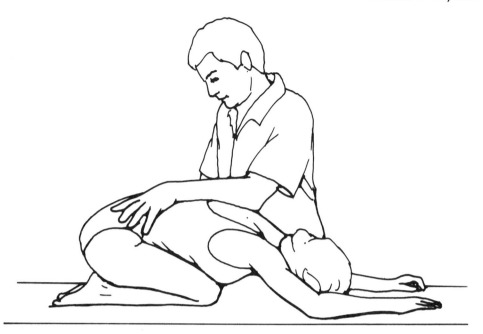

Fig. 12-11 Assisted myofascial stretch to the posterior lumbar muscles. *Patient*: Kneeling as in Fig. 12-10. *Therapist*: Once patient has assumed the position in Fig. 12-10, hand is placed firmly on the pelvis. *Technique*: The pelvis is pressed down toward the ankles. *Use*: Stretch of the myofascia.

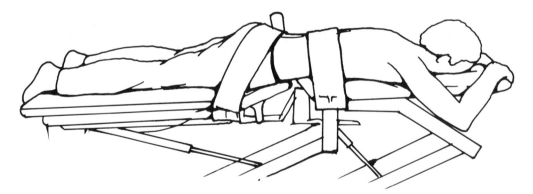

Fig. 12-12 Myofascial stretch with Paris manipulator. *Patient*: Prone lying and fixed to the table with appropriate straps. *Therapist*: Adjusts the table to put in traction, side bending, and forward bending. *Technique*: Only one side is stretched at a time. Only modest flexion is imparted. Maintain for 20 minutes. *Use*: This technique permits stretching the myofascia even in the presence of weakened ligaments and possible lumbar disc involvement since unlike the previous two methods it incorporates traction.

very little that physical therapy can do at this time other than to provide encouragement for this conservative program.

INSTABILITY

When the ligaments of the spinal segment, including the outer anulus of the intervertebral disc, the iliolumbar ligament, and perhaps the sacroiliac ligaments as well as the muscles of the low back and abdominal regions, become weakened or lose their normal tone, the result is spinal instability. Principally a ligamentous condition, it can either start as a traumatic spondylolisthesis or lead to a degenerative spondylolisthesis. The principal risk is disc rupture.

Causes

Disc degeneration
Over-strain of lumbar ligaments
Spondylolisthesis
Repeated rotary manipulation

Symptoms

Dull ache on assuming a seated position
Perhaps transient neurological signs
Inability to sit still
Pain eased by constant movement

Signs

Inability to sit still
Involuntary and even voluntary muscle guarding
Shaking or slipping in the back when performing active forward bending
"Step" displacement on standing denoting spondylolisthesis that disappears when lying down; if "step" remains it is therefore stable. Not all spondylolisthesis are unstable.
Diffulculty is straightening up after forward bending
Spontaneous "giving away" of the leg resulting in a fall

Treatment

Back school and posture
Stabilization exercises for lumbar spine (multifidus)

Isometric activities with the lumbar spine
Taping for re-education
Corset for support
Stretching out of hip restrictions
Use of viscoelastic insoles

Management

Long-term cooperation with the program is needed. Ligaments remodel at a very slow rate.
Surgery will be necessary if neurological signs advance.

Stabilization Routine

In patients with either instability or the clinical picture of repeated minor attacks of back pain, a program designed to stabilize the lumbar spine should assist. Techniques illustrated in Figures 12-3, 12-8, 12-13, and 12-14 will help. Techniques of keeping the back "rigid" while lifting, getting in and out of a car, rolling on a floor, and bouncing on a bed may all help this particular group of patients.

SPONDYLOLISTHESIS

Spondylolisthesis is a condition in which a vertebral body, usually the fifth or fourth lumbar vertebra, slips forward on the vertebra below. It affects 6 to 10 percent of the adult population and as many as 70 percent of gymnasts, power lifters, and football players. There are at least three types, each with its own principal cause.

Stress Fracture

Stress fractures occur between the two facets in the region known as the pars interarticularis. The stress is most commonly due to repetitive overload and thus is a fatigue fracture. Also possible is a sudden hyperextension injury, but this is thought to be a less frequent cause and probably follows a period of fatigue. The initial fracture produces a spondylosis, that is, a fracture without slippage. Slippage usually follows, resulting in the spondylolisthesis.

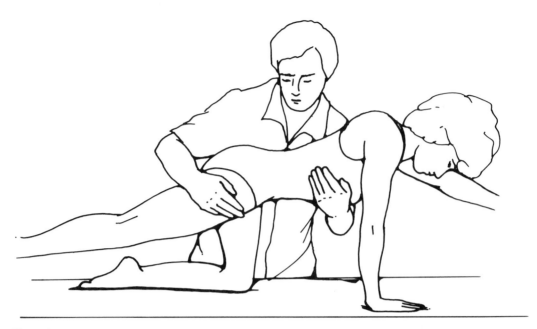

Fig. 12-13 Stabilization of multifidii group. *Patient*: Kneeling on hands and knees. *Therapist*: Positioned to support patient. *Technique*: Patient is instructed to first raise one arm, then the next, and to repeat the same with the legs. Next the patient is instructed to raise alternate arms and legs and even the arms and legs on the same side. Finally, the therapist now imparts bumps and pushes to the spine trying to get the patient off balance. *Use*: To "fine tune" and strengthen multifidii that in time will assist in regaining segmental stabilization from repeated attacks of low back pain, hypermobility, and spondylolisthesis.

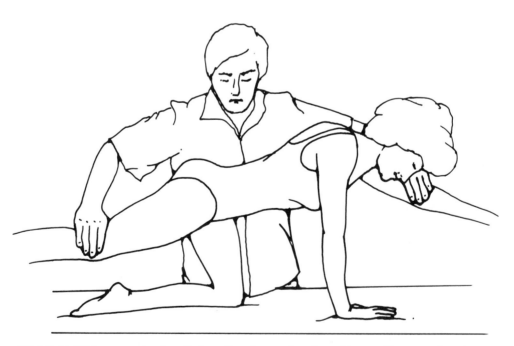

Fig. 12-14 Multifidus strengthening. *Patient*: Kneeling on hands and knees. *Therapist*: Standing at side to give resistance via opposite arm and leg. *Technique*: Press down to produce strength and in different directions to encourage stabilization similar to that in Fig. 12-13. *Use*: Strength and stabilization. The highly trained individual with well-coordinated multifidii can perform these movements even on a soft surface and move from one combination to the next.

Stretch of the Pedicles

The neural arch remains intact, but, perhaps due to adolescent obesity, the pedicle lengthens and the back has the appearance of a step, usually quite stable. There is no fracture, at least initially.

Degenerative Osteoarthrosis

Sometimes the facets degenerate and permit the cephalid vertebra to slip on the caudal articular surfaces. This may be predisposed by facet asymmetry (anomaly in the facet plane).

Causes

Each of the above types has its own particular causes, but in general, spondylolisthesis may result from:

Backward bending (gymnastic or football activities)
Obesity and disc degeneration
Congenitally asymmetrical facets

Symptoms

Dull ligamentous ache requiring a change in posture
Discomfort relieved by movement, often the very movement (e.g., backward bending) that created it
In advanced cases in which the vertebra has slipped more than one-fifth of the way across the vertebra below, neurological signs may develop

Signs

A visible and palpable step displacement appears in the low back that can be seen on standing, for in such a posture, particularly at the end of the day, the step is greater and so is the involuntary muscle guarding
Hypermobility of the involved segment along with the characteristic signs of instability (see above)
If on changing posture there is no detectable change in either the involuntary muscle holding or palpable step, then the condition is stable and does not warrant treatment other than advice on moderating activities tha might cause it to become unstable

Treatment

Support, such as a corset
Modification or reduction of activities that involve backward bending and rotation
Strengthening of abdominal and multifidii muscles
Stabilization routine (Figs. 12-13, 12-14)

SPONDYLOLYSIS

Spondylolysis is a fracture of the pars interarticularis that commonly becomes bilateral and leads to a spondylolisthesis (see above).

Causes

Stress, as in spondylolisthesis

Symptoms

Low back pain of a dull ligamentous type on assuming a static weight-bearing position. Usually detected when a patient has back pain from another source and has radiographs taken as part of the examination.

Signs

A small rotation or offset of the spinous process on the side on which the defect has occurred. This is noticed during standing.
Minor increase in involuntary muscle holding suggesting the possibility of instability. Patient should be re-examined at the end of a busy day or one that involves a great deal of sitting.

Treatment

Cessation of rotation and backward bending activities
Posture instruction
Strengthening of deep muscles

INTERVERTEBRAL DISC INVOLVEMENT

There is no standard classification of disc conditions. Certainly a classification of value to one surgeon may differ from that of another surgeon and will differ from that used by a physical therapist involved principally in nonoperative treatment. Offered here is a classification that should cover most eventualities and be of clinical value in conservative management.

In the classification set forth below, the first category having to do with disc fluid imbalance is considered to be physiological rather than pathological. However, the remaining conditions are pathological, and in general, they all have the same causes. It is of principal importance to realize that there is no such entity as a primary disc rupture (herniation). Disc pathology resulting in clinical signs and symptoms that may require and be relieved by surgery does not occur in a healthy back. Any individual who has such a condition has a history of low back pain of increasing frequency and severity. In fact, they have a typical history of a ligamentous type of back pain as described above. To avoid repetition, the causes are listed here.

Causes of Pathological Disc Involvement

Repeated postural misuse and abuse
History of ligamentous pain and segmental
    instability that was inadequately treated or
    not treated at all
Obesity

Virtually all low back surgery, in my view, is due to either the failure or denial of adequate conservative management.

Fluid Imbalance

The intervertebral disc is a hydrostatic structure into which fluids are drawn at night to be expressed out during the day and thus to complete a nutrient cycle. The force that attracts the fluid in is from the negatively charged glycosaminoglycan (GAG) molecules of the nucleus. Their mutual repulsion creates space into which fluids are drawn. Body weight during the day overcomes their force, and thus the fluids are expressed out until the forces attracting fluids in are at balance with the body weight forcing fluids out.

When a marked change of body posture is adopted, such as stooped sitting as in driving a car, the disc fluid balance is altered. The flexed position further drives fluids from the now weighted front of the disc while allowing fluids to be attracted to the now relatively unweighted posterior disc. The result is a change in the hydrostatic balance and a temporary change in the disc shape secondary to a redistribution of fluid. The individual experiences this as diffulculty in regaining the normal upright posture. This situation has in the past quite erroneously been blamed on any number of factors including muscle spasm, disc rupture, facet locking, etc. The plain fact is that this is a normal physiological occurrence.

Loss of Lordosis

Loss of lordosis is the most common form of altered intradiscal fluid imbalance.

Cause

Adopting a forced flexed posture such as when
    driving a car without adequate low back
    support
Secondary to a disc or facet condition giving rise
    to low back pain that the patient chooses to
    move away from

Symptoms

None. The condition is asymptomatic beyond the
    discomfort produced by the position.

Signs

Subject is bent over and demonstrates a loss of
    the normal lordosis.

Treatment

If the condition is not due to a disc or facet
    condition, the individual should be
    encouraged to force a return of the lordosis
    by performing what is referred to as
    "extension" exercises (Fig. 12-15).
If due to disc or facet condition, first treat the
    cause and then restore the lordosis.

Lateral Shift

Lateral shift is very similar to the previous condition but is more likely to be secondary to facet or nerve root involvement.

Cause

Facet, disc, or muscle imbalance, possibly
    postural

Signs

Bent over and to one side, usually away from the
    pain

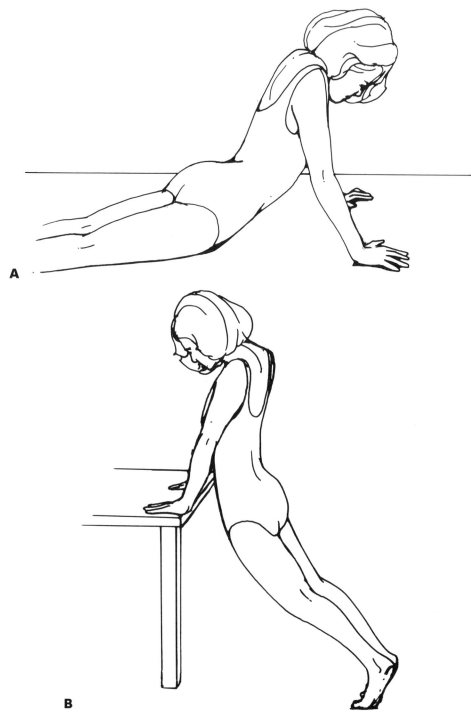

Fig. 12-15 (A) Prone press up. *Patient*: Prone lying. Does a press up while relaxing the lumbar spine and attempting to restore or exaggerate the lumbar lordosis. *Therapist*: Gives encouragement and may press down into lordosis to assist with the position. *Use*: To restore the normal lordosis. **(B)** Press up with traction. *Patient*: Stands with arms locked and holding onto a table with feet behind and back relaxed. *Therapist*: Gives encouragement and may direct the patient to oscillate the movement and sway from side to side to aid in comfort. *Use*: Can often be performed when the prone press up cannot be done owing to discomfort.

Symptoms
Minimal as the predominating symptoms are
    from the causative dysfunction

Treatment
Correct the causative pathology, then the lateral
    shift. Use a squeeze technique to correct the
    shift.

Acutely Involved Disc—Tear

An acutely involved disc with a tear is again found
on an individual with a history of low back pain
of increasing frequency and severity.

Signs and Symptoms
Sudden deep, sharp pain, perhaps accompanied
    by a tear or snap
Awareness that this is different from previous
    attacks

Treatment
Patient must immediately assume the lordotic
    position and rest lying prone. This position
    will possibly close the tear before the
    nucleus, ever willing to expand, can do so
    and escape the now ruptured anulus. The
    position will allow the outer and vascular
    anulus to heal.
Keep in lordosis by tape, corset, or other devices
    for 2 weeks.
Rest on a firm bed and sleep on the back or
    stomach to retain lordosis.

Management
With careful management, this patient will
    recover from this attack but will still need to
    be treated for the ligamentous weakness in
    the manner described above.

Painful Disc

Without Neurological Signs

Most discs that are pathologically involved tend to
be painful, but the type of pain is ligamentous as
described above. The outer anulus is the only
innervated part of the disc and so it is the only
part that can give rise to pain. Ligamentous pain
can be referred into the leg as far as the foot.

Causes
Weak ligamentous and anular fibers being
    stretched until the nociceptive fibers are
    mechanically fired.

Symptoms
Repeated attacks of low back pain of increasing
    frequency and severity
Transient neurological complaints, for example,
    numbness

Signs
Depends on the stage of the condition. Initially,
    there will be a dull ache on assuming a fixed
    position, and movement will be free and
    perhaps unstable, demonstrating a shaking
    movement on forward bending.
Passive movement testing will reveal
    hypermobility. Later, with increasing pain,
    there will be muscle guarding, increased
    sensitivity of tissues to touch and great state
    of anxiety, often fear. Instability produces
    fear.

Treatment
Stretch all tight muscles
Correct the posture
Correct tightness in the hips and in lumbar facet
    joints
Strengthen muscles, in particular, the multifidus
Practice stabilization routines
Educate the patient with back school so that he
    leads a more healthy life-style and reduce
    the stress on his back

Management
Although at this point the patient has evidence
    of disc degeneration, there is no need to
    panic provided the patient takes great care
    of his back in the future. If he does not,
    then this could well proceed to be a disc
    prolapse or herniation.

With Neurological Signs—Prolapse

Prolapse condition can only result from either the
failure or denial of adequate treatment during the
early stages of disc degeneration. Given a good
physical therapy program with adequate patient
education and commitment, this prolapse should
have been preventable.

Treatment

It will most likely to be too late to attempt the lordotic position once the nucleus has prolapsed. Any attempt to do so will narrow the intervertebral foramen, pinch and enlargen the disc protrusion, and thus add to the pressure on the already sensitive nerve root.

Acute treatment is bed rest with approximately 90° of hip and knee flexion, whatever is a position of comfort.

Some 10 to 14 days after the initiation of bed rest, it may be possible to commence positional distraction techniques, provided they are very gentle. Positional distraction is designed to open up the intervertebral foramen and to take pressure off the nerve roots. The position must be only partially assumed so as not to stretch the healing outer anulus.

At times when the traction is not being used, the patient should be lying with his back flat, and that means that the knees must be bent up and supported by pillows or by jackknifing the bed (semi-Fowler position).

About 4 weeks after onset and a good conservative program of rest and minimal activity, the patient wishing to avoid surgery is now ready for rehabilitation.

Positional distraction should be done on a twice daily basis, once at the clinic and at least once at home by the patient (Figs. 12-16, 12-17, 12-18)

Exercise to multifidus and abdominals to provide support for the trunk

A corset to give additional support while up and around

Avoid sitting and all rotational activities. Rotation can be discouraged by taping

Back school for educating the patient as to the care of his own back

At the chronic stage of treatment, there is little other than back school advice that can be given. Letting time pass and good management by the patient is all that can be done. If the severity of symptoms warrants it, the surgeon will perform surgery.

Prognosis

Most disc prolapses and herniations do not require surgery. Before 1934, surgery was not available. Correct rest and a good routine such as stated above combined with patience, education, and faith in nature's healing powers will suffice in most cases. Studies have shown that although surgery does have an initial advantage over conservative treatment, by the fourth year patients not operated on are doing significantly better than those that were. Surgery should be preserved for those rare conditions that cannot be helped by a good conservative routine. No area of orthopaedic surgery has a higher risk of failure than that of back surgery.

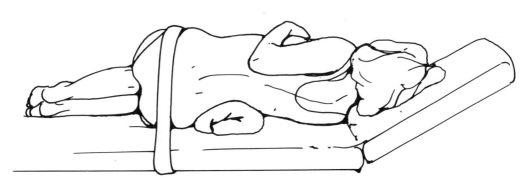

Fig. 12-16 Positional distraction. *Patient*: Side lying over pillow with affected side uppermost. The spine has been bent forward to the level and rotated to the level above to enhance the side-bending component. *Therapist*: Positions the patient and applies a strap around the pelvis to help maintain the position. *Use*: The relief of nerve root pressure by opening the intervertebral foramen, thus creating more room for the nerve root the case of a prolapse, or by pulling the bulge flat, as in the case of a herniation.

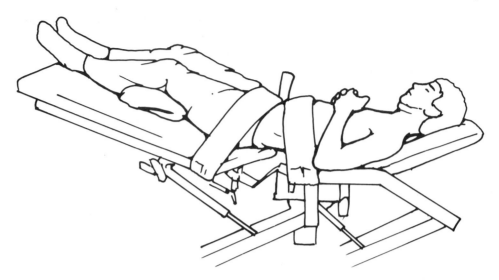

Fig. 12-17 Positional distraction on the Paris manipulator. *Patient*: Supine lying and positioned on the three-dimensional table in such a manner as to provide comfortable yet optimal side bending, forward bending, and some minimal rotation to maximally open the intervertebral foramen. Distraction is then added either by the operator or by the attachment of a standard traction device added to the foot of the table. *Therapist*: Positions the patient as described, bearing in mind the mechanics of the involved segment. *Technique*: The position itself is sufficient as a treatment and is used for only 5 minutes on the first visit. At subsequent visits, the duration is increased by 5 minutes each time until a maximum of about 45 minutes is reached. Mechanical traction, steady or intermittent, may be added. *Use*: Relief of nerve root pressure and the promotion of circulation to the nerve during the period of the distraction.

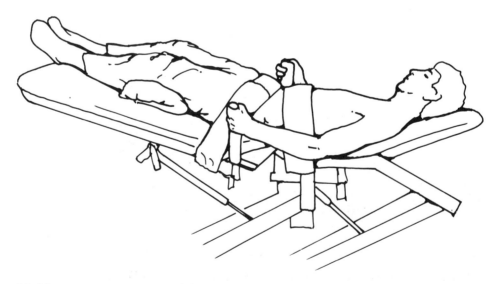

Fig. 12-18 Autotraction in positional distraction. *Patient*: Positioned and set up as in Fig. 12-18, the patient now grasps the horns on the table and imparts a steady or intermittent traction under his control. *Therapist*: May leave the patient once the session is under way. *Use*: Positional distraction with the intermittent component added by the patient addresses the need for patient involvement and may assist in gating any discomfort.

Postoperative Discs

Laminectomy and Fusion

Surgery to the spine is increasingly being recognized as a special skill not attainable by the general orthopaedic or neurosurgeon. Each surgery is carefully planned and executed according to the surgeon's perception of what is causing the symptoms and with a variety of techniques now available. After the surgery, each surgeon will be even more familiar with the condition and what was achieved at surgery. It is therefore very unlikely that the surgeon would refer the patient to a therapist without first giving a clear prescription as to treatment. Fear on the surgeon's part that therapy may harm the patient, or is an uncontrollable factor that could influence the outcome, is often sufficient reason for the surgeon not to make the referral.

Therefore, a prescription from the surgeon is warranted and indeed should be encouraged. The therapist is now a technician, albeit a skilled technician. Given the acknowledged poor results of low back surgery, the therapist would not want to be placed in a position in which he or she could be made to take the blame for an unfortunate outcome.

Treatment Principles

Minimize postoperative discomfort with TENS, acupressure

Maintain basic function with breathing exercises, lower limb passive movements

Ambulate when requested. Pool therapy may be hazardous if the pool is not properly designed and the therapy is not adequately supervised.

Before discharge, instruction in activities of daily living (ADL) back school (entire program)

Also instruction in activities of nightly living. Sexual intercourse positions that are not deemed harmful must be reviewed with the patient. This is particularly true for postfusion cases in which strips of bone are lying free over raw exposed bone and can easily invade the spinal canal through the laminal interspace should the patient (usually male) flex and extend the lumbar spine during sexual intercourse. For the

male or female patient, one safe position is to lie on the back with a pillow under the knees. The knees must not be flexed to the chest. Another safe position is side lying either facing the partner or with the back turned, but the patient must remain still and not thrust with the pelvis.

Having too often seen failed low back surgery, I believe that a major cause of this is due to inadequate instruction in ADL and, in particular, activities of nightly living. If the therapist cannot for reasons of sex, age, or sensitivity to the patient give advice on sex positions, then the therapist must request that a colleague, perhaps of the same sex as the patient, under the guise of being expert in spinal mechanics, give advice on these and related matters.

Chemonucleosis

In chemonucleosis, a proteolytic enzyme temporarily reduces the ability of the nucleus to imbibe fluid. Thus, the pressure on a weakened anulus is lowered and the bulge is reduced. Since the disc will have in effect shrunk in height there may be complications to the nerve roots exiting the foramen and thus the patient may now require a laminectomy plus a foraminectomy and fusion.

After the chemonucleosis, the disc, having lost its normal hydrostatic mechanism, will tend to be unstable and a spontaneous lateral shift at that level with secondary intradiscal fluid imbalance at other levels may ensue.

Treatment

Instruction in ADL and back school. Instruction in activities of nightly living not necessary

Encouragement to maintain the lordosis whenever seated by using such assists as a rolled-up towel, cusion, or commercially available back support

In those with a history of instability, tape may be used to encourage the lordosis, at least postoperatively

Medial Branch Rhizolysis (Facet Denervation)

Facet denervation is the procedure used by surgeons to alleviate pain arising from the lumbar facet joints. By destroying the principal nerve to the facet, facet pain is effectively blocked. Unfortunately, it is a nonspecific technique since the procedure also destroys innervation to all the posterior structures including ligaments to both the lumbar spine and sacroiliac and of course to the stabilizing muscles of the low back—the multifidus.

Treatment

Retain lordosis when seated
Avoid forward bending and rotational activities
Stabilization program as needed

THORACOLUMBAR SYNDROME

The essential pathology of thoracolumbar syndrome is hypermobility that produces midlumbar back pain and posterior lateral pain over the iliac crest and into the area of the lateral hip joint. It commonly follows spine fusion of one of the lower lumbar levels that produces the need for movement compensation at higher levels. This condition is not uncommon in women who wear fashion corsets that restrict lumbar movements and tend to produce hypermobility just above the upper margin of the corset.

Causes

A stiff low back, postfusion, myofascial restrictions, or the wearing of a corset

Symptoms

Lateral low back pain and pain over the iliac crest into buttocks
"Giving away" of the leg, resulting in a fall

Signs

Mid- or upper lumbar pain
Tenderness to palpation at the thoracolumbar junction
Tenderness to skin rolling over the iliac crest where the T12 and L1 cutaneous nerves cross it just lateral to the quadratus lumborum

Treatment

Correct all stiffness in the lower back, hips, and myofascia

Stabilize the thoracolumbar junction by exercising the multifidus in a manner that increases its agility

Management

The best management is a long-term perseverance with exercises. To prevent giving away of the leg at critical times, such as when crossing the street, walk with the leg internally rotated.

KISSING VERTEBRAE

"Kissing vertebrae" were first described by Baastrap in 1924. This syndrome occurs particularly in middle-aged portly men who are short and stocky. The condition occurs when the intervertebral discs narrow with age, thus bringing together the rather large spinous processes. These processes then impinge and set up a bursitis condition between them, hence the name kissing vertebrae.

Causes

Obesity, disc degeneration on short stocky males

Symptoms

A dull, then sharp midline low back pain that spreads to the surrounding muscles
Eased by forward bending and worsened by backward bending

Treatment

Weight loss, stretching tight myofascia, negative heels to lessen the lordosis, strengthen abdominals, stretch hip flexors, add pelvic tilt
Physician may inject into the interspinous area to deaden the painful bursa

STENOSIS

Stenosis is a narrowing of the spinal canal or intervertebral foramen or both resulting in compromise of neurological elements. This condition occurs in the population 55 years of age and older and is associated with ill health, obesity, diabetes, poor posture, and other negative life-style attitudes.

Causes

Poor posture, obesity, degenerative disc disease

Symptoms

Transient pain and neurogenic effort claudication that, unlike vascular intermittent claudication, is not immediately relieved by rest

Bizarre descriptions of pain, such as spiders crawling over the legs

Pain relieved by forward bending, which can be explained by a lengthening of the spinal canal and the opening of the intervertebral foramen

Signs

Poor health
Permanent lordosis and obesity
Myofascial restrictions in the lumbar spine
Hip contractures, poor posture

Treatment

Correct the posture and anything else that can be done improve function. Usually includes such findings as tight hip flexors and fascia lata and tight lumbar myofascia (see Fig. 9-12).

Prognosis

The prognosis is not good owing to the above health and life-style attitudes. If these can be changed, then the results may be promising. Surgery offers the best hope of relief by cleaning out the canals and fusing the spine.

13 Pelvic Girdle

Richard Nyberg

There is considerable controversy regarding the mechanical behavior of the sacroiliac joint. Much remains unknown about sacroiliac structure and function. As a result, the extent to which motion impairment or mechanical disturbance of the pelvic joints is responsible for symptoms is unclear. Unfortunately for orthopaedic physical therapy clinicians, no definite diagnostic means have been identified to incriminate symptoms as arising from the sacroiliac joints. The interpretation of symptoms and clinical signs often varies, resulting in many opinions about the exact nature of mechanical disturbance within the pelvis.

Understanding the full nature of sacroiliac disturbance, however, requires understanding the interdependent concept of the pelvic girdle system. The hips, sacroiliac, and lower lumbar spine are virtually inseparable components of the pelvis. Involvement of any one structure will directly affect the positioning and movement of the others. The sacrum, for example, is mechanically associated with the spine, whereas the ilium is aligned with and affected by the lower extremities.

The objectives of this chapter include:

Identification of the major pelvic dysfunctions—
    pubic, sacral, and ilial
A brief description of the possible causes of
    pelvic dysfunction
Listing the primary symptoms
Highlighting significant clinical signs
Identification of an appropriate manipulation
    technique for correction
A general plan of therapeutic strategies for
    overall management

Before each dysfunction is discussed individually,

a few points need clarification. First, mechanical problems of the sacroiliac will be named according to the positional fault that exists and not by the motion that is impaired. Second, joint disorders of the pelvic girdle often involve more than one type of lesion or motion problem. For instructional purposes, the pelvic dysfunctions are listed singularly; however, the clinical reality is such that the dsyfunctions usually exist in combination. Third, only mechanical conditions of the pelvic girdle are considered. Medical problems affecting the pelvis such as pelvic inflammatory disease, arthritic conditions, and pelvic fractures require medical intervention and therefore are not covered. Fourth, the relationship between cranial and upper cervical structures and the sacrum through membranous connections is accepted as a factor in pathomechanical conditions of the pelvis. Owing to segmentation of topic areas within this book, however, craniosacral relationships are not included. Fifth, the manipulation technique illustrated for each dysfunction is one of many techniques that may be used for mechanical correction. The selection of technique is determined by the nature, extent, and stage of the condition, the clinical signs identified, and the personality of the patient. Technique criteria are also based on safety, simplicity in performance, and effectiveness.

PUBIC DYSFUNCTIONS

Pubic Separation

Causes
Abnormal labor and delivery
Weak abdominals, weak hip abductors
Hip hyperabduction or external rotation

Symptoms
Symphyseal, medial hip and thigh pain
Pain with walking and stair climbing
Prolonged standing

Signs
Presence of a symphyseal sulcus (increased width)
Symphyseal tenderness to palpation
Pubic joint hypermobility
Rectus abdominus diaphysis

Manipulation Technique
Pubic compression (Fig. 13-1)
Therapist approximates ASISs

Management
Increase non-weight-bearing rest time
Avoid extreme hip abduction or external rotation
Functional integration and strengthening of the abdominals

Positions
Use pelvic binder or corset to stabilize
Strengthen hip abductors

Symphysis Compression

Causes
Spasm or tight pelvic diaphragm musculature
Hip hyperadduction or internal rotation stress
Trauma to lateral aspect of ASIS

Symptoms
Symphyseal, medial hip and thigh pain
Pain with walking and stair climbing
No pain with standing

Signs
Decreased width of symphyseal sulcus
Symphyseal tenderness to palpation
Pubic joint motion restriction

Technique
Pubic decompression (Fig. 13-2)
Therapist separates ASISs

Management
Soft tissue inhibition-stretch to pelvic diaphragm
Movement within pain tolerance is encouraged to promote pubic motion

Superior, Posterior Pubic Dysfunction

Causes
Abnormal upward force through an extended leg
Fall on an ischial tuberosity
Hip hyperflexion
Sex, pregnancy, delivery
Weak hip abductors—middle and anterior fibers especially

Symptoms
Symphyseal, medial hip and thigh pain
Pain with walking and stair climbing
Standing on the involved side

Signs
Pubic tubercle is superior and pubic bone is posterior
Tenderness over pubic tubercle
Pubic joint motion restriction or instability

Technique
Inferior and anterior pubis glide (Fig. 13-3)
Therapist mobilizes pubis inferiorly and anteriorly

Management
Rest from function if unstable
Use pelvic binder or corset to stabilize if necessary
Promote hip extension or lumbar extension when tolerated
Functional integration and strengthening of gluteus medius

Inferior, Anterior Pubic Dysfunction

Causes
Upward lift of the body with a foot fixed
Tight hip adductors
Hip hyperextension
Sex, pregnancy, delivery

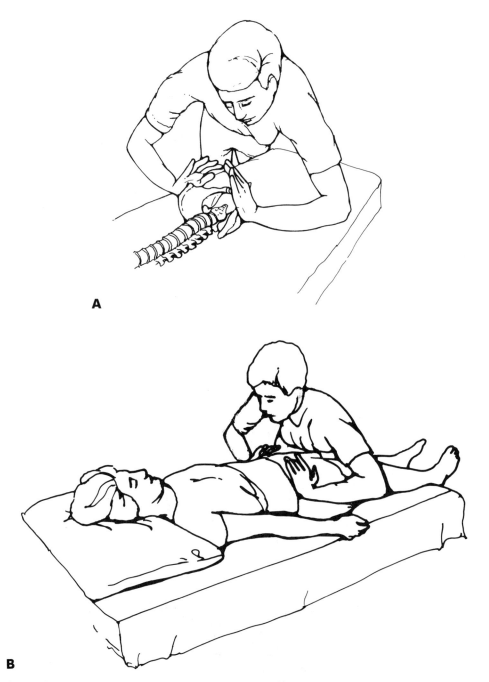

A

B

Fig. 13-1 Pubic Compression. *Patient:* Supine, legs internally rotated. *Therapist:* On one side at pelvis level facing patient. *Hand Placement:* Both hands contact the lateral aspect of the ASISs. *Force Direction:* To ASISs to approximate.

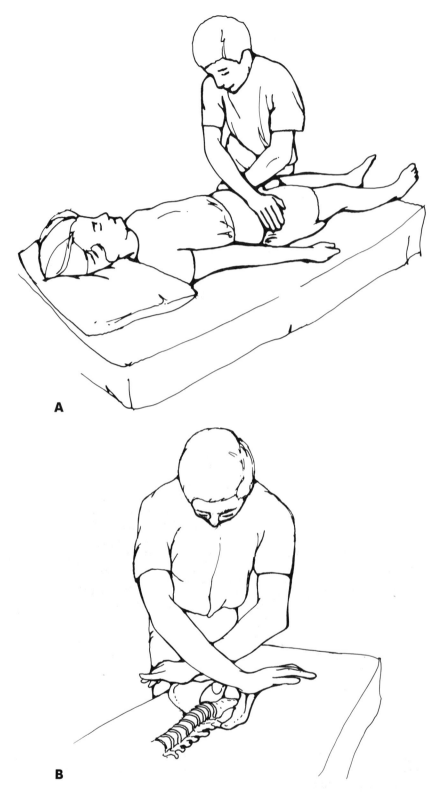

Fig. 13-2 Pubic decompression. *Patient:* Supine, with legs externally rotated. *Therapist:* On one side at pelvis facing the patient. *Hand Placement:* Arms cross so that hands can contact medial aspects of the ASISs. *Force Direction:* lateral force to ASISs to decompress.

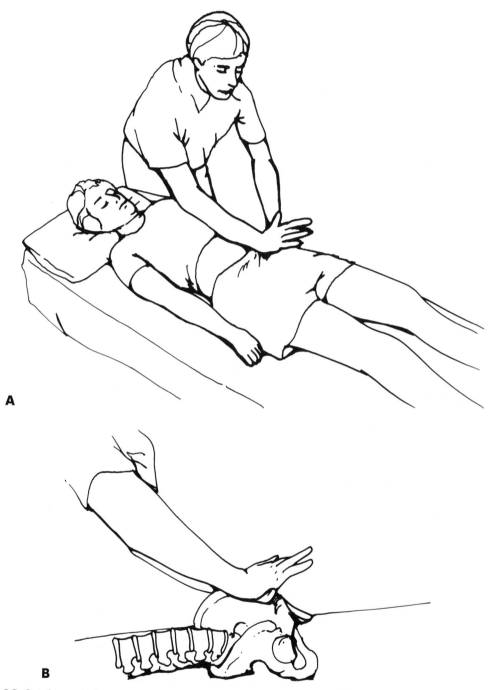

Fig. 13-3 Inferior and anterior pubis glide (left side). *Patient:* Supine. *Therapist:* On involved side at head end. *Hand Placement:* Left thumb contacts superior aspect of the left superior pubic rami and the base of the right hand contacts on top of the left thumb. *Force Direction:* Right arm applies inferior and anterior force into the left thumb to move pubis down and forward.

Symptoms
Symphyseal, medial hip and thigh pain
Pain with walking and stair climbing
Pain with hip flexion

Signs
Pubic tubercle is inferior and pubic bone is
    anterior
Tenderness over pubic tubercle
Pubic joint motion restriction
Hip adductor tendon sensitivity

Technique
Superior, posterior pubis glide (Fig. 13-4)
Therapist mobilizes pubis superiorly and
    posteriorly

Management
Promote hip flexion or lumbar flexion when
    tolerated
Soft tissue inhibition and stretch to hip
    adductors
Functional integration and strengthening of hip
    extensors and middle and posterior fibers of
    gluteus medius

SACRAL DYSFUNCTIONS

Sacral Flexion

Causes
Increased lumbosacral angle owing to structure,
    overweight, poor abdominal tone, pregnancy
Posterior sacroiliac joint ligamentous weakness
Lumbar spine hyperextension
Abnormal labor and delivery
Weak gluteus medius and maximus

Symptoms
Diffuse lumbosacral pain
Gluteal pain, occasionally sciatic pain
Pain with walking and stair climbing (especially
    down the stairs or an incline)
Pain with prolonged standing

Signs
Deep (anterior) sacral sulci and shallow
    (posterior) inferior lateral angles
Tenderness over posterior sacroilial joint
    ligaments, at Baer's point, and at the
    inferior lateral angles

Increased piriformis and psoas tone
Sacral flexion hypermobility or sacral extension
    restriction
Frequently posterior sacral swelling

Technique
Sacral extension (Fig. 13-5)
Therapist applies posterior anterior (PA) force to
    sacral apex

Management
Increase non-weight-bearing rest time
Avoid lumbar extension, promote lumbar flexion
    when tolerated
Use pelvic binder or corset to stabilize if
    necessary
Soft tissue inhibition and stretch to the
    piriformis and psoas
Functional integration and strengthening of
    gluteus medius and maximus as well as the
    abdominals

Sacral Extension

Causes
Reduced lumbosacral angle owing to structure
Flexed sitting or standing postures
Lumbar spine hyperflexion
Squatting, bending, and lifting
Coccygeal muscle spasm

Symptoms
Diffuse lumbosacral pain
Occasionally gluteal pain
Pain with walking and stair climbing (especially
    down stairs or inclines)
Pain when moving from sitting to standing

Signs
Shallow (posterior) sacral sulci and deep
    (anterior) inferior lateral angles
Less prominent PSIS
Spasm or tight pelvic diaphragm musculature
Sacral flexion restriction
L5-S1 and possibly generalized restriction in
    lumbar extension

Technique
Sacral flexion (Fig. 13-6)
Therapist applies anterior and inferior force to
    sacral base

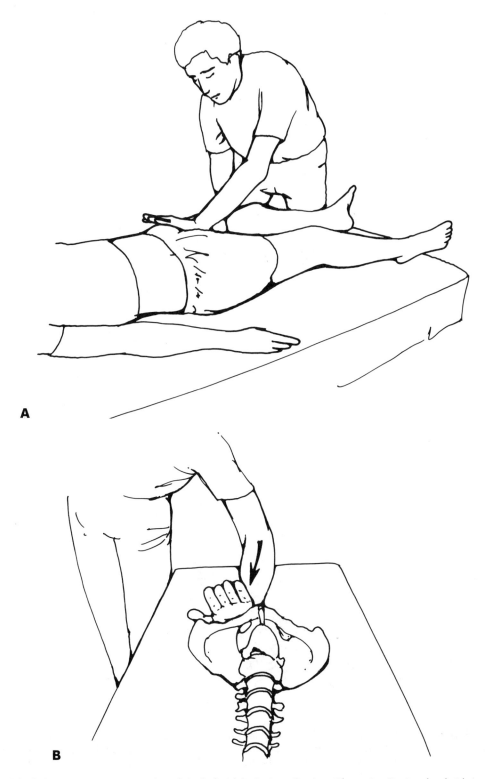

Fig. 13-4 Superior, posterior pubis glide (left side). *Patient:* Supine. *Therapist:* On involved side facing the subject at pelvic level. *Hand Placement:* Ulnar aspect of the left hand contacts the anterior aspect of the pubic body. *Force Direction:* Superior and slightly posteriorly directed force onto the left pubic body.

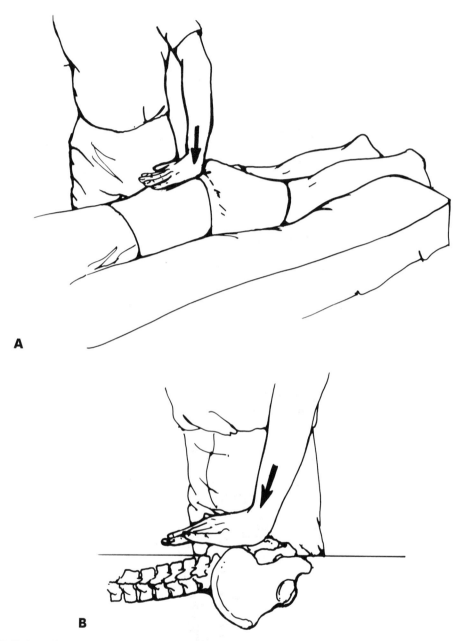

Fig. 13-5 Sacral extension. *Patient:* Prone with legs internally rotated. *Therapist:* Standing to one side of the pelvis facing the head end. *Hand Placement:* Thenar or ulnar contact on the sacral apex. *Force Direction:* Posterior/anterior force applied on the apex of the sacrum when the sacrum is felt to extend.

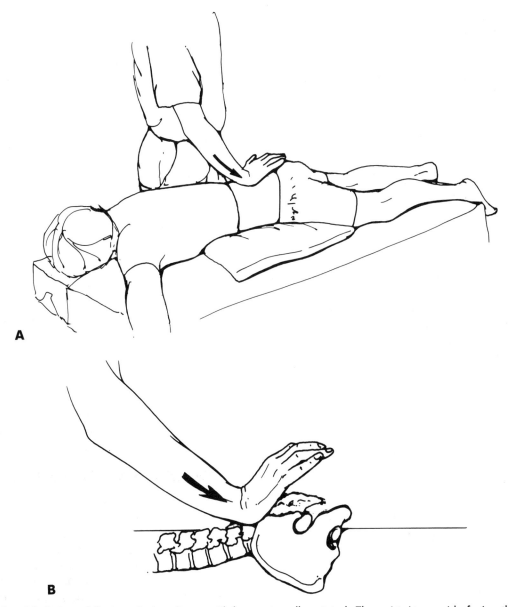

Fig. 13-6 Sacral flexion. *Patient:* Prone with legs externally rotated. *Therapist:* At one side facing the feet end. *Hand Placement:* Base of hand contacts the sacral base with the arm directed at a right angle to the base. *Force Direction:* Anterior and inferior force applied to the sacral base when the sacrum is felt to flex.

Management

Soft tissue inhibition and stretch to pelvic
   diaphragm musculature
Postural re-education to avoid flexed sitting and
   standing positions
Promote lumbar extension movements when
   tolerated

Left-on-Left Sacral Torsion Dysfunction

Four types of sacral torsion lesions exist: (1) left-
on-left sacral torsion, (2) left-on-right sacral torsion, (3) right-on-right sacral torsion, and (4) right-
on-left sacral torsion. By definition, a sacral torsion
occurs as a result of sacral rotation and tilt (side
bending) to the same side. A left-on-left sacral
torsion signifies flexion movement at the right
sacral base (movement on the left oblique axis)
and inferior movement of the left side of the
sacrum. As a result, the sacrum is positioned in
left rotation and left side bending. The causes,
symptoms, signs, and management of each type
of sacral torsion problem will vary somewhat;
however, the concepts in evaluation and treatment
of one type will carry over to the other types.
Therefore, only the most common sacral torsion
dysfunction, the left-on-left sacral condition, is
presented.

Causes

Spinal left rotation force(s)
A short left leg
Right-sided posterior sacroiliac ligamentous
   weakness
Left hip hyperflexion and/or right hip
   hyperextension
Tight left piriformis, weak gluteus medius
   (especially on the right)

Symptoms

Unilateral lumbosacral, gluteal pain
Occasionally sciatic pain
Pain with walking and stair climbing
Pain with prolonged standing, particularly if
   instability exists

Signs

Deep (anterior) right sacral sulcus and an
   inferior left inferior lateral angle

Tenderness over the posterior sacroilial joint
   ligaments, especially on the right, and at the
   inferior lateral angles
Left side bending and rotation of lower lumbar
   spine
Increased left and possibly right piriformis tone
Increased right psoas tone
Sacral extension restriction on the right and/or
   sacral flexion restriction on the left,
   restriction in sacral right side bending, right-
   sided sacral hypermobility

Techniques

Sacral right side bending (Fig. 13-7)
Therapist contacts left inferior lateral angle and
   glides left side of sacrum superior
Sacral right rotation (Fig. 13-8)
Therapist applies PA force to left side of sacral
   apex

Management

Increase non-weight-bearing rest time if unstable
Use pelvic binder or corset if necessary
Consider heel lift or arch correction on short leg
Soft tissue inhibition and stretch to piriformis or
   psoas
Functional integration and strengthening of
   gluteus medius and maximus as well as
   abdominals
Postural re-education to reduce left spinal
   rotation stresses, right hip hyperextension,
   and left hip hyperflexion

Left Unilateral Sacral Flexion Dysfunction

Four types of unilateral sacral problems occur: (1)
left unilateral sacral flexion; (2) left unilateral
sacral extension; (3) right unilateral sacral flexion;
(4) right unilateral sacral extension. A unilateral
sacral lesion exists when the sacrum rotates in one
direction and side bends in the opposite direction.
A left unilateral sacral flexion results when the left
side of the sacral base flexes (movement on the
right oblique axis) and the left side of the sacrum
moves inferiorly. The sacrum is therefore positioned in right rotation and left side bending. The
left unilateral sacral flexion dysfunction is the most
common unilateral condition and will be used as
an example for the unilateral problems.

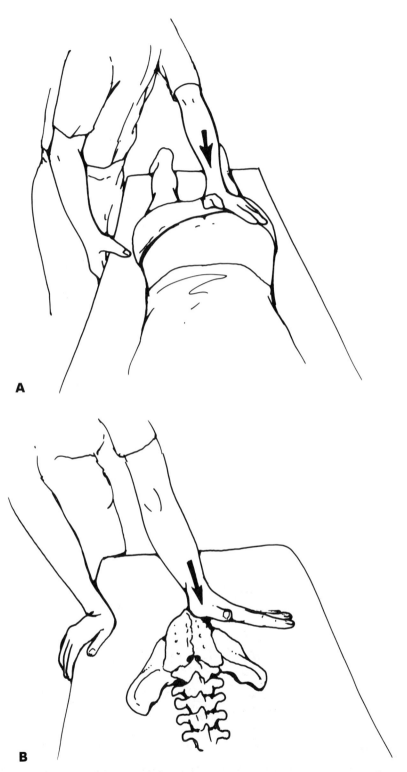

Fig. 13-7 Sacral right side bending. *Patient:* Prone. *Therapist:* On the right side of the patient at the feet end. *Hand Placement:* The thenar aspect of the left hand contacts the inferior aspect of the left inferior lateral angle. *Force Direction:* Superior, lateral force is applied to inferior aspect of left inferior lateral angle when the sacrum is felt to move superiorly on the left side.

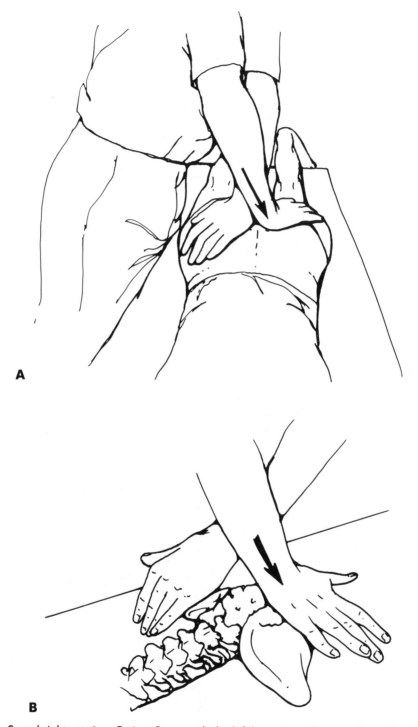

A

B

Fig. 13-8 Sacral right rotation. *Patient:* Prone with the left leg externally rotated and the right leg internally rotated (toes pointed left). *Therapist:* On the right side of the patient with the ulnar aspect of the right hand on the posterior aspect of the left inferior lateral angle. The left hand contacts over the PSIS of the right ilium. *Force Direction:* The right hand applies posterior/anterior force to the posterior aspect of the left inferior lateral angle, and the left hand applies anterior/lateral force to the right ilium for stabilization.

Causes

Spinal right rotation force(s)

A short left leg

Left-sided posterior sacro-iliac ligamentous weakness

Spasm or tight left piriformis

Weakness of the left gluteus medius

Left hip hyperextension and/or right hip hyperflexion

Symptoms

Unilateral lumbosacral, gluteal pain

Frequently sciatic pain on the left side

Pain with walking and stair climbing

Pain with prolonged standing, especially with weight bearing on the left side

Significant Clinical Signs

A deep (anterior) left sacral sulcus and an inferior left lateral angle

Tenderness over the left posterior sacroiliac ligaments and inferior lateral angles

Left side bending and right rotation of lower lumbar spine

Increased left piriformis and psoas tone

Left-sided sacral hypermobility

Right-sided sacral flexion restriction and/or left-sided sacral extension restriction

Restriction in sacral right side bending

Techniques

Sacral right side bending (Fig. 13-9)

Alternative technique: therapist contacts right sacral side and mobilizes inferiorly and medially

Sacral left rotation: therapist applies PA force to right side of sacral base (Fig. 13-10)

Management

Same as for sacral torsion except for postural re-education advice that suggests avoidance of

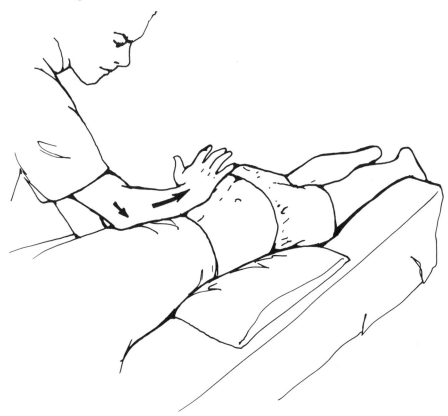

Fig. 13-9 Sacral right side bending. *Patient:* Prone. *Therapist:* On right side of patient facing feet. *Hand Placement:* The ulnar aspect of the right hand contacts the posterior aspect of the right side of the sacrum with the fingers pointed toward the feet. *Force Direction:* Inferior, slightly medial force is applied onto the right side of the sacrum by taking up tissue tension on the posterior aspect.

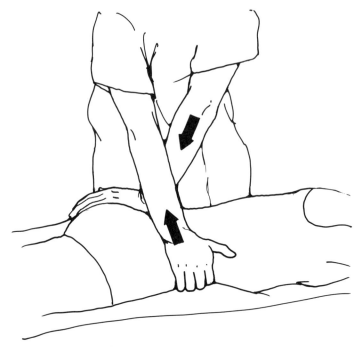

Fig. 13-10 Sacral left rotation. *Patient:* Prone with the left leg in internal rotation and the right leg in external rotation. *Therapist:* On the left side of patient facing the pelvis. *Hand Placement:* The right hand holds onto the ASIS. The ulnar aspect of the left hand contacts the posterior aspect of the left sacral base. *Force Direction:* The right hand applies posterior and slightly medial force through the ASIS for stabilization. The ulnar aspect of the left hand applies posterior/anterior force onto the posterior aspect of the right sacral base.

right spinal rotation stresses, left hip hyperextension, and right hip hyperflexion

ILIAC DYSFUNCTIONS

Left Posterior Iliac Rotation

Causes
Repeated or prolonged left lower extremity weight bearing
Direct fall onto the left ischial tuberosity
Left hamstring tightness
Left posterior sacroiliac ligamentous weakness
Left gluteus medius weakness
Left hip hyperflexion
A short left leg

Symptoms
Unilateral lumbosacral pain on the left side
Left-sided gluteal pain, occasionally sciatic pain
Pain with walking and stair climbing, especially up stairs or up inclines
Pain with flexed sitting

Signs
Left PSIS is inferior and posterior, left ASIS is superior and anterior
Left ischial tuberosity is anterior
Tenderness over the left posterior sacroiliac ligaments and medial aspect of left ilium (iliolumbar ligaments)
Tenderness over left ischial tuberosity and left inferior lateral angle (sacrotuberous and sacrospinous ligaments)
Increase in left piriformis tone
An apparent short left leg in supine position
Left iliac hypermobility or restriction in left iliac anterior rotation

Technique
Anterior ilia rotation (Fig. 13-11)

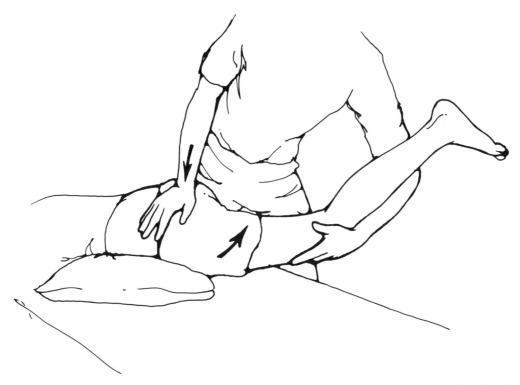

Fig. 13-11 Anterior iliac rotation—left side. *Patient:* Prone with the right leg flexed over the side of the table and the foot on floor to flatten the lumbar curve. *Therapist:* Stand at the right side of the patient at pelvic level. *Hand Placement:* The right hand is placed over the left PSIS. The left arm cradles the left leg with the hand positioned on the anterior aspect of the thigh. *Force Direction:* The left arm extends and adducts the left leg until movement is felt at the PSIS. The right arm applies anterior and lateral force to the left ilium through the PSIS while the left arm continues to extend and adduct.

Therapist extends-adducts left hip while pressing left ilium anteriorly

Management
Increase non-weight-bearing rest time if unstable
Use pelvic binder or corset for stability if necessary
Soft tissue inhibition and stretching to the left hamstring and piriformis
Promote left hip extension when tolerated
Functional integration and strengthening of left gluteus medius

Right Iliac Anterior Rotation

Causes
Right hip hyperextension
Right hip flexor tightness

Golfing
Weak abdominals and right gluteus maximus and medius

Symptoms
Right-sided lumbosacral pain, gluteal pain
Occasionally right anterior hip pain
Pain with walking and stair climbing
Occasional pain relief with walking

Signs
Right PSIS is superior and anterior, right ASIS is inferior and posterior
Right ischial tuberosity is posterior
Tenderness on the right PSIS (sacrotuberous ligament) and inferior lateral angle
Apparent long right leg in supine position

Right iliac posterior rotation restriction
Positive right Baer's point (psoas involvement)

Techniques
Posterior iliac rotation (Fig. 13-12)
Therapist contacts ASIS and ischial tuberosity
and rotates ilium posteriorly

Management
Soft tissue inhibition and stretch to right psoas
Exercise to promote right hip flexion, abduction,
and external rotation
Functional integration and strengthening of
right gluteus maximus and medius
(particularly the middle and posterior fibers)
Strengthen abdominals

Right Iliac Outflare (External Rotation)
Causes
Right hip internal rotation and/or adduction
restriction(s)
Tight hip abductors or external rotators on the
right
Fall on the lateral aspect of the right PSIS

Symptoms
Right-sided lumbosacral, gluteal pain
Pain with right hip adduction and/or internal
rotation

Signs
Right PSIS is medial and right ASIS is lateral in
relation to the midsagittal line
Right hip rotation restriction, usually internal
rotation
Tenderness over right pubic tubercle
Increased right piriformis tone
Right ilial inflare (internal rotation) restriction

Techniques
Right ilial inflare (internal rotation) (Fig. 13-13)
Therapist stabilizes sacrum on left side and
internally rotates right hip

Management
Soft tissue inhibition and stretch to the right
piriformis
Exercise to promote right hip internal rotation
and/or adduction when tolerated

Soft tissue inhibition and stretch to right hip
abductors and external rotators

Left Iliac Inflare
Causes
Left hip restriction
Left posterior sacroiliac ligamentous weakness
Fall onto the lateral aspect of the ASIS

Symptoms
Left-sided lumbosacral, gluteal pain
Pain with prolonged left leg standing
Pain with walking and stair climbing
Pain when sitting with legs crossed left over right

Signs
Left PSIS is lateral and right ASIS is medial in
relation to the midsaggittal line
Left hip restriction
Tenderness over the left posterior sacroiliac
ligaments
Increase in left piriformis tone
Weak left gluteus medius
Left iliac hypermobility

Techniques
Left iliac outflare (external rotation) (Fig. 13-14)
Therapist pulls ASIS laterally and moves PSIS
medially

Management
Soft tissue inhibition to the left piriformis
Exercise to promote left hip range of motion
when tolerated
Use pelvic binder or corset to stabilize if
necessary
Functional integration and strengthening of the
left gluteus medius
Postural re-education to reduce left hip internal
rotation stress loads on left sacroiliac

Right Iliac Upslip
Causes
Jumping or falling suddenly on an extended leg
Quadratus lumborum muscle spasm
Tight right hip adductors

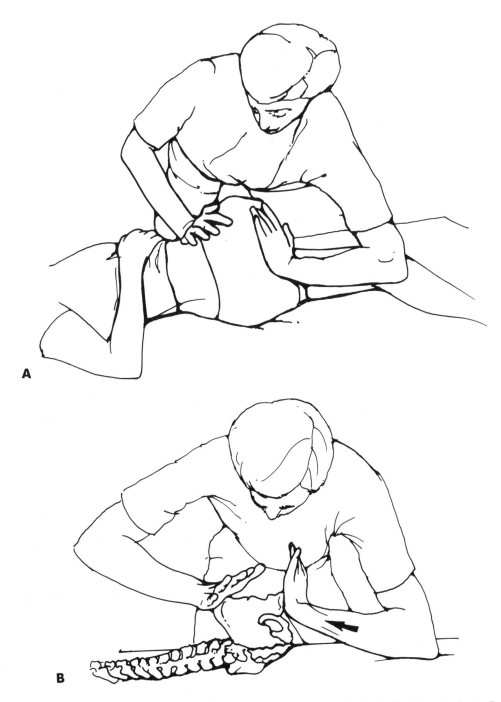

Fig. 13-12 Posterior iliac rotation—right side. *Patient:* Sidelying on the left side. The right leg is flexed until movement is felt at the PSIS. The left leg is kept extended. The upper body is rotated right to lock the entire spine. *Therapist:* Facing patient at pelvic level. *Hand Placement:* The left hand contacts the ischial tuberosity. The right hand contacts the ASIS. *Force Direction:* Turn the ilium counterclockwise by applying pressures through the ASIS and ischial tuberosity.

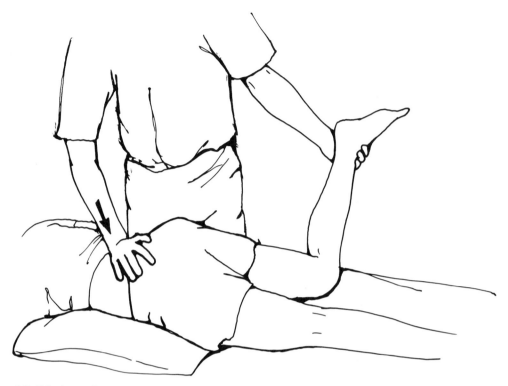

Fig. 13-13 Iliac inflare or internal rotation—right side. *Patient:* Prone. *Therapist:* To the right side of the patient at pelvic level. *Hand Placement:* The right hand applies P/A pressure to left side of the sacral base. The left hand contacts right ankle with knee flexed and internally rotates the right hip to inflare or internally rotate the right ilium.

Symptoms
Localized right sacroiliac pain
Pain during midstance of gait
Pain with right leg standing

Signs
Right ASIS, PSIS, iliac crest, pubic tubercle, and ischial tuberosity are superior
Tenderness over the right quadratus lumborum
Pain with hip compression, pain relief with hip decompression
Restriction in inferior glide of right ilium

Techniques
Inferior iliac glide (Fig. 13-15)
Therapist contacts over iliac crest and glides ilium inferiorly

Management
Soft tissue inhibitions and stretch to right quadratus lumborum
Advice to shift weight to left leg when standing
Stretch right hip adductors

Left Iliac Downslip

Causes
Short left leg
Left posterior sacroiliac ligamentous weakness
Left iliolumbar ligamentous weakness
Tight left iliotibial band
Weak gluteus medius

Symptoms
Left lumbosacral, gluteal pain
Occasionally sciatic pain

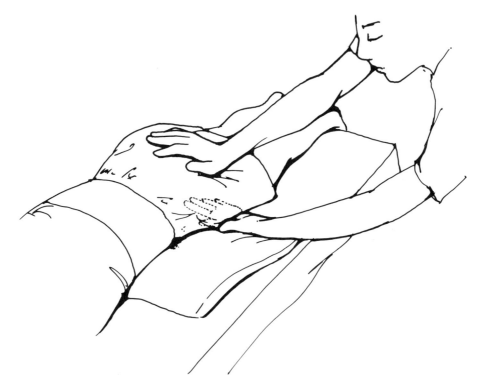

Fig. 13-14 Iliac outflare or external rotation—left side. *Patient:* Prone with the left leg externally rotated. *Therapist:* To the left side of the patient. *Hand Placement:* Fingers of the left hand contact medial to the left ASIS. Base of the right hand contacts lateral to the PSIS. *Force Direction:* The left hand pulls the ASIS laterally and inferiorly. The right hand applies medial and superior force to the PSIS.

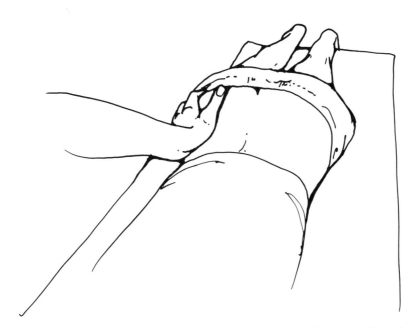

Fig. 13-15 Inferior iliac glide—right side. *Patient:* Prone. *Therapist:* To the right side of the patient at the head end. *Hand Placement:* The left hand contacts the superior aspect of the right iliac crest. *Force Direction:* The left hand applies an inferior and slightly medial force.

Pain with standing, walking, and stair climbing, especially when bearing weight on the left leg

Signs
Left PSIS, ASIS, iliac crest, pubic tubercle, and ischial tuberosity are inferior
Tenderness over left posterior sacroiliac and iliolumbar ligaments
Pain with hip distraction, pain relief with hip compression
Restriction in left hip adduction
Restriction in superior glide of left ilium
Left iliac hypermobility

Techniques
Superior iliac glide (Fig. 13-16)
Therapist contacts ischial tuberosity and mobilizes superiorly

Management
Increase non-weight-bearing rest time if unstable
Use pelvic binder or corset to stabilize if necessary
Stretch iliotibial band on left side
Functional integration and strengthening of left gluteus medius
Correct short leg with lifts
Postural advice to shift weight to right leg when standing

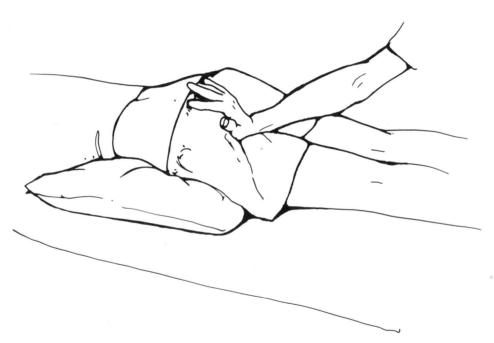

Fig. 13-16 Superior iliac glide—left side. *Patient:* Prone. *Therapist:* To patient's left side at the feet end. *Hand Placement:* Hypothenar aspect of the right hand contacts the inferior aspect of the left ischial tuberosity. *Force Direction:* The right hand applies a superior and slightly lateral force onto the ischial tuberosity.

14 Thoracic Spine

Pamela May

THORACIC OUTLET SYNDROME

A thoracic outlet syndrome results when portions of the neurovascular complex are compressed in any one of the three anatomical triangles in this region.

Causes

Functional

Hypertrophy or adaptive shortening of the scalenus anticus or medius muscles
Elevation or hypomobility of the first rib
Adaptive shortening of the pectoralis minor muscle

Congenital

Broad insertion or two-banded insertion of scalenus anticus or scalenus medius muscle
Fibrous slip running from anterior scalene to midscalene muscle
Bony exostosis of the first rib, clavicle, or transverse process of the seventh cervical vertebra
Presence of a cervical rib or fibrous band from C7

Symptoms

Arterial

Pallor, coldness, intermittent claudication
Deep ill-defined aching
Raynaud's phenomenon

Venous

Intermittent edema, venous engorgement, cyanosis

Neurological

Tingling, intermittent numbing pain in C8 and T1 distribution.
Complaints of clumsiness.
Scapular pain if dorso-scapular nerve is involved.

Signs

Forward head and rounded shoulders, protracted scapula
Elevated and or hypomobile first rib
Restricted mobility, of the upper thoracic acromioclavicular and sternoclavicular joints
Restricted myofascia in the pectoralis minor and major, scalenus anticus and medius, upper trapezius, levator scapulae, and sternoclavicular muscles
Upper respiratory breathing

Treatment

Manipulation of restricted joints including the first rib
Myofascial manipulation for tight muscles
Postural re-education with attention to head and scapular position
Instruction in diaphragmatic breathing
Home program of self-stretching and mobilizing

Techniques

Treatment for First Rib Restriction

Patient is seated with therapist standing behind (Fig. 14-1A). Place scalene muscles on slack by side bending head to side of restriction. Contact first rib posteriorly and laterally to transverse process of the T_1 vertebra with metacarpophalangeal joint

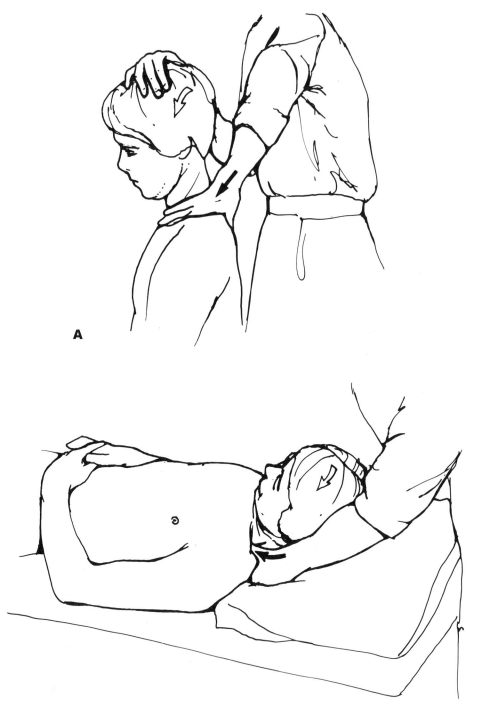

A

B

Fig. 14-1 Thoracic outlet syndrome. **(A)** Technique for first rib restriction. **(B)** Technique for elevation and inhalation restriction.

of index finger. Apply manipulation pressure in an inferior, medial, and anterior direction. Time manipulation with exhalation. Follow with a stretch to the scalene muscles.

Levels
First rib only.

Treatment for Elevation and Inhalation Restriction of the Left First Rib

Patient is supine with physical therapist at patient's head (Fig. 14-1B). Therapist places thumb on superior aspect of left first rib just posterior to clavicle. Apply inferior distraction pressure during exhalation. Repeat two to three times, taking up slack with each exhalation. Follow with scalene stretch.

Levels
Could be modified for second rib by contacting second rib just lateral to its articulation with the sternum.

FACET JOINT RESTRICTIONS

Mechanical dysfunction of the thoracic spine can be quite painful. However, it responds rapidly to treatment.

Facet Hypomobility—Thoracic Spine

Causes
As for lumbar and cervical spine

Symptoms
Pain with movement and breathing, often causing a sharp catch that stops the inhalation

Sensation of tightness in the involved region

Pain is usually well-localized posteriorly although anterior pain may be present and radicular pain may follow along the intercostal space

Discomfort in the region of the lesion, usually owing to muscle involvement secondary to the facet condition

Pain usually worse in the morning and alleviated by movement

Signs
Change in the normal kyphosis (either a flattening or an increase)

Presence of a forward head posture

Restricted segmental motion to passive motion testing

Percussion on vertebra in slight forward bending may elicit the discomfort

Tenderness on palpation in the posterior ligaments

Positional faults

A decreased space between two spinous processes usually occurs in conjunction with an increased space either above or below. If the increased space is above, then the vertebra involved is described to be in backward bending, whereas if it is below, the vertebra involved is described as being in forward bending. Since apparent positional faults are common, there must be a loss of movement for this positional fault to be in fact legitimate. Evidence of a facilitated segment includes reflex muscle response to palpation or springing of the vertebra and tenderness in posterior spinal ligaments.

Passive Motion Testing in the Thoracic Spine

There are numerous techniques performed either in sitting or prone lying.

Treatment
Manipulation of restricted segments either by direct contact on spinous or transverse processes or by isometric muscle contraction

Soft tissue manipulation

Postural re-education

Self-mobilizing and self-stretching activities to enhance and maintain improved joint and soft tissue mobility

Diaphragmatic breathing to promote improved posture and thoracic joint motion

Techniques

Treatment of T2–T3 Joint That Does Not Side Bend Right

Patient is sitting (Fig. 14-2A). Stand behind patient. Palpate to left of T2–T3 interspace with left thumb. Side bend right to level of T2–T3. Contact

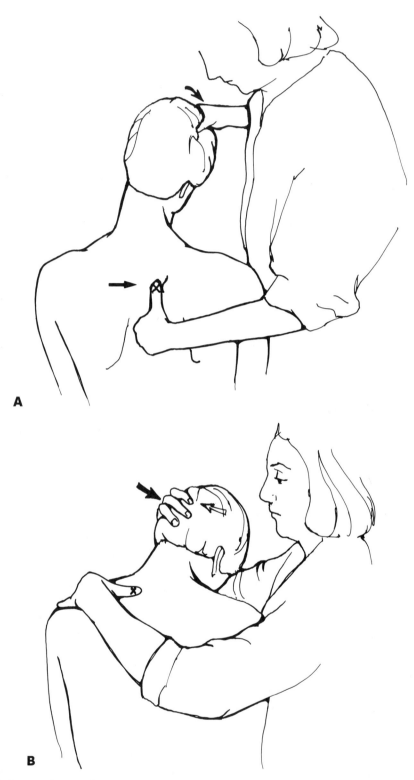

Fig. 14-2 Facet hypomobility. **(A)** Technique for T2–T3 joint with restricted right side bending. **(B)** Technique for T2–T3 joint with poor side bending and rotation right.

left lateral aspect of T3 spinous process with left thumb. Apply transverse manipulation pressure to T3 spinous process in direction of arrow. Be sure technique is performed at end range of left T2–T3 facet joint for mechanical changes. Levels: C7 to T3.

Treatment of T2–T3 Joint That Does Not Side Bend and Rotate Right

Patient is sitting (Fig. 14-2B). Stand behind patient. Forward bend, side bend right, rotate right to level of T2–T3. Contact T3 transverse process on left with your left thumb. Have patient attempt to backward bend, left rotate, left side bend against unyielding resistance of your right hand. Have patient relax, then take up slack in forward bend, right side bend, right rotation direction. Repeat two to three times. Levels: C7 to T3.

Treatment of T6–T7 Facet Joint Restricted in Forward Bending

Patient is supine with hands behind neck (Fig. 14-3A). Stand on patient's right side. Roll patient toward you with left hand. Contact transverse processes of T7 with cupped right hand; the right transverse process is contacted by your first proximal interphalangeal (PIP) joint and the left transverse process is contacted by your third PIP joint (fourth and fifth digits are flexed at all joints, second digit is in neutral, right thumb is parallel to spinous processes). Roll patient back on your right hand. Patient supports his head and neck as you forward bend him to T6–T7 level with your left hand contact on his forearms. Manipulation is performed in a posterior superior direction during exhalation as you apply pressure with left hand-forearm contact on patient's forearms. Recheck mobility before repeating technique. Technique may be used for rotation restriction by modifying hand contact on patient's transverse processes. Backward bending restrictions may be treated by altering direction of force. Levels: T3 to T10.

Treatment of T6–T7 Facets Restricted in Backward Bending

Patient is prone with pillow under abdomen to protect lumbar spine (Fig. 14-3B). T6 spinous process is contacted by your right pisiform with thumb pointing in caudal direction as you stand on patient's right side. The manipulation pressure is in an anterior direction during patient exhalation.

This technique can be modified for treatment of rotation and forward bending restrictions. Modifications for treatment of a forward bending restriction include placing the midthoracic spine in forward bending through placement of pillows and changing the pressure direction to include a superior as well as an anterior direction on the spinous processes.

To treat a right rotation restriction at T6–T7, contact the left transverse process of T6 with pisiform of right hand. Pressure is applied in anterior direction during exhalation. To enhance stretch of T6–T7 right facet joint, stabilize right transverse process of T7 with pisiform of left hand. Levels: T3 to T10.

Treatment of T6–T7 Facet Joint Restricted in Left Side Bending and Right Rotation with Isometric Technique

Patient is sitting (Fig. 14-3C). Stand behind patient. Place right arm through patient's axilla and grasp patient's lateral rib cage. Place left thumb on left lateral aspect of T7 spinous processes. Forward bend, left side bend, and right rotate to T6–T7 level. Have patient attempt to return to erect posture against your unyielding resistance. Have patient relax, then take up slack in forward bending, left side bending, and right rotation direction. Repeat two to three times. Levels: T3 to T10.

HYPERMOBILITY OF THORACIC SEGMENTS

Causes

Frequently resulting from postural and muscle imbalances, often at levels above restricted segment(s)

Trauma such as pulling, lifting, or reaching resulting in ligament and capsular sprain

Symptoms

Movement usually painless although discomfort may follow periods of increased activity

Pain usually comes on with static positions and fatigue of the muscles as a result of their protective role

Radicular pain in the associated segment

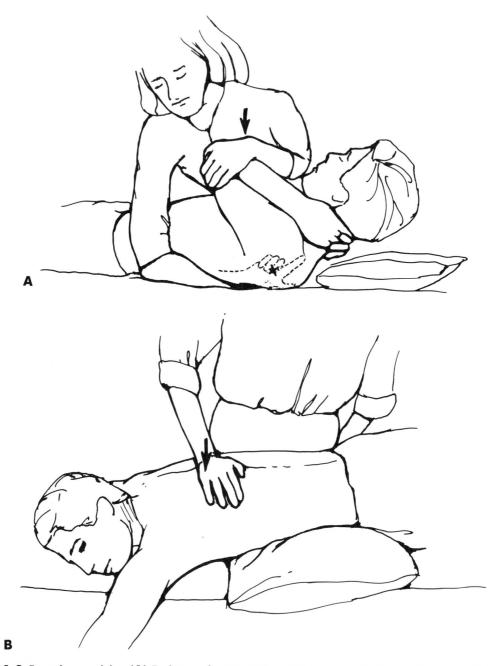

Fig. 14-3 Facet hypomobility. **(A)** Technique for T6–T7 facet joint restricted in forward bending. **(B)** Technique for T6–T7 facets restricted in backward bending. (*Figure continues.*)

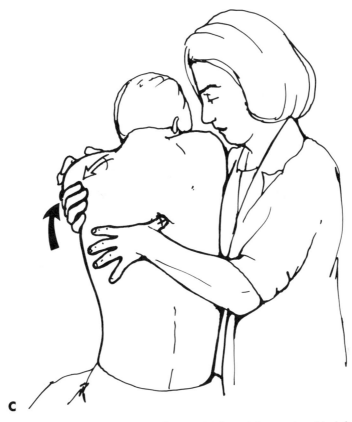

Fig. 14-3 (*Continued*). **(C)** Isometric technique for T6–T7 facet joint restricted in left side bending and right rotation.

Pain usually alleviated by short periods of gentle movement or rest

Signs

Hypomobility may be noted with passive motion testing and may present an area of hypermobility immediately above it

Palpatory changes include increased muscle tone and tenderness as well as swelling of the interspinous and superspinous ligaments (perhaps a stringy feeling in the chronic situation)

Presence of positional faults at the level of hypermobility

Treatment

Correct neighboring hypomobility

Support the involved segment

Corseting

Muscle rehabilitation of surrounding musculature

Postural re-education to reduce the strain

Diaphragmatic breathing

RIB CONDITIONS

Several articulations exist at each individual rib. Evaluation of each individual articulation of one rib is virtually impossible; however, the articulations of one rib can be evaluated as a whole. Rarely do rib hypomobilities exist without the corresponding vertebral segments being involved. Thus, anytime a rib lesion is suspected, the corresponding facet joint must also be evaluated. As a brief refresher, ribs 1, 10, 11, and 12 articulate with one vertebral body (costovertebral joint) and its transverse process (costotransverse [CT] joint). Ribs 2 through 9 articulate with two vertebral bodies plus the inferior vertebral body transverse process. In addition, ribs 1 through 7 articulate anteriorly with the sternum via synovial joints. These sternocostal and costochondral joints often become irritated. Mechanisms responsible for this will be discussed below.

Hypomobility of the Ribs

Causes
Trauma to the area such as a blow to the rib cage
Postural and muscle imbalances

Symptoms
Pain posteriorly at the costovertebral and CT joints
Occasional reference of pain laterally into chest wall
Diaphragmatic breathing will be uncomfortable with sharp pain upon deep breathing
Movement requiring rib cage excursion may be uncomfortable

Signs
Forward head and increased thoracic kyphosis
Altered breathing pattern, avoiding diaphragmatic breathing. On inhalation the anterior aspect of the ribs should move upward in the pump handle method and the lateral ribs should move upward in the bucket handle method. Palpation is by placing the fingers between the ribs in line with them.
With an inhalation restriction the rib will not move upwards during inspiration
In an exhalation restriction the rib will not descend
Tenderness present involving costovertebral joint
Restriction of motion on testing
Altered position of rib may be palpated

Treatment
Joint manipulation of restricted segments. Treat posterior joint, then retest before treating anterior joint.

Stretch of involved intercostal muscles
Postural re-education to enhance rib excursion
Self-mobilizing, self-stretching activities to enhance rib cage excursion
Diaphragmatic breathing will increase both the anterior posterior and the transverse diameter of the thoracic cavity by its influence on the ribs.

Technique

Treatment of Sixth Left Rib Restriction
Patient is prone with pillow under trunk (Fig. 14-4). Stand on patient's right side. Contact sixth left rib lateral to CT joint with your right hand, thumb pointing caudally. Stabilize opposite rib with your left hand. Manipulation pressure is in anterior caudal direction during patient exhalation. Levels: 2nd to 12th ribs.

Treatment of Exhalation Restriction, Sixth Right Rib
Patient is supine, and therapist stands at patient's head (Fig. 14-5A). With left hand, side bend and forward bend patient until you feel tension under right thumb which is on sixth rib, lateral to sternocostal joint. During exhalation, apply pressure to sixth rib in a caudal direction. Hold this new position of rib as patient inhales. Repeat two to three times. Levels: 2nd to 10th ribs. Must be more lateral for 11th and 12th ribs.

Treatment of Inhalation Restriction, Right Fifth Rib
Patient is supine, and therapist stands on the patient's right side (Fig. 14-5B). Patient's arm is straight above head. Place left hand under the patient and put tips of two to four fingers over angle of fifth rib. Have patient inhale and bring right arm forward against your unyielding resistance. Simultaneously, with left hand, pull laterally and caudally on fifth rib. Relax, take up slack at fifth rib, and repeat two to three times.

Technique must be modified to treat lower ribs (ribs 7 to 10). Patient's arm is elevated, with elbow flexed so forearm lies above head. Patient attempts to abduct arm against your unyielding resistance. Levels: 2nd to 4th ribs, with modifications for 7th to 10th ribs.

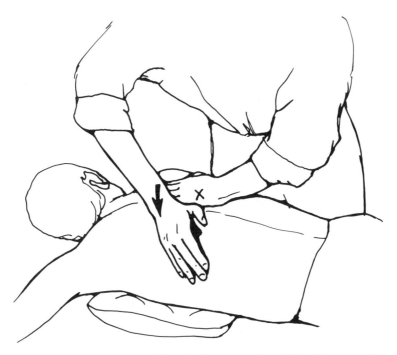

Fig. 14-4 Hypomobility of the ribs. Technique for sixth left rib restriction.

Intercostal Stretch. Restriction Between Right Ribs 6 and 7

Patient is side lying on left side (Fig. 14-6). Right arm is above head. Stand at patient's head. Place your right thumb and web space along superior border of seventh rib. Stabilize patient's right arm with your left hand. During patient inhalation, resist elevation of seventh rib. As patient exhales, apply caudal pressure to seventh rib. Repeat two to three times. Levels: 2nd to 12th ribs.

Hypermobility of the Ribs

Symptoms

Complaints of pain localized to the involved costal margin or costochondral area

Pain may initially be intermittent, aggravated by increased activity, particularly on bending or twisting, and is usually of a dull aching nature but with the possibility of sharp episodes upon a movement such as a deep breath

Presence of clicking sound or sensation, usually in the costosternal region

Signs

Protective posture

Shallow breathing

Excessive mobility on passive motion springing

Tenderness of the costochondral junction

Treatment

Correct any neighboring hypomobilities, including thoracic facet hypomobilities

Education in activities of daily living (ADL) and body mechanics to decrease the strain to the area

Gentle stretching by therapist or patient to the intercostal area to minimize soft tissue changes resulting from protective postures

Progress into full diaphragmatic breathing

Consult physician if there is a suspicion of a slipping rib and if the patient does not respond appropriately

DOWAGER'S HUMP—UPPER THORACIC KYPHOSIS

The upper thoracic kyphosis and accompanying fluid retention common in postmenopausal and

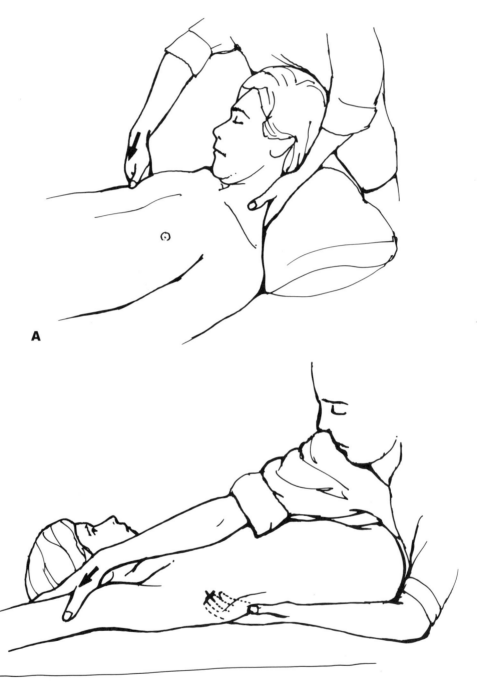

Fig. 14-5 (A) Technique for restriction in exhalation. **(B)** Technique for restriction in inhalation.

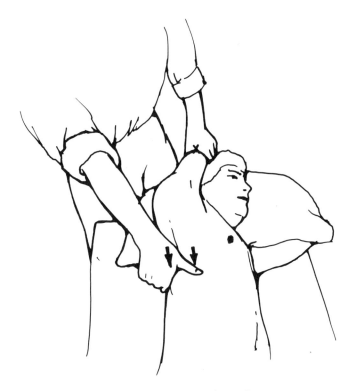

Fig. 14-6 Intercostal stretch.

somewhat osteoporotic women can occur also in women with heavy breasts or in men and women with heavy shoulders, particularly if a forward head and round shoulder posture is adopted. The result is a loss of movement in the upper thoracic region, forcing hypermobility in the lower cervical spine.

Causes

Postmenopausal osteoporosis
Heavy breasts and shoulders
Poor postural sense
Occupational

Symptoms

Minimal in the region
Tenderness and discomfort in lower cervical spine aggravated by motion or sustained positions

Signs

Loss of upper thoracic motion
Fluid swelling or tissue thickening over the upper thoracic area
Hypermobility of lower cervical joints

Myofascial restrictions similar to those found in thoracic outlet syndrome

Treatment

Manipulation to underlying stiff joints
Soft tissue manipulation
Postural correction
Exercises to maintain range

COSTOCHONDRITIS

Pathophysiology

The costochondral cartilage may become strained with persistent coughing or owing to trauma. Painful swelling results from the irritation of the cartilaginous tissues.

Causes

Trauma or persistent coughing such as in chronic bronchitis.

Symptoms

Pain on moving the trunk
Pain on coughing or deep breathing

Signs

Swelling at the costochondral junction is palpable
    and visible
Breathing pattern is shallow or guarded
Pressure on the sternum will reproduce the pain

Treatment

Gentle stretching to rib cage as a precautionary
    measure to prevent stiffness that would
    further aggravate the costochondral junction
Postural re-education
Slow, gentle diaphragmatic breathing
Light corseting such as with rib belt; use only if
    necessary for short periods
Transcutaneous electrical stimulation (TENS)
    may be of assistance in decreasing patient's
    pain

THORACIC DISC

Disc lesions in the thoracic spine are uncommon.
There is speculation that disc degeneration in the
thoracic spine is more prevalent than diagnostic
testing has revealed. When a disc lesion is diagnosed in the thoracic spine, it is usually at T7–
T11. Posterior bulging of the disc is serious in the
thoracic spine owing to the decrease in the diameter of the spinal canal at this level. Spinal cord
embarassment may occur.

Causes

Trauma such as a fall from a height when
    landing on the feet
Postural imbalances such as chronic kyphotic
    posture

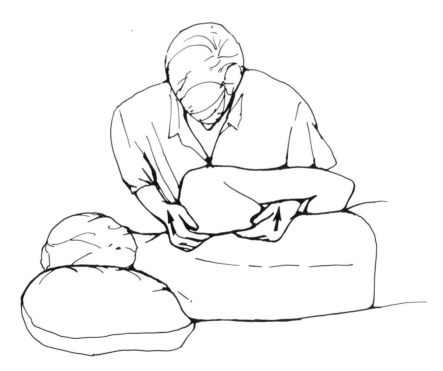

Fig. 14-7 Scapular thoracic (ST) joint stretch. *Patient:* Left side lying. *Therapist:* Face patient.
Technique: Place your right two to four fingers along superior medial scapular border. Place your left
arm through patient's right axilla and your left two to four fingers along the inferior medial scapular
border. Stabilize patient's shoulder with contact on your sternum. Move scapula in all directions to
identify myofascial restriction. Stretch in restricted directions. As muscles relax, you will be able to place
fingers on anterior medial border of scapula, which will allow distraction of scapula away from thorax.
Sustained stretches (for myofascial tightness) or repetitive movements (for ST crepitus) are appropriate
and beneficial.

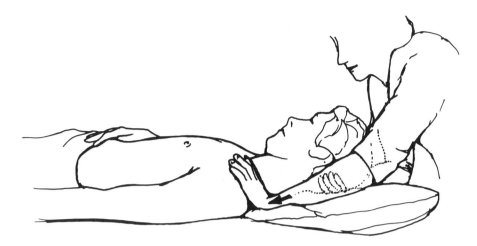

Fig. 14-8 Scalene stretch. *Patient:* Supine. *Therapist:* Stands at patient's head. *Technique:* To stretch left scalenes, place left hand (index finger and thumb) on superior aspect of left first rib. Supporting patient's head with right hand, move the patient's head to side bending right position. As patient exhales, depress the first rib, thus stretching anterior and middle scalenes. This is repeated two to three times, with more slack taken up with each exhalation. The technique can be done in a sitting position, and further stretching can be achieved with the patient's head being placed in right side bending and axial extension.

Symptoms

Possible radicular pain

Pain, usually constant, of a dull, cramping, burning nature

Occasional radiation of pain into groin

Various other findings including abdominal pain, sensory or motor disturbance, altered abdominal reflexes

Signs

Increased thoracic kyphosis

Exacerbation of patient's pain with dural stretch and aggravated more by passive rotation than by resisted active rotation

Neighboring hypomobilities

Possible upper motor neuron symptoms

Breathing tolerated without the "catching" that occurs with rib or facet lesions

Treatment (Excluding Upper Motor Neuron Signs)

Postural re-education to reduce an excessive kyphosis, resting the involved disc

Joint and soft tissue manipulations to any restricted areas in the region

Instruct in ADL, appropriate sitting and resting positions; emphasis on reducing posterior strain

Bed rest

Corseting for stabilization and resting the area may be necessary

MYOFASCIAL IMBALANCES

Postural imbalances and chronic habits permit myofascial adaptations to take place. It is thought that postural muscles tend to achieve a position that allows them a mechanical advantage in movement, but has the effect of creating an overuse syndrome, leading to hypertrophy and eventually to adaptive shortening. By contrast, phasic muscles are placed at a mechanical disadvantage that results in a weakening and strain.

Symptoms

Pain in posterior thorax, upper trapezius, or distal attachment of levator scapulae

Repetitive movement aggravates the condition

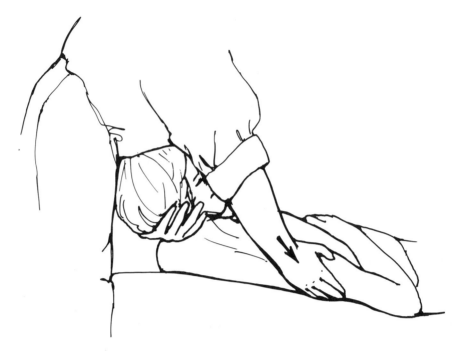

Fig. 14-9 Upper trapezius stretch. *Patient:* Supine. *Therapist:* Stands at patient's head. *Technique:* To stretch right upper trapezius, place the heel of the right hand over the patient's right acromion process. Supporting the patient's head in your left hand, place his head in a forward bending, left side bending, right rotation position. As patient exhales, depress the right shoulder girdle. Repeat two to three times, taking up more slack in the upper trapezius; with each exhalation, the therapist may choose to hold the stretch position for 30 seconds or more. Further stretch of the upper trapezius can be obtained by simultaneously distracting the head and neck with the left hand while depressing the patient's right shoulder girdle.

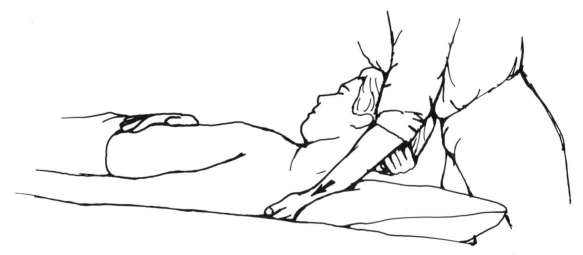

Fig. 14-10 Levator scapulae stretch. *Patient:* Supine. *Therapist:* Stands at patient's head. *Technique:* The superior medial angle of the scapula is cupped by your left hand. The patient's head is supported in a position of forward bending, right side bending, and right rotation by your right hand. A stretch of the left levator scapulae is achieved by caudal depression of the left scapula during the patient's exhalation. Repeat two to three times, taking up more slack with each exhalation.

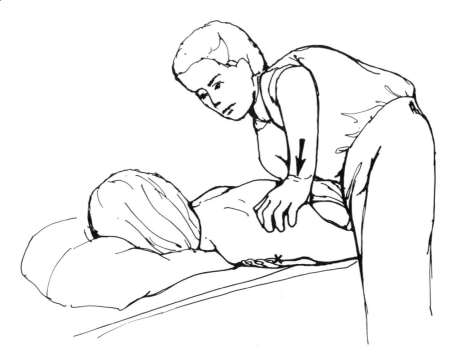

Fig. 14-11 Pectoralis minor stretch. *Patient:* Supine. *Therapist:* Stands at the patient's right side to stretch right pectoralis minor. *Technique:* Place your right hand under the patient's right scapula to stabilize shoulder girdle. Stretch the pectoralis minor through contact on the anterior aspect of the coracoid process by your left hand. Provide unyielding resistance to anterior movement of the coracoid process. Repeat two to three times, taking up slack with each repetition. A more effective stretch will be achieved by placing the patient's shoulder girdle complex off the edge of the table.

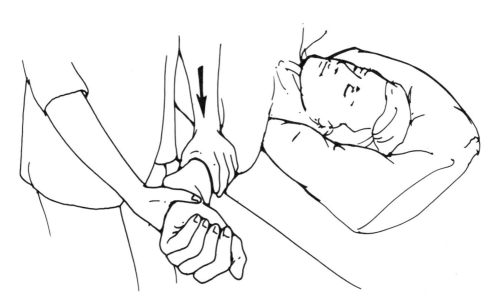

Fig. 14-12 Pectoralis major stretch. *Patient:* Supine. *Therapist:* Stands on his left side to stretch left pectoralis major. *Technique:* Resist adduction or flexion of the left arm. Be sure that the patient does not compensate during the stretch through hyperextension of the thoracic spine.

Signs (Those of Postural Change)

Forward head, internal rotation of the shoulders, protraction and outward rotation of the scapula, flattening of midthoracic kyphosis, and the presence of a dowager's hump
Possible joint hypomobility
Restricted flexibility in the following muscles:
  upper trapezius and levator scapulae: influence head position
  pectoralis major: influences glenohumeral relation
  pectoralis minor: influences scapular position
Apparent weakness and improper recruitment of lower trapezius, rhomboids, and serratus anterior

Treatment

Manipulation of restricted joints
Scapular thoracic joint stretch (effective on levator scapulae and upper trapezius tightness) Fig. 14-7
Stretch involved tight muscles
Strengthen appropriate muscles if indicated after stretching of tight muscles
Postural re-education and awareness
Home program; self-stretches
Moist heat and massage will offer relief from pain

15 Cervical Spine

Stanley V. Paris

The cervical spine, although similar to the lumbar spine in many respects, is clinically quite different in terms of treatment. Therefore, a number of the conditions affecting the lumbar spine are repeated here, along with their differences.

CERVICAL FACET CONDITIONS

Synovitis-Hemarthrosis

Causes

Wrestling, tumbling, football, falling asleep in front of television

Awkward movement or catch

Symptoms

Pain or stiffness and associated muscle guarding

Signs

Facets and ligaments tender to palpation

Muscles demonstrating involuntary holding

Treatment

Soft collar to give warmth and minimal support that will at the same time permit pain-free movement

Maintain function within comfort but nothing that would involve causing discomfort (Fig. 15-1)

At 10 days, provided there has been no aggravation of the symptoms, examine for joint restrictions (see Cervical Facet Stiffness, below) (Figs. 15-2 to Fig. 15-4)

Management

It is most important that time is permitted for the acute facet strain to settle. The optimal time appears to be 10 days. Any stretching within this period may only aggravate the condition and delay the healing process.

Cervical Facet Stiffness

Causes

Aftereffects of synovitis and or hemarthrosis

Symptoms

None. Stiff joints of themselves are not painful

Signs

Stiffness to passive intervertebral motion testing

Treatment

Manipulate to restore function so that the facets and other structures within the segment may arrest or reverse their degenerative changes and increase their tolerance to insult (Figs. 15-2 to 15-4)

Painful Entrapment of a Cervical Facet

The facet capsules are exquisitely sensitive, possessing the richest innervation of any spinal structure. Occasionally, the capsules get caught between the articular surfaces and thus prevent movement in the direction of their impingement.

Causes

Usually due to a rotation combined with backward bending

Can occur while lying in bed and gently rolling the head

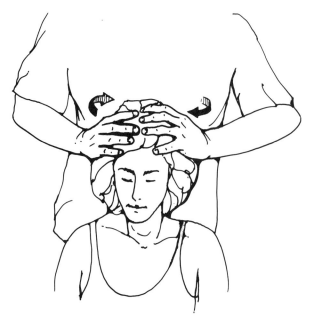

Fig. 15-1 Cervical circling—gating for the acute neck. *Patient:* Seated and well supported, preferably in an armchair. *Therapist:* Stands behind patient, placing palms and fingers of the two hands comfortably yet firmly on the cranium. *Technique:* The head is gradually moved in small circles with a diameter of perhaps 1 inch while making a track in different direction. The therapist must be sensitive to any resistance from muscle guarding and steer away from such areas. This ensures patient comfort and soon creates patient acceptance and trust. *Use:* The acute and apprehensive neck. Effect is similar to Codman's exercises at the shoulder; that is, by imparting small painless motions, the therapist can encourage (gate) a wider range of motion and help to restore function.

Symptoms
Acute pain when attempting to hold the head erect or to move in the direction of the capsule being pinched

Signs
Head held to one side
Acute tenderness to palpation of the affected facet
Muscle guarding
If the problem is on the left side of the neck, then forward bending, side bending to the right, and rotation to the right are less painful than backward bending, side bending to the left, and rotation to left, as

the latter movements tend to pinch the entrapment, while the others tend to stretch it

Treatment
Isometric manipulation (Fig. 15-2)
Traction with rotation
Maintain function after correction and treat as a facet synovitis

Mechanical Block of a Cervical Facet
Causes
Sudden force, strain, or jarring action

Symptoms
Minimal pain, occasional discomfort on effort

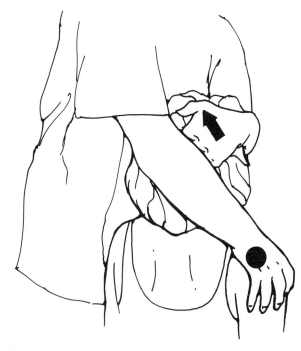

Fig. 15-2 Isometric manipulation of multifidii in the midcervical spine. *Patient:* Seated. *Therapist:* Stands to one side and supports the shoulder while holding the patient's head up against the therapist's body. *Technique:* The therapist instructs the patient to resist while a diagonal force is gradually imparted to cause an isometric contraction of the multifidii group. *Use:* Stretch of the cervical facet capsules to which the multifidii attach and more dramatically for the release of a facet capsular impingement.

Signs

Neck is held in a position that could be explained by one facet being hitched in an upward position

On palpation, the fault can be felt

Movement is restricted in the direction of the block

Treatment

Preparation of soft tissues by heat and massage

Manipulation of the joint (Figs. 15-3 and 15-4)

Active movement to retain mobility

FORWARD HEAD POSTURE

Forward head posture in or by itself is unlikely to be presented for treatment. Poor posture does have consequences in craniomandibular, upper cervical, midcervical, and upper thoracic dysfunctions, however, and should be considered as part of the syndrome in most cervical problems.

The consequences of carrying the head forward include:

Malalignment of the temporomandibular joint (TMJ) affecting occlusion

Hyperextension of the subcranial region causing compression and reduction of vertebral artery flow to brain and brain stem

Hypermobility of the midcervical region caused by slackening the ligamentum nuchae

Hypomobility of the upper thoracic region caused by locking it in forward bending

Treatment

Postural awareness by exaggerating the patient's fault in front of a mirror so he can see the trend

Axial extension techniques with finger awareness on upper lip (Fig. 15-5)

Mobilize upper thoracic spine (Figs. 15-6 and 15-7)

KISSING LAMINAE

Similar to "kissing vertebrae" in the lumbar spine, kissing laminae occur when the laminae of the midcervical spine impinge upon one another, developing bursa between them.

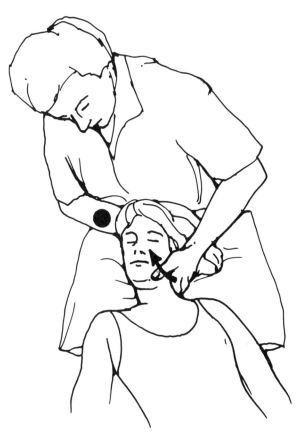

Fig. 15-3 Midcervical manipulation—facet lift up and stretch. *Patient:* Supine lying. *Therapist:* Supporting patient's head with one hand and imparting gentle rotation, the index finger of the other hand grasps the lamina and articular process of the facet joint and pulls it upward and forward along its facet plane. *Technique:* This is a gentle, relaxing, massagelike motion while the mobilizing index finger contacts first one level, then the next. *Use:* For a neck that is generally tight in either myofascia or facet without any levels demonstrating hypermobility.

Causes

Hyperlordosis of the midcervical spine secondary to a pronounced upper thoracic kyphosis (dowager's hump)

Symptoms

Pain in the midcervical region that is relieved by forward bending and aggravated by backward bending

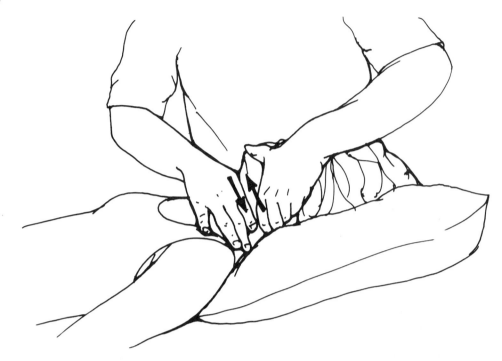

Fig. 15-4 Midcervical manipulation—reach over hold and lift up. *Patient:* Supine lying. *Therapist:* With the left hand, the therapist places the index finger on the back of the lamina and facet joint. The right hand, flexed to position the metacarpophalangeal joint of the index finger, draws across the throat to lie in front of the anterior root of the vertebra below the level where the manipulation is to take place. *Technique:* The left hand pulls up the neck via the lamina until the right hand effects a block. A stretch is then applied. *Use:* Upward slide of a midcervical facet to produce side bending and rotation to the opposite side as well as forward bending on that side.

Signs

Hyperlordosis
Tenderness to palpation

Treatment

Posture correction (Fig. 15-5)
Mobilization of upper thoracic region

MYOFASCIAL RESTRICTIONS

Myofacial restrictions most commonly occur between the neck and shoulder girdle, producing a raised shoulders posture, or between the back of the neck and upper thoracic spine, producing a forward head posture.

Causes

Forward head posture adopted, thus increasing the lordosis and permitting the myofascia to shorten
Respiratory or anxiety condition in which the shoulders are held raised
As a result of an injury to the muscles, such as in a whiplash accident, they either lose their extensibility, or adopt a shortened position or both

Symptoms

Minimal to none
Secondary changes most notable in the subcranial region, perhaps precipitating headache and craniomandibular dysfunction

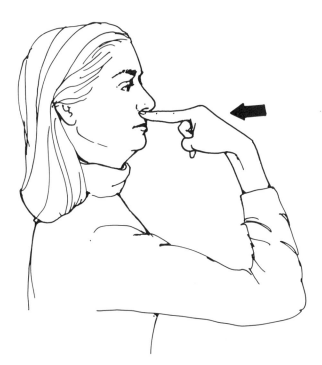

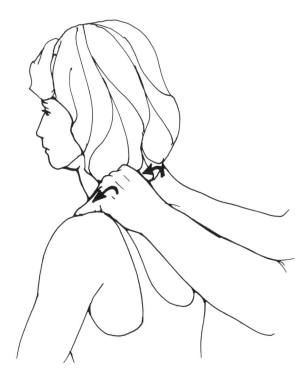

Fig. 15-5 Long-axis extension. *Patient:* Places two middle fingers on top lip with hand raised and in front. *Therapist:* Directs only. *Technique:* Patient presses back on top lip carrying head as far back as possible while keeping the hand level. The fingers are then removed, and the patient brings the head forward to the first position that is comfortable. The patient is encouraged to maintain that posital as an optimal posture for the head on the neck. *Use:* Correcting posture and developing awareness.

Fig. 15-6 Soft tissue manipulation—tissue fluid squeeze. *Patient:* Seated facing a mirror so that therapist can observe facial expressions. *Therapist:* Standing behind the patient, the therapist grasps the soft tissues at either side of the "shoal" of the neck by using the lumbrical muscles. *Technique:* The soft tissues are given a sustained squeeze of about 1 to 2 minutes to help remove any swelling from the area. *Use:* To remove soft tissue swelling that commonly accompanies the dowager's hump and in so doing to promote greater freedom of motion in the upper thoracic region.

Signs

Forward head
Loss of full-range forward bending
Side bending free

Treatment

Myofascial stretching techniques
Postural re-education
Inhibitive distraction (Fig. 15-8)

LIGAMENTOUS STRAIN—SIMPLE OVERSTRETCH OR OVERUSE

Minor strains are common among the active population, and most clear up without any problems.

Repeated too often in the presence of underlying pathology, however, they can become problems.

Causes

Wrestling
Carrying heavy objects on the shoulder
Falling asleep while a passenger in a car or in front of television, and resting with the neck stressed

Symptoms

Pain, restlessness, muscle holding

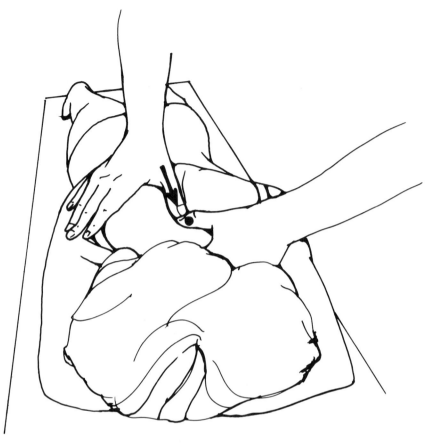

Fig. 15-7 Upward slide of upper thoracic facets. *Patient:* Prone lying. *Therapist:* Standing, the therapist places a thumb on the transverse process of an upper thoracic vertebra and reinforces this with a second thumb that will deliver the mobilizing force. *Technique:* The mobilizing force is delivered along the plane of the facet joints. *Use:* To improve forward bending on that side as well as side bending and rotation to the opposite side.

Signs

Pain on full-range motion, or in direction of injury
Tenderness of facets or ligaments to palpation

Treatment

Postural re-education
Soft collar or plastic corset support
Movement within the range of comfort

Prognosis

The prognosis is excellent, with complete recovery from the condition within a few days.

LIGAMENTOUS SPRAIN AND RUPTURE— WHIPLASH

The use of the term *whiplash* is generally held in disfavor as the word denotes a motion that may not in fact have occurred. Acceleration and deceleration are probably better terms and would include some of the other causes of violent trauma to the cervical ligaments such as being struck on the head by the boom of a yacht, or by a step or ledge during a fall.

Any forces sufficient to damage cervical ligaments will have also have quite possibly damaged the facets, intervertebral discs, muscles, and per-

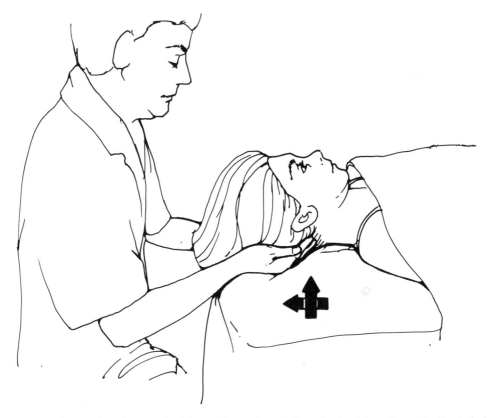

Fig. 15-8 Subcranial and cervical inhibitive distraction. *Patient:* Supine lying. *Therapist:* Seated, the therapist rests the backs of the hands on the table and places the ends of the middle fingers on the inferior nuchal line of the patient's occiput. *Technique:* The fingers lift the head up so that the occiput is entirely supported by the fingers. A long-axis distraction is then applied. As the tension in the neck changes, the fingers take up the slack. Treatment is from 2 to 4 minutes. Initially, the patient's eyes are open, but at later treatments the eyes may be closed and relaxation suggestion used.

haps the trachea, esophagus, brain stem, internal ear mechanism, eyes, and vertebral arteries as well as the cervical sympathetic nerves.

In all cases, the therapist must be alert to the possibility of odontoid fracture or upper cervical ligamentous rupture. A safe rule to follow in this area is: "If muscle guarding is present, do not remove it."

Causes

Motor vehicle accidents
Any head trauma of sufficient violence, such as falls, being struck by a yachting boom, football

Symptoms

Pain of a diffuse and variable nature
Dizziness, vomiting, blurred vision, imbalance, difficulty in gait, visual and hearing changes

Signs

Restriction of movement and muscle guarding
Defensive behavior, fear and anxiety, awkwardness

Treatment

Rigid brace at least of the Philadelphia type
Although physical therapy in the form of traction and movement may bring relief, one

should remember that traction and movement were the very nature of the injury, and although physical therapy may enable the patient and the doctor to think that something is being done, it is in fact only giving temporary relief to the patient through gating while delaying recovery of these ligaments. Immobilization is the rule for ligamentous injuries and injuries of other serious soft tissue structures and should be applied here.

There is no use for traction
After 6 weeks begin active movements
After 10 weeks begin gentle mobilization

SPONDYLOSIS

Spondylosis is a segmental degenerative disease of the cervical spine and is rather like disc disease in the low back. It occurs in the older population (45 years and older), whereas in low back disc disease problems occur principally between 28 and 50 years of age.

Spondylosis involves degeneration of the disc vertebra interface, particularly in the region of the lateral interbody articulations. The result is the formation of osteophytes.

Causes

Misuse and abuse
Poor posture, forward head, round shoulders
Upper thoracic kyphosis with loss of mobility in that region, forcing hypermobility and thus osteophytes in the midcervical region

Symptoms

In advanced cases, there may be neurological problems, with pain reference to the neck and arms

Signs

Mostly radiological, showing narrowed foramen and reduced disc space with the presence of osteophytes at the lateral interbody articulation

Treatment

Mobilize the upper thoracic region (Figs. 15-6, 15-7)
Posture
Positional distraction to remove nerve root pressure (Fig. 15-9)
Avoid bending the neck backward or rolling it around

MYELOPATHY

Advanced degenerative changes beginning with spondylosis may, if they begin to involve structures of the spinal canal, namely, the cord, destroy portions of that cord, leading to myelopathy. Myelopathy is often confused with other neurological conditions such as multiple sclerosis.

Causes

Spondylosis that progresses unchecked

Signs

Weakness in all extremities, most noticeably the legs
Vague weaknesses in various parts of the body

Symptoms

Minimal
Often mimicking multiple sclerosis or other spinal cord diseases

Treatment

Posture
Surgery to remove the offending osteophytes and then perhaps to perform a fusion
Avoid bending the neck backward or rolling it around

DISC DISEASE

Disc disease is rare in the neck and is most often confused with spondylosis.

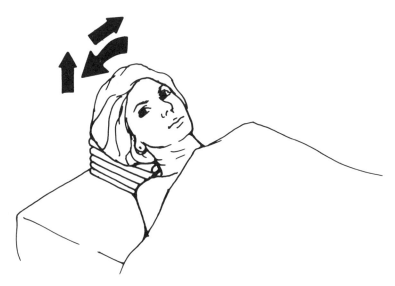

Fig. 15-9 Positional distraction of the midcervical spine. *Patient:* The patient is placed on a series of books or magazines that increase the angle of forward bending until the movement just arrives at the segment to be distracted. *Therapist:* Places hand on the neck opposite the painful side and then bends the neck over the hand and may rotate it slightly away to gain maximal opening of the foramen. *Use:* Relieve nerve root pressure.

Causes

Degenerative changes, spondylosis
Trauma

Symptoms

Interscapular and arm pains with neurological symptoms

Signs

Same as those for spondylosis
Neurological signs

Treatment

Posture
Mobilization of upper thoracic region (Figs. 15-6, 15-7)
Positional distraction (Fig. 15-9)

INSTABILITY OF THE CERVICAL SPINE

Instability of the cervical spine is a serious condition that may accompany rheumatoid arthritis. It has been said that if a rheumatoid arthritic patient lived long enough, he would eventually die of spinal cord injury owing to instability of the ligaments in the upper cervical spine.

Causes

Rheumatoid arthritis
Hypomobility of the upper thoracic spine
Forward head posture
Repeated traumas

Symptoms

Dull achy pains
Transient neurological complaints

Signs

Forward head
Restricted upper thoracic motion
Involuntary muscle holdings
Hypermobility on passive motion testing

Treatment

Mobilize upper thoracic spine (Figs. 15-6, 15-7)
Posture
Brace or corset

No full-range exercises, although isometrics may help

Management

Great caution must be exercised. The cervical spine is a very mobile structure, prevented from excessive motion by the integrity of its ligaments. If these ligaments are affected by disease or by trauma, then this very important protective mechanism is interrupted and spinal cord injury and death may result.

16 Subcranial Region

Stanley V. Paris

MYOFASCIAL RESTRICTIONS

Myofascial restrictions commonly result from subcranial problems and should be dealt with before treating the underlying problems.

Causes

Forward head posture
Upper cervical facet strain

Symptoms

Tightness and dull ache

Signs

Forward head
Limited nodding, backward bending free, and
    side bending slightly limited
Radiologically, an increase in the upper cervical
    lordosis

Treatment

Inhibitive distraction (see Fig. 15-8)
Manual traction
Musclle stretching

Management

PNF techniques should not be used to stretch the myofascia in this region, because the forces that these muscles develop can create segmental strains.

SUBCRANIAL LIGAMENTOUS RUPTURE—WHIPLASH

The subcranial area is most critical after whiplash because of the possibility of fracture of the odontoid process or rupture of the alar ligaments, both of which can be missed on radiographic examination. Should either of these events have occurred, it is possible for the patient to rotate the subcranial region to such a degree that the spinal cord will be compromised, possibly to life-threatening results. This unfortunate event occasionally occurs after motor vehicle accidents when the victim may be handled without adequate support being provided. The presence of any muscle guarding in this area after trauma should be a sign that the body provides its own protection, and in no way should an attempt be made to remove such muscle guarding during the first 6 weeks after injury.

Causes

Motor vehicle accidents
Yachting accidents (struck by boom)
Falls, wrestling

Symptoms

Pain and stiffness

Signs

Muscle guarding and restrictive motion
Whenever muscle guarding is observed, it should
    be considered to be fulfilling nature's work
    and must not be relaxed until it is certain
    that there is no fracture or ligamentous
    rupture

Treatment

If fracture is present, the treatment is
    hospitalization and surgical management
If severe strain is present, four to six weeks of
    rigid support is advisable
Radiographs may miss a fracture and cannot
    detect ruptured ligaments

LIGAMENTOUS INSUFFICIENCY—RHEUMATOID ARTHRITIS

Laxity of the subcranial ligaments is rarely due to stress and strain but rather is caused by systemic conditions such as rheumatoid arthritis. The danger is that the individual will be lacking in the usual restraints to excessive movement and that a sudden or forceful motion may cause the atlas to rotate too far on the axis and as a result cause spinal cord damage sufficient to cause death.

Causes

Rheumatoid arthritis
Genetic hypermobility

Symptoms

None other than dull ache or occasional
  headache

Signs

Positive alar-odontoid integrity test. (This test is
  not illustrated here due to the fact that it
  should be carefully described and taught in
  a classroom setting.)

Treatment

Surgical fusion of atlas to axis

VERTEBRAL ARTERY SYNDROME

Causes

Genetic
Arteriosclerosis of the carotid or internal carotid
  arteries, thus placing a greater burden on
  the vertebral artery

Symptoms

Dizziness, nausea, ringing in the ears, blurred
  vision, faintness on performing or adopting
  head positions that occlude the vertebral
  artery

Signs

None except when performing the vertebral
  artery test which causes nystagmus, slurring
  of speech, unequal pupil dilation, slowness
  of response to verbal inquiry

Treatment

Head postures
Activities of daily living and activities of nightly
  living

ACUTE FACET STRAIN

Causes

Motor vehicle accidents, wrestling, poor posture

Symptoms

Stiffness and discomfort
Sometimes painful block owing to capsular
  impingement

Signs

Stiffness and muscle guarding
Restriction of active movements

Treatment

Leave alone for 10 days until injury settles down
Manipulation and range of motion (see Fig. 15-1)

FACET STIFFNESS OR BLOCK

Facet restrictions and even blocks are very common. They cause little if any discomfort and may go undetected for years before secondary problems bring them to the attention of the patient. Secondary problems includes headache, localized pain, and scoliosis.

Causes

Trauma causing facet strain
Muscle guarding the injured joints until they
  stiffen

Symptoms

Minimal discomfort
Headache

Signs

A loss of restriction of subcranial movements
such as back bending, side bending, forward
bending, and rotation
Each of these movements is tested both actively
and passively and found to be limited
Scoliosis (see below)

Treatment

Manipulation. The techniques in the subcranial
area require careful instruction and are
considered to be at an advanced level of
practice. Under no circumstances should
thrust techniques be employed.

HEADACHE

The topic of headache, its classification, and treatment is too extensive for comprehensive presentation in this text. However, the following is presented for the reader's consideration.

Causes

Stress
Dysfunction in the cervical and upper thoracic
spines
Craniomandibular dysfunction
Cranial dysfunction

Symptoms

Headache

Signs

Many, including mood changes

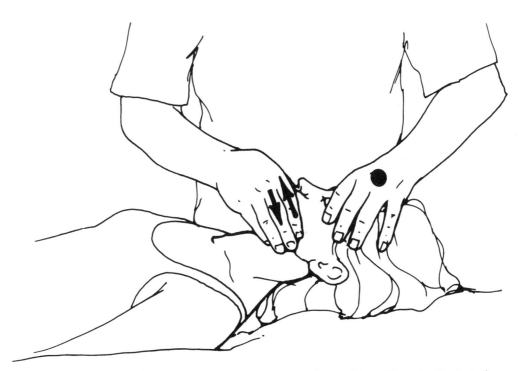

Fig. 16-1 Cranial manipulation by maxillary swing. *Patient:* Supine lying. *Therapist:* Contacts the maxilla between the thumb and middle finger, taking care to grasp above the roots of the teeth and support the forehead with the other hand. *Technique:* The maxilla is first pressed upward and outward to one side and then to the other. *Use:* Sinus stimulation for drainage.

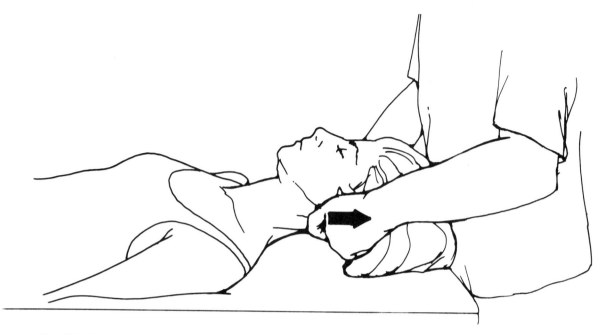

Fig. 16-2 Cranial manipulation by mastoid lift. *Patient:* Supine. *Therapist:* While seated or standing behind patient, the therapist grasps the mastoid processes with the hood of the index finger. *Technique:* Long-axis extension is applied. *Use:* Cervical traction and cranial release.

Treatment

Correct any dysfunctions in the causative areas
listed above.

Management

The headaches that physical therapists are most
able to help are those that have a history of trauma,
show a strong association with other cervical pain,
or can be initiated by emotional or physical stress.

SCOLIOSIS

Like headache, scoliosis is a vast subject warranting
extensive presentation. It receives only a brief
introduction here.

Causes

Orthopaedic surgeons look principally for short
leg, hip disease, vertebral anomalies, and
muscle dysfunction
Physical therapists may in addition consider
sacroiliac displacement and subcranial faults

Symptoms

Minimal

Signs

Side bending and rotation deformity

Treatment

Depends on extent of curve. Physical therapy has
not made many inroads in this area because
we have been unable to prove that we can
offer anything of benefit.

CRANIAL DYSFUNCTIONS

The fact that the cranium is not a solid structure
is gaining gradual recognition. Indeed, the cranium consists of a number of bones that are
movable throughout life. Some of the conditions
related to the cranium such as headache may either
arise there or be referred to this region, thus
complicating the understanding of the cranium in
the production of symptoms.

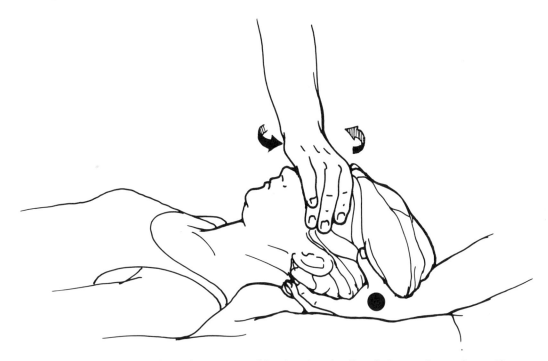

Fig. 16-3 Cranial manipulation by rotation of forehead on hindhead. *Patient:* Supine lying. *Therapist:* Supports the posterior occiput with one hand while extending the thumb and middle finger of the other hand to grasp the forehead. *Technique:* The hand on the forehead exerts a rotational strain in first one direction and then the other. *Use:* Cranial motion for sinus conditions and perhaps headache.

Sinus

The sinuses are well-known sites of pain. The observed response to pressure applied to them provides a clue to treatment.

Causes

Familial, allergy, climate, and injury

Symptoms

Facial pain
Stiffness
Headache

Signs

Rare, although a discharge may be observed

Treatment

Postural drainage
Diathermy and ultrasound have been used in the past but are now the subject of controversy as to their possible effect on the eyes and the pituitary gland
Manipulation frequently stimulates the sinus to drain and may bring temporary relief (Figs. 16-1–3).

17 Temporomandibular Joint

Steven L. Kraus

Temporomandibular joint (TMJ) dysfunction is an abnormal condition of the TMJ that results from neither a developmental abnormality, disease, or trauma sufficient to cause a fracture or dislocation. TMJ dysfunction involves the capsule and/or intracapsular structures. TMJ dysfunction can be a complication of any one or a combination of the preceding disorders. TMJ dysfunction, however, can also occur as a separate entity. In an average clinical setting, the most common disorder of the TMJ will be dysfunction. Reviewed in this chapter are the more common dysfunctions of the TMJ. Such dysfunctions can also occur separately or in any combination with each other.

ANTERIORLY DISLOCATED DISC WITH REDUCTION

When the patient is in a maximum intercuspated position (back teeth are together), the disc is anteriorly dislocated to the condyle. During opening of the mouth, the disc relocates itself to the condyle, and upon closing the mouth, the disc dislocates anteriorly to the condyle.

Cause

The primary cause for the disc to dislocate anteriorly to the condyle is the elongation of the collateral ligaments, the slope of the articular eminence, the elasticity of the superior stratum, and tone of the upper head of the external pterygoid muscle. The shape of the condylar head and disc are other variables that will contribute to an altered position of the disc on the condyle.

The tissue that is primarily responsible for relocation of the disc on the condyle during opening is the superior stratum.

Symptoms

If painful, pain will be felt in the region of the TMJ on the side of involvement with possible reference of pain into areas innervated by cranial nerve V. Pain will increase or be altered during functional and parafunctional (bruxism) movements of the mandible.

Signs

During mandibular opening, there will be a "click" or "snap" and then during closing another click or snap; this is the reciprocal click. The opening click will usually occur at the beginning or middle range of opening, whereas the closing click will occur toward the end of the closing.

Treatment

If pain or hindrance in function warrants treatment, a common treatment is an anterior repositioning appliance or a nonrepositioning appliance applied by a dentist (Fig. 17-1). The dentist should be adequately trained in the use of such an appliance and have a good clinical understanding of this dysfunction. Physical therapy modalities to decrease pain and any associated muscle guarding will enhance the effectiveness of the appliance. If either appliance is not successful in maintaining proper disc-condyle positioning, and the pain or hindrance in function is significant to the patient and clinician, then an oral surgery consultation is indicated.

Management

Management may best be accomplished by the normalization of muscle tone and function. If a

415

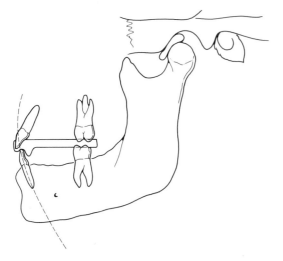

Fig. 17-1 An anterior repositioning appliance in the treatment of an anterior disc dislocation that reduces. (Razook, SJ: Nonsurgical management of TMJ and masticatory muscle problems. p. 130. In Kraus SL (ed): TMJ Disorders: Management of the Craniomandibular Complex. Churchill Livingstone, New York, 1988.)

satisfactory and stable disc-condyle position has been achieved, specific occlusal work in selected cases may be indicated. Otherwise, periodic use of an intraoral appliance and physical therapy may be the best management of this dysfunction. Physical therapy to help in relaxation of muscle tone of the jaw and cervical muscles through patient education and exercises as well as the use of modalities should be beneficial.

Prognosis
Satisfactory to good

ANTERIORLY DISLOCATED DISC WITHOUT REDUCTION

During all movements and positioning of the mandible, the disc remains anteriorly dislocated to the condyle.

Cause

This dysfunction has the same cause as discussed above for an anterior disc dislocation that reduces, regarding the mechanism that caused the disc to dislocate. The disc, however, stays anterior to the condyle during all jaw movements because of an increase in muscle guarding of the mandibular elevator muscles and/or elongation of the superior stratum.

Symptoms

If painful, pain will be felt in the TMJ on the side of involvement with possible reference of pain into areas innervated by cranial nerve V. Pain increases during functional and parafunctional movements of the mandible.

Signs

In the initial stages (less than 6 months), joint noises will not be heard during mandibular movements. The mandibular opening will be less than functional opening (25 mm) with deflection to the side of involvement. Deflection to the side of involvement during protrusive mandibular movement will be seen, and lateral mandibular movement will be decreased to the opposite side of the involvement.

In the chronic stage (greater than 6 months), the disc has been "shoved" further anterior to the condyle. Mandibular dynamics will not be as restricted as was seen in the acute stage. However, joint noises of crepitus are present throughout full opening and closing.

Treatment

If pain or hindrance in function warrant treatment, apply manual intraoral techniques of distraction and translation to the involved side (Fig. 17-2). Once the disc is relocated on the condyle, usually confirmed by a "snap" and normal mandibular dynamics, place cotton rolls between the molars and proceed immediately with what was the treatment discussed for an anterior disc dislocation that reduces. If unsuccessful in relocating the disc and the pain or hindrance in function is significant to the patient and clinician, a nonrepositioning appliance or oral surgery is indicated.

Management

Once the disc is relocated on the condyle, management of the disc-condyle position is the same as for anterior disc dislocation that reduces.

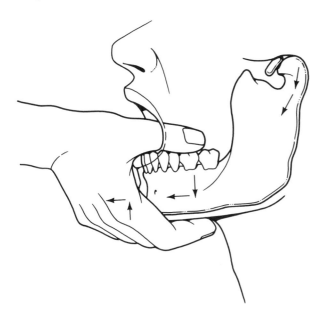

Fig. 17-2 Intraoral technique of distraction and translation used in an attempt to "recapture" an anterior disc dislocation that does not reduce. (Kraus S: Temporomandibular joint. In Saunders D: Evaluation, Treatment and Prevention of Musculoskeletal Disorders. Duane Saunders, Minneapolis, MN, 1985, with permission.)

Prognosis

Satisfactory to good

HYPOMOBILITY SECONDARY TO CAPSULAR TIGHTNESS

Capsular tightness is a result of the intermolecular cross-linking—adhesions of collagen fibers. A capsule may be partially or totally tight.

Causes

Capsular tightness may result from trauma, immobilization, and acute or chronic inflammatory processes.

Symptoms

If painful, the pain will be felt over the side of involvement with possible reference into areas innervated by cranial nerve V. Pain will increase during functional and parafunctional movements of the mandible.

Signs

If a complete capsular tightness is present, mandibular opening will be less than the functional opening with deflection to the side of involvement. Deflection to the side of involvement during protrusive mandibular movement will be seen, and lateral mandibular movement will be decreased to the opposite side of the involvement.

Treatment

Modalities to decrease pain and increase extensibility of the capsular tissue are offered. This may be accomplished with heat and ultrasound while tongue blades are placed intraorally. Intraoral arthrokinematic techniques are then applied to further enhance capsular extensibility (Fig. 17-3).

Management

Patient will need to be instructed in a home treatment program (heat and tongue blades) to maintain what capsular extensibility is accomplished during the treatment session. Capsular tightness resulting from acute or chronic inflammatory processes will require a prolonged management program.

Prognosis

Poor to excellent, depending on cause

HYPERMOBILITY (SUBLUXATION)

By agreement, subluxation is said to occur when the condyle moves anteriorly to the crest of the articular eminence onto the articular tubercle.

This condition occurs readily in an asymptomatic population. However, in the presence of other dysfunctional TMJ conditions, hypermobility may perpetuate the problem. Depending on the frequency and duration of subluxing, subluxation can cause pain and other TMJ dysfunctions.

Causes

Hypermobility is caused by predisposing osseous structures of the TMJ and capsular-ligamentous laxity.

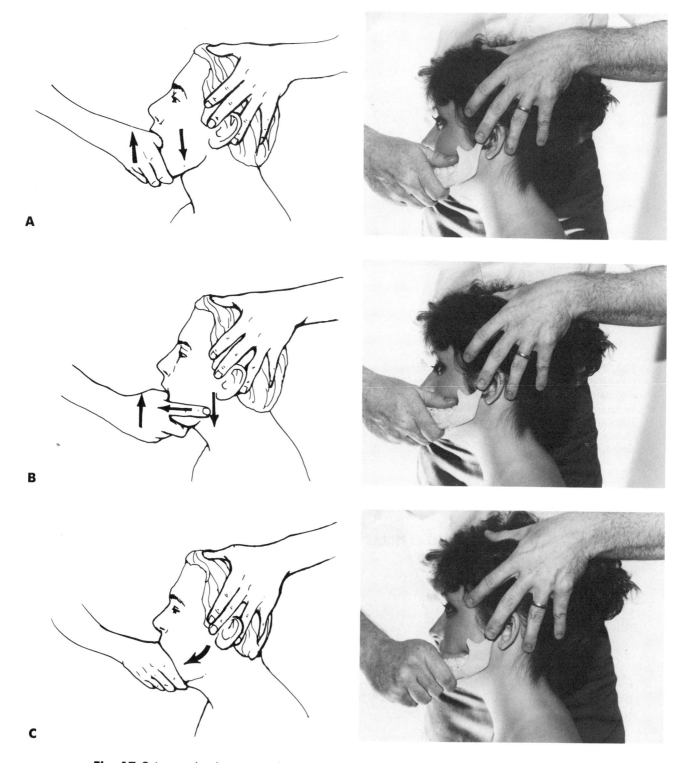

Fig. 17-3 Intraoral techniques used in the treatment of capsular tightness. Notice that techniques A and B are the same techniques used in the treatment of an anterior disc dislocation that does not reduce. The difference in the techniques is the range, amount, and duration of the force rendered. **(A)** Distraction. **(B)** Distraction with translation. **(C)** Lateral glide (joint play). (Kraus SL: Temporomandibular joint. In Saunders D: Evaluation, Treatment and Prevention of Musculoskeletal Disorders. Duane Saunders, Minneapolis, MN, 1985, with permission. Photos from Kraus SL: Physical Therapy Management of TMJ Dysfunction. p. 139. In: Kraus SL (ed): TMJ Disorders: Management of the Craniomandibular Complex. Churchill Livingstone, New York, 1988.)

Symptoms

If painful, pain will be over the TMJ on the involved side with possible reference of pain into areas innervated by cranial nerve V. Pain will increase or may only be present at the end of opening.

Signs

If subluxation occurs unilaterally, the mandible during opening will deflect abruptly to the opposite side of the involvement at the end of opening. At the beginning of closing, the mandible will abruptly swing back to midline.

Treatment

Educate the patient as to what point in jaw opening subluxation occurs. Treatment is to instruct the patient on exercises that will not open the mouth wide enough to produce the subluxation. Modalities such as heat, ice, and ultrasound will be beneficial if this condition is painful.

Management

Patient awareness and cooperation is essential.

Prognosis

Good to excellent

STRAIN

Any force through the mandible having sufficient repetitive impact, magnitude, duration, and direction can cause deformation of the pain-sensitive tissues such as the capsule, disc, and retrodiscal tissues.

Causes

Strain may be caused by micro- or macrotrauma with or without sufficient increase in muscle activity. Such trauma contributes to capsulitis and/or retrodiscal inflammation.

Symptoms

Pain occurs on the side of involvement in the area of the TMJ with possible reference of pain into areas innervated by cranial nerve V. Pain increases during functional and parafunctional movements of the mandible.

Signs

Patient may be hesitant to move the mandible because of pain. Depending on the degree of intracapsular edema, the patient may also be unable to bring his back teeth together on the side of involvement owing to the edema.

Treatment

Treatment consists of modalities to decrease pain and muscle guarding. Ice, heat, or ultrasound can be applied to the TMJ, depending on amount of edema present. Electric stimulation to the mandibular elevator muscles can help in muscle relaxation. If inflammation persist, a nonrepositioning appliance applied by the dentist may be beneficial.

Management

Management goals are to decrease inflammation and normalize muscle tone.

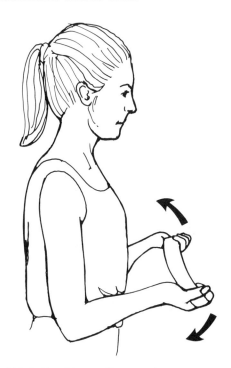

Fig. 17-4 Shoulder girdle strengthening excercise. This exercise helps to improve tone for the shoulder girdle external rotators and scapular retractor muscles. The starting position is holding an elastic tubing palms up, elbows to the side, and bent 90° with good head-neck posture. Patient is instructed to pinch the shoulder blades together slightly while externally rotating at the glenohumeral joint. The patient is asked to breathe out so he will not be holding his breath.

Prognosis

Good to excellent, in approximately 2 to 4 weeks depending on the magnitude of the trauma

MUSCLE IMBALANCE OF THE CERVICAL SPINE

The reader should not assume that muscle imbalances of the cervical spine are caused by TMJ dysfunction or vice versa. A brief overview of the management of cervical spine muscle imbalance is included here because of the frequently associated muscle hyperactivity and accompanying symptoms observed in both the mandibular and cervical spine areas. Mandibular and cervical spine muscle hyperactivity can occur in the absence of any TMJ involvement. When the TMJ is involved, however, treatment should always include the control of muscle hyperactivity. Clinical observations demonstrate that when cervical spine muscle imbalances are managed, more efficient control over mandibular muscle hyperactivity is often achieved. Therein lies the importance of considering muscle imbalances of the cervical spine in the management of the symptomatic TMJ. For a more detailed explanation of the cervical spine influencing the temporomandibular region, the reader is referred to Kraus SL: Cervical spine influences on the craniomandibular region. In Kraus SL (ed): *TMJ Disorders: Management of the Craniomandibular Complex*. Churchill Livingstone, New York, 1988.

The term muscle imbalance is referred to in this section as altered muscle tone, which is demonstrated by some muscles as an increase in tone, and in others as a decrease in tone. Muscle imbalances secondary to neurobiological and nutritional diseases and to trauma will not be a part of this discussion.

Clinically, a high percentage of muscle imbalances have an insidious onset. Trauma, of course, would further compound the pre-existing muscle imbalances. Muscle imbalances can involve other tissues of the spine such as the disc, facet joints, capsules, and nerves. Muscle imbalances and other tissue involvement (joints, disk, connective tissue) secondary to the muscle imbalances contribute to the altered afferent input to the central nervous system (CNS). Such altered afferent input to the

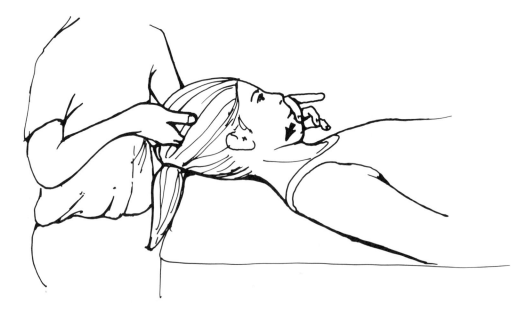

Fig. 17-5 Anterior cervical strengthening exercises. Patient is taught how to tuck the chin in. From this chin-tuck position the patient is asked to raise his head 4 to 6 inches off the table/floor. Pausing only slightly, the patient lowers his head to the mat, keeping the chin tucked in. It is important to inform the patient not to clench or hold his breath while doing the exercise.

SITTING - RISING

Chairs should have:
- wheels (if possible)
- unyielding straight back
- up/down adjustment of seat (if possible)

- low back support (Discuss with physical therapist.)
- armrests which do not prevent you from getting close to your work area.

- Reading material should be at eyelevel (if possible)
- **Do not look** down at your work by moving your head, neck, and shoulders forward. Look down by moving your head on your neck only.
- Keep chest up always.

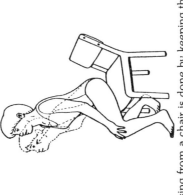

Correct position - solid; incorrect - dotted. Do not sit with head, neck, and shoulders forward.

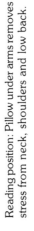

Reading position: Pillow under arms removes stress from neck, shoulders and low back.

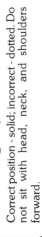

Rising from a chair is done by keeping the chest up (solid), and **NOT** with chest down (dotted).

Fig. 17-6 Chest awareness. Misuse of the cervical spine and associated muscles can easily occur during various daily movements and positions. A very simple, effective way for the patient to become more aware of proper movement and positioning of the cervical spine is to instruct the patient to maintain and initiate movement, keeping the chest up and chin slightly tucked in. This will be beneficial when getting up and down from a sitting position, standing or sitting, or during other functional activities involving head-neck positioning. (Kraus S: Cervical Spine Mobility. Stretching Charts Inc. Tacoma, WA, 1987, with permission.)

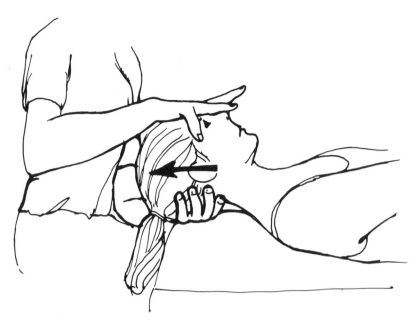

Fig. 17-7 Manual traction is a nonspecific traction applied to the cervical spine. The bottom hand placement is on the occiput so that the middle finger and thumb are "hooking" the mastoid processes. It is not advisable to pull through the mandible. The traction is applied along the longitudinal axis of the body. The poundage of pull using manual traction is immaterial. Instead, the amount is based on the patient and tissue(s) response.

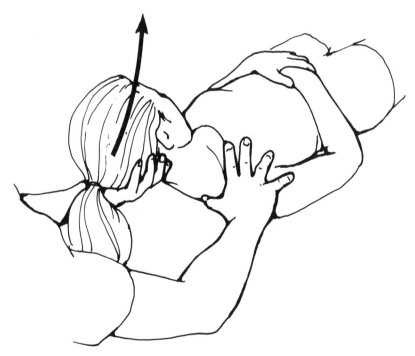

Fig. 17-8 "Upper arc" stretch. This technique is directed toward the posterior lateral cervical muscles and soft tissues. The active hand on the head supports the occiput, similar to the manual traction hold, and the other hand stabilizes the shoulder. The active hand will rotate the chin-nose away from the side of the stabilizing hand; at the same time the head-neck is taken into an up and forward diagonal direction. Care should be taken to avoid excessive side bending. Additional stretch can be achieved by the stabilizing hand pushing down on the shoulder. When areas of "tightness" are located, the stretch can be maintained or a hold relax contraction can be applied.

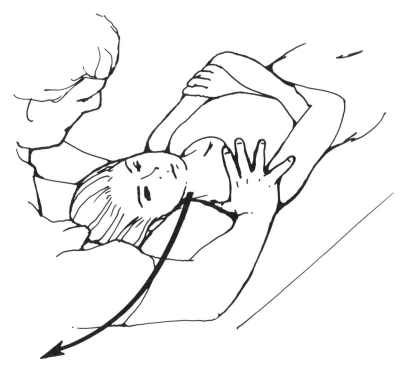

Fig. 17-9 "Lower arc" stretch. This technique is directed toward the anterior lateral cervical muscles and soft tissues. The active and stabilizing hands are the same as in Figure 17-8. The difference is that the active hand will rotate the chin-nose toward the side of the stabilizing hand, and at the same time the head-neck is taken into a down and back diagonal direction. Care should be taken to avoid excessive sidebending. When areas of "tightness" are located, the stretch can be maintained or a hold relax contraction can be applied.

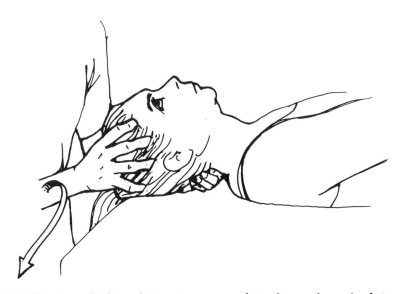

Fig. 17-10 "Melting" stretch. This technique is more specific to the muscles and soft tissues that are tight in the area of a segment. One hand cradles the neck, with the tip of the index finger making specific contact in an articular pillar of the cervical column. The active hand grasps the cranium. With moderate traction from both hands, the active hand directs the head into a down and back diagonal direction; allowing the chin-nose to rotate, side bend, and extend to the side of the index finger of the hand that is cradling the neck (the "melt").

CNS is believed to contribute to symptoms of the cervical spine and those referred to the head and upper extremities.

Symptoms can be extremely variable from patient to patient and within the same patient. Complaints of stiffness, tiredness, aching, tingling, numbness, vertigo, and nausea are all possible symptoms seen clinically that can respond well to the treatment of muscle imbalances and of the associated tissues of cervical spine dysfunction. The clinician will always be alert to the need for a medical consultation if such symptoms persist.

Causes

Muscle imbalances may be caused by misuse of cervical musculature by (1) occupational hazards; (2) lack of self-awareness during sitting, standing, and movements; (3) lack of specific exercises; (4) improper sleeping postures. Muscle imbalance may also result from emotional or environmental stressors.

Symptoms

Symptoms can be extremely variable but classically the patient will complain of tension-tightness, limitation in neck movement, and various referred pain to the head, upper extremities, and midback.

Signs

Posterior cervical/shoulder girdle muscle tone will be increased with associated myofascial trigger points as observed during palpation. Patient will often position his head classically in a forward head posture.

Treatment

Treatment modalities should be delivered to the tight musculature. The patient should be taught postural re-education exercises (Figs. 17-4 to 17-6). Manual therapy techniques are applied to the tight muscle and soft tissues (Figs. 17-7 to 17-10). Cervical and lumbar supports are provided as needed.

Management

Once the patient has been given freedom of movement (better mobility of muscle, soft tissue, joints) in the cervical spine and correct instructions on how to maintain better muscle function through exercises and supports, and if the patient has the opportunity or creates the opportunity to follow through with exercises, then management is often the patient's responsibility. Because of the various environmental and emotional stresses we are all faced with, periodic re-evaluation and treatment by the therapist is suggested.

Prognosis

Good to excellent

18 Extremity Dysfunction: Principles of Management

Catherine E. Patla

Joint movement is more easily examined in the extremities than in the spine; as a result, more attention can be paid to subleties of movements such as accessory motion and joint play. Additionally, the technique of extremity manipulation is somewhat different from the nonthrust stretch techniques that are more commonly used on the spine. These will be more fully explained below (see Classification of Extremity Joint Motion). Also, the evaluation of the extremities takes a slightly different form, which is presented here (see Extremity Evaluation, below). One topic important to extremity evaluation, but omitted from the evaluation of the spine, is end feel.

CLASSIFICATION OF EXTREMITY JOINT MOTION

Examination Movements

Examination movements are those that may be examined by the clinician to detect the presence of joint dysfunction.

Classical Movements

Classical movements are those movements that form the more traditional description of movement and that can be measured by the goniometer, for example, cardinal plane movements.

Active Joint Movements

Active joint movements are those motions that take place within the joint as a result of voluntary muscle action.

Passive Joint Movements

Passive joint movements are those motions in which a joint is passively moved through a range of motion by the therapist. They are used to contrast with active motion and to determine the nature of resistance at the end of the range (see end feel).

Accessory Movements

Those motions that accompany (are accessory to) the classical movements and are essential to normal full range and painless function are called accessory movements.

Joint Play Motions

Joint play motions are movements not under voluntary control that occur only in response to an outside force. Examples are diverse and include the additional passive range that exists at the end of all active ranges and such actions as the forward glide of the distal tibia and fibula on the talus during heel strike.

The therapist can use these motions to detect the joint's ability to relieve and absorb extrinsic forces.

Component Motions

Component motions take place in a joint complex or related joint to facilitate a particular active motion. For instance, with glenohumeral external rotation there is an associated anterior glide of the humeral head; with knee extension there is an associated anterior glide of the tibia.

Component motions may be used to detect those dysfunctions in the joint complex or related joint that may be interfering with active motion.

End Feel

End feel is that sense of resistance to motion at the end of range that is identified by the examiner when imparting to the joint either a classical or accessory movement. During manipulation, the end feel is constantly monitored for its response to treatment and its transition from abnormal to normal.

Since a joint can be moved actively (classical movement) only in a limited number of directions, and yet must in daily use perform in an infinite number of directions (accessory motion), the directions in which end feels can be tested are also infinite. Practically speaking, therefore, the test is confined to the classical directions of active movement and to some selected accessory motions, depending on the individual patient's perceived joint needs.

Normal End Feels

Soft tissue approximation
    The joint feels soft and spongy, for example, elbow or knee flexion
Muscular
    Elastic reflex resistance with discomfort, for example, straight leg raising or frontal abduction of the shoulder
Ligamentous
    Firm arrest of movement with no give or creep (creep is a time-dependent phenomenon), for example, abduction of the extended knee
Cartilaginous
    Sudden stop but not hard, for example, extension of the elbow
Capsular
    Firm arrest of movement with a slight creep, for example, hyperextension at the elbow

Abnormal End Feels

Capsular
    Abnormal creep resistance
    Proportionate in a characteristic pattern
      (1) chronic inflammatory—harsh, tight arrest
      (2) acute inflammatory—painful with induced muscle guarding

Adhesions and scarring
    Sudden sharp arrest in one direction, for example, common at the inferior aspect of the glenohumeral joint
Bony block
    Sudden hard stop short of normal range, for example, myositis ossificans or fracture within a joint
Bony grate
    Roughing, grating, for example, advanced chondromalacia
Springy rebound
    Slight bouncing back, rebound, for example, luxated meniscus at the knee
Pannus
    Soft crunchy squelch, for example, common at elbow extension
Loose
    Ligamentous laxity, for example, second-degree ligament injury, rheumatoid
Empty
    Boggy, soft, not limited mechanically, for example, synovitis, haemarthrosis
Painful
    Considerable report of pain before end range is reached, for example, end feel is thus lacking in resistance other than the patient's protective or evoked splinting. Suspect neoplasm abscess.
Muscle
    Abnormal elastic resistance, for example, muscle guarding, contracture

Treatment Movements

Manipulation

Manipulation is the skilled passive movement of a joint. In this regard it is different from *range of motion*, which relates to the movement of limbs (osteokinematics) and not to the movement of joints (arthrokinematics).

Experienced manipulators have at their discretion a great variety of methods. The most commonly used techniques in the extremities include the following.

Graded Oscillations

Grade I. Small oscillatory motion at the beginning of range. Effect is principally neurophysiological.

Grade II. Larger oscillatory motion in the middle of joint range. Effect is principally neurophysiological.

Grade III. Large-amplitude motion going up against the end of available range. Effect is neurophysiological with some crude mechanical effects.

Grade IV. Small amplitude of motion at the end of available range. Effect is neurophysiological and if applied along the joint plane or at right angles to it, it is a mechanical effect as well.

Progressive Oscillations

Here a series of oscillations is given at increasing depths, or with increasing pressure against the end feel or barrier. This has an effective mechanical effect with some neurophysiological effects.

Sustained Stretch

Sustained stretch is one of the more common methods in which the barrier is engaged and a steady force is applied and maintained for 2 to 10 seconds. It has mostly a mechanical effect.

Intermittent Stretch

Perhaps the most common technique of all is the application of a stretch to the barrier that is alternately applied for 1 second, released for 1 second, and then applied again three to ten times. This stretch is principally mechanical with some comforting neurophysiological effects.

Distraction

Traction is a force applied to a limb. Only if it is delivered to a joint at right angles to its plane and while in the loose-pack position will distraction result.

Distraction I. A very slight traction force is applied to barely unweight the joint surfaces.

Distraction II. The articular surfaces are distracted until the slack of the capsule is engaged.

Distraction III. The capsule is stretched by one of the above stretch techniques.

Steps of the Extremity Evaluation

1. Pain assessment
2. Initial observation
3. History & interview
4. Structural inspection–position
5. Palpation for–condition
6. Joint active range
7. Joint passive range and end feel
8. Muscle selective tissue tension
9. Muscle length and myofascia
10. Muscle strength
11. Special tests
12. Movement analysis
13. Palpation for–tenderness
14. Neuromuscular & neurovascular
15. Radiological
16. Assessment
17. Treatment plan
18. Explanation and prognosis

COMMON EXTREMITY DYSFUNCTIONS

Capsule Restriction

Capsule restriction is caused by an alteration of the collagen fibers or water content of the connective tissue of the capsule that results in functional loss of movement actively and passively.

Causes

Restriction occurs with nonspecific trauma to capsule, for example, bursitis, tendinitis, postfracture, postimmobilization, or with joint strains followed by end ranges of joint, active or passive movements, not carried out functionally.

Symptoms

There is some loss of functional active motions in all the joint movements.

Pain may be reported at end range of all the joint movements.

Signs

Active and passive motions are limited in same directions. Active and passive movements follow a particular pattern of restriction. Patterns are specific for each joint (see particular joint).

Pain comes on as active or passive end ranges are approached.

End range resistance is an abnormal firm creep resistance.

All passive accessory motions are limited; amount of limitation is relative to the classical passive motions.

Treatment

Manipulate accessory motions.

Use modalities, such as diathermy, ultrasound, and moist heat, for maintaining the lengthened capsule. Moist heat is preferred only if the capsule is minimally covered by dense connective tissue, for example, fingers or toes.

Management

Tendinitis and bursitis are often present with a tight capsule. Treat the tendinitis and bursitis to the level of low reactivity or moderate reactivity before treating capsule for mechanical effects (grades III, IV, or prolonged stretch).

Address posture and functional movements within achieved active range by patient education and advancement of home program.

Gradually begin to strengthen surrounding muscles, once active range has been improving progressively for approximately 4 weeks after manipulation and once proper posture can be maintained.

Identify the occupational and functional stresses that may be contributing to capsule irritation.

Given the event of capsule trauma and subsequent inability to move the joint through the full ranges of motion, compensations of muscles and other joint positioning are likely to ensue. Pay attention to evaluating and treating compensations over a long period of time.

A long-standing tight capsule or a highly reactive joint may take several months to treat. As long as the range of motion and function gains are observed, then therapy is warranted. A home program of stretching is necessary. After 4 to 6 months, strong stretching, designed to cause the connective tissue elements to yield, may be employed.

When range of motion, both active and passive, and function have plateaued, then manipulation treatments must be stopped as further passive stretching may stimulate the connective tissues such that further proliferation tightening occurs (Wolf's Law of Connective Tissue Response to Stimulus). Should this be the case, the patient is placed on a home program of maintaining pain free movement within the range while avoiding stressing the end range.

Prognosis

The last 5° to 10° of movement of all planes may be limited and subjectively described as a pulling *restriction* during functional activities. This range may be the goal of treatment.

Capsule Instability

Capsule instability exists once the connective tissue of the capsule has been taken to the yielding (or necking) point.

Causes

A force or direct trauma placed on a joint either near or at the joint's close-pack position or excessive distractive or rotary stress placed on the joint near its end range may cause capsule instability.

Symptoms

Joint is unstable in functional position or movements.

Signs

Specific classical and accessory motions are hypermobile, and the patient adopts a compensatory posture.

Treatment

Stabilize by taping or use of an assistive device. Strengthen musculature supporting the joint. Educate the patient in posture and occupational, functional, and sport activities to avoid positions and stresses at which the joint is vulnerable to further hypermobility, subluxation, or dislocation.

Management

Patients may require long-term follow-up for continued assessment of home program.

Prognosis

The prognosis is fair to excellent depending on patient's ability to avoid unstable positions of the joint.

Tendonitis

Over-stress situations may result in swelling of a tendon. The presence of swelling, and then adhesion formation, is believed to interfere with the normal tendon fiber gliding during muscle contraction, which then leads to decreased range of motion and pain.

Tendons have very poor corollary blood supply compared with that of other soft tissues. Under conditions of over-stress, the tendon is vulnerable to sprain injury with perhaps subsequent poor healing because of the insufficient blood supply.

Causes

Occupational, functional, or sport over-stress
Over-stress to tendon brought on by either strength or endurance weakness of the primary muscle or surrounding musculature
Tight muscles or tight capsule
Bony impingement
Poor posture
Poor body mechanics

Symptoms

Pain on active motion
Highly reactive conditions show pain at rest

Signs

Active motion reproduces pain in particular movements. Active movements are painful in the direction of the anatomical functioning of the tendon. A painful arc may be observed, especially if the tendon is being mechanically impinged.

Passive stretching of the tendon reproduces pain. Full passive motion should exist.

Resisted isometric contraction produces patient's complaint of pain yet otherwise demonstrates normal strength. This is the most reliable sign.

Palpation may reproduce pain, but not all tendons can be specifically palpated.

Treatment

Transverse friction massage
Use of modalities to decrease inflammation, such as ultrasound, iontophoresis, phonophoresis, interferential and high-voltage stimulation
Stretching exercises to tendon and muscle followed by specific strengthening of muscle tendon involved
Educate in posture and body mechanics
Stretch tight myofascia
Strengthen weak muscle
Manipulate restricted accessory motions

Management

Transverse friction massage treatment should be effective in treating tendinitis by the third or fourth treatment session. A decrease of symptoms and improvement of functional active movements can be observed after the first treatment session. If the changes are not occurring, than any or all of the following are at fault: (1) the treatment is being carried out inappropriately; (2) functional, occupational, or sport stresses remain; (3) any of the original causes persist.

Prognosis

Excellent
Poor for bony impingement

Ligamentous Sprain

Biomechanically, ligaments sprain under sustained load much sooner than the capsule or muscle. Once a yield or sprain has occurred, ligamentous laxity may result. Additionally, the strain that injured the ligaments may have resulted in intra-articular serofibrinous exudate and thus result in the formation of adhesions that will alter mechanics and affect range.

Causes

Too much strain leading to sprain, as in occupational, functional, or sport-related activities

Symptoms

Pain, particularly with sustained static loading
Altered active motion
With laxity, leg or arm giving way under sustained loading

Signs

For restriction (or scarring):
   Limited active and passive motion
   Passive accessory motions are limited,
      especially joint play
For laxity:
   Joint instability exists in classical and accessory
      passive motions
   Active motion may or may not demonstrate
      instability

Treatment

For restriction:
   Transverse friction massage
   Use of heat modalities
   Manipulate accessory motion(s) restrictions
   Instruction of home stretching exercises
   Postural and body mechanics education
   Education for occupational and functional po-
      sitioning and perhaps support of extremity
      for a stressful activity
For laxity:
   Stabilize by assistive device(s), if necessary
   Postural and body mechanics education
   Education for occupational and functional po-
      sitioning and movement
   Muscle strengthening and endurance training

Management

Make certain that the patient understands the activities that require use of assistive devices and those activities that should be avoided under conditions of ligamentous laxity. Weekly assessment is necessary as the patient regains the ability to perform more strenuous daily and functional activities.

Prognosis

For restriction, the prognosis is dependent on the nature of the restriction in regard to the scarring or the amount of damage that has occurred with the sprain.

For laxity, there is a moderate to excellent prognosis if the joint can be stabilized during activities that place stress on the joint. A poor prognosis exists when either the assistive device or the muscle strength and endurance cannot be maintained during functional or sports activities.

Bursitis

Bursae are vulnerable to over-stress and subsequent swelling owing to their anatomical presence at joints and between tendons or muscles. Too often a diagnosis is made as "bursitis" without a thorough evaluation to differentiate among bursa, tendon, or muscle dysfunction and without sufficient attention given to identifying the cause of the irritation.

Causes

Occupational, functional, or sport over-use; tight, weak, or fatigued muscles; tight capsules; bony impingement; structural asymmetries; poor posture; or poor body mechanics may all contribute.

Symptoms

Active motion is painful or limited.

Highly reactive conditions may cause pain at rest, especially with pressure placed on the bursa, as in side lying (with the shoulder bursa compressed).

Signs

Active motion may show painful arc. Active motion produces pain in particular movements. Limitation of functional movement is in the direction of either anatomical compression by a bony impingement or compression via tendon, muscle, or fascia plane.

Passive motion, which compresses bursa through soft tissue pulling or approximation, may reproduce the pain.

Resisted isometric contraction may produce pain in a highly reactive condition.

Deep palpation for provocation on the bursa reproduces the symptoms of pain and is the best differential sign.

Treatment

Modalities that may be useful to decrease the inflammation are ultrasound, interferential, iontophoresis, or phonophoresis.

Educate the patient in posture, body mechanics, and stresses to avoid.

Stretch tight muscles and myofascia, strengthen weak muscles, and manipulate tight capsule.

Management

Given that the cause of the inflammation has been eliminated, in three to four treatment sessions the symptoms should be decreasing and functional gains should be showing. Physiologically and scientifically, the use of modalities has not shown unequivocal success in diminishing or eliminating "calcium deposits." Clinical success has often been reported.

Prognosis

Excellent

Adhesions

Physiologically, adhesions originate from swelling resulting from an accumulation of serofibrinous exudate, present from either joint or soft tissue damage. Adhesions may form within 72 hours of injury and may remain vascular up until the seventh to the tenth day. Adhesions have the potential to become thicker and larger as exudates are allowed to accumulate.

Causes

Sprains to joint or periarticular structures may cause adhesions.

Symptoms

Painful restrictions are felt in one direction of active movement.

Signs

Active and passive classical motions are limited in the same (one) direction.

Accessory passive motion is limited in the same directions corresponding to the passive classical motion.

End range resistance is a firm arrest of movement short of normal range. No creep is present.

Treatment

After initial trauma, keep joint actively moving within pain-free range. Manipulation is performed after 10 days of tolerated active motion.

Management

Following manipulation, the joint must be kept moving functionally within the range of comfort.

Prognosis

The prognosis is excellent.

Intra-Articular Fluid

After trauma to a joint, swelling of a synovitic nature is observed any time from 30 minutes to several hours after injury. By contrast, hemarthrosis is detected by observable swelling almost immediately following the injury.

Causes

Sprain may induce collection of intra-articular fluid.

Symptoms

Throbbing sensations may be reported. Patients may report feeling of warmth. Haemarthrosis is considered more painful than synovitis.

Signs

Active range of motion is limited.

Passive classical motion is not limited mechanically. If synovitic, passive movements are quite free and painless. If hemarthritic, passive movements are sluggish and uncomfortable.

Normal muscle strength may be inhibited.

Swelling is palpable and often observable.

Treatment

Reduce the fluid state by placing ice on the injury for a short time (10 minutes maximal); elevate and compress by wrapping. Modalities such as interferential or high-volt stimulation may be useful.

Eliminate stresses from joint (for example, weight-bearing, muscle contraction).

Management

Given a history and joint observations that suggest haemarthrosis, consultation with a physician should be sought.

Muscle strengthening (isotonics and isokinetics) should not be started until fluid state has been eliminated. Isometrics should be performed if the isometric contraction is pain free.

If haemarthritic, full range motions should not be attempted for 10 days for fear of rupturing adhesions while they are still vascular, resulting in further interstitial or intra-articular bleeding.

Prognosis

The prognosis is excellent once the stress of trauma and the cause of swelling have been removed and all other stresses (weight bearing, muscle contraction) have been carefully monitored and controlled.

Extra-Articular Fluid

After trauma to periarticular structures, swelling occurs at the site of trauma.

Causes

Functional, occupational, or sport activities may induce production of extra-articular fluid.

Symptoms

Minimal, moderate, or high reactive level of pain may be present depending on degree of injury. Patients may report a throbbing sensation and limitation of functional activities.

Signs

Either active or passive classical motions may be limited depending on the structure injured.

Observable and palpable swelling occurs at the site of injury. Swelling may be diffuse and therefore may be observed or palpated at locations other than at the original area of injury.

Joint or periarticular structures may feel warm.

Treatment
Ice, elevation, compression
Interferential or high-voltage stimulation or both
Intermittent Compression
Conventional massage
Eliminate stresses (weight bearing, movement, muscle contraction)

Management

Avoid placing stresses on injured structures, i.e., weight bearing, muscle contraction. Allow 10 days rest for minimal injury and up to 3 weeks rest for healing of tears.

Prognosis

Excellent once stress of trauma has been removed and all other stresses have been carefully monitored.

Osteoarthrosis

Osteoarthrosis is degeneration of hyaline cartilage.

Causes
Poor posture
Occupational or functional stresses, sport trauma
Obesity
Intra-articular fracture

Symptoms
Painful active movements
Stiffness in joints with static positioning

Signs
Active motion limitation with moderate to advanced conditions; otherwise, full range of motion exists
Range of motion painful
Painful weight bearing under sustained static loads in moderate to advanced states
Limited passive classical motion owing to pain
Limited accessory passive motion
End range resistance has a quality of grating or roughness

Treatment
Eliminate joint stresses (weight, poor posture, and stressful occupational, functional, and sport activities)
Reduce stresses on the joint by stretching tight muscles, fascia, and capsule
Maintain active motion by stationary bicycling at low resistance
Use of shoe cushions to decrease weight-bearing stresses
Use of a cane to take some stress off the lower extremity joints

Management

Long-term follow-up is important to monitor anatomical and everyday stresses while evaluating status of home program.

Prognosis

Present studies show that continuous passive motion and treatment that results in a redistribution of forces can replace worn-out hyaline with fibrous cartilage.

Bony Impingement

In bony impingement, joint mobility is limited owing to either periosteal approximation or loose bodies within the joint.

Causes

Postfracture with subsequent callus formation
Trauma resulting in bone chip or loose bodies

Symptoms

Limitation of end range of motion with or
without pain

Signs

Limited active and passive classical and accessory
motions
End feel is hard and range of motion is short of
normal

Treatment

Reduction of the loose body by manipulation
No other possible conservative treatment

Management

Patient education to maintain available range
and adopt good postures to prevent muscle
and capsule restriction.

Prognosis

Poor for achieving full motion and function

Peripheral Nerve Entrapment

Many peripheral nerves are vulnerable to impingement somewhere along their anatomical routes. The impingement may be due to osseous canal narrowing, bony compression, muscle, tendon, or fascia approximation, or postural compression. Ischemic reactions can occur from these impingements leading to pain, parasthesia, and motor or sensory deprivation or loss.

Causes
Postfracture
Postimmobilization
Occupational, functional, sport over-stress
Poor posture
Poor body mechanics
Pregnancy
Obesity

Symptoms
Functional loss of active motion
Specific or nonspecific location of pain
Numbness or diminished loss of sensation
Weakness of muscle strength

Signs
Diminished or lost motor or sensory changes
Restricted active motion
Restricted classical and accessory passive motions
Tight muscles
Tight fascia
Tight capsule
Poor posture
Structural asymmetries
Swelling of periarticular structures or joint

Treatment
Treat dysfunctions identified, such as
  Manipulate restricted accessory motions
  Stretch tight muscles and fascia
  Use of modalities for swelling, such as
    ultrasound, iontophoresis, phonophoresis,
    interferential, high voltage stimulation,
    and cryotherapy
  Use of modalities for pain, such as
    transcutaneous electrical nerve stimulation
    (TENS), interferential, high voltage
    stimulation, cryotherapy, and compression
    of joint (by taping or wrapping)
  Educate in posture, body mechanics, reduction
    of over-stressful activities, and positions

Management

Evaluation and treatment may aggravate symptoms at first, but the increase of symptoms suggests that the cause is being addressed. Look for a gradual improvement in functional activities. If paresthesia exists, the positive effect of treatment will be a reduction in the parasthesia before motor changes improve. Further consultation with a physician may be necessary if motor changes do not improve.

Prognosis

The prognosis depends on the amount of damage to the nerve caused by the compression and swelling. The prognosis is better the sooner the compression or swelling can be eliminated.

Meniscal Impingement

The exact pathophysiology of meniscal impingement is unknown, but it is speculated that the mobility of the meniscus is impaired owing to a present or past history of swelling from either trauma or surgery or that the mobility is decreased secondary to an abnormal postural position. The condition is most common at the knee and may also occur at the head of the radius in a small population. Impingements of the meniscus may occur secondary to sprains or strains of the joint capsule, tears of the meniscus, or loose bodies in the joint.

Causes

Meniscus is entrapped by adhesion formation resulting from swelling or caused by an awkward postural position or movement.

Symptoms

Nonspecific location of pain
Nonspecific or specific position of joint that brings on pain
Functional loss of movement somewhere within the range of motion
Present or past history of joint swelling

Signs

Active and passive classical motions may be painfully limited in the same direction. Many times the active and passive classical motions may not be limited, especially with low reactive conditions.

End range resistance is most distinguishing as the differential evaluation sign. End range resistance has a springy rebound quality.

Palpable intra-articular swelling may be present.

Treatment

Manipulate in direction of restricted accessory motion.

Management

Discuss functional and occupational stresses that may have caused condition.

Prognosis

Excellent unless a tear of meniscus exists or a loose body is present in the joint.

Decreased Mobility of Fat Pad

Fat pads function to cushion soft tissue and protect joint margins. Many fat pads are attached to the capsule and function to protect the capsule during active movements.

Causes

Trauma leading to intra-articular or extra-articular swelling that then leads to adhesion formation around or within fat pads
Tight capsule as a result of trauma or immobilization

Symptoms

Decreased functional mobility
Frequent muscle sprains or tendonitis

Signs

Possible decrease in active motion
Possible pain at end range of active motion that either stretches or compresses the meniscus
Classical and accessory motions produce pain at end range of motion that either compresses or stretches the fat pad
End range resistance of a soft and crunchy squelch

Treatment

Manipulate fat pad
Manipulate capsule if tight
Stretch tight muscles

Management

Given that each synovial joint has at least one muscle that attaches to the capsule, these muscles may be useful to help move the fat pad via a pull on the capsule.

Prognosis

Excellent

Postfracture

Bones normally heal in 6 to 8 weeks.

Causes

Direct trauma

Symptoms

Decreased functional mobility
Joint stiffness
Possible pain on weight bearing
Coordination loss

Signs

Possible decrease in classical and accessory motions
Possible joint capsule tightness, intra-articular adhesions, muscle contracture, hard end feel short of normal
Possible muscle weakness
Possible gait deviations

Treatment

If normal healing occurs, at 6 weeks vigorous manipulation is appropriate for tight capsule or adhesions if patient can tolerate
Muscle re-education, gait re-education

Management

Movement is important as soon as possible postimmobilization.

Prognosis

The prognosis is excellent, especially when joint structures have not been involved in the trauma and normal healing of bone has occurred. Callus formation may limit goals of active and passive range of motion and gait changes may ensue.

Pain

In a highly reactive condition, pain may limit all ranges of movement actively and passively and may limit the therapist's ability to perform a differential evaluation. In this situation, the therapist may not be able to identify any one particular dysfunction.

Causes

Varied physical or emotional disruptive events
Mechanical or chemical stimuli

Symptoms

Subjective report of amount and intensity of pain

Signs

Inability to identify a particular dysfunction because of pain with the joint evaluation, muscle evaluation, ligamentous evaluation, and movement and gait evaluation

Treatment

Grade I and II oscillations in osteokinematic or arthrokinematic movements
Heat, cold, electrical stimulation, TENS, or biofeedback

Management

If after four treatment sessions the level of reactivity has not decreased and the therapist still cannot identify and treat any one particular dysfunction, then further medical consultation must be sought.

Prognosis

Once physical or emotional stresses have decreased, prognosis is excellent to begin treatment of a particular dysfunction.

Myofascial Tightness

Myofascial tightness occurs when mobility of myofibers on one another is impaired or the connective tissue mobility within the fascial plane is impaired.

Causes
Poor posture
Occupational or functional sprains or strains
Extra-articular fluid

Symptoms
Nonspecific feeling of body tightness or stiffness
Incidence of soft tissue or joint injuries with
  stressful activities

Signs
Active or passive classical or accessory motions
  limited
Palpable abnormal firmness of muscle in fascial
  planes
Altered smoothness of rhythm of active motion,
  particularly with repetitive movements
Postural changes

Treatment
Massage and stretching
Postural education
Active exercises and stretching exercises

Management
Pay attention to joint strains that may occur from
  stretching exercises

Prognosis
Excellent

Muscle Injury

Muscle injuries, just like any other soft tissue
injuries, are manifested in various forms. Overuse
conditions may be reported as soreness the day
after performing a running activity. Moderate to
major strains may exist in which contraction of a
muscle continues to be painful for several days
after activity. Specific identification of the muscle
involved and the strength and endurance deficit,
along with the patient's functional needs, is essential to proper education, treatment, and management.

Causes
Over-stress in occupational, functional, and sport
  activities
Direct trauma

Symptoms
Decrease of functional activities
Painful movement or lack of movement

Signs
Active joint motion decreased, particularly at end
  ranges
Passive classical motion not limited
Passive stretching of muscle may reproduce
  discomfort
Resisted isometric contraction is the best
  differential (selective tissue tension)
Strength deficits
Endurance deficits
Reflex changes
Sensory changes
Swelling
Palpation for condition may identify any of the
  following: firmness of muscle, tenderness of
  muscle, gap in muscle

Treatment
Over-stress as in "weekend warrior sprains":
  Rest from activity from 1 to 2 days
  Transverse friction massage or conservative
    massage
  Isometric and gentle isotonic contractions
  Gradual movements, such as with a quadriceps
    sprain, continued walking but avoiding
    hills, ramps, and stairs
Minor to moderate strains:
  Rest from activity for 1 to 2 weeks after injury,
    continue active motion within pain-free
    range of motion
  If after 2 weeks active range of motion is full
    and pain free, then begin gentle
    progressive muscle strengthening
  Resume gradual vigorous exercises in
    moderation
Major strains:
  Supportive or assistive device, non-weight
    bearing for 3 weeks, no active range of
    motion for 3 weeks, but institute isometric
    contractions several times during the day
  Begin active or active assistive joint range of
    motion after 3 weeks of rest. When active
    range of motion is full and pain free,
    begin gradual progressive isotonics and
    increased weight bearing.

Transverse friction massage and conventional massage may be useful after the 3 weeks of immobilization.

Partial tear:

Immobilization for 3 to 5 weeks for healing

Begin active–assistive range of motion and passive exercises; gradually go into active movements and only in pain-free positions

Begin isotonics and progressive resistive exercises as tolerated but in moderation

Complete tear:

Physician management is essential. The medical decision may be to avoid surgical repair of the tear and to work with physical therapy. Education and training to a muscle or muscle group to assist in compensation for the injured muscle is a possible approach.

Management

Given the event of muscle trauma and subsequent need to rest or immobilize muscle, compensation of other muscles or joint positioning is likely to ensue. Pay attention to evaluating or treating compensations over a long period of time.

Prognosis

If no more damage has occurred, the prognosis is excellent, but with a partial to complete tear, rehabilitation may require a minimum of 6 months to almost 2 years for full recovery.

Muscle Contracture

Loss of sarcomere number is the physiological problem with pathologically shortened muscles.

Causes

Contracture is often caused by muscle immobilization secondary to events such as fracture, intra-articular, extra-articular, or periarticular structural damage.

Symptoms

Restricted active motion and decreasing functional loss are seen.

Signs

Active and passive motions are limited in the same direction to almost the same degree.

End range resistance is firm stop; no rebounding resistance is felt at end range, which is common with normal muscle extensibility.

Treatment

Static stretching for a minimum of 20 minutes in a lengthened position and massage to muscle fibers.

Management

Serial splinting or casting is useful to maintain static stretch, particularly during hours when resting at home. Patient may need to build up to 20 minutes time, depending on level of reactivity. Maintaining the static stretch for several hours at a time is desirable. Resplinting or casting at acquired new range is the management goal. Only begin strengthening program once a plateau has been reached in muscle length gains.

Prognosis

The prognosis is fair to excellent depending on the presence of scarring, adhesion, and the patient's tolerance to static stretch.

19

Upper Extremity

Catherine E. Patla

SHOULDER—GLENOHUMERAL JOINT

Capsule Tightness

Capsule tightness of the shoulder has been frequently termed "frozen shoulder." The term is not a diagnosis but rather a description of the limitation presented by the patient's lack of functional use. Scientific evidence in the areas of pathology, physiology, and epidemiology has not established definitive cause and effect relationships for the clinical problems. Retrospective studies investigating this clinical problem have shown that capsule dysfunction predominantly occurs in women 50 years of age and older who have sustained various types of injuries to the shoulder, from a noninvasive strain to a more serious trauma such as a fracture or dislocation.

Causes

Nonspecific trauma to capsule, for example, bursitis, tendonitis, postfracture, postimmobilization

Joint strains followed by end ranges of joint not being carried out either actively or passively

Immobilization of the shoulder from either fracture or subluxation/dislocation

Symptoms

Some loss of functional active movements in all joint movements but particularly in external rotation

Discomfort at end range of all joint movements

Signs

Active and passive classical motions are limited in the same direction. The pattern of restriction is as follows: greatest limitation of external rotation, less limitation of abduction, and least limitation of internal rotation. Scapular mobility is often not restricted.

Pain occurs as active and passive end ranges are approached.

Accessory movements are limited in all directions, especially anterior and inferior glides.

End range resistance of classical and accessory motions has an abnormal creep resistance.

Muscle tightness exists.

Treatment

Manipulate restricted accessory motions. The directions of movements are lateral distraction, anterior glide, posterior glide, and inferior glide. Use of rate of the movement will depend on operator's intent as to the desired effect of the treatment and on the reactivity level of the patient (Figs. 19-1 to 19-4).

Patients are instructed in home program of self-mobilization or isometric manipulation to coincide with the arthrokinematic movements performed under treatment.

Muscle tightness may exist, particularly of internal rotators (teres major, subscapularis, and latissimus dorsi), pectoralis group, levator scapula, and scaleni group. The patient may require manual stretching of these muscles and/or may be placed on a home program.

For maintaining the lengthened capsule, use modalities such as diathermy, ultrasound, or moist heat (moist heat is preferable only if the capsule is minimally covered by dense connective tissue such as is found in the fingers or toes).

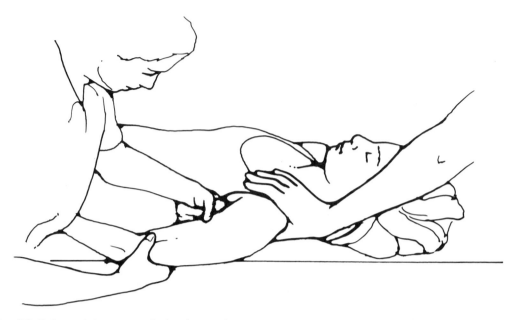

Fig. 19-1 Lateral distraction of glenohumeral joint. *Patient:* Supine. The arm is positioned in approximately 30° of abduction on the table. *Therapist:* Standing. One hand contacts the distal humerus to stabilize it, and one hand contacts the proximal medial aspect of the humerus. An assistant contacts the proximal clavicle and scapula to stabilize them. *Technique:* The proximal hand exerts a lateral force. *Use:* A joint play necessary for all glenohumeral motions.

Management

Refer to management section under the general category of capsule tightness in Chapter 18.

Prognosis

Refer to prognosis section under the general category of capsule tightness in Chapter 18.

Capsule Instability

Capsule instability after trauma typically occurs to the anterior aspect of the capsule. Anterior capsule instability is often caused by trauma occurring when the arm is positioned in abduction and external rotation. The capsule is especially vulnerable at the end ranges of these positions. Capsule instability, in the presence of subluxation or dislocation, is often present after a neurovascular accident, that is, a stroke. The capsule instability occurs very early after the neurological insult. The result often is that the glenohumeral superior ligaments become unstable owing to lack of adequate muscle tone to maintain the scapula in a neutral position. In particularly, the rhomboids lose adequate strength and endurance. Once the scapula has rotated either upward or downward, the superior glenohumeral ligaments become vulnerable to over-stretching. The shape of the rib cage may predispose the rotation direction. The patient's position when sitting and using an armrest that is at an inappropriate height may also contribute to ligament stretching. The patient with neurological injury also requires adequate shoulder complex stability when assuming upright positions. Management is required to maintain a neutral scapular position for these patients.

Causes

Force or direct trauma placed on a joint either near or at the joint's close-pack position or excessive distractive or rotary stress placed on the joint

Symptoms

Unstable joint in functional position or movements

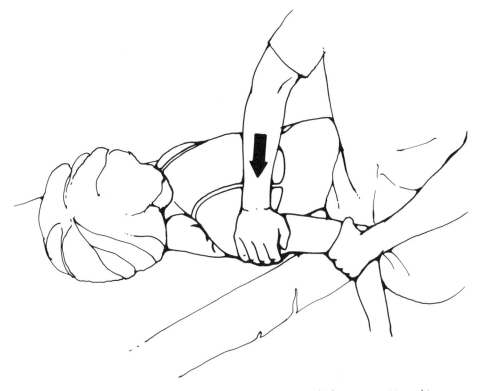

Fig. 19-2 Anterior glide of glenohumeral joint. *Patient:* Prone with the arm positioned in approximately 30° of abduction on the table. A folded towel is placed on the anterior aspect of the clavicle and chest. *Therapist:* Standing. One hand contacts the distal humerus to stabilize it, and one hand contacts the posterior aspect of the glenohumeral joint. *Technique:* The forearm exerts an anterior glide through the hand on the posterior joint surface. *Use:* A component motion necessary for glenohumeral external rotation, extension, coronal abduction, and horizontal abduction.

Signs

Hypermobility of external rotation and anterior glide

Presence of compensatory active range of motion in the shoulder complex and surrounding joints

Compensatory posture

Treatment

Stabilize by wrapping or assistive device

Strengthen musculature supporting shoulder joints, and perhaps also the proximal and distal joints

Education in posture, occupational, functional, and sports activities to avoid positions and stresses where the joint is vulnerable to further hypermobility, subluxation, or dislocation, for example, the close-packed position (external rotation and abduction)

Management

Patients may require long-term follow-up for continued assessment of home program

Prognosis

The prognosis is fair to excellent depending on the patient's ability to avoid unstable positions of the joint and on the amount of instability that is present.

Tendonitis

The supraspinatus tendon is the most frequently irritated tendon of the superior tendons of the glenohumeral joint. The vulnerability of this ten-

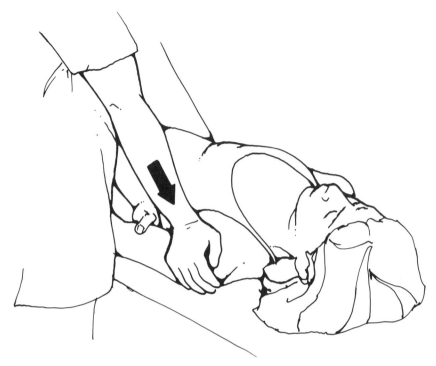

Fig. 19-3 Posterior glide of glenohumeral joint. *Patient:* Supine with arm positioned in approximately 30° of abduction on the table. *Therapist:* Standing. One hand contacts the distal humerus to stabilize it, and one hand contacts the anterior aspect of the glenohumeral joint. *Technique:* The forearm exerts a posterior glide through the hand contact on the anterior aspect of the joint. *Use:* A component motion necessary for glenohumeral internal rotation, sagittal flexion, and horizontal abduction.

don to inflammation is due to its anatomical location. With the arm at the side, torque is placed on the glenohumeral joint but particularly on the supraspinatus tendon. The position of the arm at the side decreases, or may even obliterate, the blood supply to this tendon.

Causes

Occupational, functional, or sport stresses that require repeated use of the arm overhead (as in swimming) or with the arm kept at the side or moved in a horizontally adducted position (as with a mail clerk)

Over-stress to the tendon brought on by either strength or endurance weakness of the muscle(s), tight muscle(s), tight capsule, bony impingement (owing to abnormal configuration of the acromium or acromioclavicular ligament)

Poor posture, especially the forward head, kyphosis, and shoulder complex protraction

Poor body mechanics

Symptoms

Pain or limited active motion

Pain at rest with highly reactive conditions, particularly when lying on the side of the dysfunction or when sitting in a chair with the armrest too high

Limitation of function with elevated diagonal movements

Signs

Active motion produces painful arc with coronal abduction. The "empty beer can" test is positive, that is, internal rotation with diagonal abduction.

Full passive classical motion of coronal and diagonal abduction should exist.

Passive stretching of supraspinatus tendon may reproduce patient's complaint of discomfort.

Resisted isometric contraction of external rotation and both diagonal and coronal abduction reproduce patient's complaint of pain.

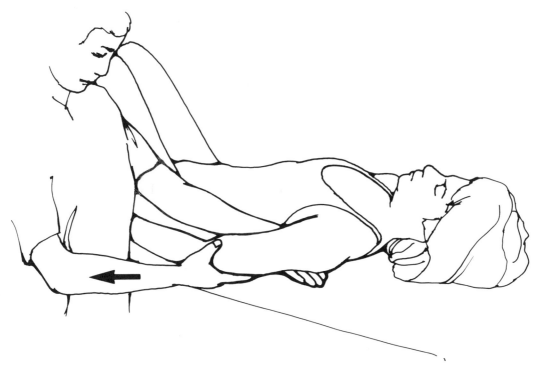

Fig. 19-4 Inferior glide of glenohumeral joint. *Patient:* Supine with the arm positioned in approximately 30° of abduction. *Therapist:* Standing with the web space of one hand contacting the scapula neck to stabilize it, while one hand contacts the distal humerus. *Technique:* The forearm exerts an inferior force through the distal humerus hand contact. *Use:* A component motion necessary for diagonal abduction, coronal abduction, and sagittal flexion.

Palpation of the supraspinatus muscle, as close to the joint line as the deltoid muscle permits, may be useful in discriminating the muscle fiber irritation versus the tendon irritation.

Treatment

Transverse friction massage to the supraspinatus tendon (Fig. 19-5)

Use of modalities to decrease the inflammation such as ultrasound, iontophoresis, phonophoresis, interferential and high-voltage stimulation

Educate in posture and body mechanics

Stretch tight muscles

Strengthen weak muscle

Manipulate tight capsule

Management

Refer to management under general category of tendonitis in Chapter 18.

Once inflammation has resided and objective signs have decreased, observe for muscle inbalance, which is very common after a tendonitis. Unless strength and endurance of all the shoulder complex musculature and the surrounding joints is addressed, then the tendonitis may occur again.

Infraspinatus Tendonitis

Infraspinatus tendonitis is not as common as supraspinatus tendonitis.

Causes

Refer to general tendonitis and supraspinatus tendonitis in Chapter 18.

Symptoms

Pain and functional limitation with external rotation and perhaps even with internal rotation or coronal abduction

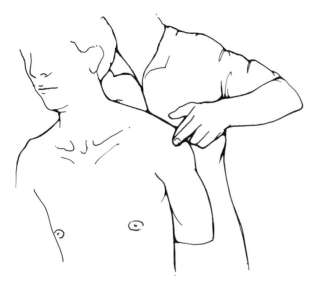

Fig. 19-5 Transverse friction of supraspinatus tendon. *Patient:* Sitting with arm positioned in internal rotation, extension, and adduction. *Therapist:* Standing with the index finger contacting the supraspinatus tendon. The middle finger is placed on the dorsal surface of the index finger. *Technique:* Transverse massage is applied. *Use:* Increase mobility of the supraspinatus tendon.

Signs

A painful arc on active coronal abduction may exist.

Resisted isometric contraction of external rotation is painful. The testing position is done with the patient's arm at the side with the elbow held at a right angle. The resistance to external movement is applied above the wrist so that the wrist and elbow are not incriminated. Be careful that the patient is not abducting the arm while resisting the external rotation.

Palpation may not be useful as a differential test because of the overlying deltoid musculature.

Treatment

Transverse friction massage may not be possible because of inability to palpate the tendon directly. For further treatment refer to tendonitis section in Chapter 18.

Management

Refer to tendonitis section in Chapter 18.

Prognosis

Refer to tendonitis section in Chapter 18.

Biceps Tendonitis

The exact etiology of biceps tendonitis, just as with other tendonitis, is not always known. Observation indicates that it may be caused by such activities as gymnastics in which the arms are repeatedly brought over the head and the elbow is maintained in various static positions. Another causative activity is knitting (which requires a sustained position of the elbow, hand, and shoulder while vigorously using the supinator-pronator and internal rotators).

In the early 19th century, medical authors speculated that one of the causes of capsular tightness was a trauma leading to an irritation of the long head of the biceps tendon, which then led to decreased use of the shoulder and a resultant tight capsule. Attention was given to the intra-articular attachment of the biceps tendon.

Cause

Refer to section on tendonitis in Chapter 18.

Symptoms

Pain occurs on active and functional arm elevation. For other symptoms, refer to tendonitis section in Chapter 18.

Signs

Pain and loss of rhythm occur with arm elevation, particularly when the arm is brought down to the side from the elevated position.

Resisted isometric contraction of coronal abduction of the arm with arm at the side reproduces the patient's complaint. If resisted flexion and extension at the elbow do not hurt, then test resisted abduction with the elbow kept into extension versus with it kept in flexion. If the long tendon of the biceps at the glenoid origin is in dysfunction, then the previous differentiation of elbow positioning (constant length phenomena) will show that the painful reaction only occurs with the elbow kept in extension.

When resisted contraction of elbow flexion and shoulder coronal abduction is strong and painful, an irritation of the tendon somewhere other than at the origin may be possible.

Yergason test for incriminating a problem of the tendon at the bicipital groove should be performed.

Palpation may also reproduce symptoms.

Treatment

Massage tendon with transverse friction while it is stretched. Refer to treatment under previous tendonitis dysfunctions, this chapter.

Management

Refer to previous tendonitis dysfunctions, this chapter.

Prognosis

Refer to previous tendonitis dysfunctions, this chapter.

Bursitis

The most common bursal areas to be involved in bursitis in the shoulder complex are the subdeltoid and the subscapularis.

Causes

Occupational, functional, or sport over-stress to bursa that, if not a direct trauma, may be brought on by either strength or endurance weakness in muscles, tight muscles, tight capsule, or bony impingement

Poor posture

Poor body mechanics

Symptoms

With subdeltoid bursitis, active arm elevation is painful or limited in function.

With subscapularis bursitis, active horizontal adduction is painful or limited in function; arm elevation, internal rotation, and external rotation may also be painful or limited.

Lying on the side of the dysfunction may be uncomfortable.

Signs

Clinically, four different patterns have been re-

ported for subdeltoid bursitis that may show up as examination findings. These patterns represent clinical observations and are not based on scientific analysis, and it would only be anatomical speculation to describe the etiology. The four patterns are as follows:

1. Full active arm elevation with occasional discomfort at midrange; no definite painful arc exists; resisted movements do not hurt.
2. Full active arm elevation with discomfort at midrange; definite painful arc exists; resisted coronal abduction reproduces discomfort.
3. Limited and painful active elevation; painful arc exists; changing pattern of pain on resisted coronal abduction.
4. Gross limited and painful active elevation; too painful to interpret a painful arc; resisted coronal abduction does not give a consistent interpretation, that is, pain sometimes occurs on resistance testing while other times no pain occurs on resistance testing; some limitation of passive abduction.

Deep palpation for provocation at the anatomical area of the bursa reproduces pain and is the best differential test.

Treatment

Treatment modalities that may be useful to decrease inflammation are ultrasound, interferential, iontophoresis, or phonophoresis.

The patient should be educated in posture, body mechanics, and stresses to avoid.

Stretch tight muscles and myofascia, strengthen weak muscles, and manipulate tight capsules.

Management

Given that the cause of bursitis has been eliminated, in three to four treatment sessions the symptoms should be decreasing and functional gains should be developing. Physiologically and scientifically, the use of modalities has not shown unequivocal success in diminishing or eliminating "calcium deposits." Clinical success has often been reported.

Prognosis

The prognosis is excellent.

Adhesions

The inferior capsule redundancy is an area where adhesions frequently develop. Adhesions are also likely to form in the anterior aspect of the capsule, particularly after immobilization secondary to a subluxation or a dislocation.

Causes

Adhesions are caused by trauma to joint or peri-articular structures that results in serofibrinous exudate with subsequent laying down of collagen, resulting in adhesions or scarring.

Symptoms

Painful restriction and limitation of motion occurs in one direction of movement.
With inferior adhesions, diagonal and coronal abduction is painful or restricted.
With anterior adhesions, external rotation and coronal abduction are painful or limited.

Signs

Active and passive classical movements are limited in the same one direction (refer to symptomatic motions above).
Accessory passive motion of inferior glide is limited with inferior adhesions, and anterior glide is limited with anterior adhesions.
End range resistance is a firm arrest of movement short of normal range. No creep consistency of resistance is felt.

Treatment

After the initial trauma, keep the joint actively moving within the pain-free range. Gentle manipulation is performed after 10 days of tolerated active motion. If condition is low to moderate reactive, manipulation should either stretch out or break adhesions.

Management

The joint must move functionally within the acquired range after manipulation. Use of ice may be useful after manipulation to decrease the possibility of swelling.

Prognosis

The prognosis is excellent.

Peripheral Nerve Entrapment

Suprascapular Nerve

The suprascapular nerve is vulnerable to entrapment at the suprascapular notch. Trauma such as a forceful horizontal adduction of the arm or falling on the outstretched arm with the arm adducted may injure the nerve at the scapular notch. The transverse scapular ligament, maintaining the nerve at the notch, may be injured by trauma, and hence the nerve may be unstable in the notch. Nerve dysfunction at the notch may cause a bone-nerve approximation, thus causing an ischemic reaction in the nerve.

The suprascapular nerve is motor in function. Sensory fibers innervate the deep tissues and the capsule of the glenohumeral joint and hence pain is deep and poorly localized.

Causes

Suprascapular nerve entrapment is caused by trauma to the arm such that the arm is placed in a position of forceful horizontal adduction, thereby traumatizing the nerve against the scapular notch. A fracture such as Colles' fracture may lead to the not so uncommon secondary problem of shoulder pain and stiffness after the wrist fracture.

Symptoms

Almost all the ranges of shoulder motion are restricted to various degrees owing to pain or lack of mucle power.
Pain at rest and pain when lying on the side of the dysfunction may be typical, particularly in a high reactive condition.

Signs

Active motion limitation may occur in musculature derived from C5 and C6 nerve roots.
Passive classical and accessory motions are not limited but may be difficult to evaluate secondary to pain.
Muscle testing may show specific weakness of C5 and C6 musculature depending on the nature of the compression and how long the compression has been present.
If the entrapment has been present for a sufficient time, there will be atrophy of the supraspinatus and infraspinatus muscles.
In situations in which specific motor weakness cannot be identified, the differential

evaluation may be very difficult because a branch of the suprascapular nerve innervates the shoulder joint capsule and another branch innervates the acromioclavicular joint. Both of the joints can be expected to be highly reactive. Hence, even passive range of motion evaluation may be difficult to carry out.

Treatment

Medical management may consist of injection for inflammatory process to the nerve or surgical intervention to stabilize the nerve at the notch.

Conservative management may work toward decreasing the inflammatory process at the suprascapular notch by such modalities as interferential or high-voltage stimulation or ultrasound.

Emphasis should be placed on occupational and functional stresses, particularly in avoiding the position of horizontal adduction of the arm. Wrapping with Ace bandages or taping to the scapula may be useful to control excessive movements of the scapula and hence decrease irritation of the nerve.

When the high reactive state has resolved, specific strengthening to C5 and C6 nerve root musculature is warranted.

Management

Specific identification of the suprascapular nerve entrapment can be difficult. Medical analysis, with tools such as electromyography (EMG) or nerve conduction tests, may be useful to qualify and quantify the dysfunction. The condition is often very painful and debilitating to functional activities. Expect a very long rehabilitation process not only in regard to specific treatment of the inflammation and strength, but also in adaptation to new postures and new functional motions, which may be necessary.

Prognosis

The prognosis is fair to excellent depending on how extensive damage to the nerve is.

Dorsal Scapular Nerve

The dorsal scapular nerve is a motor nerve that has distributions to the levator scapulae and the rhomboideus minor and major. It is vulnerable to impingement at the anatomical triangle formed between the scalenus medius and scalenus anticus muscles with the first rib.

Causes

There are three general causes of impingement of the dorsal scapular nerve. They are:

1. Hypertrophy of the scalenus medius muscle.
2. Abnormal insertion of the scalenus medius muscle on the first rib.
3. Hypertrophy of the scalenus anticus muscle.

Symptoms

The major complaint is of pain. The pain distribution may be reported along the medial border of the scapula on the affected side, but most likely it will be reported as diffuse pain that radiates down the lateral surface of the arm and forearm.

Another symptom is functional loss of shoulder or cervical active motion or both owing to pain or loss of strength.

The patient may place the hand on top of the head as a mechanism to relieve pain.

Signs

Diminished scapula rhythm may exist on the side of entrapment.

Depending on the extent of the entrapment, specific active shoulder motion may be limited in the distribution of the C5 and C6 nerve roots. Otherwise, nonspecific strength weakness may be seen as a result of a painful shoulder-cervical complex.

Classical and accessory passive motions are not limited but may be unable to be evaluated owing to pain.

Specific palpation is not confirmatory owing to the typical referral of any pain that is present.

Forward head posture is often present.

Cervical active mobility is often limited, especially in side bending, rotation to opposite side, and backward bending.

Tendinitis or bursitis may be present due to abnormal active motion and/or rhythm

Treatment

Occupational and functional postures need to be assessed as a possible primary cause of the scalenus hypertrophy.

Education and postural instruction are often the initial steps of treatment. If the condition is highly reactive, such that patients cannot assume a normal head posture, gentle progressive manual treatment will be needed to work out tightness of muscles or myofascia. The gentle treatment may consist of use of a heat modality followed by massage or myofascial stretching. Assistive devices such as taping or a cervical collar may be useful to take the stress off the area or off the muscles during functional or occupational activities.

Management

If the condition has been present for a long time, the extent and frequency of clinical treatment may be long-standing. Patients may require a great deal of help to understand the activities that are performed during the day and night that place stress on the nerve or tighten the muscles.

Prognosis

The prognosis is fair to excellent depending on how extensive damage to the enrve is.

THE WRIST

Capsule Tightness

Causes

Capsule tightness may occur secondary to fracture and subsequent immobilization, involving the carpals, radius, or ulna, or it may occur secondary to immobilization of wrist or elbow.

Symptoms

Some loss of functional active movements may exist in all the joint movements.
Pain may be present at the end of range of all the joint movements.

Signs

Active and passive classical motions are limited in both flexion and extension to about the same degree.
Pain comes on as active or passive end ranges or both are approached.
End range resistance is an abnormal creep resistance.
Passive accessory motions are all limited and are limited relative to the passive classical motions.

Treatment

Manipulate restricted accessory motions. Wrist flexion requires dorsal glide of the proximal carpal row and volar glide of the distal carpal row;

extension is the reverse of flexion (Figs. 19-6 to 19-8).

Use heat to aid in the elongation of collagen such as diathermy, ultrasound, or moist heat.

Management

With high or moderately reactive patients, a day or night splint may be useful in protecting the joint against excessive movement stresses. COBAN (a commercial product similar to an Ace wrap) is useful in decreasing positional discomfort.

Be certain to evaluate individual carpal bone mobility since any dysfunction in the mobility of individual carpal bones may result in limitation of the classical range of motion, both flexion and extension, and adduction and abduction.

Prognosis

The outcome will depend on the type of fracture and subsequent postfracture scarring of the capsule.

Discharge from therapy is warranted once active and passive motion measurements and functional capabilities have plateaued.

Malalignment of Carpal Bone

The most common subluxation-dislocation of the carpal bones is of the lunate bone. The malalignment occurs in a volar direction owing to normal anatomical weakness of the surrounding ligaments.

Causes

Any direct trauma or forceful movement of the wrist causing the wrist to be placed in full extension may cause the lunate bone to be forced further into an anterior (or volar) direction. Malalignment may occur secondary to a Colles' fracture or to fracture of the scaphoid bone.

Symptoms

Discomfort or sharp pain may occur when the wrist is placed in full extension. Functional activities such as pushing up from a chair or weight bearing with the wrist in extension (on all fours) may be compromised, or there may be inability to perform repeated or

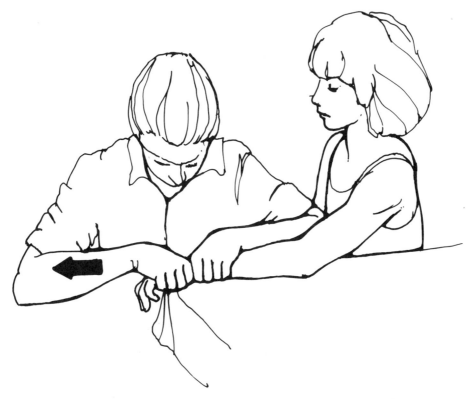

Fig. 19-6 Distraction of the wrist, proximal carpal row. *Patient:* Sitting with the forearm pronated and supported on the table. *Therapist:* One hand contacts the distal radius and ulna to stabilize; the web space of the other hand contacts the proximal carpal row. Wrist is held at approximately 0°. *Technique:* The forearm exerts a distraction force (perpendicular to the articulation of the radius and ulna) through the hand contact on the proximal row. *Use:* A joint play necessary for all wrist movements.

quick functional activities requiring the wrist to be placed at the end ranges of wrist extension.

Limitation of active flexion or extension of the wrist may be present.

The patient may report paresthesia or altered wrist strength.

A volarly placed lunate may put compression on the neurovascular bundle at the carpal tunnel. Hence, median nerve compression symptoms may be reported.

Signs

Some loss of functional active motion of wrist flexion and extension (especially extension at the end range) may be present

Active abduction and adduction (especially at the end ranges) may be limited.

Passive classical motion may be limited in the same parameters as active motion.

End feel is abnormal, particularly the end ranges of wrist extension, abduction, and adduction. The abnormal end feels may typically be any of the following: bone on bone (hard abnormal), tight creep, or painful.

Passive accessory motion limitations are typically seen between either lunate and triquitrum or lunate and capitate. Rarely are there restrictions of movements between lunate and scaphoid.

If the lunate is volarly placed such that the neurovascular bundle is compromised, then signs of median nerve compression (sensory or motor or both) may be present. The patient may also show signs of circulatory insufficiency.

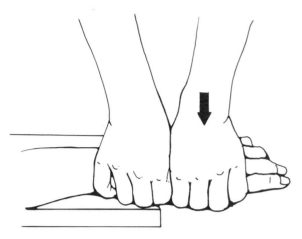

Fig. 19-7 Volar glide, proximal carpal row. *Patient:* Sitting with forearm pronated and supported on the table. *Therapist:* Standing with one hand contacting the distal radius and ulna to stabilize, while other hand contacts the dorsal aspect of the proximal carpal row. Wrist is held at approximately 0°. *Technique:* The forearm exerts a volar glide through the hand contact on the dorsal proximal carpal row. *Use:* A component motion necessary for wrist extension.

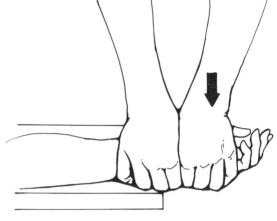

Fig. 19-8 Dorsal glide, proximal carpal row. *Patient:* Sitting with forearm supinated and supported on the table. *Therapist:* Standing with one hand contacting the distal radius and ulna to stabilize, while the other hand contacts the volar aspect of the proximal carpal row. The wrist is held at approximately 0°. *Technique:* The forearm exerts a dorsal glide through the hand contact on the dorsal carpal row. *Use:* A component motion necessary for wrist flexion.

Treatment

Manipulate accessory motion restriction(s).

Manipulation in one direction for one articulation during each visit is a useful treatment approach as better assessment of the outcomes of the manipulation treatment can be made.

Use of ice for short durations (maximum of 10 minutes) may be useful after manipulation, especially if manipulation was performed as a grade IV or prolonged stretch technique.

Prognosis

The prognosis is excellent if the malalignment is due to adhesion formation and manipulation can affect this adhesion restriction.

The prognosis is poor if malalignment results in hypermobility of the ligaments. If the ligaments are hypermobile, then the outcome of manipulation shall be nil. Further physician management may be necessary to treat the instability. Use of wrapping and assistive devices may be a conservative alternative to treat instabilities.

Tenosynovitis—De Quervain's Disease

Tenosynovitis of the abductor pollicis longus and extensor pollicis brevis tendons is involved in De Quervain's disease. The tendonitis is often quite limiting to functional activities, and has been seen in persons whose occupation or sport activities involve strenuous hand and thumb activities.

Causes

Occupational, functional, or sport over-stress resulting in excessive or vigorous flexion and adduction of the thumb or extension and abduction of the thumb

Over-stress to the tendon(s) brought on by either strength or endurance weakness of the muscle(s); tight muscles; tight capsules

Poor posture

Poor body mechanics

Symptoms

Pain or limitation of active thumb extension and abduction and possibly pain on active wrist extension

Pain on full flexion and adduction of the thumb along with simultaneous flexion of the wrist

Patients highly reactive conditions have pain at rest

Signs

Positive Finkelstein test (flexion and adduction of the thumb along with slight adduction and flexion of the wrist)

Pain with resisted isometric contraction of abductor pollicis longus, extensor pollicis brevis, and possible wrist extension

Painful deep palpation of the extensor and abductor tendons

Treatment

Rest from function and activities with use of splint for at least 5 days. If the above signs are still present to the same degree as in the initial evaluation, then a more vigorous treatment approach may be necessary, such as transverse friction massage to tendon with tendon kept taut during the treatment. Use of ice before and after treatment may be necessary for anesthetic effect. Use of splint after treatment is necessary. Keep tendon moving within its sheath by instruction of active nonresistant exercises.

Once painful contraction has decreased, the use of strengthening exercises is imperative.

Management

If the above treatment approach is not successful, physician management via injection of the tendonitis may be useful for positive outcome of physical therapy intervention.

Prognosis

The prognosis is excellent.

Ligamentous—Ulnar Collateral Ligament

The ulnar collateral ligament is frequently restricted after trauma to or immobilization of the wrist joint.

Causes

Restriction may occur secondary to immobilization after reduction of a Colles'

fracture or fracture in the distal aspect of the ulnar side of the wrist.

Trauma to the ulnar border of the wrist resulting in observable or nonobservable swelling may cause tightness.

Symptoms

There is pain and often limitation of functional movement of the wrist. Activities that require weight bearing to the wrist such as sustained holding of an object or pushing or pulling with the hand and arm are often difficult or painful. Patients with highly reactive states may report pain at rest.

Signs

Active motion may be limited in wrist movements, particularly ulnar and radial deviation.

Active supination may be limited.

Passive classical motion shows reproduction of pain with radial deviation.

All passive classical wrist movements may be limited, and supination may also be limited.

End range resistance may be any of the following: bony, painful, or firm creep.

Passive accessory movements show limitations of proximal carpal row mobility, particularly to the radial direction. Ulna-meniscus-triquetrum accessory movement may be limited. If the latter accessory movement is limited, then both active and passive motion of supination will be limited.

Palpation to the ulnar collateral ligament is tender.

Treatment

Use manipulation technique for soft tissue stretching of the ulnar border.

Use transverse friction massage over the ligament's attachments, proximal and distal, and over the middle of the ligament.

Management

When the ulnar border is tight, the soft tissue manipulation stretching technique is the most useful technique immediately postimmobilization.

Prognosis

The prognosis is fair to excellent depending on the amount of adhesions and scarring present in the ligament.

Peripheral Nerve Entrapment

Carpal Tunnel

The entrapment of the median nerve at the anatomical carpal tunnel of the wrist may be caused by bony malalignment, soft tissue hypertrophy, or swelling. Many times the diagnosis of carpal tunnel syndrome is made without a thorough evaluation of the median nerve at all of the following areas: the elbow (pronator teres syndrome), the three thoracic outlets, and all of the cervical and first thoracic joints and nerve roots. All of the former joint complex areas may contribute to a carpal tunnel complaint. Occasionally, the patient's primary complaint of discomfort may be at the hand and wrist, and yet the primary problem may be proximal to the carpal tunnel, even as far away as the cervical spine. Dysfunction at the carpal tunnel specifically is addressed here.

The median nerve is both motor and sensory in distribution. The muscles innervated are the first and second lumbricales, the opponens pollicis, and the abductor pollicis brevis. The skin sensory distribution is over the radial half of the midpalm area and continues distally to the palmar surfaces of the first three and one-half digits. The distribution continues over the dorsum of the digits to the distal interphalangeal joints.

Causes

Various problems may contribute to the carpal tunnel syndrome such as:

Occupational, functional, or sport over-stress to the wrist

Chronic over-sprain to the flexor surface of the wrist leading to subsequent observable or nonobservable swelling

Bony compression via malalignment of the lunate bone

After reduction of a Colles' fracture or fracture of the distal ulna

Restricted mobility of the pisiform caused by tightness of any of the following: flexor-

extensor retinaculum, ulnar collateral ligament, pisohamate ligament, flexor carpi ulnaris tendon, abductor digitus minimus tendon

Distal retention of fluid, particularly present during the last trimester of pregnancy

Symptoms

Pain or limitation of active wrist flexion or extension may exist.

Patients with highly reactive conditions may experience pain at rest, particularly night pain. The night pain is often so severe as to disturb sleep.

Functional movements are often limited owing to joint movement pain or to lack of normal hand strength.

Observable swelling may be present at the wrist.

Altered finger sensation and strength may be present.

Signs

Phalen's position of the wrist may produce pain and median nerve numbness (maintaining full wrist flexion).

Movement of wrist extension and flexion may be limited and painful.

Classical and accessory motions should have a full range unless there is bony impingement by the lunate, unless swelling is so great as to limit mobility, or unless the pisiform is restricted owing to tightness of any of the six soft tissue attachments on it.

Tinel sign may be positive, especially if the nerve is regenerating.

Palpation of the carpal tunnel produces tenderness and perhaps reproduction of paresthesia of median nerve distribution.

Asymmetric muscle contraction of wrist and long finger flexors with median nerve innervation may be weak and painful.

Objective sensory changes in the median nerve distribution may be reported.

Treatment

Modalities to decrease inflammation may be useful, such as ultrasound, interferential, high-voltage stimulation, iontophoresis, or phonophoresis.

A splint, and especially a night splint, may be useful when the splint is made such that the wrist is maintained in a neutral and slightly ulnar-deviated position.

An ace wrap or COBAN may be useful.

If malalignment of the lunate bone is present, then manipulation is indicated.

If soft tissue tightness exists in any of the following: extensor or flexor retinaculum, ulnar collateral ligament, flexor carpi ulnaris, abductor pollicis longus, or pisohamate ligaments, then manipulation of the pisiform bone or soft tissue stretching techniques with massage or both are indicated.

Educate the patient in posture and body mechanics.

Stretch tight muscles and strengthen weak muscles but only after the inflammation and irritation of the carpal tunnel area have decreased to a state of low reactivity.

Management

To identify the abnormal stresses placed on the wrist, the patient's functional activities should be carefully monitored, particularly sleeping positions. As the condition improves to a state of low reactivity, the use of a splint may be useful as the patient begins to increase activities.

Physician management may consist of use of anti-inflammatory medication or injections to aid in the outcome of physical therapy management.

Prognosis

The prognosis is fair to excellent depending on the damage done to the nerve as the result of the initial problems. Reduction of parasthesia, even minimal, is a good sign that conservative management is helpful. Do not be too alarmed if the patient's symptoms increase with the initial first or second therapy intervention. The increase of symptoms may in fact show that pressure has been taken off of the nerve and that a subsequent release phenomenon is occurring.

Ulnar Nerve Entrapment

The ulnar nerve is vulnerable to entrapment at Guyon's tunnel. The tunnel is formed by the bony margins of the pisiform bone, the hook of the hamate, and the triquetral bone, forming the floor of the tunnel. The roof of the tunnel is formed by the volar carpal ligament and the palmaris brevis muscle (if present). The frequency of ulnar nerve entrapment in this anatomical area has been reported to be fairly common in long-distance bicyclists and people who put pressure on this area, as with use of a cane. The ulnar nerve has both motor and sensory distribution. The muscles innervated are the palmaris brevis, abductor digiti minimi, flexor digiti minimi, opponens digiti minimi, lumbricales, interossei, flexor pollicis brevis, and the adductor pollicis. The sensory distribution is the skin area of the ulnar half of the fourth digit and the whole of the fifth digit palmarly and dorsally to just proximal of the metacarpophalangeal joints.

Causes

Over-stress, typically by compression forces sustained to the ulnar palmar border of the hand, as in occupational, functional, or sport-related activities

Postfracture of the ulnar border of the carpal bones, fracture of the distal ulna, malalignment of the ulnar border bones

Dysfunction of the volar carpal ligament or palmaris brevis muscle

Symptoms

Pain, numbness, or lack of muscle strength of hand or fingers

Atypical limitation of active motion of fingers or wrist

Functional limitations due to parasthesia or strength impairment

Signs

Full-range active motion that may be limited owing to lack of muscle power

Limited classical and accessory motions at any of the carpal bones previously mentioned; tightness between the articulations

Palpable swelling.

Palpable tenderness over the palmar aspect of the tunnel, although even tenderness is present within normal persons.

Muscle weakness of the ulnar nerve distribution, depending on the extent of the entrapment

Treatment

Positioning, postural, and functional education to avoid over-stress to the tunnel

Manipulation if carpal bone tightness exists

Use of modalities such as: interferential, high-voltage stimulation, iontophoresis, phonophoresis, or ultrasound to decrease inflammation

Management

Identify those activities and positions that can lead to over-stress at Guyon's tunnel.

Prognosis

Excellent as long as the problem is not related to abnormal ligamentous laxity

FINGERS

Capsule Tightness of the Metacarpophalangeal, Proximal Interphalangeal, and Distal Interphalangeal Joints

Mobility of the three joint areas of each finger is often observed in physical therapy to be restricted after immobilization and surgery. Scarring of the skin can limit joint mobility. Scarring of the synovial sheath and tendon can also limit joint mobility. Isolated capsular tightness is yet another possible dysfunction restricting mobility in these joints. Capsular tightness is discussed here.

Causes

Postimmobilization

Post surgery

Symptoms

Functional loss of active finger mobility

Pain with functional movements

Signs

Some loss of all active and passive classical movements of the fingers

Limited passive accessory movements in all directions

Pain reported at the end range of all available motions

End range resistance is an abnormal creep resistance

Diminished muscle strength and coordination

Treatment

Manipulate restricted accessory motions (Figs. 19-9 to 19-12)

Begin strength and coordination training once lengthening of the capsule plateaus

Management

Avoid working with muscle strengthening until the capsule has been lengthening by using the manipulation techniques consistently for about 3 weeks. Muscle strengthening too early may work

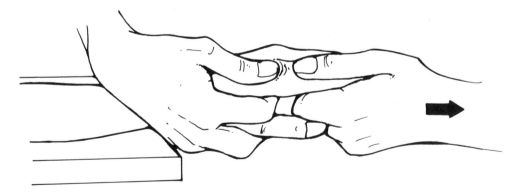

Fig. 19-9 Distraction of the metacarpophalangeal joint. *Patient:* Sitting with forearm pronated and hand supported on the table. *Therapist:* Sitting with one index finger and thumb contacting the volar and dorsal surfaces of the proximal joint to stabilize, while the other index finger and thumb contact the volar and dorsal surfaces of the distal joint. The joint is held at approximately 20° of flexion. *Technique:* The forearm exerts a perpendicular force, relative to the distal articulation surface, through the distal finger contacts. *Use:* A joint play necessary for all metacarpophalangeal movements.

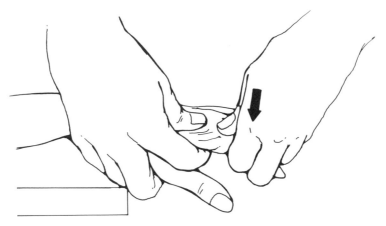

Fig. 19-10 Volar glide, metacarpophalangeal joint. *Patient:* Sitting with the forearm pronated and hand supported on the table. *Therapist:* Standing with one thumb and index finger contacting the dorsal and volar surfaces of the proximal joint to stabilize, while the other thumb and index finger contact the dorsal and volar surfaces of the distal joint. Joint is held at approximately 20° of flexion. *Technique:* The forearm exerts a volar glide through the finger contact on the dorsal distal joint surface. *Use:* A component motion necessary for metacarpophalangeal flexion.

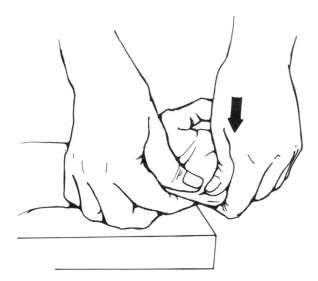

Fig. 19-11 Dorsal glide, metacarpophalangeal joint. *Patient:* Sitting with the forearm supinated and hand supported on the table. *Therapist:* Standing with one thumb and index finger contacting the volar and dorsal surfaces of the proximal joint, and the other thumb and index finger contacting the volar and dorsal surfaces of the distal joint. Joint is held at approximately 20° of flexion. *Technique:* The forearm exerts a dorsal glide through the finger contact on the volar distal surface. *Use:* A component motion necessary for metacarpophalangeal extension.

against the desired manipulation effects. During the time that manipulation is carried out, the patient is instructed in functional finger and hand motions to accentuate the results of manipulation.

Prognosis

Fair to excellent depending on the nature of the capsule restrictions

ELBOW

Capsule Tightness

Capsule tightness is a fairly common condition of the elbow, particularly after immobilization.

Causes

Capsule tightness of the elbow is caused by immobilization resulting from either fracture or soft tissue injury.

Symptoms

Some loss of functional active movements in all the joint motions may occur.

In highly reactive conditions, pain will be present at the end range of all the joint motions.

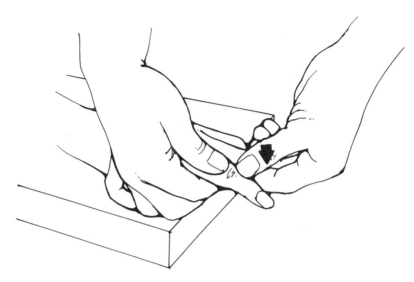

Fig. 19-12 Unicondylar glide, proximal interphalangeal joint. *Patient:* Sitting with forearm pronated and hand supported on the table. *Therapist:* Standing with one thumb and index finger contacting the dorsal and volar surfaces of the proximal joint surface, while the other thumb and index finger contact the lateral condylar dorsal and volar surfaces of the distal joint. The joint is held at approximately 20° of flexion. *Technique:* The forearm exerts a volar glide through the thumb contact on the lateral distal surface. *Use:* A joint play necessary for all proximal interphalangeal joint movements. The other three unicondylar glides are not shown.

Signs

Active and passive classical motions are limited in the same direction. Flexion is more limited in motion than extension. Limitations of pronation and supination may be present, with limitation greatest at supination.

Passive accessory motions are limited in all directions, particularly with cephalic and caudal movements of the radius, lateral mobility of the radial head, and ulna distraction.

Pain comes on as the active and passive end ranges are approached.

End range resistance is an abnormal creep resistance.

Treatment

Manipulate restricted accessory movements (Figs. 19-13 to 19-16).

Management

Be certain to pay attention to end range resistance, especially after fracture or dislocation. If the end range resistance is a bony or hard resistance short

of the normal range, then consider that postfracture callus formation is restricting mobility. The abnormal bone restricts the physical therapist's goal to increase the joint motion.

Prognosis

The prognosis is fair to excellent depending on the nature of the capsule tightness and the ability of the patient to maintain functional mobility.

Muscle Dysfunction after Trauma

Retrospective studies show that myositis ossificans (bone in the muscle) occurs in persons who have sustained a supracondylar fracture of the humerus, a dislocation of the elbow, or a trauma of the brachialis muscle.

Causes

The trauma to the brachialis muscle may result from a dislocation or fracture of the humerus, radius, or ulna. Radiographs may not confirm the presence of myositis ossificans. Some researchers report that the ossification does not show up on radiograph as late as 1 month postinjury.

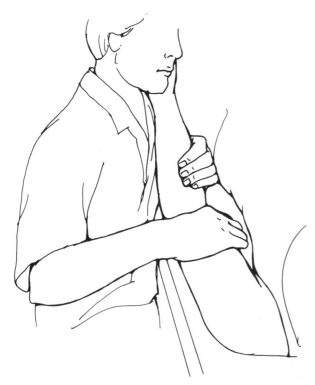

Fig. 19-13 Ulna distraction. *Patient:* Supine with arm supported on the table. *Therapist:* Standing with one hand contacting the anterior distal surface of the humerus to stabilize; the other hand contacts, with all four finger pads, the anterior proximal surface of the ulna. Joint is held at approximately 70° of flexion and 10° of supination. *Technique:* The forearm exerts a perpendicular force, relative to the ulnar surface, through the contact of the fingers on the ulna. *Use:* A joint play necessary for all movements of the elbow.

Symptoms

There may be pain and limitation of active functional movements, particularly elbow extension.

Pain may be present at rest.

Signs

Active motion is limited in both flexion and extension. Supination or pronation or both may be limited.

Passive classical and accessory motions are not limited as long as postfracture callus formation is not limiting motion.

Resisted isometric contraction shows an increase of pain with flexion.

With advanced conditions of ossification, palpation of the bony mass is possible. In less advanced conditions, palpation produces tenderness, particularly at the anterior surface of the elbow.

Treatment

If the initial problem is a muscle injury, the only treatment should be resting the elbow in flexion by use of either a splint or a cast. Active motion is only performed periodically in the day and only in a pain-free range. After 2 to 3 weeks, the splint should be gradually adapted so that the elbow can assume positions closer to extension.

In advanced cases in which ossification is well formed, no treatment is useful for increasing range of motion and function. Many investigators report that this particular condition should be dealt with by education about and avoidance of stressful and functional activities. These researchers believe that the bony mass may disappear spontaneously in the course of 2 years, especially if the area is not stressed. Excision of the bony mass has not been shown to be the best intervention.

Management

Patients must be instructed in use of the splint and particular avoidance of any stressful activities of the shoulder, hand, and arm.

Prognosis

A fair to excellent prognosis may be expected depending on the etiology and the treatment approach. The earlier the intervention with resting and stress avoidance, the better the outcome.

Extensor Mechanism Tendonitis

The tendons that are typically dysfunctional on the radial side of the elbow are either the extensor carpi radialis brevis or the extensor carpi radialis longus. Dysfunction of one or both of these tendons is often labeled "tennis elbow." The use of this term is quite inappropriate since the term does not differentiate between tendon dysfunctions and other dysfunctions that may cause the complaint. Some other problems may be caused by radial head meniscus, radial nerve entrapment, capsule tightness, loose body, or postfracture. The term tennis elbow also does not in itself suggest

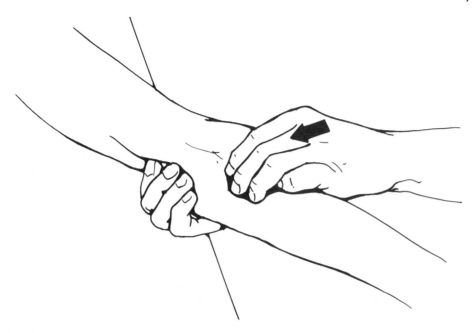

Fig. 19-14 Anterior glide, radial head. *Patient:* Supine with arm supported on the table. *Therapist:* Standing with one hand contacting the posterior distal surface of the humerus and the posterior proximal surface of the ulna to stabilize, while one thumb contacts the posterior surface of the radial head and two finger pads contact the area of the anterior radial head. The elbow is held at approximately 70° of flexion and 10° of supination. *Technique:* The forearm exerts an anterior glide force through the thumb contact on the radial head. *Use:* A component motion of elbow flexion and a joint play of pronation.

any mechanism of treatment since all of the latter dysfunctions are treated differently from a tendonitis. Tendonitis of the two tendons is discussed here.

Causes

Tendonitis may result from occupational, functional, or sport over-stress, for example, poor techniques in tennis playing, inadequate hand grip on tennis racket, inappropriate racket string tension; over-stress to tendons brought on by either strength or endurance weakness in muscles, tight muscles, restricted myofascia, tight capsule, or bone impingement; poor posture; or poor body mechanics.

Symptoms

Pain occurs with activities requiring motions of wrist, as in flexion and, perhaps, extension, along with elbow extension. Pain is often present with these active motions. Patients with highly reactive conditions may have pain at rest.

Signs

Active motion of elbow extension, wrist extension, and second or third finger extension is painful and may be limited.

Active wrist flexion and elbow flexion may be limited or painful or both, particularly in highly reactive conditions caused by stretching.

Highly reactive conditions may be painful just with elbow extension, and because of pain, the patient cannot even flex the wrist while the elbow is kept extended.

Resisted isometric contraction reproduces the patient's complaint of pain. All isometric contractions are performed with the elbow in full extension while the therapist resists wrist extension and resists separately third and second finger extension (Fig. 19-17). To differentiate between the brevis and the longus tendons, the operator selectively isolates the fingers. The resistance of extension of the third finger with reproduction of pain incriminates the brevis tendon.

Palpation to the epicondyle and to the supracondylar ridge may discriminate between the brevis and longus tendons. Palpation is misleading because of referred tenderness.

Palpable swelling may be present at the above-mentioned anatomical sites.

Treatment

Use transverse friction massage.

Use modalities to reduce inflammation such as ultrasound, iontophoresis, phonophoresis, interferential, and high-voltage stimulation.

Perform stretching exercises for the tendon once the reactivity has decreased and the patient can actively fully extend the elbow and partially flex the wrist and fingers without discomfort. Once stretching exercises have been done for approximately 1 week, then begin strengthening with both concentric and eccentric contractions.

Educate the patient in posture and body mechanics, and in proper arm and body mechanics in occupational and sport activities.

Strengthen weak muscles, manipulate tight capsule, and stretch tight myofascia.

A circumferential band below the elbow may be useful to redistribute the muscle force to the tendon as sport and functional activities resume.

Management

Refer to the management section under general category of tendonitis in Chapter 18.

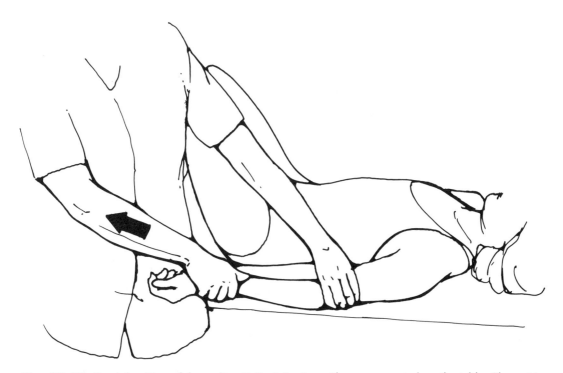

Fig. 19-15 Caudal motion of the radius. *Patient:* Supine with arm supported on the table. *Therapist:* Standing with one hand contacting the anterior distal surface of the humerus, while the other hand contacts the distal radius with the golfer's grip. The elbow is held at approximately 70° of flexion and 10° of supination. *Technique:* The forearm exerts a caudal force on the distal radius hand grip. *Use:* A component motion necessary for elbow extension and wrist flexion.

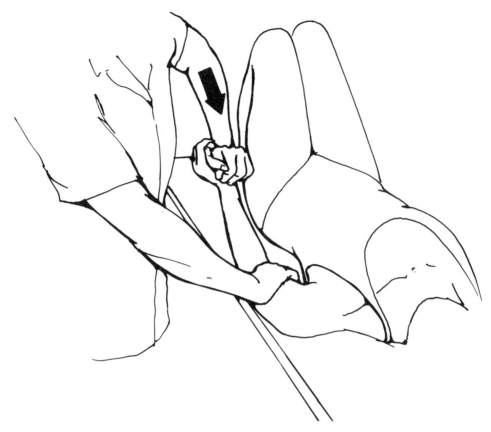

Fig. 19-16 Cephalic motion of the radius. *Patient:* Supine with arm supported on the table. *Therapist:* Standing with one hand contacting the anterior distal surface of the humerus to stabilize, while the other hand contacts the thenar eminence with the sawmiller's hand grip. The elbow is held at approximately 70° of flexion and 10° of supination. *Technique:* The forearm exerts a cephalic force through the thenar eminence hand contact. *Use:* A component motion necessary for elbow flexion and wrist extension.

Be certain to look for other dysfunctions after the inflammation and discomfort has receded. Typical dysfunctions that may be present are muscle weakness with eccentric contraction, lack of extensibility of muscle or tendon, and myofascia restrictions.

Prognosis

The prognosis is fair to excellent depending on the amount of swelling present and the subsequent damage to the tendon fibers.

Flexor Mechanism Tendonitis

Tendonitis of the flexor tendon mechanism at the ulnar border of the elbow is often referred to as "golfer's elbow." The frequency of golfers acquir-

ing this dysfunction is quite high. Just as stated above for tennis elbow, the terminology does not suggest dysfunction of any particular structure nor suggest treatment. Tendonitis of the flexor tendon is discussed here.

Causes

Occupational, functional, or sport over-stress, such as, poor hand grip on the golf club
Over-stress of tendon brought on by either strength or endurance weakness of muscle, tight muscle, tight myofascia, tight capsule
Poor posture or poor body mechanics

Symptoms

Pain or limitations with functional activities requiring elbow flexion and wrist flexion
Pain at rest with highly reactive conditions

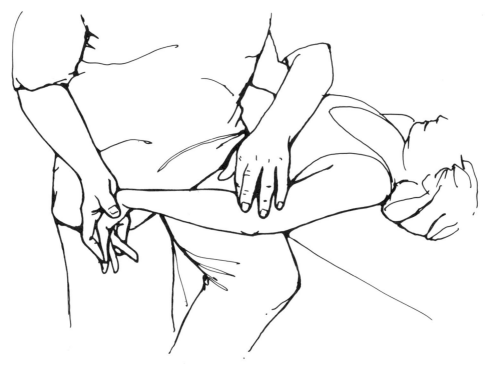

Fig. 19-17 Stretch of extensor carpi radialis brevis tendon. *Patient:* Supine with arm supported on the thigh of the operator. *Therapist:* Sitting on the edge of the table, one finger palpates the extensor carpi radialis brevis tendon, and one hand monitors the position of the patient's elbow, hand, and middle finger. *Technique:* Maximal stretch to the tendon is with full elbow extension, full wrist flexion, and full middle finger flexion. *Use:* Increases mobility of the tendon fibers.

Signs

Pain or limitations with active elbow flexion and wrist flexion

Limitations or pain with elbow extension and wrist extension in highly reactive conditions

Pain with passive positioning of elbow extension and wrist extension owing to tendon stretching

Pain from resisted isometric contraction of wrist flexion and pronation

Pain from palpation at medial epicondyle (palpation misleading because of referred tenderness)

Treatment

Transverse friction massage

Use of modalities to decrease inflammation such as ultrasound, iontophoresis, phonophoresis, interferential, and high-voltage stimulation

Stretching exercises for tendon

Strengthening exercises to muscle once full motion is pain free

Education in posture and body mechanics

Education in body mechanics during sport activity

Stretch tight muscles and myofascia

Strengthen weak muscles

Manipulate tight capsules

Management

Refer to management section under general tendonitis category in Chapter 18.

Prognosis

Refer to extensor mechanism tendonitis above.

Biceps Tendonitis

For biceps tendonitis, refer to the tendonitis section under Shoulder—Glenohumeral Joint, above.

Olecranon Bursitis

The olecranon bursa is the most frequently irritated bursa at the elbow joint. Two other bursae that are also vulnerable to irritation are the superficial epicondylar bursa and the radiohumeral bursa. The olecranon bursa is discussed here.

Causes

Occupational trauma, functional, or sport overstress may cause olecranon bursitis.

Symptoms

Pain limits full functional movements of the elbow, particularly flexion.

Patients with highly reactive conditions may experience pain at rest.

Pain occurs when pressure is placed on the posterior aspect of the elbow, as in resting the bent elbow on a table top.

Signs

The end range of active extension may be limited or painful. Active flexion may be limited or painful.

Passive extension may be painful when stretching the elbow extensors.

Resisted isometric contraction of the anconeus or triceps may irritate the inflamed bursa and reproduce pain.

Deep palpation of the olecranon produces tenderness.

Functional activities such as leaning the elbow on a table or a quick flexion movement at the elbow, particularly with resistance applied into wrist flexion, may reproduce pain.

Treatment

Modalities to decrease inflammation may be useful, such as ultrasound, interferential, iontophoresis, or phonophoresis.

The patient should be educated in posture, body mechanics, and stresses to avoid.

Stretch tight muscles and myofascia, strengthen weak muscles, and manipulate tight capsule.

Management

Refer to management section under general category of bursitis in Chapter 18.

Prognosis

The prognosis is excellent.

Peripheral Nerve Entrapment

Median Nerve

The entrapment of the median nerve at the elbow is often referred to as "pronator teres syndrome." The entrapment can occur as the median nerve passes through the pronator teres muscle. Resultant sensory or motor dysfunctions depend on the amount and extent of compression. The sensory area includes the radial side of the palm and the palmar side of the first, second, and third digits and half of the fourth digit. The distribution also extends over the tips of the fingers to the dorsum skin to the distal interphalangeal joints. The muscles innervated are the pronator teres, flexor carpi radialis, palmaris longus, flexor digitorum sublimis, flexor pollicis longus, and flexor digitorum profundus. The motor dysfunction may be present as abnormality of strength in regard to turning the wrist (pronation) or flexion of the wrist, partial loss of flexion in the fingers, and loss of opposition of the thumb.

This syndrome can mimic a carpal tunnel syndrome in regard to the subjective complaints (see Carpal Tunnel, above).

Causes

Direct trauma may cause this syndrome, either by continued static pressure in the area or as a direct blow. The term "honeymoon paralysis" is used to describe the entrapment. The partner's head rests against the upper forearm of the other partner, which may lead to compression of the nerve.

Fracture of the humerus, radius, or ulna may give rise to abnormal pressure on or trauma to the nerve.

Frequently the cause is repeated forceful pronation along with forceful finger flexion in functional activities.

Symptoms

Pain or limitation occurs when actively turning the wrist in either direction.

The fingers may be numb.

Loss of strength of fingers and wrist may exist.

Signs

Pain or limitation of elbow pronation may occur.
Passive supination reproduces pain.
Resisted isometric contraction of pronator teres reproduces pain.
Palpation may produce tenderness at the anterior flexor surface of the elbow.
Altered sensation in the median nerve distribution of forearm, arm, or hand may exist.
Muscle weakness of median nerve distribution of forearm and hand may exist.

Treatment

Modalities to decrease inflammation may be useful, such as ultrasound, interferential, iontophoresis, or phonophoresis.
Deep massage is given to the pronator teres muscle.
Contract-relax technique is applied to pronator teres.
Stretch tight myofascia.
Educate patient in body posture, body mechanics, and stresses to avoid.

Management

Patients may not know exact positional or functional etiology and do not often report elbow or forearm discomfort. The major complaint of discomfort and lack of function is at the wrist and distally into the fingers. Because of this description, a carpal tunnel is often diagnosed.

Prognosis

The prognosis is fair to excellent, depending on the extent and amount of compression.

Radial Nerve

The radial nerve is vulnerable to entrapment as the nerve passes under the fibrous edge of the extensor carpi radialis brevis muscle and then through a slit in the supinator muscle. The radial nerve in this anatomical area is both a sensory and a motor nerve. The superficial radial nerve is the skin sensory nerve, and the deep branch of the radial nerve is the motor nerve (often termed the posterior interosseous nerve). The superficial radial nerve passes over the extensor carpi radialis brevis, thereafter running down the forearm under the brachioradialis muscle. The deep branch passes through the body of the supinator to the posterior aspect of the forearm. The superficial radial nerve innervates the skin over the radial side of dorsum of the wrist and hand and then terminates in the dorsal digital nerves. Sensation is afforded to the dorsal surface of the radial three-and-one-half digits. The deep branch of the radial nerve innervates nine muscles: extensor carpi radialis brevis, supinator, extensor digitorum communis, extensor digiti quinti, extensor carpi ulnaris, extensor pollicis longus, extensor pollicis brevis, abductor longus pollicis, extensor indicis proprius.

Entrapment of the radial nerve can mimic a tennis elbow or, as with entrapment of the superficial branch of the nerve, De Quervain's disease.

Causes

Occupational, functional, sport over-stress
External trauma to proximal aspect of the forearm
Displaced fracture of the radial head
Repeated forceful supination, extension of the wrist and fingers

Symptoms

Pain or limitation of pronation or supination or both
Pain or limitation of wrist and finger extension
Numbness in fingers
Impaired elbow, wrist, or finger strength

Signs

Painful movement or lack of full movement of extension of wrist and fingers or supination of the elbow
Pain at rest in highly reactive conditions
Full passive classical and accessory motions
Passive pronation reproduces pain
Pain with passive extension of the elbow with simultaneous flexion of the wrist and third digit flexion
Pain caused by resisted isometric contraction of supinator and resisted contraction of the extensor carpi radialis brevis (by positioning the elbow in extension along with resisting wrist extension and third finger extension)
Palpation tenderness at the anterior radial head, but not definitive owing to referred pain
Decreased sensation of radial nerve distribution
Muscle weakness of radial nerve distribution

Treatment

Modalities to decrease inflammation, such as ultrasound, interferential, iontophoresis, or phonophoresis

Contract-relax techniques for supinator or extensor carpi radialis brevis

Deep massage to supinator and extensor carpi radialis brevis

Stretch myofascia

Management

If condition is not influenced by the above treatment, then injection by a physician may decrease inflammation.

Ulnar Nerve

The ulnar nerve is vulnerable to entrapment in its osseous groove behind the medial epicondyle. The nerve is held in the groove by a fibrous expansion of the common flexor origin. This entrapment site has been called the "cubital tunnel." The ulnar nerve is both sensory and motor. The sensory portion supplies the dorsal ulnar side of the hand and the fourth and fifth digits along with the ulnar side of the palm. The motor aspect supplies the flexor carpi ulnaris and the ulnar half of the flexor digitorum profundus.

Causes

Direct trauma

Postfracture

Dysfunction of the osseous groove, as in a shallow groove, or a dysfunction in the fascial covering over the groove

Symptoms

Awkwardness and clumsiness of hand and wrist

Disturbed sensation of the fourth and fifth digits

Unrelenting thoracic back pain

Signs

Active motion of the wrist and particularly the fingers limited owing to muscle strength or pain

Active limitation of wrist flexion, fourth and fifth finger flexion and adduction

Pain with elbow flexion or extension

Pain with passive classical motion of either flexion or extension of the elbow

Pain with passive wrist extension and fourth and fifth finger extension

Resisted isometric contraction of the flexi carpi ulnaris and the flexor digitorum profundus may show weakness

Interosseous weakness of the fourth and fifth digits (earliest sign)

Disturbed sensation to fourth and fifth digits

Decreased sensation to pinprick in the fourth and fifth digits

Pain from palpation of the ulnar nerve at the humeral groove

Palpation tenderness of the thoracic area without significant dysfunction findings

Treatment

Modalities to decrease inflammation, such as ultrasound, interferential, iontophoresis, or phonophoresis

Educate in posture, body mechanics, and stresses to avoid at the posterior aspect of the elbow

Management

Given that the etiology may be a result of narrowing of the groove or due to disturbance of the fascial covering of the groove, physician management may be warranted.

Prognosis

Fair to excellent depending on the amount and extent of compression to the nerve

Radial Head Meniscus

Studies of cadavers have shown that approximately 17 percent of the population has radial head menisci. Neither the function nor the etiology of dysfunction of the meniscus is known at this time. Dysfunction may result in a misdiagnosis of tennis elbow.

Causes

Occupational, trauma, functional, or sport overstress such that the elbow is repeatedly forced into extension and the wrist into flexion

Symptoms

Pain or limitation of elbow extension

Functional movements limited because of pain.

Signs

Active elbow extension painful but not always limited in motion

End range passive classical motion of extension painful but not always limited

End range resistance of extension produces a springy rebound resistance

Accessory motion, particularly anterior and posterior glides of the radial head, is restricted and produces a springy rebound resistance

Pain with accessory movement of the radial head

Palpation tenderness of the radius-humerus joint line

Treatment

Manipulate meniscus

Management

Use of ice after manipulation to control swelling

Prognosis

Excellent unless meniscus is a loose body

Lower Extremity

Catherine E. Patla

ANKLE

Capsule Tightness

Reference to the ankle in this section is to the joint areas of the mortise (talocrural joint) and subtalus (hindfoot).

Causes

Immobilization secondary to fracture or soft tissue damage may cause capsule tightness.

Symptoms

Symptoms of capsule tightness may include the following: active limitation of ankle movement, usually with pain; pain on weight bearing; difficulty in walking or inability to walk on even or uneven terrain; inability to run.

Signs

Active motion of plantar flexion and dorsiflexion are limited and painful. Plantar flexion shows greater limitation than dorsiflexion

Passive classical motion is limited and painful in the same pattern as active motion.

End range resistance is an abnormal creep resistance in both the dorsiflexion and plantar flexion end range.

Passive accessory motion is limited and may be painful in talus glides, talus distractions, tibia glides, calcaneus glides, and calcaneus distraction.

Palpation may produce tenderness along the joint lines. Palpation is not incriminatory because of referred tenderness, which is typically expected in the entire ankle area.

Palpation may detect swelling.

Alterations in gait may be present.

Treatment

Manipulate restricted accessory movements (Figs. 20-1 to 20-5).

Management

Direct careful attention to observing deviations in gait.

Once manipulation treatment is showing progressive improvement in the range of motion and functional gait, begin strengthening exercises to anterior, posterior, medial, and lateral compartments.

Prognosis

The prognosis is fair to excellent depending on the cause of the capsule tightness and the ability to regain extensibility of the collagen fibers.

Tendonitis Tendo Achilles

Causes

Tendonitis tendo Achilles may result from occupational, functional, or sport over-stress; alteration of typical walking or running cycles; or alteration of footwear or surface terrain.

Symptoms

Pain may occur at the heel with weight-bearing, either with walking or running.

In highly reactive states, the heel or midcalf may be painful with non-weight-bearing.

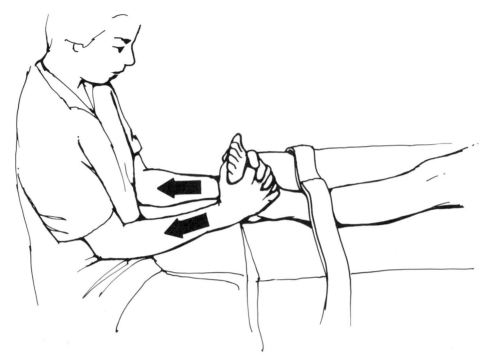

Fig. 20-1 Talus distraction. *Patient:* Supine with the leg straight and supported on the table. *Therapist:* Sitting with little fingers contacting the dome of the talus, the thumbs supporting the plantar surface, and the fingers contacting the dorsal surface of the midtarsal area. The ankle is held at approximately 5° of plantar flexion. A strap is used to stabilize the distal tibia and fibula. *Technique:* Both forearms exert a perpendicular force, relative to the concave surface of the tibia and fibula, through both little fingers contact on the talus. *Use:* A joint play necessary for all ankle motions.

The patient may complain of heel or calf pain with activities requiring dorsiflexion or weight-bearing on the ball of the forefoot.

The patient may complain of pain at the heel or calf with flat shoes versus no complaint of pain with shoes with higher heels.

Signs

Active motion of dorsiflexion increases pain, particularly on harder surfaces and with flatter shoes.

Pain may limit full plantar flexion and full dorsiflexion.

Passive classical motion is full and pain-free in plantar flexion, but dorsiflexion is limited and painful.

End range resistance of dorsiflexion is muscle resistance and it is painful.

Resisted isometric contraction of gastrocnemius and soleus reproduces pain. Resistance evaluation is also performed by having the patient demonstrate one-leg weight bearing while rising on the ball of the foot several times.

The tendon or muscle belly of the gastrocnemius muscle is tender to palpation. Palpation for the condition may detect swelling.

Alterations in gait may be observed.

Treatment

Deep transverse friction massage is applied to tendon or muscle belly.

Strenuous activity such as running and walking on ramps and prolonged weight bearing in flat shoes or bare feet is avoided during the period when treatment is being administered

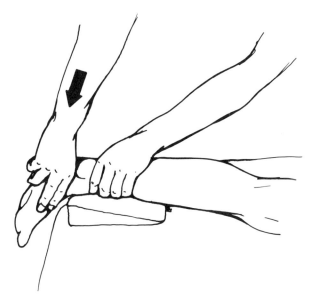

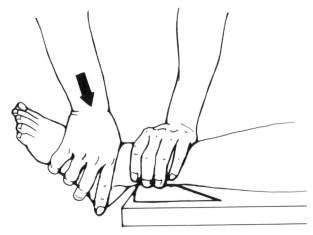

Fig. 20-2 Anterior glide of the talus. *Patient:* Prone with the distal tibia and fibula supported on a wedge. *Therapist:* Standing with one hand contacting the posterior distal surface of the tibia and fibula to stabilize, while one web space contacts the area of the posterior talus. The ankle is held in approximately 5° of plantar flexion. *Technique:* The forearm exerts an anterior glide force through the web space contact on the posterior talus area. *Use:* A component motion necessary for plantar flexion.

Fig. 20-3 Posterior glide of the talus. *Patient:* Supine with the distal tibia and fibula supported on a wedge. *Therapist:* Standing with one hand contacting the anterior distal surface of the tibia and fibula to stabilize, while one web space contacts the dome of the talus. The ankle is held at approximately 5° of plantar flexion. *Technique:* Forearm exerts a posterior glide force through the web space contact on the dome of the talus. *Use:* A component motion necessary for dorsiflexion.

and as long as resisted plantar flexion is painful.

Modalities to decrease inflammation may be useful, such as ultrasound, interferential, iontophoresis, or phonophoresis.

Management

The patient should be questioned thoroughly regarding history of previous steroid injections to the tendo Achilles. Several steroid injections can damage the collagen. Careful avoidance of manual stretching must be adhered to if patient has a history of steroid injections.

Non-weight-bearing status may be necessary during the initial treatment period to take stress off the healing tendon.

Prognosis

The prognosis is excellent.

Posterior Tibial Tendonitis

Tendonitis of the tibialis posterior is often termed "shin splints." The term "shin soreness" or "shin splints" is frequently used among athletes to describe pain in the leg after trauma. The term cannot particularly refer to the tibialis posterior muscle-tendon, for dysfunction may exist in the peroneal muscle-tendon group or the tibialis anterior muscle-tendon.

Causes

Occupational, functional, or sport over-stress causes posterior tibial tendonitis.

Symptoms

Active movement of inward motion of the foot may be painful or limited.

Functional gaits, such as walking or running, may be painful or limited.

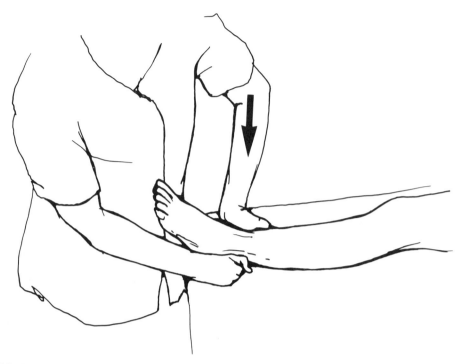

Fig. 20-4 Posterior glide of the distal tibia. *Patient:* Supine with the leg straight and supported on the table. *Therapist:* Standing with one thenar eminence contacting the posterior surface of the fibula to stabilize, while one palm contacts the dorsal distal surface of the tibia. *Technique:* The forearm exerts a posterior glide force through the palm contact on the tibia. *Use:* A joint play necessary for all motions of the ankle.

Signs

Active motion of inversion is painful or limited. Active motion of eversion may be painful or limited.

Passive classical motion is painful in eversion.

Passive motion in inversion may be limited and painful.

End range resistance is of either a painful response or abnormal muscle quality.

Resisted isometric contraction reproduces pain with inversion.

Palpation for reproduction of tenderness is performed throughout the muscle and tendon area to locate the site of greatest tenderness.

Treatment

Transverse friction massage is applied.

Use modalities to decrease inflammation, such as ultrasound, iontophoresis, phonophoresis, interferential, and high-voltage stimulation.

Educate the patient in posture and body mechanics.

Educate and train the patient in gait for walking, using ramps and stairs, and running.

Management

Frequent irritation of the tendon may be occurring because of structural deformities of the hindfoot such as in a talipes valgus deformity (pronated hindfoot). The problem causing the talipes valgus should be identified and may be structural, abnormal muscle tone, myofascial restrictions, joint instability, or joint tightness. Dysfunctions should be looked for all the way up the kinetic chain to the spine.

Prognosis

The prognosis is excellent.

Ligamentous

Anterior Talofibular Ligament

The anterior talofibular ligament is frequently injured. As with all ligaments after injury, the ligament may be restricted in mobility or may be hypermobile. Hypermobility of this ligament often results in what many call an unstable mortise or ankle joint.

Causes

Occupational, functional or sport over-stress that points the foot down and inward may injure this ligament.

Symptoms

With hypermobility, the patient reports an unreliable ankle that gives out often, with a momentary sharp pain followed by swelling of the ankle for 1 or 2 days afterward.

With a tight ligament, there may be limitation or pain when pointing the foot down and inward.

The anterior aspect of the ankle may be painful to palpation for provocation, and swelling may be present there.

Signs

With hypermobility, only with the presence of swelling is limitation of dorsiflexion, plantar flexion, inversion or eversion observed. With conditions other than swelling, active motion of inversion and plantar flexion is greater than normal and may be painful at the abnormal end range. Active motion on weight bearing may produce a complaint of pain (e.g., raising up leg on the ball of the forefoot without shoe support) and inability to maintain balance. Passive motion of inversion and plantar flexion is greater than normal.

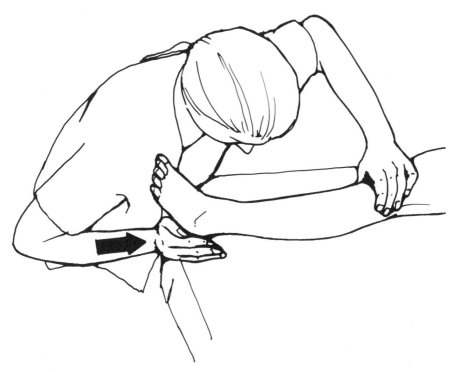

Fig. 20-5 Cephalic motion of the fibula. *Patient:* Supine with the leg straight and supported on the table. *Therapist:* Standing with one hand palpating the proximal fibula and one thenar eminence contacting the lateral surface of the calcaneus. The therapist's shoulder contacts the plantar surface of the foot to assist in stabilization. *Technique:* The forearm exerts a cephalic force to the fibula through the thenar eminence contact on the lateral aspect of the calcaneus. *Use:* A component motion necessary for dorsiflexion.

With ligament tightness, active inversion and plantar flexion are limited. Patient demonstrates difficulty in standing on one leg on the ball of the foot without shoe or arm support.

With restricted mobility, inversion and plantar flexion are limited or painful.

Passive accessory motion is most incriminatory.

With hypermobility, too much motion is felt with medial and lateral glides of the talus, and posterior and anterior glides of the talus may show hypermobility.

With ligament tightness, restriction is seen with the following: medial and lateral glides of the talus, anterior and posterior glides of the talus, and talus distraction.

End range resistance often shows a slight abnormal resistance such as laxity or swelling with a hypermobile ligament and abnormal creep or pain with a tight ligament.

Structural observance may show talipes varus or talipes valgus of the hindfoot. The position of the structural aspect of the hindfoot is dependent on where the injury has occurred and the overall body type and lower kinetic chain structure.

Palpation often produces tenderness over the ligament.

Treatment

If hypermobility of the ligament exists, then support to the hindfoot and forefoot by orthoses is indicated.

If hypomobility of the ligament exists (caused by adhesions or scarring), then treatment is manipulation of resisted accessory movements. Transverse friction massage may be useful.

After rehabilitation for either of these ligament dysfunctions, the patient is placed on a balance board once low reactivity and functional movement are maintained.

Management

The unstable mortise is many times more difficult to identify, whereas the ligament that has adhesions is much easier to identify, especially with accessory motion evaluation.

Prognosis

For hypermobility, the prognosis is fair to good depending on the ability to stabilize. For hypomobility, the prognosis is good to excellent depending on the length of the previous adhesion period.

Calcaneofibular Ligament

The calcaneofibular ligament is one of the most frequently injured ligaments, along with the anterior talofibular ligament. Hypomobility of this ligament is discussed here.

Causes

Occupational, functional, or sport over-stress may result in forced foot inversion.

Symptoms

Turning the foot inward may be painful or limited.

There is functional loss or pain with weight bearing, normal gait, walking on ramps, and running.

Swelling and pain occur at the lateral side of the ankle.

Signs

Active motion is painful and limited in inversion.

Patients with highly reactive states have limited and painful inversion and eversion. They may also demonstrate pain or limitation in plantar flexion and dorsiflexion.

Passive classical motion may be limited or painful in inversion and eversion.

Passive accessory motion is painful or limited in talus distraction, medial and lateral glides, and anterior and posterior glides. Anterior and posterior glides of the distal fibula may be limited and painful.

End range resistance is abnormal creep, painful or empty (swelling).

Palpation of the ligament produces tenderness.

Treatment

See Anterior Talofibular Ligament, above.

Management

See Anterior Talofibular Ligament, above.

Prognosis

See Anterior Talofibular Ligament, above.

Anterior Compartment Syndrome

The exact etiology of anterior compartment syndrome is often very vague, and often the exact dysfunction is difficult to evaluate. The frequency of discomfort in the anatomical area of the anterior compartment, especially among athletes, has led to a very general impression that tightness and discomfort are the result of a dysfunction of the anterior tibialis muscle. The bellies of the anterior tibialis, extensor hallucis, and extensor digitorum muscles are confined in this space. The tibia and fibula, the interosseous membrane, and the superficial fascia are also contained in the anterior space. The anterior tibial artery transverses this anatomy. Increased swelling, increased blood flow, and hypertrophy of any of the muscles listed above may compress the anterior tibial artery. The occlusion of the artery, along with the primary problem, can lead to temporary paralysis of any of the muscles. An abnormal sensation of pins and needles in the inner four toes may be experienced because of compression of the superficial peroneal nerve as it exits through the fascial foramen. Without medical attention given to this compromise of blood flow, the possibility exists of irreversible paralysis because the nerve and blood vessels may become damaged by the continued pressure. Particular attention is given to continued redness of the skin, to pulse rate, and to ability to extend the toes and dorsiflex the ankle. If any of these symptoms become worse, physician management (and perhaps even surgery to divide the fascia) is warranted to prevent ischemic necrosis, contracture, or a complete paralysis.

Causes

Occupational, functional, or sport over-stress, that is, direct trauma over the anterior compartment, may cause this syndrome.

Symptoms

Throbbing pain or sharp pain in the anterior compartment of the leg may be brought on by walking or running activities.

The patient is unable to extend the toes or dorsiflex the forefoot.

There is continued redness of the skin along with a pulsating feeling in the anterior aspect of the leg.

The toes and foot are discolored.

Palpable swelling occurs in the anterior compartment of the leg.

Signs

Active motion of extension of the toes is limited or painful. Active motion of dorsiflexion of the ankle is limited.

Passive classical motion is painful or limited with dorsiflexion or plantar flexion or both. Depending on the etiology, passive motion could be full and painless.

Depending on the etiology, end range resistance might be normal, painful, or empty (swelling).

Resisted isometric contraction of any of the three muscles (anterior tibialis, extensor hallucis, or extensor digitorum) may be interpreted as painful and weak, painless and strong, or painful and strong.

Palpation elicits tenderness in the anterior compartment and is often specific in identifying the site of dysfunction.

Observation may show redness of the skin, swelling of the anterior compartment area, or even discoloration of the foot or toes.

The pulse of the dorsal foot may be compromised. Be certain to evaluate the pulse in the weight-bearing and non-weight-bearing position and to compare the pulse with exertion versus nonexertion.

Treatment

In the more severe cases, rest the anterior compartment from function by use of non-weight-bearing status.

Modalities for inflammation may be useful during the non-weight-bearing state.

In the less reactive conditions, deep massage to the muscle bellies and myofascia may be useful.

In severe cases, physician management is sought to aid in discussion for a treatment approach.

Educate the patient in gait (walking and running), posture, and body mechanics.

Stretch or strengthen muscles as appropriate only after all symptoms are reduced and swelling and blood compromise have been resolved.

Management

For the most severe cases not requiring physician attention, daily evaluation is important even if home visits must be made. A seemingly moderate case can advance very quickly to a severe case without the patient realizing the severity.

Prognosis

The prognosis is poor to excellent depending on the etiology.

Peripheral Nerve Entrapment

Interdigital Nerve

The interdigital nerve is vulnerable to entrapment between the third and fourth toes, in the web space of the metatarsal heads. The entrapment is quite common and is often misdiagnosed as a Morton's neuroma. A neuroma may eventually form with compression but is not likely to be the source of the original discomfort. The entrapment is also referred to as "electrician's toe" because of the vulnerability of foot posture when the metatarsophalangeal (MTP) joint is hyperextended, which is common among electricians or even painters who stand still on ladders for a great deal of time. The interdigital nerves are sensory nerves to the toes. The sensory supply is to the tips and the plantar and dorsal surfaces of the toes.

Causes

A direct downward force against the dorsum of the foot may compress the ligament against the nerve.

Static positions may hyperextend the toes at the MTP joints. High-heeled shoes incline the forefoot down and force hyperextension of the toes.

Irregular push-off caused by shoes, gait in walking or running, or terrain may force the toes into hyperextension.

Entrapment may occur secondary to a hallux valgus formation in which the second and fourth MTP joints are compromised and may possibly be forced into a hyperextended position.

A tight or shortened gastrocnemius-soleus may maintain the hindfoot in plantar flexion, causing hyperextension of the MTP joints.

Any trauma to the foot may cause the toes to go into hyperextension, as in descending a stairway or awkwardly coming off of a curb.

Symptoms

Burning pain, sharp pain, or even throbbing pain may be reported on the plantar surface of the foot or may even be felt on the dorsal surface of the foot.

Sensation disturbances of the third and fourth toes may exist.

In the most severe cases, there is radiating pain up the leg and even to the level of the hips.

Gait, as in walking and running and especially descending stairs and ramps, may be very painful or impaired.

Signs

Active motion is not limited mechanically but may be limited through pain in extension of toes. Plantar flexion of the toes may eliminate discomfort slightly or even totally.

Passive classical motion is full mechanically but may be painful in hyperextension.

Passive plantar flexion may relieve discomfort to some extent.

Passive accessory motion is often abnormal, with either pain or tightness in the anterior or posterior glides of the third and fourth MTP joints.

End range resistance may be either painful or empty (swelling).

Deep specific palpation on the plantar surface between the third and fourth metatarsal heads reproduces pain and is very uncomfortable.

Pinprick in the inner web space between the third and fourth toes may show alteration of sensation.

Treatment

A metatarsal bar or a longitudinal bar on the third and fourth plantar surfaces of the metatarsal bones may decrease pressure. Any orthosis in the metatarsal area that supports and increases plantar flexion is desired.

Correct structural abnormalities, such as a pronated foot or a talipes valgus of the hindfoot.

Stretch tight gastrocnemius and soleus muscles and tight myofascia.

Use modalities to decrease inflammation.

Educate the patient in posture and body mechanics.

Instruct the patient in walking and running gaits.

Manipulate if accessory motions are restricted.

Management

During the conservative treatment approach, and especially if the condition is highly reactive, use of a non-weight-bearing status may be helpful to better evaluate the outcome.

Prognosis

The prognosis is fair to excellent, depending on the amount of ischemic damage to the nerve.

Posterior Tibial Nerve

The posterior tibial nerve is vulnerable to entrapment at the osseous fibrous tunnel made up of the posteroinferior aspect of the medial malleolus and the laciniate ligament covering the neurovascular bundle. The neurovascular structures in this tunnel include not only the posterior tibial nerve but also the tendons of the tibialis posterior, extensor hallucis longus, and extensor digitorum longus. Entrapment at this area is often referred to as "tarsal tunnel syndrome." The posterior tibial nerve is both motor and sensory in distribution. The posterior tibial nerve branches into three nerves beyond the malleolus, and these nerves are responsible for supplying the skin of the plantar surface of the entire foot and the plantar and opposing dorsal surfaces of the toes. Muscle weakness is shown by loss of flexion at the MTP joint and extension at the interphalangeal joints, that is, the intrinsic musculature is affected.

Causes

Posterior tibial nerve entrapment is frequently seen as a secondary complication of fracture of the malleolus, talus, or calcaneus. It may be caused by complications after inappropriate casting of fractures. It can also occur with excessive pronation of the hindfoot.

Symptoms

Bringing the foot actively inward is painful and often limited.

Pain occurs on full weight-bearing along with deviations in gait in walking or running.

A burning, throbbing, or dull sensation on the sole of the foot may be present.

Signs

Active motion may be painful or limited in motions of the ankle including plantar flexion, dorsiflexion, and inversion and eversion.

Passive classical motion of eversion and plantar flexion may be painful or limited owing to stretching.

Passive accessory motions may show limitations of the following: anterior or posterior glides of the tibia, talus lateral and medial glides, anterior and posterior glides, calcaneus medial and lateral tilts and anterior and posterior glides.

End range resistance may be painful or show abnormal muscle resistance, particularly in eversion.

Resisted isometric contraction may produce painful weakness of flexion of the MTP joint or extension of the interphalangeal joints.

Palpation may identify the specific area of tenderness along the osseous fibrous tunnel or along the sole of the foot. Palpation produces tenderness at the neurovascular area.

Altered sensation may be present on the sole of the foot and the dorsal tips of the toes.

Weight bearing may reproduce pain.

Gait shows deviations in avoidance of pressure on the medial side of the calcaneus and avoidance of talipes valgus of the hindfoot.

Swelling may be palpable.

Alterations in gait may be seen.

Treatment

If the entrapment is due to abnormal foot mechanics or posture pronation then orthoses or correcting the positional fault or both are advocated.

Modalities to decrease inflammation may be useful.

Massage, including deep friction massage, to the laciniate ligament and lower aspect of the vascular bundle, may be helpful.

Management

When prolonged compression has been placed on this osseous fibrous tunnel such that ischemic necrosis, paralysis, or contracture has occurred, then physician consultation and management is necessary.

Prognosis

The prognosis is fair to excellent depending on the extent of the ischemic condition.

Deep Peroneal Nerve

The deep peroneal nerve is vulnerable to entrapment on the dorsal aspect of the foot. The nerve is both motor and sensory. The sensory distribution is to the web space between the first and second toes. The motor innervation is to the extensor digitorum brevis and the first dorsal interosseous muscle. The lateral branch of this nerve, which is the higher branch, innervates the extensor brevis muscle, and the medial branch, or more distal branch, innervates the interosseous muscle.

Causes

Entrapment may result from a direct blow on the dorsal aspect of the forefoot, or footwear or a cast that puts pressure on the dorsal aspect of the foot.

A strong plantar flexion and inversion force applied to the foot may cause injury to various parts of the peroneal nerve.

Abnormal osseous position as in an anterior direction of the cuboid bone or the cuneiform bone or the second metatarsal shaft may injure the nerve.

Symptoms

Pain may occur at the large toe if the medial branch is involved, or there may be nonspecific pain in the dorsal aspect of the foot if the lateral branch is involved.

The patient has difficulty in walking with inability to extend the toes.

Forcefully pointing down the foot as in plantar flexion will increase the pain.

The gait often shows a limping pattern with reported discomfort.

Signs

Active motion limitation with or without pain occurs in extension of the toes.

Passive classical motion may produce pain with forceful end range plantar flexion of the foot and toes. However, this position may not selectively incriminate the peroneal nerve and may also indicate any problems of the peroneal nerve proximal to the ankle joint.

Passive accessory motion may be limited in anterior and posterior glides of the cuboid and cuneiform bones.

End range resistance may be painful in all motions.

Resisted isometric contraction may show painful weakness of the short extensors, which may be more observable by having the patient extend the toes against resistance when the ankle is at complete dorsiflexion.

Palpation pressure along the course of the nerve should identify the location of dysfunction and should incriminate the deep peroneal nerve versus the more proximal superficial peroneal nerve.

Abnormal sensation is reported to pinprick within the web space of the first and second toes dorsally.

Gait demonstrates limping and deviations.

Treatment

Modalities to decrease inflammation may be useful.

Accessory movement limitations require manipulation.

Correction of structural malalignment is necessary.

Management

Long-term follow-up may be necessary to assess functional, occupational, and sports gait.

Prognosis

The prognosis is fair to excellent depending on the extent and amount of ischemic or mechanical damage.

Superficial Peroneal Nerve

The superficial peroneal nerve is vulnerable to entrapment in the distal portion of the leg as it goes through the opening in the deep fascia in its descent down the leg. The nerve is purely sensory at this point. The sensory distribution covers the lower one-third of the lateral aspect of the leg and the dorsal aspect of the first, second, third, and fourth toes minus the cleft and web space between the first and second toes.

Causes

Forceful plantar flexion motion or inversion of the ankle and foot, direct trauma to the region, or tightly laced boots in this region may entrap the nerve.

Symptoms

The patient complains of burning or sharp pain, usually of a superficial nature, in the region of the nerve distribution.

Signs

Active motion is full and pain free except perhaps for the end range of plantar flexion and inversion.

Passive classical motion is full and pain free except perhaps in the position of plantar flexion and inversion.

Palpation produces tenderness along the region of the anatomical distribution, particularly at the fascial opening and emergence of the nerve.

Sensation to pinprick may be altered in the area of sensory distribution.

Gait demonstrates limping, often with discomfort.

Treatment

Modalities to decrease pain and inflammation may be useful.

Superficial or deep massage may be useful to break up tightness in fascial area.

A lateral heel wedge may be used to increase the eversion posture of the foot or to relax the fascial or lateral aspect of the leg.

Management

If the above managements are not effective in decreasing the symptoms, then physician management is necessary.

Prognosis

The prognosis is fair to excellent depending on the damage to nerve caused by the compression.

HIP

Capsule Tightness

Unlike any other peripheral joint, the hip is unlikely to be moved through the full range of motions in daily functional activities. An increase of hip tightness and degeneration of the hip is reported to be more predominate in Western cultures. People in Western cultures tend to be more sedentary in jobs and life styles, whereas people in Eastern cultures are more active and rarely have to assume a sitting position as part of a job. The early stages of hip joint degeneration show marked capsule and muscle tightness. Hip capsule tightness is discussed here.

Causes

Rarely is the hip joint immobilized, but immobilization can result in capsule restrictions. Disuse of the full end ranges of hip motion, as with lack of exercise and a predominantly sedentary life-style can, cause capsule tightness, as can structural or muscle asymmetries of the spine, hip, or lower extremity.

Symptoms

Stiffness is felt in the spine, hip, or lower extremity joints, particularly after the patient has assumed a static position.

Pain, stiffness, or limitation are seen in functional movements. Quality or quantity of walking is altered because of stiffness or pain.

Pain on weight bearing may be present.

Signs

Active and passive classical motions are limited in the same movements. The limitation is in flexion, abduction, and medial rotation. Some patients may show more limitation of extension than flexion.

A positive Scouring test may be present.

Passive accessory motions are limited in all

directions. The greatest limitation felt is in inferior glide and lateral distraction.

End range resistance is either a abnormal creep or muscle resistance.

Tightness of muscles is typical, particularly the following: tensor fascia, rectus femoris, adductors, and piriformis.

The iliotibial band is often tight (see Knee, below).

Treatment

Manipulate restricted accessory motions (Figs. 20-6 to 20-11).

Stretch tight muscles and myofascia.

Strengthen weak muscles after stretching program is completed.

Educate the patient in functional movements, stretching activities, posture, and body mechanics.

Teach the patient the proper way of walking for exercise to the hip.

Management

Working with the general population to prevent hip tightness and resultant osteoarthrosis is imperative. Too often in physical therapy the patients with hip complaints are seen only in advanced conditions of osteoarthrosis.

Prognosis

The prognosis is fair to excellent depending on the collagen pathology and on the ability of the patient to alter his life-style to a less sedentary one.

Osteoarthrosis

Degeneration of the hip joint is the result of connective tissue tightness of the hip or spine and a sedentary life-style. (see Hip, Capsule Tightness, above). In the previous section is found a description of osteoarthrosis in total. The only difference is that in the most advanced cases of osteoarthrosis,

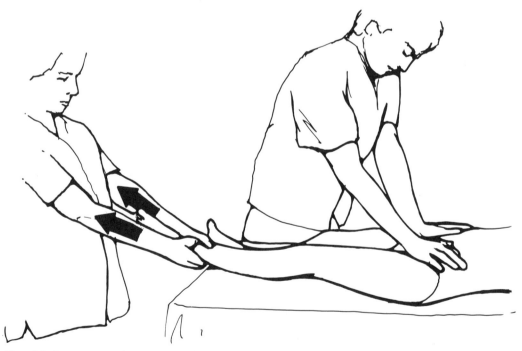

Fig. 20-6 Long-axis distraction of the hip. *Patient:* Supine with the leg supported on the table. *Therapist:* Standing with hands contacting the distal tibiofibula. Assistant supports the patient's iliac crests. The hip is placed in the loose-pack position. *Technique:* Both forearms exert a long-axis distraction force by leaning into the therapist's body. *Use:* A joint play necessary for all motions of the hip.

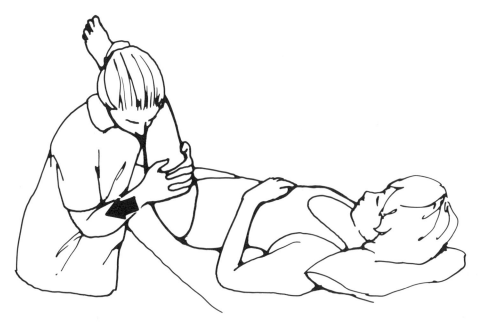

Fig. 20-7 Inferior glide of the hip. *Patient:* Supine with the leg supported on the table. *Therapist:* Standing with both hands contacting the anterior proximal aspect of the femur. The patient's leg is supported on the therapist's shoulder and the hip is placed in the loose-pack position. *Technique:* Forearms exert an inferior force through the hand contacts on the femur and by the therapist leaning back into his or her body weight. *Use:* A component motion necessary for hip flexion and abduction.

all the above descriptions occur to a much greater extent.

Psoas Bursitis

Causes

Functional, occupational, or sport over-stress may cause psoas bursitis.

Symptoms

Pain is reported in the groin or anterior thigh area.

Pain may also be reported solely at the area above the patella.

Signs

Active motion of flexion with adduction reproduces the pain.

Passive classical motion of flexion with adduction reproduces the pain. Passive lateral rotation may produce discomfort.

Palpation may produce specific pain reproduction in the anterior groin, but this area is most uncomfortable to palpation even in normal individuals.

Psoas muscle strength is normal, but muscle or myofascia may be tight.

Poor posture is another sign.

Treatment

Modalities that may be useful to decrease inflammation are ultrasound, interferential, iontophoresis, or phonophoresis.

Stretch tight muscle and myofascia.

Educate the patient in proper standing and sitting postures.

Management

The physician may inject the bursa to decrease the inflammation.

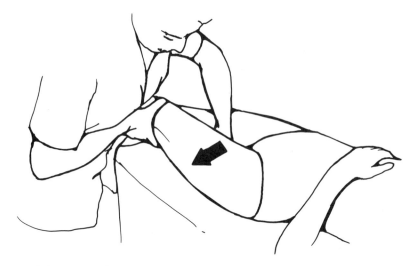

Fig. 20-8 Lateral distraction of the hip. *Patient:* Supine with the leg supported on the table. *Therapist:* Standing with one hand contacting the distal lateral surface of the femur to stabilize, while the other hand contacts the proximal medial aspect of the femur. The hip is placed in the loose-pack position. *Technique:* The forearm exerts a lateral force through the proximal hand contact. *Use:* A joint play necessary for all motions of the hip.

Prognosis

The prognosis is excellent.

Greater Trochanter Bursitis

Bursitis at the greater trochanter is the most common bursitis at the hip joint.

Causes

Causes include functional, occupational, and sport over-stress; muscle or myofascial tightness; structural asymmetry; and poor posture. With runners, inadequate shoes or running surfaces may be factors.

Symptoms

Pain exists when in the sidelying position.
Pain may be present during standing, walking, running, or sitting.
Patient may be able to point to the lateral hip as a source of pain.

Signs

Active and passive classical motions are full, but adduction may be limited by pain.
Sometimes contraction of the piriformis produces some discomfort, but the contraction does not reproduce the specific pain.
Muscle and myofascial tightness is present.
Palpation tenderness at the greater trochanter is the differential test.
Poor posture or inadequate shoes for walking or running activities may be observed.

Treatment

Modalities that may be useful to decrease inflammation are ultrasound, interferential, iontophoresis, or phonophoresis.
Stretch tight muscles and myofascia.
Educate the patient in posture, movement, and equipment with functional, occupational, and sport endeavors.

Management

During the evaluation, careful attention must be paid during the palpation. All parameters of the greater trochanter must be specifically palpated. All the tendinous attachments must be specifically palpated.

The physician may inject the bursa to decrease the inflammation.

Prognosis

The prognosis is excellent.

Peripheral Nerve Entrapment

Lateral Femoral Cutaneous Nerve

Entrapment of the lateral femoral cutaneous nerve is often termed "meralgia paresthetica." The entrapment site of the nerve is at the anterior superior spine where the nerve passes through the inguinal ligament. The nerve has a sensory distribution. The nerve branches anteriorly and posteriorly below the inguinal ligament. The anterior branch innervates the skin of the anterior and lateral thigh as far as the knee. The posterior branch innervates the skin posteriorly and laterally from the trochanteric area to the middle of the thigh.

Causes

Obesity of the lower abdominal area and the thigh

Direct trauma to the area

Static or forced adduction of the leg

Shortened leg on the opposite side of the complaint

Forced pelvic tilt or backward bending of the spine

Abnormal tone of abdominal or hip muscles

Abnormal iliac fascia

Dysfunction of the inguinal ligament

Symptoms

Burning, numbness, or abnormal skin sensations of the anterolateral or posterolateral thigh

Back pain

Signs

Full active and passive classical motions of the hip and spine except with muscle or myofascial tightness

Painful end range of active or passive hip adduction

Pain with pelvic tilt

Pain produced by palpation

Abnormal tone of abdominal muscle

Short leg on the opposite side

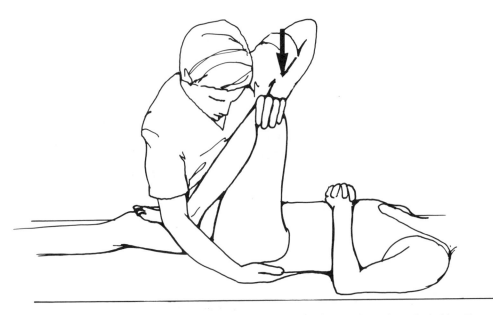

Fig. 20-9 Posterior glide of the hip. *Patient:* Supine with the leg supported on the table. *Therapist:* Standing on the opposite side of the table with one hand contacting the posterior ilium to stabilize, while the other hand contacts the flexed knee joint and holds the femur in the flexed and adducted position. *Technique:* The forearm exerts a posterior lateral force through the hand contact on the distal femur (knee joint). *Use:* A component motion necessary for hip flexion and internal rotation.

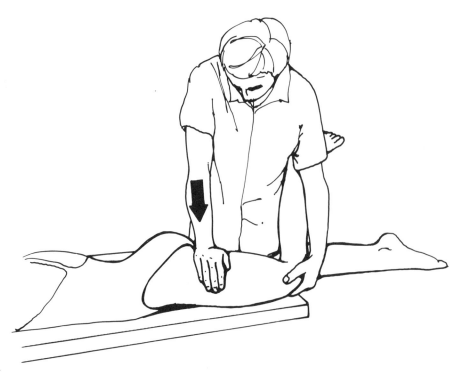

Fig. 20-10 Anterior glide of the hip. *Patient:* Prone with leg supported on the table. *Therapist:* Standing on the opposite side of the table with one hand contacting the anterior distal aspect of the femur to hold the femur in extension and rotation, while the other hand contacts the proximal posterior aspect of the femur. *Technique:* The forearm exerts an anterior force through the proximal hand contact. *Use:* A component motion necessary for external rotation and extension.

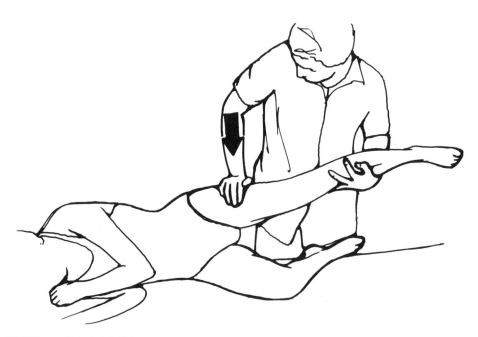

Fig. 20-11 Medial glide of the hip. *Patient:* Sidelying on opposite side of the hip to be treated. *Therapist:* Standing behind the patient with one hand contacting the proximal tibia to support the leg in the loose-pack position, while the other hand contacts the proximal lateral aspect of the femur. *Technique:* Forearm exerts a medial force through the proximal hand contact. *Use:* A component motion necessary for abduction and flexion.

Treatment

Modalities that may be useful to decrease inflammation are ultrasound, interferential, iontophoresis, and phonophoresis.

With a pelvic tilt or a short contralateral leg, use a temporary heel lift to take pressure off the nerve and fascia.

Treat the lumbar spine (see Ch. 12, Lumbar Spine).

Educate the patient in posture and body mechanics.

Management

Physician may use injection to decrease the inflammation. Physician may need to assist with referral to dietetics.

If a heel lift is used to work with the pelvic tilt or the contralateral short leg, monitoring of the patient's need for this heel lift over time is important. Too often heel lifts are prescribed and used even after the problem is resolved.

Prognosis

The prognosis is poor to excellent depending on the etiology of the entrapment.

Sciatic Nerve

(See Ch. 12, Lumbar Spine).

KNEE

Patellofemoral Degeneration

Degeneration of the articular surface of the patella or femur is often termed "chondromalacia." The term means "cartilage bad" and therefore does not identify the problem or the treatment.

Causes

Direct trauma to the patellofemoral joint

Functional, occupational, and sport over-stress

Structural asymmetry in spine, pelvis, or lower extremity

Increased Q angle

Tightness of muscle, fascia or capsule of spine, pelvis, and lower extremity joints

Overweight

Poor posture

Symptoms

Deep nonspecific knee pain (sometimes the patient can specifically identify pain at the patella)

Pain or limitation of active knee motions

Limping or discomfort with walking, particularly when using stairs and ramps

Swelling present around the patella

Signs

Pain or limitation of active knee motions

Pain or limitation with passive classical knee motions

End range resistance of classical knee motions may be limited due to pain or pannus, although the end feel may be normal

Passive accessory motion of the patella may or may not be limited in motion

End range resistance of the passive accessory motions may be either normal or abnormal (depending on the cause)

Positive Scouring and Compression tests

Resisted isometric contraction of the quadriceps may produce pain especially when testing within 30° to 90° of knee flexion

Asymmetrical weakness of quadriceps or hamstrings

Palpation tenderness along the margins of the patella or at the patellar facets

Palpable swelling

Abnormalities in gait, walking and running

Difficulty using stairs and ramps

Inability to squat or inability to maintain a squatting position

Treatment

Use of modalities to decrease inflammation

Avoid excessive weight bearing to aid in decreasing the inflammation

Manipulate restricted accessory motions (Figs. 20-12 to 20-15)

Stretch tight muscles and myofascia

Decrease structural asymmetry stresses by using orthoses or functional assistive devices

Strengthen weak muscles

Educate the patient in stresses to avoid, particularly stresses placed on the knee joint between the range of 30° to 90°

Instruct the patient in low-resistance stationary bicycling

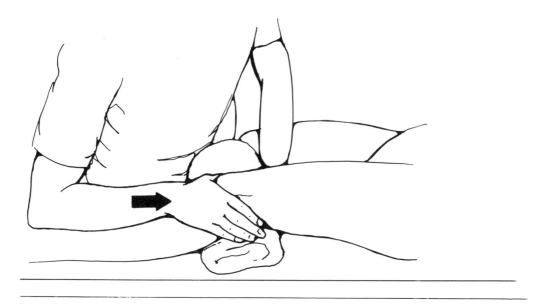

Fig. 20-12 Cephalic glide of the patella. *Patient:* Supine with the leg supported on the table. *Therapist:* Standing with the web space of one hand contacting the inferior aspect of the patella. A support is placed under the knee to maintain the joint in flexion. *Technique:* Forearm exerts a cephalic force through the hand contact on the inferior patella. *Use:* A component motion necessary for knee extension.

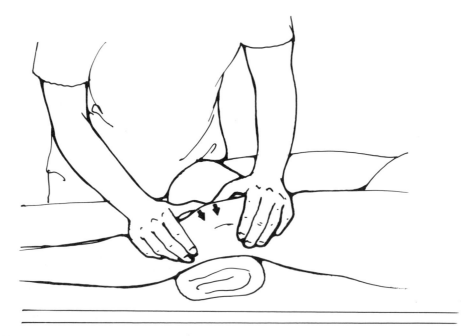

Fig. 20-13 Lateral glide of the patella. *Patient:* Supine with the leg supported on the table. *Therapist:* Standing with distal thumbs contacting the medial side of the patella. A support is placed under the knee to maintain the joint in flexion. *Technique:* The thumbs exert a lateral force. *Use:* A joint play necessary for all motions of the knee.

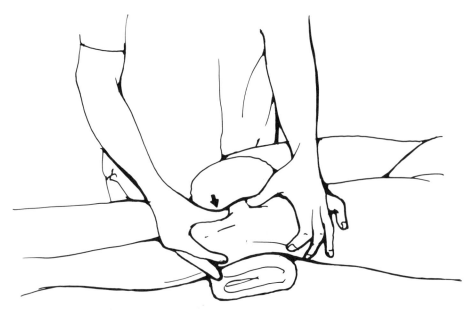

Fig. 20-14 Longitudinal axis rock of the patella. *Patient:* Supine with leg supported on the table. *Therapist:* Standing with the thumb pads contacting the anterior-superior and anterior-inferior surfaces. A support is placed under the knee to maintain the joint in flexion. *Technique:* One thumb exerts a gentle posterior force, while the opposite thumb monitors movement. *Use:* A joint play necessary for all motions of the knee.

Educate the patient in avoidance of functional, occupational, and sport stresses

Management

As of yet, no scientific evidence has shown that conservative treatment can reverse the degenerative pathology. Observation shows that conservative treatment may be able to prevent further degeneration.

Physician management may be necessary to aid in dietetic referral for the overweight patient.

Many times this condition necessitates a alteration in life-style, occupation, or sports to prevent further stresses on the joint.

Prognosis

The prognosis is poor to excellent depending on the cause and when conservative management was initiated.

Tibiofemoral Capsule Tightness

Knee capsule tightness is a common clinical occurrence.

Causes

Knee capsule tightness occurs with nonspecific trauma to the capsule, such as bursitis, tendonitis, postfracture, and postimmobilization, or it occurs with joint strains followed by end ranges of joint active or passive movements not carried out functionally.

Symptoms

Some loss of functional, active knee movements may occur.

Pain may be present at the end ranges of all the active movements.

Alterations in gait may exist.

Signs

Active and passive classical motions are limited in the same direction.

Active and passive classical motions follow a pattern of restriction that is slight limitation of extension (e.g., 5° to 10°) and gross limitation of flexion (e.g., 90° or more).

Pain comes on as the active and passive motions are approached.

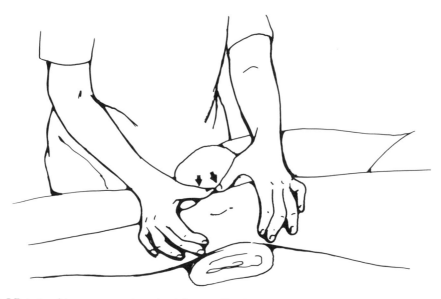

Fig. 20-15 Lateral transverse axis rock of the patella. *Patient:* Supine with the leg supported on the table. *Therapist:* Standing with the thumb pads contacting the medial anterior surface of the patella. A support is placed under the knee to maintain the knee in flexion. *Technique:* The thumbs exert a gentle posterior force through the thumb pad contacts. *Use:* A joint play necessary for all motions of the knee.

End range resistance is an abnormal creep resistance.

Passive accessory motions are limited and may be painful in the following movements: tibia distraction, anterior and posterior glides of the tibia, anterior and posterior glides of the femur, unicondylar glides of the tibia, and anterior tilt of tibia.

Passive accessory motions of the patella are often limited in mobility. Passive accessory motions of the proximal tibio-fibular joint may be limited.

Palpation may produce tenderness along the joint line.

Muscle tightness is often present, particularly of the hamstrings and popliteus.

Myofascial tightness is often present, especially within the quadriceps mechanism, the iliotibial band, and the patellar retinaculum.

Alterations in gait and functional mobility of the lower extremity may be present.

Treatment

Manipulate restricted accessory movements (Figs. 20-16 to 20-22)

Instruct patient in home program of stretching exercises

Stretch tight muscles and myofascia
Strengthen weak muscles
Instruct in gait, walking and running
Educate in posture and proper body mechanics

Management

See Capsule Tightness, Treatment, above.

Once low reactivity is present, a balance board is useful for proprioceptive and nocioceptive stimulation.

Prognosis

The prognosis is fair to excellent depending on the pathology of the collagen and connective tissue makeup.

Quadriceps Tendonitis

Quadriceps tendonitis is commonly seen in adolescents involved in competitive sports.

Causes

Functional, occupational, or sport over-stress
Asymmetries of structure or muscle pull in the lower extremity

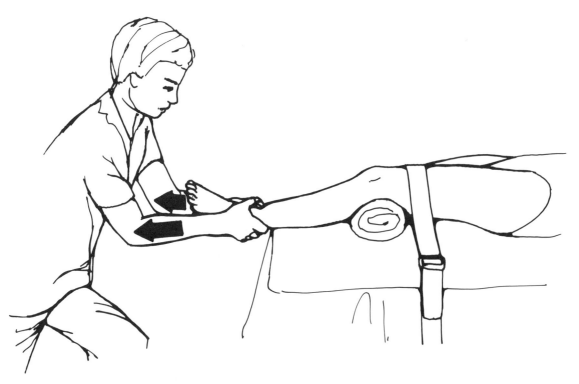

Fig. 20-16 Tibia distraction. *Patient:* Supine with the leg supported on the table. *Therapist:* Standing with both hands contacting the distal tibia and fibula. A support is placed under the knee to maintain the joint in approximately 20° of flexion. A strap is placed across the distal femur and around the table to stabilize. *Technique:* The forearms exert a pull perpendicular to the tibial articular surfaces through the distal hand contact by leaning into the therapist's body weight. *Use:* A joint play necessary for all motions of the knee.

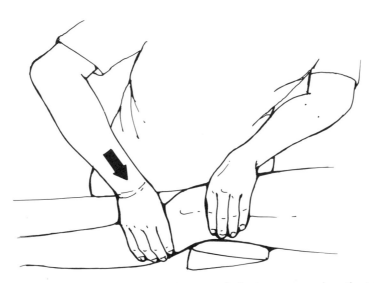

Fig. 20-17 Posterior glide of the tibia. *Patient:* Supine with the leg supported on the table. *Therapist:* Standing with one hand contacting the anterior distal surface of the femur to stabilize, while the other hand contacts the anterior proximal surface of the tibia. A support is placed under the distal femur to stabilize and maintain the joint in approximately 20° of flexion. *Technique:* The forearm exerts a posterior force through the proximal tibia contact. *Use:* A component motion necessary for knee flexion.

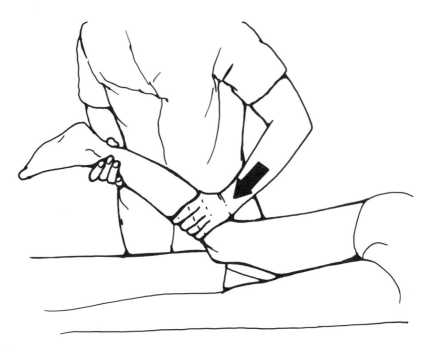

Fig. 20-18 Anterior glide of the tibia. *Patient:* Prone with the leg supported on the table. *Therapist:* Standing with one hand contacting the distal tibia to support the knee in approximately 20° of flexion, while the other hand contacts the posterior proximal surface of the tibia. A support is placed under the distal anterior surface of the femur to stabilize. *Technique:* The forearm exerts an anterior glide through the hand contact on the posterior surface of the tibia. *Use:* A component motion necessary for knee extension.

Symptoms

Limitation or pain with active knee motions
Pain with weight bearing
Alterations or pain with walking or running

Signs

Active knee extension is painful and may be limited
Active flexion is limited and painful
Passive classical flexion is uncomfortable at end range
Resisted isometric contraction is the best differential test to reproduce the pain symptoms
Palpation to identify specific area of inflammation
Myofascial tightness often exists
Muscle weakness often exists
Alterations of gait, walking or running
Structural asymmetry, such as excessive pronation

Treatment

Use of modalities to decrease inflammation, such as ultrasound, interferential, iontophoresis, or phonophoresis
Transverse friction massage
Stretch tight muscles and myofascia
Strengthen weak musculature
Use of assistive device (orthosis) to alter structural asymmetry
Instruct in gait, walking and running
Educate in proper sports surfaces and shoes
Educate in proper body mechanics

Management

Use a circumferential band above or below the patella to redistribute the muscle force to the tendon as sports and functional activities resume.

Prognosis

Excellent once the cause has been eliminated.

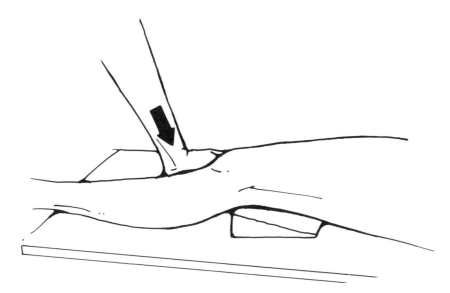

Fig. 20-19 Posterior medial unicondylar glide of the tibia. *Patient:* Supine with the leg supported on the table. *Therapist:* Standing with proximal palm contacting the anterior medial surface of the tibia. A support is placed under the femur to support the femur and to maintain the knee in approximately 20° of flexion. *Technique:* The forearm exerts a posterior force through the hand contact on the medial tibia. *Use:* A component motion of internal rotation and flexion.

Pes Anserine Bursitis

Inflammation of the pes anserine bursa occurs more commonly than it is identified. Patient symptoms and complaint often lead to a diagnosis of chondromalacia.

Causes
Functional, occupational, or sport over-stress
Alterations in sport pattern
Direct trauma

Symptoms
Diffuse knee pain, often reported to be inside the knee
Limitations or pain with functional active knee motions
Alterations in functional mobility of the lower extremity

Signs
Limitation or pain with active knee motions
Resisted isometric contraction of any of the three muscles may be uncomfortable
Palpation of the bursa reproduces pain.

Treatment

Modalities may be used to decrease the inflammation, such as ultrasound, interferential, iontophoresis, or phonophoresis.

Management

See Ch. 18, Bursitis.

Prognosis

Excellent

Iliotibial Band Friction Syndrome

The iliotibial band is vulnerable to a friction irritation at the femoral epicondyle.

Causes
Functional, occupational, or sport over-stress
Alteration of sport pattern, such as change of shoes, change of ground surface or terrain
Tightness of muscles
Weakness of muscles
Structural asymmetry

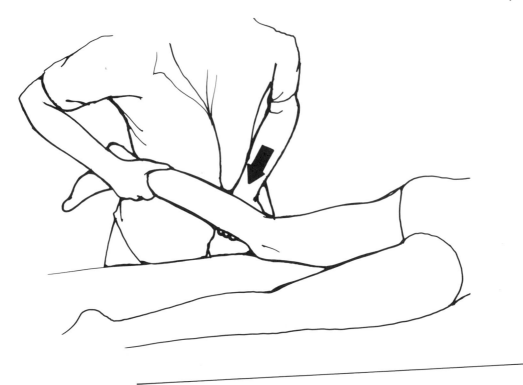

Fig. 20-20 Anterior lateral unicondylar glide of the tibia. *Patient:* Prone with the leg supported on the table. *Therapist:* Standing with one hand contacting the distal tibia and fibula to maintain the knee in approximately 20° of flexion, while the other hand contacts the posterior proximal lateral surface of the tibia. *Technique:* The forearm exerts an anterior force through the hand contact on the posterior lateral surface of the tibia. *Use:* A component motion necessary for internal rotation and flexion.

Symptoms

Deep knee pain often felt once the activity is initiated or sometime into the activity

Pain limits the amount of functional activity

Signs

Deep palpation of the femoral epicondyle

The femoral epicondyle should be palpated with the knee in different positions. The testing should be done in at least three knee positions. The three positions are: 0° to 10° of extension, flexion from 100° to full flexion, and midrange.

Iliotibial band tightness

Muscle tightness, such as tensor fascia, adductors, hamstrings, or peroneal group

Myofascial tightness

Muscle weakness

Structural asymmetry, such as pronation, hip anteversion, or tibial torsion

Treatment

Modalities to decrease the inflammation, such as ultrasound, interferential, iontophoresis, or phonophoresis

Transverse friction massage

Stretch tight muscles and myofascia

Strengthen weak muscles

Correct or alter structural asymmetry, if possible

Educate in over-stresses, particularly in sports, terrain, and equipment

Management

Once the inflammation has receded, monitor the functional and sports stresses.

Prognosis

Excellent

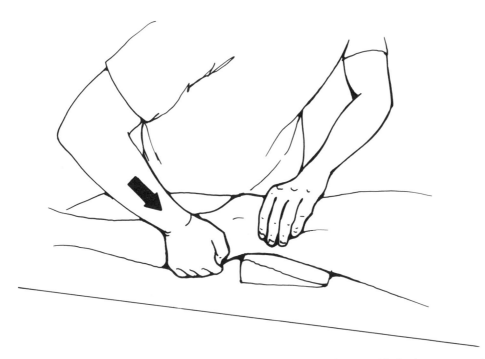

Fig. 20-21 Posterior lateral unicondylar glide of the tibia. *Patient:* Supine with the leg supported on the table. *Therapist:* Standing with one hand contacting the anterior distal surface of the femur to stabilize, while the other hand contacts the anterior proximal lateral surface of the tibia. A support is placed under the distal femur to stabilize and maintain the knee in approximately 20° of flexion. *Technique:* The forearm exerts a posterior force through the hand contact on the anterior lateral surface of the tibia. *Use:* A component motion necessary for external rotation and extension.

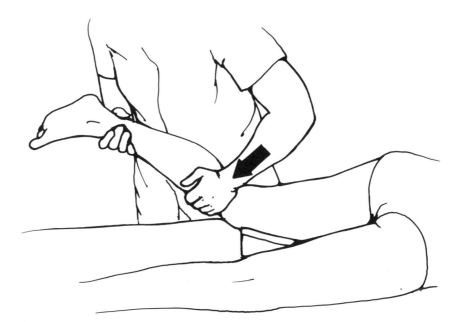

Fig. 20-22 Anterior medial unicondylar glide of the tibia. *Patient:* Prone with the leg supported on the table. *Therapist:* Standing with one hand contacting the distal tibia to support and maintain the knee in approximately 20° of flexion, while the other hand contacts the posterior proximal medial surface of the tibia. A support is placed under the distal femur to stabilize. *Technique:* The forearm exerts an anterior force through the hand contact on the posterior medial surface of the tibia. *Use:* A component motion necessary for external rotation and extension.

Cruciate Ligament Instability

The most common cruciate ligament instability is that of the anterior cruciate ligament. Once the trauma is forceful enough to tear the ligament, a dysfunction of the meniscus and/or the capsule usually occurs. With anterior cruciate instability, a rotary instability often ensues. Posterior cruciate instability is not so common. With posterior cruciate instability, a straight instability exists. The following section does not attempt to isolate the instabilities with etiology or signs.

Causes

Functional, occupational, or sport over-stress, usually of a rotary or straight force

Symptoms

Giving way of the knee during functional or sport activities
Pain or swelling

Signs

For the anterior cruciate: positive anterior draw sign, positive Lachman sign, positive for rotary stressing
For the posterior cruciate: positive posterior draw sign, positive Sag test, positive Godfrey test
Swelling
Muscle weakness

Treatment

Use of modalities to treat the swelling
Muscle strengthening
Use of assistive device for sport or occupational function

Management

Physician management is necessary to assist with treatment approach and goal setting.

Ligamentous Sprains

Collateral Ligament

The collateral ligament involved in trauma may result in limited mobility owing to adhesion formation. The medial collateral ligament is more commonly injured than the lateral collateral ligament. The medial collateral ligament is discussed here.

Causes

Functional, occupational, or sport over-stress, usually as a valgus stress

Signs

Limitation and pain of active knee flexion
Alterations of gait; using stairs may be painful or altered

Symptoms

Limitation and pain of active and passive classical motion of flexion
  Active and passive classical motion of extension is usually full unless swelling is present
Valgus end range resistance is a tight creep or painful
Passive accessory motion of valgus is limited or painful
Deep palpation of the ligament produces discomfort
Swelling palpable
Gait deviations

Treatment

Transverse friction massage
Passive stretching of knee flexion
Use of heat modalities to aid in lengthening
Instruction in exercises to encourage knee flexion
Instruction in gait, use of stairs

Management

Once range of motion of flexion is improving, daily treatment may be necessary to continue the extensibility of the ligament fibers. Active movement in the new range is imperative.

Prognosis

The prognosis is fair to excellent depending on the nature of the ligamentous adhesions.

Meniscus

With the advancement of arthroscopy for the diagnosis and treatment of meniscal dysfunction, physical therapists are treating fewer primary meniscal tears. Conservative treatment is involved more with postarthroscopy evaluation and treatment. However, meniscal sprains do occur that require conservative treatment. This treatment is discussed here.

Causes
Functional, occupational, or sport rotary stress to the knee

Signs
Limited or painful active knee motions

Swelling

Limitation or pain with functional, occupational, and sport activities

Symptoms
Limitation or pain with active knee motions

Passive classical motions limited

Passive, classical, end range of tibial rotations are often painful

End range resistance is a springy rebound, or if swelling is present then an empty end feel is felt

Painful muscle contraction often exists

Intra-articular swelling is palpable

Palpable tenderness in area of coronary ligaments

Alterations in gait and functional movements

Treatment
Transverse friction massage to area of coronary ligaments

Modalities to decrease the inflammation, such as ultrasound, interferential or high-voltage stimulation

Take pressure off of the meniscus by eliminating or decreasing weight bearing

Manipulate meniscus if mobility is limited

Educate in gait and functional movements

Management
If above treatment approaches do not alter the symptoms, then a consultation with a physician is necessary to determine whether a meniscus tear is present.

Prognosis
Excellent

Peripheral Nerve Entrapment

Common Peroneal Nerve

The common peroneal nerve rests against the fibula neck and continues to descend down the leg by piercing through an opening in the peroneus longus muscle and then branching into the superficial and deep peroneal nerves. The nerve is vulnerable to entrapment at the fibular neck and at the emergence through the muscle. The nerve is both motor and sensory in distribution. The muscles innervated are the peroneus longus, peroneus brevis, tibialis anterior, extensor digitorum longus, extensor hallucis longus, peroneus tertius, and extensor digitorum brevis. The sensory distribution to the skin is the area of the distal one-third of the leg and the dorsal surfaces of the first to fourth digits.

Causes
Direct pressure on the nerve

Fibular fracture

Forceful inversion and plantar flexion trauma to the foot and ankle

Excessive hindfoot supination with functional plantar flexion positions of the foot, for example, ballet dancers

Symptoms
Pain in the lateral aspect of the leg and the foot

Muscle weakness of the leg or foot

Altered gait

Signs
Limited active motion of foot and ankle

Altered skin sensation

Muscle weakness

Myofascia tightness

Gait deviations

Tenderness to palpation of the nerve

Excessive inversion of the calcaneus or plantar flexion of the cuboid or fifth metatarsal

Hypermobility of passive accessory motions of the cuboid, third cuneiform, and the fifth-fourth metatarsal

Treatment
Lateral heel wedge to maintain an everted hindfoot

Wedges to stabilize the hypermobility of the forefoot

Use of modalities to decrease inflammation, such as ultrasound, interferential, iontophoresis, or phonophoresis

Massage muscles and myofascia

Strengthen weak muscles

Instruct in gait
Instruct in functional, occupational, sport
    stresses to avoid

Management

Continuously evaluate function and structure of the lower extremity.

Prognosis

Fair to excellent depending on the etiology.

Saphenous Nerve

The saphenous nerve is vulnerable to entrapment in the subsartorial canal, or Hunter's canal, at the distal medial aspect of the thigh, above the knee joint. A dense sheet of fascia covers the canal. The fascia attaches to the vastus medialis and the adductor longus and magnus. The sartorius muscle covers the dense fascia, and the two connective tissues move together. Contraction and tone of these four muscles can affect the fascia and hence the canal space. The saphenous nerve is sensory in distribution. The distribution is to the skin of the medial aspect of the knee and leg, with articular branches to the knee.

Causes

Direct trauma
Functional, occupational, and sport over-stress,
    for example, excessive tibial torsion,
    especially internal tibial torsion
Excessive pronation of the ankle or internal
    rotation of the hip
Hypertrophy of the above-mentioned muscles
Tightness of the above-mentioned muscles
Tightness of the fascia

Symptoms

Knee pain
    Patient may or may not be able to discern
        specifically the medial side of the knee as
        painful.
Pain or limitation in using stairs and ramps

Signs

Pain or limitation in active motions of the knee,
    hip, or ankle
Tenderness to palpation at Hunter's canal
Fascial tightness at the canal
Muscle imbalance, that is, tightness or
    hypertrophy or weakness
Altered skin sensation
Structural deviations, such as pronation of the
    hindfoot, tibial torsions, femoral torsions
Gait deviations

Treatment

Massage muscle and fascia
Stretch muscles
Use of modalities for pain or to decrease
    inflammation
Use of orthoses to correct, if possible, structural
    asymmetry
Instruct in gait
Instruct in stresses to avoid, for instance resting
    the muscles in a non-weight-bearing status

Management

Entrapment of the saphenous nerve is not frequently identified by diagnosis.

Prognosis

Fair to excellent depending on the cause.

21 The Child with Orthopaedic Problems

Ann F. VanSant

Infants and children with disorders of the musculoskeletal system have distinctly different physical therapy problems from those demonstrated by adults. First and foremost, infants and children are growing and rapidly developing. This fact should guide and direct all physical therapy for this population. Obviously, infants should not be compared with adults when undertaking evaluation and treatment. Too often, however, adult standards of physical function are applied to the still growing and developing child. Maturity of posture and movement cannot be expected until late into the teenage years. When working with children, remember that control over body musculature is still not fully developed. Evaluation and treatment procedures that require relaxation and isolated muscle function such as manual muscle testing must be applied with regard for the normal course of development of neuromuscular control. Standards against which children's performance is judged must be adjusted to reflect this fact.

Second, when working with a child with an orthopaedic problem the therapist must realize that the child is both an individual and an integral part of a family. The child must be evaluated and treated with this idea in mind. Children eventually become self-reliant, and accept responsibility for their own physical health. Physical therapists should work with parents to foster development of self-responsibility. Until the child is able, families assume responsibility for their child's health and well being. Therefore, families need to be involved to the greatest extent possible in decision making concerning their child's physical therapy.

Another characteristic that differentiates musculoskeletal problems in children from those seen in adults is that many syndromes that affect children do not necessarily have pain as a presenting symptom. When pain is present, pain relief becomes the first priority in treatment. However, the common basis of all pediatric orthopaedic physical therapy practice is a concern with prevention and correction of motor habits that lead to deformity. In fact, the word orthopaedics reflects this idea: ortho-, meaning straight, and -paedic, a suffix meaning child. The very term orthopaedics describes the prevention and correction of musculoskeletal deformities in growing and developing children.

PHYSICAL THERAPY EVALUATION FOR THE INFANT AND CHILD

Physical therapy evaluation of children with orthopaedic problems includes both subjective and objective information. Subjective data should be gathered concerning the present problem, its history, and the family history related to the condition. In addition, information is needed concerning the present function of the family and the child within the family so that appropriate regard may be given to the social ramifications of physical therapy intervention. Ultimately, a chief complaint should be obtained from a responsible family member if the child is too young to articulate his

495

own difficulty. Chief complaints emanating from parents of children with orthopaedic problems often center on the physical appearance of the infant or child, or on a failure of physical function, such as delay in achievement of motor milestones. For those disorders in which pain is a symptom, crying, fussiness, or other descriptions of discomfort are observed or presented by parents as the chief complaint. Traditionally, subjective data is gathered primarily to delineate the symptoms of the problem. However, for physical therapy, subjective information is also critical to determine the personal and social strengths of the child and family. In treatment these strengths can be tapped for the benefit of the child.

Objective information is the cornerstone for defining the child's problem in biomechanical, neurological, motor developmental, or functional terms. Deformity is commonly perceived and evaluated within a biomechanical perspective. Physical therapists who work with children must also be concerned with neurological and developmental aspects of deformity. For example, a dislocated hip produces obvious deformity that may be delineated through measures of leg length, range of motion, and assessments of muscle power. This same deformity may lead to habitual use of specific postural and movement patterns as a compensation for the deformity. The preference for compensatory motor patterns results in a limitation of the variety of motor patterns expected of the normally developing child.

A test of motor pattern development may more fully delineate the orthopaedic problem. It is important to remember that tests of motor development status are tests of functional abilities for children. Just as adults are examined with regard to functional abilities, the functional tasks of childhood are assessed through developmental tests. At first this idea my seem unusual, yet the developmental milestones and tests of motor abilities in infants and children represent functional achievements of childhood.

Although deformity commonly presents in subjective assessment as a complaint about appearance, deformity may lead to delay or failure to achieve motor milestones and therefore represent the absence of functional ability that is normal for the child's age group. Parents may report no difficulty with achievement of major motor milestones; however, the first or only child particularly warrants developmental assessment as parents may have no standard against which to judge their child's progress. Failure to include assessment of each of these major aspects of a child's function may lead to errors in defining the problem and subsequent failure in selecting appropriate treatment procedures. For these reasons, factors other than those required to analyze biomechanical aspects of orthopaedic problems must be evaluated when working with children.

General Considerations

When evaluating an infant or child, remember that children are more comfortable with their parents than with a stranger. Rather than being an impediment to evaluation, parents are essential to the full understanding and demonstration of the condition. Therefore, keep the parents involved during the testing and evaluation process. The child should have an opportunity to become familiar with any equipment that will be used for testing, such as goniometers or balance boards. Some extra attention to ensure trust and comfort on the part of the child is well worth the time. The child who is upset or fearful will not perform in a customary manner, making the test results unreliable.

Your impression of the child's nature is important for deciding which procedures to administer first. The child who has been actively clamoring for attention may do well with more active tasks initially. The initially shy child may need more explanation of the order and process of evaluation and additional parental involvement to ensure trust and comfort. In any instance, the process and role that the child will play should be fully explained to the child and parents.

Preliminary data including the child's name and nickname, sex, date of birth, and present age should be obtained and recorded. Although apparently trivial, the present age and date of birth should be concordant. The year of a child's birth sometimes may be misreported and asking the child's present age helps to detect and resolve this problem.

Subjective Data

The process of obtaining subjective data for the initial evaluation of an infant or child is discussed below. For therapists working in a health care setting in which they do not represent the primary entry point into the health care system, much of this information may have already been gathered by a primary health care worker and would be available in the child's medical record. If a child is brought to physical therapy for the first time by a parent, the process described below is appropriate, although one may eliminate gathering details of past medical history if they are available in the child's medical record. In examining children for the first time in a school or hospital without the benefit of a parent being present, the medical record is the starting point. Other professionals such as nurses or teachers are also invaluable sources of information concerning the child's general problems and demeanor.

An appropriate way to begin the history taking is to ask the parent, "What have you noticed that doesn't seem right?" Listen carefully and with your full attention to the response. If both parents are present, both should be given an opportunity to answer and add to the other's remarks. This gives you an opportunity to learn of differences in observation and perception of the problem by the parents and to determine who is the primary caretaker for the child. The initial inquiry should be followed with further questions: (1) when the problem was first noticed; (2) if it came on suddenly or gradually; (3) once noticed, were the signs there constantly or did they seem to come and go; (4) has the problem gotten worse or better; (5) what seems to help or make it worse; and (6) was there any particular incident that accompanied the onset of the problem, such as illness or injury.

This last question is a good transition from present to past history. Inquiries concerning the child's birth history and health history are important. Determine whether the child was born on time and whether there were any complications with pregnancy or delivery of the child. Breech presentation and premature rupture of the membranes are often associated with congenital deformity. Determine how many other children there are in the family, including their ages. Any past or current medical problems should be noted by inquiring about the health of each of the major body systems: neurological, including major sensory systems; circulatory; pulmonary; gastrointestinal; and urinary.

You may begin family history taking by asking if any member of the family has any major health or medical problems. In examining the child with orthopaedic dysfunction, you should inquire specifically about muscle, bone, joint, or nervous system problems in family members.

As the history and chief complaint are being gathered, notice the child in interaction with the parent. Parents may demonstrate the child's difficulty during this time by showing you the affected area or asking the child to perform the troublesome task, such as demonstrating the posture of the foot or having the child walk. As the parents describe and demonstrate their concerns, observe the child's reaction. Do you detect shyness, or an outgoing nature? Is the child talking during the process and clamoring for attention? These opportunities to observe the child in action are invaluable assists for selecting and determining the order in which you administer more specific evaluation procedures.

Objective Data

Observation and physical inspection of the child is the beginning of objective evaluation. As mentioned previously, subjective information gathering gives the therapist an opportunity to gain a general impression of the child. When you first begin to focus your attention on the child, observe the posture, or the manner in which the parent is holding the infant or child, and the overall activity level.

For infants that are not yet walking, a postural assessment is an excellent way to begin the objective evaluation. Posture, of course, is age related. That is, different postures are expected at different ages. By observing an infant's or child's posture, you are performing both a developmental and a biomechanical assessment. For infants who are not yet standing, postural assessment is accomplished by observing the preferred or habitual posture. In babies, one begins by noting the manner in which the parent holds and handles the infant. Where are the hands placed while supporting the child? Up high under the cervical and occipital region, or lower down near the axilla and upper thoracic spine? Is the child sitting with the trunk unsupported, with the parent's hands primarily in contact with the pelvis or thighs of the child? Parent intuitively provide infants and children with the support they need. As the child develops the ability to control his posture, parental assistance decreases. Thus, a hand placed in the lower thoracic region indicates that the infant is controlling the upper thoracic and cervical regions.

Has the parent been primarily restraining the child from activity, keeping him in a quiet sitting posture?

Does the parent change the child's posture, perhaps placing the child on the floor?

What position does the parent or child select, that is, standing, sitting, or lying on back or stomach?

When the child is on his own, does he move about, change general postural patterns? For example, does he get up on hands and knees, roll over, sit up, or pull to standing?

Postural Considerations

Normal Postural Patterns of Infancy

An alternating pattern of postural symmetry and asymmetry is characteristic of the first year of life. Early in the first trimester, with the exception of the head being rotated toward one side, symmetry is expected in trunk and limb position. About the age of 2 to 4 months, an asymmetrical resting posture is expected in the upper extremities. This has often been characterized as the period when the asymmetrical tonic neck postural pattern is evident. Yet it is most important to remember that although this postural pattern is evident in the infant's behavior, the head or limbs may be frequently seen moving out of the characteristic reflexive pattern. The infant then begins again to demonstrate symmetry in postural patterns, with the head tending to return to a midline position with respect to the body. Arms and legs are used simultaneously and symmetrically in the supine infant when reaching for the feet or in a propped sitting posture as the child approaches the fifth month. When the infant is placed sitting, you should note the posture of the head. Is it held forward with respect to the long axis of the body or in line with the body, a posture that appears later? When the infant held in sitting, is the trunk inclined forward; are the lower extremities flexed and laterally rotated allowing the lateral aspect of the thighs and legs to contact the support surface?

Flexion of the spine gradually is replaced with an extended posture proceeding from the cervical to the lumbar spine over the course of the first 6 to 7 months. By observing the infant's axial posture in the sagittal plane, you may judge the relative development toward an extended vertical posture. It is not uncommon for the infant to extend the trunk in brief repetitive bursts of activity while being held in sitting. However, without full development of the ability to right to the vertical and balance the trunk, the infant does not sit without support. The inability to sit erect is often attributed to what has been called "weakness" in the trunk. Infants may well be weak when compared with an adult model of strength. Yet until the central nervous system has developed the action patterns of balanced flexion and extension necessary to maintain the trunk in a vertical posture and the processes that enable selection and control of the joint motions required for proper performance on a manual muscle test, it seems inappropriate to judge an infant as weak.

Normal Postural Patterns of the Toddler and Pre-School-Aged Child

If the child is a pre-schooler, is he actively moving about? Look particularly for variability in body action.

Does the child walk and climb about, get up and down from a seated or squatting position in a variety of ways?

Does there seem to be but one way the child performs a given activity?

Does the child seem to favor a part of the body, tending to limp or not to use that part in functional activities?

Normal Postural Patterns of the School-Aged Child

The school-aged child is more reserved in demeanor when in a clinical setting. Yet even when the child is sitting or standing, the frequency of bodily movements is greater than that seen in adults. Swinging the legs, or wrapping them around the chair, bringing the feet up onto the chair seat, gripping the chair with the hands, folding and unfolding the arms are quite common behaviors. Active inspection of the room and its occupants and objects is to be expected.

Growth and Anthropometric Measures

Measures of height and weight should be performed on all children and adolescents. Body segment length and girth provide objective documentation of many disorders of the musculoskeletal system. Often orthopaedic disorders accompany growth disorders and orthopaedic dysfunction may lead to atrophy or growth disturbance in affected body segments. Length and girth measures should be obtained for all body segments that show orthopaedic or functional problems.

Height and Weight

You will need a flexible steel tape measure and an accurate scale to obtain measures of height and weight and should refer to standard growth charts included in Appendix 21-1 to this chapter to compare your measures with the norms for the child's age.

Measuring Height and Weight

Procedures for obtaining height appear obvious, yet one must remember that the measures should be obtained in a way consistent with the standards against which the child will be judged. In most instances, an infant's height is expressed in terms of crown–rump length with the infant positioned supine. Children should take their shoes off before their standing height is obtained unless the standard height chart indicates that the standards were taken on children wearing shoes. Similarly, when obtaining weight, know the procedures used to obtain the standards for comparison before taking the measure. It is wise to record the time of day

that your measures were taken. This will enable replication of the measures in a most consistent manner.

When comparing a child's stature to standard anthropometric norms, remember that in conventional growth studies the left extremities are measured. In physical therapy applications, both right and left sides are measured for length and girth to compare an affected part with its unaffected counterpart. To obtain reliable segment length and girth measures, one must ensure that the position of the segment is appropriate and then carefully and precisely palpate bony landmarks.

Leg Length Measures

Although it is quite common to gather anthropometric measures on the lower extremities, the principles of obtaining similar measures on other body segments do not differ from those used for the lower extremity. Careful palpation leading to precise identification of bony landmarks is the key to obtaining reliable measures.

Measuring Leg Length

When obtaining lower extremity length, first ensure that the lower extremities are in a neutral position without obvious rotation, abduction, or adduction. Inspect the extremity from the saggital plane to determine whether there is a resting posture of hip flexion. A flexed hip effectively shortens the extremity, as do adduction and abduction. When a neutral position of the lower limb cannot be obtained, use the most superior tip of the greater trochanter as a proximal point of measure. To reliably locate the greater trochanter, rotate the extended limb from the neutral position medially and laterally with your fingertips moving distally from just below the iliac crest until you palpate the greater trochanter rotating beneath your fingers. Use your fingertips to locate the most proximal tip of the trochanter and anchor your tape at this point. If the ASIS is being used as a landmark, place your hands over the lateral aspect of the iliac crests while facing the child. Carefully move your hands anteriorly and inferiorly, all the while palpating the crests as your hands move over them. Use both of your thumbs to locate the anterior superior iliac spines and run them gently but firmly along the course of the spines. Make a habit of consistently anchoring the steel tape over the most cephalic point on the spine, so that you can be consistent on future measures. Similarly, if the medial malleolus is being used as the distal landmark, use your index finger to palpate the distal border of the malleolus and run the tape to the most distal projection in order to ensure a consistent landmark for your measures. Similar techniques can be used with other bony landmarks.

Measure of Flexibility

Range of motion varies with age. Adult standards are not appropriate for young children. There have been few studies of normal flexibility in infants and children using conventional cardinal plane measures. Data that are available are reported in Appendix 21-2 and should be used in place of conventional adult norms.

When traditional cardinal plane norms are not available other flexibility measures can be substituted. This is but one more area in great need of normative studies.

General Considerations of Flexibility

Flexibility in Infants

In very young infants, normal paths of motion of the joints do not conform to cardinal planes. That is, prenatally and for a period postnatally, infants move primarily in diagonal paths that cut across all three cardinal planes. By first observing an infant's habitual posture, you can define the habitual path of motion. Inspect the position of the limb segments because infants have a tendency to hold the extremities in the plane of movement (Fig. 21-1). Do not force the limbs from this movement plane to make cardinal plane measures.

In the lower extremities, a hip flexion, slightly abducted and externally rotated posture is normal. This is an active posture. Unfortunately, this state of the musculature is sometimes referred to as passive tone. Remember that the infant's musculature is actively producing this posture. Passive movement out of this position should be accomplished gently and without force. The hips of a newborn are stable within the normal excursion

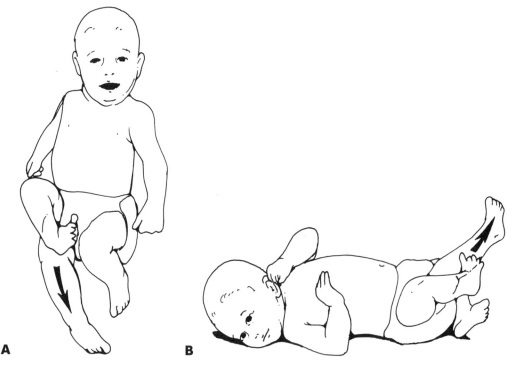

Fig. 21-1 Infant kicks—(**A**) down and (**B**) across.

of the joint, but forcing the hips into the extreme ranges of extension, adduction or abduction, or medial or lateral rotation can cause harm. Symmetry of passive hip movement is a most important criterion of normalcy. The hips can be moved simultaneously to assess symmetry.

Range of motion in the knees and feet also differs from that of older persons. When the hips of the young infant are in their normal resting posture of flexion, the knees usually cannot be extended beyond 90°. There is sufficient dorsiflexion of the foot on the leg such that the dorsum of the foot comes into contact with the anterior aspect of the leg. These differences in lower extremity range of motion do not represent pathology. Physical therapy is not indicated to increase range of motion in the hips and knees. In time, the effect of gravity and the infant's active movements will bring passive movement into the more commonly expected ranges for older age groups.

In the upper extremities, the scarf sign is often used to assess the passive range of adduction of the arm across the chest. In a somewhat nontraditional way, the position of the elbow is noted with respect to the sternal notch. Normally the infant demonstrates resistance to moving the elbow beyond this position. The elbows may not quite reach a position of 180° of extension. Again, symmetry of passive movement of the right and left extremities is an important criterion of normalcy.

Most pathology of the musculoskeletal system is evident in asymmetries, or deviations from the normally flexed posture, during this early postnatal period. For example, a clubfoot deformity is notable by the absence of the expected degree of dorsiflexion. Torticollis is evident in the asymmetrical head position characteristic of this condition, and hip dysplasia is commonly evidenced by asymmetry not only in hip posture but in active and passive movements as well.

Flexibility in Children

Owing to the absence of cardinal plane norms, one may resort to the use of more functional tests of flexibility. Flexibility has been the concern of physical educators who have used techniques other than goniometric methods to assess the child's "flexibility" (see later discussions).

Muscle Strength—The Integrity of Muscle Innervation

The traditional assessment of "strength" in children is complicated by the young child's inability to isolate action in one muscle from action in other muscles. Traditional methods of strength testing require the individual to perform isolated joint movement within one of the cardinal planes of the body. As is well known, muscles course across the cardinal planes running between their origin and insertion. Each muscle, if contracted in isolation, would by nature of its anatomical attachments produce movement in all three planes. From a neural control perspective, cardinal plane movements require the cooperation of groups of muscles to carefully control the direction and path of the limb within the specified plane. Indeed, one must remember that cardinal planes are abstractions that were applied to the anatomical and kinesiological sciences to make communication more precise. They were not invented to reflect the natural function and control of muscles by the central nervous system. The ability to control a limb movement by keeping the body segment traveling within a specified mechanical plane is a complex task of neural control. Feedback from sensory receptors must be analyzed and interpreted to provide corrective signals to the musculature to keep the limb from deviating out of the specified plane of movement.

From a developmental perspective, the child's ability to discriminate, analyze, and translate sensory feedback into control of action gradually develops over the period of early childhood. To expect an infant or young child to perform isolated joint actions within the cardinal planes is inappropriate. Children neither understand nor appreciate the need to perform a movement within a cardinal plane. In simple terms, the mechanical model of human movement on which manual muscle testing is based is irrelevant to the young child's interests and capabilities.

One can, however, judge the integrity of innervation to the musculature by designing tests that evoke active movement and thus contraction in various muscle groups. In the tradition of manual muscle testing one can note the following:

Whether the resultant contraction produced
    movement opposing the force of gravity.
Whether that movement was carried through the
    age appropriate range of movement.
The plane in which the movement occurred.

Thus, one can develop a baseline measure of the ability of the musculature to produce power sufficient for antigravity function.

Testing the Integrity of Innervation in Infants

Observation and Palpation
The simplest and most noninvasive method to determine if muscles are innervated is observation of the infant's spontaneous active movements. By spending time watching and then palpating the musculature of interest, one can note both the nature and extent of movement and by deduction determine which muscle groups are innervated. This procedure is effective, however, only when the infant is awake and responsive.

The Stretch Position
Positioning and holding the infant in the stretch position for the muscle group of interest is a means of determining active muscle power. For example, if the knee extensors are being examined, gently move the leg into a fully but not forcibly flexed position and hold the extremity in this position for a short period of time. Awake and alert infants normally react to being held at the end of their passive range by actively moving out of the restricted position, or actively contracting the muscles during attempts to move them into a stretch position. This procedure relies on the integrity of the stretch reflexes.

Reflex Testing
The third method of determining the integrity of innervation of musculature is through the use of age-appropriate reflex testing. Numerous infant reflexes have been delineated in terms of the general age range in which they are normally observed, the reflexogenic zone, the adequate stimulus, and the predicted response. Charts provided in Appendices 21-3A and 21-3B may be used to select a movement pattern response that by deduction would involve the use of muscles of interest to the examiner. The adequate stimulus is then applied to the appropriate reflexogenic zone, and the response or failure of response can be used to determine the integrity of innervation.

A final method that can be used in conjunction with any of the above procedures involves light stroking over the belly of the muscle you are testing. Skin receptors generate sensory signals that through reflexive pathways facilitate the underlying musculature. Young infants are responsive to this form of stimulation to evoke muscle contraction.

Testing Muscle Power in Young Children

By their very nature, toddlers and pre-school-aged children are bundles of activity. As with infants, observation of active movements often preclude the necessity of performing detailed assessments of muscle power. Again, attempts to have the young child move within cardinal planes are thwarted by the child's ability to understand the traditional test instructions and the child's inability to precisely control and isolate muscle function.

From a developmental and neurological perspective, tests of isolated joint action can be used to judge the relative maturity of the nervous system. For example, rotation of the forearm into pronation and supination and isolated finger-lifting tasks are used to judge neural maturity. The presence of associated reactions, for example, the linkage of forearm rotation with glenohumeral abduction and adduction and medial and lateral rotation, is the mark of an immature nervous system. It is believed that only with full development of the cortical spinal pathways and associated central connections does the individual have the potential to isolate muscle action. Experience in observing the performance of preschool-aged and school-aged children attempting these tasks reveals that children in these age groups are unable to isolate such joint actions until they are nearly in their teens. According to the standards for muscle testing, these associated reactions would be considered substitutions. It is important to understand that the associated reactions are the natural response to requests to perform such tasks, and it is possible that even in adults performance of isolated joint action may be a learned phenomenon. Experience with children also suggests that they are bored by such tasks and question the reasons why they are required to do them.

With these considerations in mind, one may approach the task of testing muscle power in those children who have sufficient language to be able to discriminate body parts, such as the foot, knee, or hand and who can move to visual targets such as your hand. Testing time should be limited for young children and when boredom is apparent. For this reason, it is important to have identified the general musculoskeletal problems and prioritized the body regions that need to be tested before embarking on muscle testing. If several body regions require testing, the evaluation should be spread over several sessions.

Sensory Evaluation

Traditional tests of sensory integrity, like muscle tests, assume a fully mature nervous system. Often the ability to understand the directions associated with sensory tests depends on developmentally advanced language processes. Anyone who has performed a test of sensory function in a patient with receptive aphasia will appreciate the language processes associated with sensory testing. Yet the examination of sensory systems is a most important part of the evaluation of a child with musculoskeletal dysfunction. The methods of testing again must be adapted to the capabilities of the infant or child.

Examining Sensation in Infants

Touch, proprioceptive stimuli such as stretch, joint movement, and pressure, and nondamaging thermal stimuli may be applied to determine whether a body region is innervated with sensory pathways. Similarly, the special senses may be examined by using auditory, visual, and olfactory stimuli. Infants frequently respond to such stimuli through reflexive motor responses. Appendix 21-4 lists the various sensory modalities tested by traditional tests of infant reflexes. This may serve as a starting point for the selection of appropriate stimuli and standards for judging the integrity of the sensory modalities. Facial expressions of startle, attention,

or discomfort are also common in response to various stimuli. Attention to stimuli may be exhibited as a shift in gaze and quieting of body movement. A failure to respond, or continuation of ongoing activity in a body region removed from the source of stimulation, are indicative of lack of sensation. One should repeat stimulation if there is any question of attributing a response or lack of a response to a stimulus.

Motor Development

The orderly sequence of acquiring postural and movement abilities describes the natural process by which infants and children achieve functional independence. In most instances, motor sequences list in order and describe with varying degrees of detail the tasks expected at progressive ages. Theoretically, it has been commonly proposed and therefore often regarded as fact that the motor tasks of an early age are a prerequisite to achievement of the motor tasks of a later age. This general thesis has been used frequently in physical therapy to justify the ordering of teaching the infant or child tasks within a treatment plan. However, since within a normal population of infants and children there are instances when tasks are achieved in other than commonly reported sequences, the thesis that early tasks are prerequisite to later tasks is untrue.

There are important reasons for assessing motor development other than to determine the order of treatment activities. Developmental sequences outline "appointments with function." The child's gradual acquisition of the abilities to align and maintain the body with respect to the force of gravity, to move the body from one general posture to another, to be stable within a postural configuration, to move the body from one point to another in the environment, and to accomplish activities while maintaining a static or dynamic posture represent measures of both development and functional ability.

Many tests of motor development are available to the physical therapist. The two recommended here are easily administered, are reliable when conducted according to procedures outlined in their accompanying test manuals, and are commonly used. The fact that they are common tests is an advantage if a child you are treating is ever transferred to another part of the country.

One of the simplest tests to administer is the Gross Motor Test included in the Gesell Developmental Schedules. The overall purpose of the schedules is to estimate intellectual potential based on measures of infant and child maturity. There are five schedules measuring the maturity of five skill areas: gross motor, fine motor, language, personal-social, and adaptive. The test covers the age ranges of birth to 72 months or 6 years and samples a broad range of behaviors at specific age levels. It is important that the most recent revision of this test be used, as the age levels and sequences, particularly in the gross motor area, have changed from earlier editions. In addition, more recent versions of the schedules have been standardized on more representative samples of the population of infants and children in the United States.

The second recommended test that is easy to administer is the Bayley Scales of Infant Development.

POSTURAL DISORDERS IN INFANTS AND CHILDREN

One of the most common reasons children are taken to an orthopaedist stems from variations in posture that parents detect. The parents report their concerns about the child's appearance. For those parents with toddlers and preschool-aged children, their concerns are often with what might be considered normal age-related postural variations seen when the child is standing. Frequently their complaints center around the appearance of the child's lower extremities. For example, parents are concerned about apparently flat feet, in-toeing and out-toeing, knock knees, and bow legs. Often, education of the parents to the normal range of postural variation and how posture changes with age may be the definitive treatment for these problems. However, this does not preclude thorough physical therapy evaluation of the toddler or preschool-aged child to determine if the parents have detected a problem that falls outside the limits of normalcy.

When parents of preambulatory infants, older school-aged children, or adolescents complain of their child's appearance, the complaint is more likely to be related to a problem outside the range of normalcy. Abnormalities in these age groups usually present as parental complaints of asymmetry of posture. These complaints, when followed with a detailed physical therapy evaluation, often reveal problems that require physical treatment of the child. For example, congenital torticollis, subluxation or dislocation of a hip, and scoliosis can present as parental concern with asymmetry of posture.

In the following sections, postural disorders most frequently encountered in infants, children, and adolescents are presented. Common disorders and their physical therapy evaluation and treatment are presented by body region: the axial region, shoulder girdle and upper extremities, and lower extremities. Within each region, disorders are presented according to the age group in which they commonly appear. Thus, in the section on postural disorders of the axial region, congenital torticollis appears before idiopathic scoliosis, as the former is usually treated during the period of infancy or early childhood, while the latter is a disorder encountered predominantly in the older school-aged child or teenager.

Postural Disorders of the Axial Region

Congenital Muscular Torticollis

Congenital muscular torticollis is caused by fibrosis in and contracture of the sternocleidomastoid (SCM) muscle. In the majority of infants the right SCM is affected. The postural abnormality is also termed "wryneck," and the exact etiology is unknown. Congenital torticollis is associated with difficult delivery and breech presentation. An uncommonly high percentage of infants with congenital torticollis also have dislocated hips. The condition is more common in girls than in boys.

Common Subjective Findings
The problem is usually detected in the newborn nursery, although mild contractures may go unnoticed until later. In these instances, the problem is discovered by the mother as a tendency of the infant to look and to hold the head to one side. This may particularly be a problem during feeding. The mother may notice that the child demonstrates

difficulty turning toward and maintaining contact with one breast, but not the other. As noted above, a difficult delivery or breech presentation is not uncommon in the history.

Objective Procedures

Observe the infant in the mother's arms, in the crib, or on another supporting surface, taking note of the frequency of spontaneous movement and the range and relative distribution of movements across the limbs. Directing your attention to the axial region, note particularly if the infant orients or turns the head toward you or the mother's face when talking to the infant from positions directly in the midline and to the right and left of the infant. You or the mother should be close to the infant's face when this is evaluated, at a distance of approximately 12 inches.

Postural Evaluation

Observe the infant in the supine position first. It is common for normal infants to demonstrate a tendency to posture with the head turned to the right. As right SCM involvement is most common, the observed posture in infants with congenital muscular torticollis is typically characterized by lateral flexion or tilting of the head to the right with rotation of the face and chin to the left. The normal infant postures with the head rotated to the side without lateral flexion; therefore, in the case of left SCM involvement, the habitual posture of lateral tilting of the head to the left with chin rotated to the right helps discriminate between the normal and abnormal head posture.

While the infant is in the supine position, take time to observe the posture of the trunk and extremities. Symmetry is the norm in the newborn period. Since infants with torticollis often have a history of breech presentation, it is important that you screen the whole body for any other postural deformities. Pay particular attention to the hips, which may be subluxed or dislocated in infants with a history of breech presentation.

The young infant with torticollis cannot be placed prone with the head located in a midline position. When placing a normal newborn infant prone with the face on the support surface, one can expect the infant to momentarily lift and turn the head to free the face. The infant with torticollis lies with the face slightly rotated to the left with lateral flexion to the right. The infant is rarely successful in moving out of this posture but may struggle, fuss, and cry, appearing to protest and express discomfort. You can, however, support the infant in the prone position by placing one of your hands under the abdomen and the other over the thoracic spine on the back. Ensuring that the head and face are free from support, note the symmetry of asymmetry and frequency and range of head lifting. While the infant is prone, inspect the trunk and shoulder girdles for symmetry. Infants and children with Sprengel's deformity demonstrate a supine posture similar to that of infants with torticollis. Sprengel's deformity is a bony malformation and elevation of one scapula. You should inspect the scapulae for a relatively equal vertical posture. If one scapula is positioned higher than the other, you should palpate them to determine the relative size of the scapulae. In infants with Sprengel's deformity, the involved scapula is smaller. There may also be a fibrous band or bar of bone running transversely from the upper third of the medial border of the scapula to one of the lower cervical vertebrae.

The hips should also be inspected for signs of subluxation or dislocation in the prone position. Most characteristically, hip instability presents with asymmetrical gluteal and thigh creases.

The asymmetrical posture of the head and neck may also be observed when the infant is held in a sitting posture.

Growth and Anthropometric Measures

Infants with muscular torticollis do not necessarily demonstrate growth disturbances. However, if left untreated, these infants may begin to demonstrate facial asymmetries that eventually result in bony deformity. In addition, a scoliosis of the lower cervical and upper thoracic spine may develop. The best way to document the presence or absence of facial asymmetry is with a photograph.

Flexibility

Although particular attention should be directed to the neck and upper limb girdle areas, a general evaluation of limb flexibility should be carried out. As the SCM is contracted, limitations in passive and active movement of the neck are to be expected. These include rotation toward the involved side, lateral flexion away from the involved side, and extension of the middle and lower cervical spine. When the infant is passively moved into the position reversing all three motion components of the SCM, it may be possible to palpate the fibrous-like tissue in the muscle belly. Palpation is usually possible in the first two postnatal weeks. Remember, muscles synergistic to the SCM may also shorten as an adaptation to the infant's habitual posture.

Testing the Integrity of Muscle Innervation

Weakness is not a primary sign of torticollis. Failure of antagonistic musculature to move the neck through a full active range may be due primarily to reflexive inhibition of the antagonists when excessive stretch is put on the SCM. If, however, the SCM is not treated early in the infant's life, noncontractile fibrous tissue may replace muscle tissue and a true weakness of the affected muscle may result.

Sensory Evaluation

With the exception of expressions of discomfort when the affected SCM is elongated, sensory evaluation is expected to be within normal limits.

Motor Development Evaluation

As stated previously, normal postural and movement patterns expected of a term infant are affected. Postural alignment of the head in the supine, prone, and supported sitting positions is altered by habitual asymmetrical posture and a decreased range and frequency of turning the head toward the involved side. Head lifting when prone may be absent, and asymmetry of head righting is noted when the child is pulled up from the supine position. The response to the stimulus for the rooting reflex may be diminished when the infant is expected to turn toward the involved side.

Treatment Objectives

Symmetry of postural alignment of the head and neck by the age of 4 to 6 months

Full and equal range and frequency of active head and neck movements by the age of 4 to 6 months

Treatment Guidelines

Parents need to be involved in the treatment of the infant on a daily basis

Mother and father need to be instructed in treatment procedures. Home visits may be necessary.

Parents and infant should be followed on a 3- to 5-day follow-up interval until you are absolutely sure that they are performing the stretching exercises appropriately.

Cardinal plane stretching exercises are not as efficient as a single diagonal stretching exercise that takes into account all three motion components of the SCM.

The shoulder should be stabilized with one hand while the other hand is used to laterally flex, rotate, and extend the neck (Fig. 21-2).

The easiest way to incorporate treatment into the mother's and infant's daily routine is to have the stretching exercise performed at each diaper change.

Suggestions should be given regarding arranging the crib so that the infant is encouraged to turn toward the affected side when the parents or caretakers approach. When playing with the child, or during feeding, rotation toward the midline and beyond should also be encouraged. Attractive toys or, better still, an individual's face will interest the infant and can be used to encourage tracking with the eyes that will lead the head to midline and beyond. These suggestions should also be extended to the

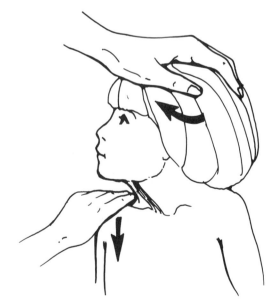

Fig. 21-2 Stretch position for torticollis.

infant's day care center or babysitter if the child is not at home during the day.

The Older Infant and Young Child with Congenital Torticollis

Although less common, there are instances of children who either did not receive or did not benefit from early treatment of their torticollis. In the untreated case, replacement of contractile tissue with fibrous tissue within the affected muscle is expected. Such cases are likely to become surgical candidates, and physical therapy assumes a role in their preoperative and postoperative management.

The surgical procedure is most commonly a resection of approximately 1 inch of the involved SCM at either the proximal or distal attachment. The proximal attachment is more commonly resected in girls, as the cosmetic result is more acceptable. Resection of the distal attachment represents a less difficult surgical procedure and therefore is usually elected in young boys. In protracted cases, usually children not treated until adolescence, both the proximal and distal attachments may be surgically removed.

Postoperatively, the child may be placed in soft canvas head halter traction with the chin rotated toward and the head laterally tilted away from the involved side. To maintain this overcorrected posture, counter-traction is applied in a downward direction to the shoulder on the involved side. Two to three days postoperatively, physical therapy may be started to attain symmetry of posture and to further increase mobility of the upper axial region toward an overcorrected position that will enable active movements of rotation toward, and lateral flexion away from, the involved side.

Symmetry of posture and movement in the axial region is the objective of treatment and should be attained in the natural age-related posture and movement patterns of the child. For example, if one is working with an infant of 6 to 7 months of age, righting reaction can be used to achieve the objectives of treatment. The common symmetrical postures for this age include sitting, the hand-knee position when prone, and supported standing. Active movements involving the upper axial region include tracking of objects and individuals to both sides of the body in each of these relatively symmetrical postures, rolling to the prone or supine position by turning the face in the direction of the roll, coming from a prone or hand-knee position to side-sitting by using rotation of the axial region, and pulling up to sitting from supine with manual assistance. Each of these activities can be incorporated into the infant's physical therapy program.

Kinesiological analysis of rolling and rotational form required to achieve a sitting posture allows selection of the direction of rolling emphasized in treatment to achieve automatic yet active movement toward the overcorrected positions. For example, a child with involvement and surgical resection of the right SCM will require activities to encourage rotation of the face toward the right with lateral flexion toward the left (Fig. 21-3). Evoking a rolling pattern from supine that requires the infant to track an object moving up and over the right shoulder will effectively incorporate the movement components leading away from the preoperative habitual posture.

In older children, orthopaedic management may include casting the head, neck, and trunk in the overcorrected position or the use of a modified Buckminster Brown brace that holds the child in an aligned symmetrical posture. In both cases, the child is usually permitted to be up and about, gradually resuming full activities after 1 week.

When the brace is used, it may be removed for exercise and bathing, but is otherwise worn during waking and sleeping hours. The advantage of management in a brace is that the child is held in the symmetrical posture that is one of the ultimate objectives of treatment. The exercise program is important for the achievement of movement patterns, particularly away from the previous habitual posture.

The child managed in a cast will be held in the overcorrected position for 4 to 8 weeks. This presents a more formidable physical therapy problem owing to failure to experience symmetry of posture and bidirectional movement for a protracted period postoperatively. Additional restrictions of mobility may result, and atrophy of muscle may compound an already difficult situation. If there is ever a question concerning whether bracing or casting will be used postoperatively, remember that bracing management presents the opportunity for a more rapid achievement of the objectives of physical therapy and a decreased risk of secondary loss of mobility and muscle power.

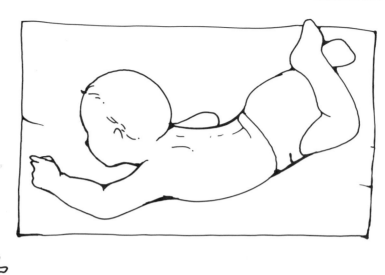

Fig. 21-3 Encouraging active movement to affected side.

In all of these cases, although most particularly in the case of casting in the overcorrected position, it is important to assess and monitor the function of the accessory nerve. Lengthening of the shortened structures on the involved side by overcorrection particularly places the nerve at risk for traction injury.

Finally, the young child with surgical correction of torticollis represents a formidable physical therapy challenge since the child is neither interested in nor possesses the sensory discrimination or motor control required for exercise involving isolated joint actions. Until the child reaches the older school-aged years, corrective postural exercise is not valued by the child and therefore becomes the goal of the parents and physical therapist and not necessarily the child. Under such circumstances, the assistance of the parents is critical, and management of an exercise program must continue under direct supervision. Children of this age need help in appropriate performance of corrective movement. Repetitive assistive exercise utilizing manual guidance and visual cues can be applied in a gentle yet disciplined atmosphere that recognizes and understands the absence of the child's committment to a program of self-improvement. Self-awareness of one's posture and appearance only become a concern on which the child acts in later childhood and adolescence.

Idiopathic Scoliosis

Common Subjective Findings

Postural asymmetry is the common complaint that is the presenting symptom of idiopathic scoliosis. Parents or teachers may be the first to detect the spinal curvature by noticing a "high shoulder." Owing to the modesty of preadolescents, they are rarely observed in less than full dress by the parents. Only in the summer do they shed sufficient clothing for the discerning parental eye to detect the beginnings of asymmetry. For that reason, emphasis on early detection and screening for scoliosis has been given attention in the lay press and is included in an increasing number of school health and physical education programs. This increased public awareness is responsible for larger numbers of early referrals for evaluation and treatment of girls with scoliosis.

Prepubescent and adolescent girls are critically concerned with their appearance. Although they themselves may not be the detectors of the postural abnormality, once their attention is drawn to the problem, they become acutely aware, concerned, and anxious over their condition at the age when so much of their self-esteem is based on physical appearance. With the greatest incidence of idiopathic scoliosis appearing in this volatile period of the human lifespan, the successful treatment is to a large degree dependent on the adolescent's ability to take responsibility for her own well-being and the ability of the physical therapist to establish a helpful yet trusting and adultlike respect for the adolescent. Parental concerns about their child's posture may be met with seeming indifference on the part of the child, when this attitude likely reflects only the struggle for independence from parental control. Parents cannot force their concerns and attitudes on the adolescent, and neither can the physical therapist. It is the expectation of adultlike behavior and treating the adolescent as an adult that often provides the encouragement for the individual to assume an adultlike responsibility for her own health problems. In my experience, this type of relationship is necessary for successful physical therapy for idiopathic scoliosis or any postural problem in this age group.

During subjective evaluation, address your questions to the adolescent, not primarily to the parents. Parental observations, concerns, and questions are important and should be gathered at the end of the subjective interview of the child. This procedure of concerning yourself first with the patient and her symptoms, impressions, and concerns is critical to the establishment of effective rapport in later treatment efforts.

It is important to establish what the adolescent has noticed about her posture, whether she has experienced pain or discomfort, or any other unusual sensations.

Objective Findings

A thorough evaluation of the child with an axial postural problem should begin with a postural evaluation. Standing posture should be analyzed from the front, back, and side views. Only a minimal amount of clothing should be worn to enable a thorough inspection of body alignment. A bathing suit is ideal. When your patient is undressed, you may also observe the skin and determine whether there are cafe au lait marks, which are a sign of neurofibromatosis, a disease of neural tissues that is often accompanied by a relatively progressive form of scoliosis that frequently requires surgical spinal fusion.

When examining standing posture, be aware that it takes several minutes for the individual to settle into her habitual posture and that standing in a stationary position for too long a period is likely to cause feelings of being light-headed or dizzy. Watch carefully the color of the lower legs and feet for evidence of pooling of the blood and decreased venous return that can hallmark the problem of temporary circulatory insufficiency. Interrupt the evaluation process periodically and allow the individual to move around a bit before resuming your analysis, and when the static standing posture is reassumed, do not forget to again allow time for the patient to settle into the habitual posture.

Always begin the postural analysis by aligning the individual so that a plumb line appears to fall through the center of mass of the body. A plumb line is a must. To achieve this when examining from the side view, ask the individual to move or move the plumb bob until it corresponds with a line bisecting the proximal tip of the greater trochanter, which can be marked either by causing erythema or by marking with a skin pencil over the most proximal point of the trochanter. Using this arrangement, the plumb line practically, although not with perfect accuracy, should bisect the center of mass from the side view. When viewing the front of the individual, have the plumb line bisect the umbilicus, and from the rear view, mark a point on the skin that is equidistant from the PSISs and at the same vertical level.

After ensuring that the plumb is aligned properly, ask your patient to assume as natural a posture as possible. Begin your observation at the head and work downward to the feet.

Finally, a forward bending test is carried out as a part of the postural analysis. Kneeling or sitting behind the individual, with your eyes at the level of the waist, have your patient bend forward until the spine is approximately parallel with the floor. The rotatory components of the deformity in a structural scoliosis make a unilateral "rib hump" apparent. This is the differential sign of structural scoliosis.

I have never been able to complete a thorough postural evaluation, examining from the side, front, and back, in less than 45 minutes. To hurry the process reduces the reliability of your findings that form the basis for the treatment of postural stereotypes. The careful analysis of posture will also lead you to the selection of appropriate flexibility and muscle power tests to establish the baseline for defining the musculoskeletal problems and devising subsequent treatment.

Normal Postural Patterns of Later Childhood and Adolescence

Coming out of the period of early childhood, the older child is considered to have a stabilizing posture. A mild thoracic kyphosis with protracted scapulae and a slightly forward head is common throughout childhood and into adolescence. Two important aspects of postural change from early to later childhood involve a decrease in apparent lordosis with protrusion of the abdomen and a decrease in the tendency to stand in genu recurvatum. The earlier appearing lordotic posture with hyperextended knees is often considered a passive posture in that the child seemingly makes little effort to actively combat the force of gravity. As the child moves to the period of adolescence, the inclination of the pelvis (as measured by the angle of the line connecting the anterior and posterior superior iliac spines with respect to a horizontal line) decreases from approximately 35° to 40° to approximately 20°. The decrease in the anterior tilt of the pelvis is the primary characteristic of the stabilizing posture. These major changes in standing posture are seen by inspecting the posture from the side.

Common Postural Findings in Idiopathic Scoliosis

There are quite typical signs of idiopathic scoliosis that are evident through postural analysis. These signs, however, are typical of most forms of scoliosis, and therefore the differentiation of a functional scoliosis from a structural curvature in a clinical examination is dependent on the forward bending test. When viewing the posture from the front and back, one rarely finds an individual without some small but noticeable asymmetries of scapular or pelvic posture. Such a detailed and discriminating inspection of an individual's posture, particularly in a screening situation, can lead to an impression that major problems exist, unless the examiner offers reassurance.

Growth and Anthropometric Measures

The following measures should be taken: sitting and standing height, length of the body when standing, upper and lower extremity lengths (please refer to Appendix 21-1).

Measure of Flexibility

The postural evaluation as indicated above will direct you toward appropriate flexibility measures. For example, the lordotic posture that accompanies idiopathic scoliosis necessitates measures of hip flexibility, particularly determination of the presence of hip flexion contractures. Utilize the Thomas test position and, to ensure reliability, have the individual hold one thigh as firmly as possible against the abdomen as the other thigh is lowered toward the examining table. With one of your hands positioned under the posterior crest of the ilium, concentrate on determining the point at which the crest moves away from its position of firm contact with your hand.

Be sure to have your patient positioned such that the knee extends beyond the edge of the table to prevent a knee flexion posture that contributes to a false measure of hip flexion contracture. When the knee extends beyond the end of the table, one may also flex and extend the knee, observing the change in hip flexion posture to assess the relative contribution of the rectus femoris to any limitation of hip extension.

Another common finding in the postural evaluation of the scoliotic is pelvic obliquity. Habitual posturing with the brim of the pelvis in an oblique rather than horizontal plane leads to compensatory shortening of musculature about the pelvis and hip, particularly of the adductors on the high side and the abductors on the low side. Careful stabilization of the pelvis is necessary to differentiate tensor fasciae latae tightness on the lower side of the pelvis, which is often the site of abductor tightness. With the patient in sidelying, with the back at the edge of the examining table, bring the upper thigh back into extension. Exerting downward pressure on the lateral brim of the ilium, to hold the pelvis in position, allow the thigh to lower into adduction and carefully observe for both lateral rotation of the thigh and extension of the knee. Failure of the thigh to drop into adduction, lateral rotation of the hip, and extension of the knee are all signs of tensor fasciae latae tightness.

Testing the Integrity of Muscle Power

Manual muscle testing in its traditional form many be applied to the older child or adolescent. Again, however, a word of caution is indicated. Many of the test requirements are not common activities performed on a routine basis. For this reason, it is possible that the individual is "learning" the motor patterns that are necessary for isolated joint action and thus for successful performance of the test. As relationships between postural alignment and muscle power have not been demonstrated, it is possible that improvements in muscle testing scores after programs to strengthen muscles are in fact reflections of motor learning. To the extent that manual muscle testing reflects awareness and control of alignment between body segments, both of which can be learned, it is a useful documentation of progress in patients with postural problems.

Common findings in muscle tests are asymmetries of performance. This is not unexpected as habitual asymmetrical postural patterns will preferentially require certain muscles to act within a shortened range while others perform from a lengthened postition. These findings are particularly true for the trunk musculature. Be aware that it may be impossible for your patient to assume the symmetrical starting position for the majority of the tests of trunk strength owing to limitations of flexibility.

Sensory Evaluation
In definitive evaluation, a screening of sensory systems is indicated to rule out scoliosis secondary to neural system dysfunction.

Functional Activities of the Older Child and Adolescent
You should inquire whether there are any limitations in functional ability. Although normal self-care and daily living activities are usually not affected in cases of idiopathic scoliosis, you should remember and inquire about the wider range of physical endeavors common in the adolescent. These include participation in sports and dance. The adolescent may reduce participation in these activities because of self-consciousness over appearance or anxiety over the effect of physical activity on the condition itself.

Treatment Programs for Idiopathic Scoliosis
The treatment of scoliosis includes exercise, bracing with exercise, neuromuscular electrical stimulation with implanted or surface electrodes, and surgical correction or stabilization of the spinal deformity. The role of physical therapy varies with each of these treatment modalities, but there is indication for physical therapy management in each instance.

Exercise: With and Without Bracing. The objective of an exercise program for scoliosis, whether or not bracing is employed, is symmetry of posture. The common regimen of exercises developed to be used in conjunction with bracing is based on the notion that an imbalance of muscle strength is responsible for the asymmetrical posture that over time led to bony deformity. This regimen had its foundation in Williams' flexion exercises designed to strengthen the trunk musculature and to reduce lumbar lordosis and the anterior tilt of the pelvis. The posterior pelvic tilt is at the heart of each exercise. Indeed, the posterior pelvic tilt is the postural set from which each exercise in the regimen is performed.

Effective instruction in the exercise regimen requires, as previously mentioned, an attitude of self-responsibility and motivation on the part of the patient. There is no substitute for these attitudes. In addition, the sensory ability to discriminate the position of the pelvis, scapulae, and spine will ultimately determine the success of the program. In cases in which your patient does not demonstrate self-motivation and responsibility, or in which the ability to discriminate relative postural alignment within the axial region is not demonstrated, the effectiveness of the program is diminished.

The Pelvic Tilt with Knees Flexed. The posterior pelvic tilt in a supine hook-lying position is the first exercise taught, and until it is possible for your patient to perform this action with ease at will, other aspects of the exercise program should be delayed. Instruct your patient in this exercise in your first treatment session. First demonstrate the posterior pelvic tilt to your patient. Have her place her hand beneath your lumbar spine and feel the pressure you place with your back against her hand as you slowly and firmly perform the tilt. Place your hand under the patient's lumbar spine while she is lying with the legs extended. Have her curl up into flexion by bringing both knees to the chest, and repeat this activity while she concentrates on the sensation of pressing her lower back into your palm. Repeat until she is able to reliably detect the increase in pressure that signifies flattening of the lumbar spine. After teaching this sensation, have her assume hook lying, and with both hands grasping over the ASISs and around the lateral aspect of the pelvis, move the pelvis posteriorly until it contacts the support surface. Repeat this activity, having your patient verify the sensation of firm contact against the mat.

Notice if your patient automatically begins to assist with the movement. Acknowledge her assistance if present, or if absent, instruct your patient to help a bit in the performance of this movement. Continue to guide and assist the patient to ensure proper performance, but when possible, begin to decrease the firmness of your contact and guidance until you are providing only light tactile contact. At this point, have the patient perform independently and critically observe her performance for symmetry and smoothness of execution. Give her verbal feedback on the quality of execution: concentrate on only one aspect at a time, keep your feedback concise, and if possible use your hands again to give targets that she may move to. First emphasize speed—she should perform slowly. Then emphasize symmetry, and after ensuring symmetrical performance, move on to the smoothness of performance. Determine whether your patient is holding her breath during trials, and if so, remind her that she should breath normally. Often patients will stop inhalation and exhalation during initial attempts to learn a new task. Presumably this might allow greater concentration on the task, as the natural tendency when learning a new task is to block all movement except that requested. If your patient continues to hold her breath, engage her in conversation that will automatically bring about exhalation during the performance of the task.

It is possible that this will be the only exercise taught. Occasionally, you will encounter an individual with good discriminatory abilities who quickly learns to perform the tilt accurately and reliably. These individuals may proceed to learning to perform the posterior pelvic tilt in the supine position with the legs extended and when standing. Do not instruct the patient in more than three exercises on the first session.

The Pelvic Tilt with Knees Extended. When teaching the pelvic tilt with the legs extended,

gradually progress the patient from the hook-lying position by having her perform two to three trials at each of a series of progressively more extended hip and knee postures. Pay attention to performance in each position, and ask your patient if she believes she has performed the exercise correctly. This is an excellent way to determine the accuracy of her kinesthetic sense. After determining the quality of performance that she detected, give accurate feedback about your observations. This critical interchange will ultimately assist her in establishing an accurate kinesthetic memory trace that will be the basis for self-monitoring of her performance.

The Pelvic Tilt when Standing. When teaching the pelvic tilt in the standing position, begin against a wall. This ensures a surface that the lumbar spine can contact for sensory feedback. Again, use your hands to manually assist your patient's performance, and after gradually discontinuing this assistance, use verbal feedback to correct and improve the qualities of speed and symmetry. Once you are satisfied with her performance against the wall, have the patient attain and then hold the posterior tilt isometrically, and step away from the wall.

The Prone Posterior Pelvic Tilt. The prone posterior pelvic tilt is a more difficult task to teach. Again, using your hands to manually assist in the movement of flattening the lumbar spine is important. Ask the patient to concentrate on lifting the ASISs from the surface while pressing the pubic symphysis against the surface. You will note a tendency for the entire trunk to move into flexion as the tilt is performed. After your patient is able to elevate the ASISs and press the symphysis against the surface, she needs to begin to learn to confine the action of spinal flexion to the lumbar area. Ask her to keep the upper part of her trunk flat against the surface and just move the lower part of the trunk when performing the tilt. This is a difficulty activity as you are requiring her to dissociate the upper and lower trunk musculature that most commonly act together in reinforcing the same action. Whenever a task is difficult, take time to observe whether your patient is again holding her breath. If so, you will need to reinforce with her the need for regular breathing during this activity. Successful performance of the pelvic tilt in the prone position without accompanying flexion of the thoracic spine is a prerequisite to performance of the following activity.

Prone Pelvic Tilt with Thoracic Extension-Hyperextension. After the patient has accomplished the dissociated pelvic tilt in the prone position, it is time to teach thoracic extension while maintaining lumbar flexion. This exercise is designed to combat the tendency toward thoracic flexion that accompanies idiopathic scoliosis. After moving the patient into a position of lumbar flexion, ask your patient to hold this posture while she elevates the shoulders and upper chest. Pay close attention to the paravertebral musculature and vertebrae during this activity, noting the most caudal spinal level demonstrating extension. Use your fingertips to point out to your patient how far down the spine she is able to extend. If necessary give tactile cues to assist her in learning to produce extension more caudally. She should be attempting to reverse thoracic flexion beyond the level of the apex of thoracic flexion that you noted in your postural evaluation.

Chest Expansion. While your patient is holding a pelvic tilt in the standing position, use your hands to provide manual cues while teaching a symmetrical pattern of chest expansion during inhalation.

Pelvic Tilt Push-ups. A push-up, with the fulcrum at the knees rather than at the toes, while holding a pelvic tilt, is taught first. Often you will need to perform this activity yourself to demonstrate it. After your patient has obtained and is holding the prone posterior pelvic tilt, you can assist in keeping her spine straight by placing one hand under the abdomen and the other over the spine in the lower thoracic region and maintaining contact while she performs the push-up. Begin gradually with this activity, again assuring yourself that the patient is able to perform correctly before adding this to the home program. Three push-ups are not an unreasonable starting point for those who are out of condition. Adding just one push-up per week until ten can be performed usually results in success and keeps your patient demonstrating progress. The key to correct performance is the ability to keep the posterior pelvic tilt and the remainder of the spine straight while

doing the push-up. After about 2 weeks of ten repetitions of the modified push-up, it is time to move to a standard push-up while maintaining the posterior tilt. As with the initial trials of the modified push-up, beginning attempts should be closely monitored and manual assistance should be provided to keep the spine straight. Replace one or two of the modified push-ups with standard push-ups each week until ten standard push-ups can be performed in succession.

Hamstring Flexibility. In the long sitting position, work to assure 90° of hip flexion with the knees extended. The objective of this activity is to enable your patient to move smoothly and effortlessly into a pelvic posture in which the ASISs are inclined approximately 15° below a horizontal line through the PSISs. Have the patient work to attain this posture actively. If she spends upwards of 23 hours a day in a brace or body jacket that has a posterior pelvic tilt incorporated into its design, this activity is a must.

Activities Performed while Wearing the Brace or Body Jacket

These two activities are taught while the brace or body jacket is being worn.

Pad Pull-away. In the standing position, have your patient first assume a posterior pelvic tilt. While she holds the pelvic posture, have her laterally shift away from the corrective pad over the apex of the primary curve and then derotate, reversing the posterior rotatory component contributing to the rib hump. Initially this activity should be taught as a three-step sequence with each successive postural adjustment being added to the previous step. Commands might be as follows: first the pelvic tilt, hold it, now the lateral shift and hold, and now rotate. This series will eventually become a smooth one-step correction of all three components of the scoliotic posture. Although this activity begins as an exercise performed as a part of the complete program, the goal is to have this maneuver performed several times each half hour, much as a postural adjustment normally occurs automatically and without conscious effort. After she is performing well, instruct your patient to perform this activity whenever the brace feels uncomfortable. Indeed, the effectiveness of bracing likely lies in the mild discomfort it produces that ensures active postural adjustment to relieve areas of constant pressure. The contact of the corrective pads is always there as a reminder, and if they are appropriately placed, they will ensure proper performance of the pad pull-away.

Active Distraction. Active distraction is another activity performed with the assistance of the brace. After the patient first assumes a posterior pelvic tilt while standing in the brace, have the patient who wears a Milwaukee brace grab the front upright bar with both hands. While pulling downward on the bar, she should actively straighten the upper spine, becoming taller. Visual imagery often assists the patient to understand this postural activity. The images of lengthening the neck or having a skyhook attached to the crown of the head are often helpful. Tactile cues may also be used in the latter case. Ensure that the cervical spine is extended and that there is sufficient flexion at the atlanto-occipital joint to keep the face vertical and the mouth horizontal. As with the pad pull-away, this activity starts as a part of the exercise program and when performance warrants, the patient should be instructed to use this activity throughout the day to relieve discomfort.

Postural Disorders of the Hip

Hip disorders are among the most complex and challenging for the orthopaedist working with children and represent a large portion of pediatric orthopaedic cases. Because the hip joint has such an important role in locomotor function, a hip disorder can be a major disabling condition. Orthopaedists treat hip problems as aggressively as possible at the earliest sign of dysfunction. In the growing child, this is an important principle since it not only allows the problem to respond to external means of correction but allows the maximal corrective influences of the growth process. In the sections that follow, the most common conditions that are observed to affect the hip of the growing child are examined. A developmental ordering of the conditions has been applied. The first condition discussed is that of congenital hip dislocation: an abnormality normally detected in the neonatal period or during early infancy. In-

formation concerning the detection and treatment of muscle imbalance about the hip follows. This problem usually becomes a concern of physical therapists early during the first year of life for children with chronic neuromuscular problems such as cerebral palsy or paraparesis as a result of myelodysplasia.

The condition of Legg-Perthes disease is presented next, since this problem usually presents in early childhood. Finally, the traumatic slipped capital femoral epiphysis is addressed as a problem of later childhood or early adolescence.

Congenital Dislocation of the Hip

Congenital dislocation of the hip (CDH) can present at birth as a frank dislocation or as a more subtle abnormality that may or may not be detected in early infancy. The less obvious abnormality is characterized by a subluxed or dislocatable hip that is not frankly dislocated. Being less easily detected, the subluxed or dislocatable hip can be more harmful than the frank dislocation since recognition of the abnormality and subsequent treatment may be delayed.

The cause of frank congenital dislocation is unknown but is usually associated with other congenital abnormalities such as arthrogryposis, wryneck, clubfoot, and others. There is evidence of a genetic predisposition to CDH; laxity of the soft tissue structures about the hip is also thought to play a role in the etiology, as is breech presentation. The condition is more common in girls than in boys.

After a closed or open reduction of the hip by an orthopaedist, the hip will be casted or splinted in a position of flexion and abduction (Fig. 21-4). This position ensures proper alignment between the femoral head and the acetabulum, such that the femoral head is receiving maximal coverage by the acetabulum. Additionally, soft tissue structures that have been stretched as a result of the malalignment will have an opportunity to shorten to an appropriate length.

In the past, wide abduction and an extreme degree of internal rotation were used to ensure seating of the femoral head in the acetabulum. However, an increased incidence of avascular necrosis of the femoral head was associated with such positioning. This extreme posture has been aban-

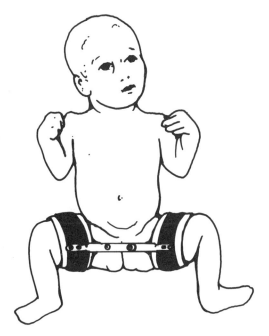

Fig. 21-4 Child splinted in flexion and abduction.

doned in favor of a more moderate position of flexion and abduction.

Closed reduction involves manipulation of the hip without surgical intervention. Surgical myotomy of the adductors and open reduction may be required when the range of movement does not allow the surgeon to reduce the dislocated hip. Open reduction is more likely in the dislocated hip that is not detected early in infancy.

Common Subjective Findings
Parents or nurses may detect some difficulty diapering the infant, particularly when trying to spread the thighs apart. The care giver may also notice that one leg appears longer than the other, or other examples of postural asymmetry of the lower limbs may be detected.

Objective Findings
With the infant supine and the diaper removed, inspect the area about the hips visually. Note any asymmetry of inguinal creases. With the infant's knees flexed to 90°, simultaneously flex both hips to a 90° angle. Position yourself such that your eyes are at the level of the knees. There is obvious shortening of the thigh on the dislocated side. *Do not forcibly extend the hips*, but gently bring the

lower extremities toward extension. Compare the width of the pelvifemoral junction. A widening of this area is to be expected on the side of the dislocation. Using both hands, palpate both trochanters with your fingertips as the thumbs rest gently over the infant's thighs (Fig. 21-5) and note the relative height of the most proximal aspect of the greater trochanter. A high-riding trochanter is an objective sign of a frank dislocation. Turn the infant prone and inspect the gluteal and thigh creases and gluteal dimples. On the dislocated side, the gluteal crease will extend further laterally and be higher than the crease on the normal side and the number of thigh creases will be increased.

The same asymmetries are present to a lesser degree in the infant with a subluxation. One should be aware, however, that *hips of newborns are easily dislocated* and that positive although transient signs of dislocation are not that uncommon. Some of the most common objective findings are an occasional false-positive. This is likely a result of aggressive evaluation of the normal yet fragile hip of the newborn infant. Early detection and treatment of hip dislocation is very important however, and false-positive findings should not be a deterrent to an effective screening system.

Normal Postural Patterns of Infancy
As noted above, the asymmetry of the postural alignment of the hips is readily apparent in the unclothed infant. The limb on the side of the dislocated hip is held in flexion and external rotation. A newborn with a dislocated hip when held in a sitting or standing position will demonstrate an asymmetrical weight-bearing pattern: dropping or listing toward the affected side. If not treated, the asymmetry will result in compensatory postural patterns and a reduction in the variability of postural patterns. There is no evidence of delay of development of postural milestones such as sitting and standing.

Growth and Anthropometric Measures
Some growth disturbance of the involved limb is expected if the hip is not treated. The favoring of the unaffected hip will promote relative overgrowth of the sound lower extremity when compared with the less favored affected extremity. An objective assessment of the relative use of the two

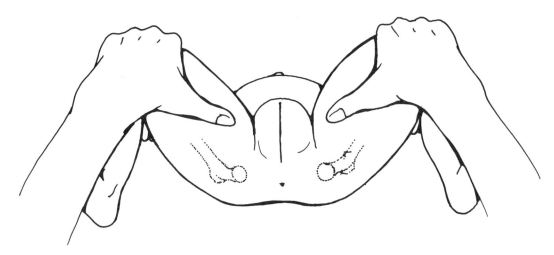

Fig. 21-5 Examination of pelvifemoral junction in detecting congenital dislocation of the hip.

limbs after correction of a dislocated hip should include length and girth measures.

Measures of Flexibility

When obtaining measures of range of motion, *care should be exercised not to force the infant's hips into movement ranges expected of adults.* Infants do not have the same excursion of hip movements, particularly in extension. This is likely due to the cartilaginous architecture of the hip as well as the prenatal posture. *Infants do not move in cardinal planes.* Careful observation of the infant during an active state should reveal both the plane and the normal excursion of that infant's hips. Flexibility is reduced on the dislocated side. Limitations to be expected include a decrease in the degree of hip extension compared with that of the sound hip, profound limitation of rotations, and a limitation of abduction. All limitations are due to the location of the femoral head, which is positioned above the acetabulum and directed anteriorly.

Testing the Integrity of Innervation in Infants

Although there is no expectation of neurological involvement in the infant with a hip dislocation, because this condition is not uncommonly associated with other congenital anomalies it is wise to perform a rapid screen of reflexive function of both lower extremities, particularly if there is a history of breech presentation.

Sensory Evaluation

Sensory function would be expected to be within normal limits unless there is a history of breech presentation or associated congenital abnormalities as may accompany a frank dislocation. The reflexive test that reveals absence of motor responses should be followed by careful assessment of an infant's facial responses or general activity level when sensory stimuli are applied. For example, an infant who does not appear to have detected a stimulus applied to the lower extremity may require a more detailed sensory evaluation. Such testing requires that the therapist be cognizant of the infant's behavioral state, and to be valid the test may need to be repeated more than once.

Motor Development

Observe and note the spontaneous movement patterns of the lower extremities such as kicking to determine whether there is asymmetry of range and frequency of movement. Movement patterns involving hip extension and abduction will not be carried through their full range on the dislocated side. Movement patterns elicited in reflexive tests may also be asymmetrical when comparing right and left sides. For example, the pattern of extension with abduction normally observed in the initial phase of the crossed extension reflex will be compromised. There is no evidence, however, that the child with CDH will demonstrate delay in the achievement of motor milestones such as rolling or getting to sitting.

Treatment Objectives

Referral for appropriate orthopaedic treatment.

Instruct family in the physical management of the infant during the period of orthopaedic treatment.

Full active mobility of the affected hip within 3 months of the termination of orthopaedic treatment.

Postural symmetry about the pelvis and hip during sitting, standing, and walking.

Treatment Guidelines

Screening. Physical therapists working in pediatrics in a general hospital should assure themselves that all infants are being screened for frank dislocation and that a system of referral for orthopaedic evaluation is in place. Determine whether newborns are screened routinely for dislocated hips in your setting. The referral system should ensure that infants suspected of having a subluxation or a hip that is dislocatable are provided proper orthopaedic evaluation and follow-up. Orthopaedists will usually have attempted to make this a routine procedure. Determine what the referral system is and whether it is effective. It is most important that all infants are screened. It is of less importance who performs the screening as nurses, pediatricians, or physical therapists may be competent to carry out this function. Encourage cooperative arrangements that ensure the very best and prompt care for the infant. The longer treatment is delayed, the more invasive and complicated the correction becomes. A hip that may be easily reduced and splinted in the newborn period if left untreated may develop an adduction contracture and require surgical release and reduction followed by casting.

Cast and Skin Care. If an infant's hip is casted or splinted as a form of treatment for dislocation or subluxation, the family needs instruction in cast management and care. Adhesive tape should be applied along the edges of the cast to protect the skin. The skin should be inspected daily to examine for rashes or abrasions.

A fussy infant may be experiencing discomfort from the cast or splint. In the case of a splint, instruct the family to remove the appliance and inspect the skin immediately. In the case of a cast, they should inspect the edges and if possible feel under the edges of the cast for foreign objects. The family should be instructed to guard against small objects being dropped accidentally inside a cast. Any instance such as this should be treated as an emergency. Steps should be taken to remove the object as soon as possible, even if it means taking the child to the orthopaedist to have the cast removed and reapplied.

Positioning. Many removable appliances have been developed to accomplish positioning in flexion and abduction after reduction of the hip. Their relative merits are constantly being weighed, and usually the availability and orthopaedist's experience with one or the other device determines which treatment is applied.

The Pavlic harness (Fig. 21-6) is a common device that prevents hip extension while allowing other hip movements. Because mobility is not as restricted in the Pavlic harness, this has become a more preferred positioning device. Abduction splints and Frejka pillows (Fig. 21-7) are also still widely used to accomplish the corrected posture.

Explain to the family the importance of varying the infant's posture throughout the day and during sleep. Provide suggestions for positioning the infant or child. Demonstrate the use of wedged pillows to support the infant in prone, supine, and sitting positions (Fig. 21-8A, B, and C). The infant's posture should be varied as frequently during the period of immobilization as it would be if the child were not casted or splinted.

Mobility. Full active mobility of the hip is of greatest importance when the infant or child has been immobilized or when initial treatment has been delayed beyond the period of early infancy. In these instances, the possibility of contracture of soft tissue structures about the hip is greatly increased. Most notably, the adductors are shortened. For the infant, mobilization is best accomplished by training the family members to engage the infant in active play. An extremely effective method of mobilization is through swimming or active play in the bath.

Encouraging activity in the bath or in a pool is particularly effective after removal of a cast. Al-

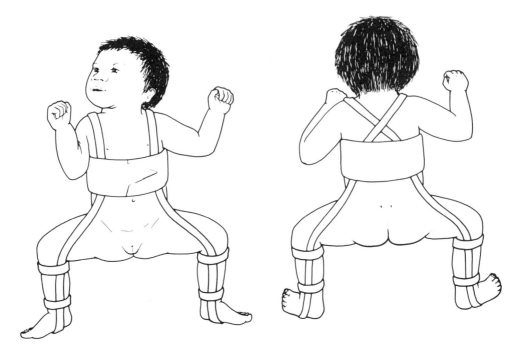

Fig. 21-6 The Pavlik harness prevents both active and passive extension of the hips but permits all other movements and thereby helps to stimulate the development of the reduced hip. (From Tachdjian MO: Congenital Dislocation of the Hip. Churchill Livingstone, New York, 1982.)

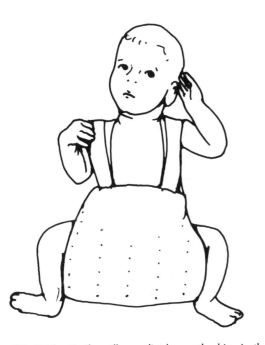

Fig. 21-7 The Frejka pillow splint keeps the hips in the stable position of flexion and abduction while still allowing some active movement of the hips.

lowing the child to actively kick and stretch out is much more effective than a program of passive stretching exercise under the control of a therapist or parent.

After immobilization in flexion and abduction, activities should be designed that encourage hip extension. Adduction range need not be specifically encouraged as the child will gain adduction mobility as a result of self-initiated activities. Design interactive games with the infant that require or encourage use of the involved hip in extension. If the infant is under 9 months of age, use prone activities to encourage active hip extension. Basic elements of proprioceptive neuromuscular facilitation are particularly effective in eliciting the movement pattern of extension, abduction, and internal rotation in infants. Manual contacts over the extensors and stretch to the muscle groups active in the extension pattern are effective in facilitating the infant's active movements in the direction desired. If the baby is over 1 year old, standing up from the prone position should be encouraged. Movement through the positions of plantigrade and an abducted squat are used as the

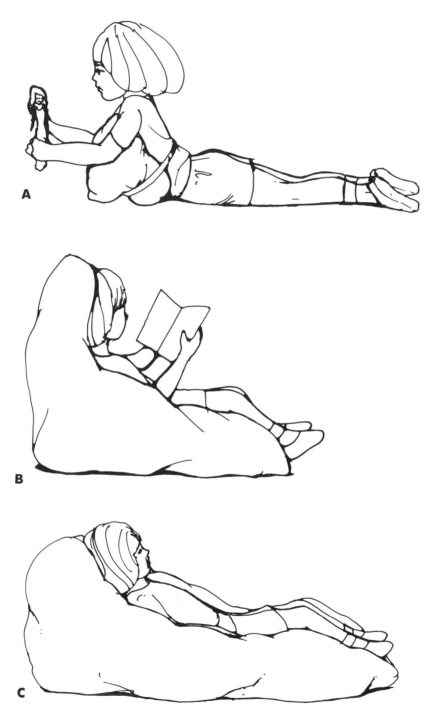

Fig. 21-8 A young girl demonstrates the use of wedge pillows and the positioning that can be used to support the infant while prone **(A)**, supine **(B)**, and sitting **(C)**.

child moves up to stand in extension and abduction. It is important to discover and employ the hip extension activity most enjoyed by the infant as that will be the one most practiced. Take advantage of the child's natural preference for activity to gain mobility quickly.

Postural Asymmetries. Depending on the age of the infant, posture should be examined in the sitting and standing positions after removal of the cast or splint. Asymmetries are usually indicative of residual tightness of soft tissue structures and deserve particular attention. The principles outlined above should be followed to elicit active participation of the infant in activities designed first to ensure mobility needed for postural symmetry and then to encourage symmetry of performance. Symmetry refers not only to the ability to maintain midline alignment but also to the ability to perform basic postural functions equally well with the right and left sides of the body. This includes sitting or standing and balancing over the right and left side. These abilities are gained only by practicing them. If there is an inability to maintain a level pelvis when bearing weight on the right leg, the only effective process of remediation is practice of that task. Strengthening exercises of hip abductors in infants and young children are futile. Since the pattern of muscle activation for the task of unilateral stance is quite dissimilar to the pattern of muscle activation involved in the traditional strengthening activities, one would be foolish to expect a strengthening program to be an effective procedure for accomplishing the goal of having hip abductors active during unilateral stance, particularly in this population of children. The infant or child needs to be encouraged and assisted to maintain a level pelvis while standing on the right foot. Again, games and activities that will engage the child in interaction with another person are most effective in accomplishing such treatment objectives.

Neuromuscular Pattern Imbalances Leading to Hip Deformity

Children with chronic neuromuscular conditions such as cerebral palsy or myelodysplasia or conditions characterized by chronic pain such as rheumatoid arthritis are all at risk for orthopaedic deformities. These deformities are traditionally attributed to muscle imbalance, muscle spasticity, or muscle spasm. It is important to recognize, however, that the imbalance of muscular forces is not confined to agonist-antagonist relationships about a single joint. Children with these chronic disabling conditions have stereotypic dominant patterns of posture and movement that lead to deformity. The problem must be viewed as an imbalance involving a synergy of muscle action within a limb. Often, dominant patterns of posture and movement encompass the body as a whole. The etiology of such patterns of imbalance cannot be attributed to the muscle or even the motor neuron. These stereotypic postural and movement patterns result from more complex central nervous system influences that involve multiple levels of the spinal cord and, in the case of the child with cerebral palsy, multiple levels of the brain. The term *neuromuscular pattern imbalance* is a more accurate reflection of the pathokinesiological features of the most common orthopaedic problems encountered by pediatric physical therapists.

Children with cerebral palsy and with myelodysplasia present with posture and movement patterns that predispose them to hip subluxation. If not treated, hip dislocation may result. These posture and movement patterns are characteristic and most frequently comprise flexion and adduction of the hip. Hip flexion and adduction are integral components of the set of postural and movement patterns that dominate these children's motor behavior.

Owing to the absence or reduced frequency of extension and abduction patterns, the flexors and adductors may not be exercised through their full length on a daily basis. This situation leads to contracture. If this pattern of flexion and adduction goes unarrested, bone deformity results. In addition, a reduction in overall activity level and abnormalities of motor development that delay the onset of weight bearing on the lower extremities also lead to growth retardation in the long bones.

Common Subjective Findings

Children identified as having cerebral palsy and those at risk for neurological dysfunction are commonly under physical therapy management at an early age. As a result, it is the therapist who commonly voices the first subjective findings. Increasing difficulty in maintaining abduction and extension of the hips with neutral or external rotation is the usual hallmark of impending orthopaedic problems. Parental complaints will concurrently center on difficulty getting the legs apart for dressing or diapering.

In the case of the child with myelodysplasia, the parents may note that the child's knees tend to be increasingly difficult to separate, particularly during diapering. They may also report that the child is increasingly intolerant of the prone position. The preferred posture becomes sitting with the hips flexed, adducted, and internally rotated (Fig. 21-9).

Parents of the child with chronic pain will also report that the child is intolerant of the prone position and prefers postures that incorporate hip flexion and adduction.

Objective Findings

In such cases, the signs of hip subluxation or dislocation outlined above may be present. Always examine the child for these signs.

Dominant Patterns about the Hip in Cerebral Palsy Syndromes. Children with the spastic cerebral palsy syndromes such as hemiplegia, diplegia, and quadriplegia are predisposed to hip deformities. This is also true during the natural evolution of the neurological condition through a dystonic syndrome to a spastic diplegia or quadriplegia. Hip deformity rarely develops in children with a primary syndrome of athetosis or ataxia.

Except during the period when a dystonic syndrome is evident, the dominant postural and movement pattern of the lower limb involves flexion, adduction, and internal rotation about the hip joint with accompanying knee flexion and ankle plantar flexion. During the dystonic period, hip and knee extension are more predominant, resulting in postural alignment of the lower extremities in hip extension, adduction, and internal rotation with knee extension and ankle plantar flexion. Infants and young children evidencing this dystonic cerebral palsy syndrome are usually not able to stand and walk. The dominant postural pattern is most pronounced when the child is supine or held in standing.

Dominant Hip Patterns in Myelodysplasia. Children with myelodysplasia will present pattern imbalance about the hip that ranges from partially innervated hip flexors toward increasing dominance of the hip flexors, adductors, and internal rotators that is unmatched by the hip extensors,

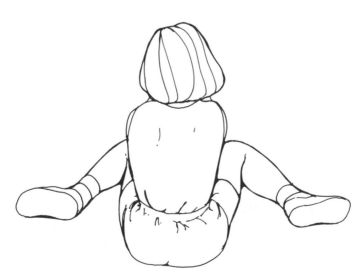

Fig. 21-9 Subjective finding in a child with myelodysplasia—the "television position" of sitting.

abductors, and external rotators. The knee extensors and ankle dorsiflexors are more active in children with lower level spinal lesions than are the knee flexors and ankle plantar flexors. The pattern of hip flexion, adduction, and internal rotation remains evident even in children with the lowest level spinal lesions. This is because the hip extensors, abductors, and external rotators are innervated through spinal structures with a lower level than those innervating their antagonists.

Dominant Hip Patterns in Chronically Painful Conditions. In young children with chronic hip pain, such as that evidenced in rheumatoid arthritis, the dominant postural pattern of the hip is characterized by hip flexion, adduction, and external rotation.

Growth and Anthropometric Measures

Not uncommonly there is growth retardation, particularly in the lower extremities, as a result of decreased mobility and lack of weight-bearing activities. Include leg length measures as a routine part of your evaluation. Measure from both the anterior superior iliac spine to the distal tip of the medial malleolus and from the most proximal tip of the greater trochanter to the distal tip of the medial malleolus. Take great care in ensuring accurate identification of bony landmarks before taking measures.

Measures of Flexibility

Be constantly on guard for decreasing flexibility. Use age-appropriate norms when evaluating hip flexion range of motion (see ranges provided in Appendix 21-2). Anticipate decreased range of movement into hip abduction and extension and a tendency for increased range in medial rotation and decreased range in external rotation in the children with cerebral palsy and myelodysplasia. The child with chronic pain will have a limited range into internal rotation. Commonly one hip is more restricted than the other.

Testing the Integrity of Innervation

The Child with Cerebral Palsy. Sensory and motor nerves are expected to be intact in children with cerebral palsy. Any decrease in reflexive responsiveness would be attributed to brain dysfunction.

The Child with Myelodysplasia. In children with myelodysplasia, expect a lack of integrity of innervation owing to abnormal development of the spinal cord and spinal nerve roots. Reflexive testing is the most efficient means to document the neural impairment in infants with myelodysplasia. There is decreased reflexive responsiveness below the level of the lesion. Observe spontaneous movement patterns to determine whether they are representative of and congruent with innervation patterns determined through reflexive testing.

Using light pinches, examine the movement patterns that are evoked when these stimuli are applied around the circumference of the limb. Because of "local sign" properties of the flexor withdraw reflex, potentially harmful stimuli can be used to evoke withdraw patterns that are not just composed of flexion movements. By application of gentle pinches around the circumference of the lower limbs, innervation patterns will be revealed. If innervation is intact, the infant will pull away from the source of the stimulus. The pattern of muscle action will involve different muscles depending on the site of stimulation and the initial position of the limb. The form of the movement will reveal which muscles are innervated. Thus, a pinch over the adductors when the limb is flexed may result in knee extension and a relaxation of the adductors, while the same stimulus applied to an extended limb may result in hip and knee flexion.

A predictable pattern of innervation results from lumbar level lesions. These are evidenced in innervation of the hip flexors and adductors and, with lower level lumbar lesions, knee extensors and medial hamstrings. The hip extensors and abductors do not begin to be able to compete with the degree of hip flexor and adductor innervation until the lesion involves only the cauda equina. Even in these instances, pattern imbalance may result in deformity that must be corrected by surgical means.

The Child with Chronic Pain. In children with chronic pain, sensory and motor nerves are intact. Any decrease in reflexive responsiveness might be attributed to an ongoing active attempt to prevent movement that causes pain.

Sensory Evaluation

The Child with Cerebral Palsy. Sensory nerves are expected to be intact in children with cerebral palsy. Processing of sensory information by brain centers is likely to be impaired. Such problems are perceptual in nature rather than attributed to basic sensory functions.

The Child with Myelodysplasia. By the time the child with myelodysplasia is beginning to develop deformities of the hip, the sensory deficit should be well documented. Reflexive functions will be affected, and the infant and young child with myelodysplasia will need to be safeguarded from harmful situations that would normally be detected and evoke protective responses.

If a sensory evaluation has not been completed on an infant you are treating, begin with reflexive testing. Absence of motor response to stimuli does not necessarily imply absence of sensory function. The deficit resulting from the congenital abnormality may involved interneurons or motor neurons with sensory conduction to the central nervous system and possibly to higher brain structures that are intact. For this reason, direct your attention to the face of the child you are examining, and particularly note quieting or shifting the gaze that might follow application of cutaneous stimuli. Gentle pinches may evoke facial grimaces or fussing.

When conducting the definitive sensory evaluation allow sufficient time to follow the distribution of sensory nerve roots, beginning above the documented level of disruption of the spinal cord and moving caudally. Check all nerve root distributions for responses to light tough, pinprick, and heat. A laboratory test tube filled with very warm water should be used to test responses to heat.

Motor Development

Observe and note the spontaneous postural and movement patterns of the lower extremities, especially those about the hips. Pay particular attention to the relative frequency of flexion and adduction patterns as compared with extension and abduction patterns about the hip. In the case of children with cerebral palsy, expect the developmental milestones to be delayed. Children with myelodysplasia that is uncomplicated by hydrocephalus should accomplish a large majority of developmental milestones of the first three trimesters within the normally expected time frame. However, the movement and postural patterns used to accomplish the developmental tasks are not those commonly observed.

In most cases of neuromuscular pattern imbalance, there is a tendency to maintain the hips in a posture of flexion and adduction beyond the first trimester of infancy. Determine whether this tendency is seen in all positions: prone, supine, and when the infant is held in sitting and standing. Watch for an extension and abduction pattern of kicking in the prone position. Observe the supine to prone rolling pattern and note the lower extremity movement patterns used to accomplish the task. Look particularly to see whether one leg pushes into abduction and extension as the body rolls away from that extremity. This movement pattern should be observed during the late second or third trimester. Observe the child sitting to see whether the legs are widely abducted or whether they are held together in adduction. Stand the child and observe postural alignment in standing. The normal postural pattern, secondary standing, that appears during the second trimester is not likely to be observed. The normal pattern is characterized by hip extension and abduction. Expect the child with neuromuscular dysfunction to stand in adduction with some degree of hip flexion. Extension and abduction may only be attained in a therapeutic setting after a period of handling or may be built in to a positioning device such as a prone stander. Try to determine, when the child is removed from therapy or from a positioning device, if the postural pattern is one involving hip flexion and adduciton.

Treatment Objectives

Ensure that the family understands how neuromuscular disorders can lead to bone deformities.

Instruct family and other caretakers in proper range of movement techniques that ensure continued flexibility and normal length of the hip flexors and adductors particularly.

Promote postural and movement patterns of the hip that include extension and abduction.

Encourage weight bearing on extended and abducted hips.

Continually monitor for signs of hip subluxation or dislocation and refer for orthopaedic evaluation and follow-up if hip range of motion decreases.

Provide supportive and postoperative care that ensures return to full activity as soon as practicable after any corrective orthopaedic procedure.

Treatment Guidelines

Explain to the family how dominance of flexor and adductor postural and movement pattern predispose their child to hip subluxation and dislocation. Explain the effects of this deformity on functional abilities. Enlist their ideas and suggestions to ensure that the child's hip flexibility stays within acceptable limits. Encourage the family to select an orthopaedist who will evaluate and follow the child's hip development. Be ready to offer suggestions of orthopaedists who work with children in your community.

Teach the family to provide passive range of motion to maintain hip flexibility. Have the family member use a Thomas position for ranging into hip extension and ensure that the lumbar spine is flat against the support surface when taking the thigh into extension (Fig. 21-10). If the child is in day care or preschool program, ensure that the caretakers are also instructed in these procedures and work with the family to ensure that someone assumes responsibility for this aspect of the child's care. Offer to teach the caretaker the same procedures in the presence of a family member.

As appropriate, utilize positioning devices such as wedged cushions for sitting and lying that keep the lower extremities abducted. Encourage the

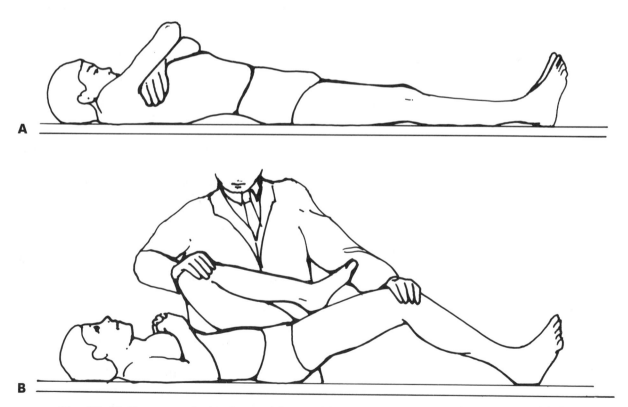

Fig. 21-10 Thomas test for hip flexion deformity. **(A)** When the patient is lying supine, a hip flexion deformity can be masked by an increase in the lumbar lordosis. **(B)** Passive complete flexion of the opposite hip straightens out the lumbar spine and reveals the true extent of the hip flexion deformity.

family to define a period of each day for the child to be in a position that promotes as much hip extension as possible. This could be done prone or standing, depending on age of the child and the interests and abilities of the family.

In treatment sessions, begin moving the child into and through postural and movement patterns that require hip abduction and extension.

Have the child roll by first flexing the lower extremity, bringing the foot into a position to push against the supporting surface, and then pushing down on the foot with the hip moving into extension and abduction with the knee flexed to effect the roll (Fig. 21-11).

Have the child play by pivoting in the prone position using an extension and abduction lower extremity pattern to push the body about.

Encourage standing from a squat position that ensures hip abduction and neutral rotation in the start position (Fig. 21-12).

Encourage a variety of sitting postures that incorporate hip abduction: long and short sitting with hip abduction (1), side sitting with one hip abducted and externally rotated and the other in slight abduction and internal rotation (b), and tailor sitting with both legs abducted and externally rotated (c) (Fig. 21-13).

Standing with the lower extremities in abduction and extension and a neutral degree of rotation is a critical activity. Be sure that the child has such an opportunity on a daily basis. Standing frames which ensure proper alignment of the lower extremities in young children with myelodysplasia

are available through orthosis suppliers (Fig. 21-14). The standing frame was designed as a preliminary orthosis to the parapodium. The parapodium enables the child with paraparesis secondary to myelodysplasia to stand with the lower extremities extended and with slight abduction and neutral rotation of the hips without the need for upper extremity support (Fig. 21-15). This device is useful for a wide variety of disabilities in which the objective is to enable upright activities with appropriate alignment of the lower extremities.

Prone standers are also readily available from commercial suppliers (Fig. 21-16). Prone standers can be used to enable children to stand with their lower extremities in abduction and extension. Like the parapodium, the prone stander allows the child to have the upper extremities free to engage in play or school activities. These devices when available should be used to assist with early institution of weight bearing in the child with neuromuscular pattern imbalance.

Reassess the child on a monthly basis and ensure that the family receives orthopaedic consultation when range of movement decreases or if there are any signs of subluxation about the hip.

If a child develops a deformity, only orthopaedic surgery can correct the problem. Less severe deformities may respond to myotomy or tenotomy. These soft tissue surgeries are designed to effectively lengthen shortened muscles. The procedures are done to prevent progression of the deformity and to reduce the deforming forces. If done early in life, and if followed by corrective growth forces, soft tissue procedures may promote correction of mild bony abnormalities. The older the child and the greater the deformity, the less likely a muscle procedure will be effective in promoting correction

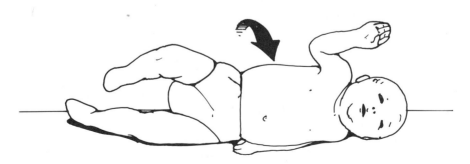

Fig. 21-11 Rolling on floor.

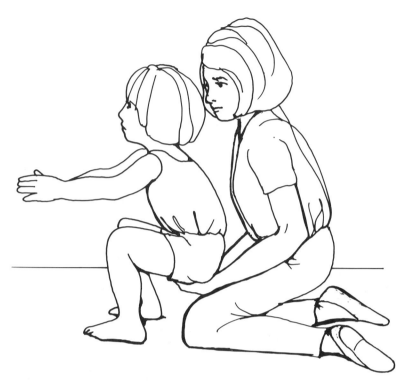

Fig. 21-12 Standing in squat position.

of deformity. In older children and in children with severe deformities, osteotomy is necessary to correct the deformity. For children with subluxed or dislocated hips, valgus and anteversion deformities of the femoral neck are quite common. Muscle lengthening, varus, and derotation osteotomies are quite common. Plates and pins are often inserted to hold the bones in proper alignment until the osteotomy heals. Sometimes muscles are transplanted to achieve a balance of muscle power about the hip. Transplantations are not very effective in children with reduced abilities for motor control, such as those seen in cerebral palsy. Transplantation procedures are more common and effective for children with myelodysplasia. Do not expect a young child after muscle transplant to be able to selectively control the transplanted muscle. Transplant procedures that work best in children are those in which the transplanted muscle acts as a tether to prevent an unwanted movement. The Sharrard procedure is an example of a muscle transplantation that can effectively result in a abduction tether. In the Sharrard procedure, the psoas is detached from its insertion on the lesser trochanter and passed through an osteotomy in the pelvis to a new attachment on the greater trochanter. The flexor is redirected to become an abductor that might balance adduction in the child with a preoperative dominance of flexion and adduction.

In the case of myotomies and tenotomies, casting may or may not be employed postoperatively. If the surgeon advocates early mobilization, removable plaster splints or bivalve casts might be provided for the child. These are used as positioning devices, particularly at night during sleep. Early

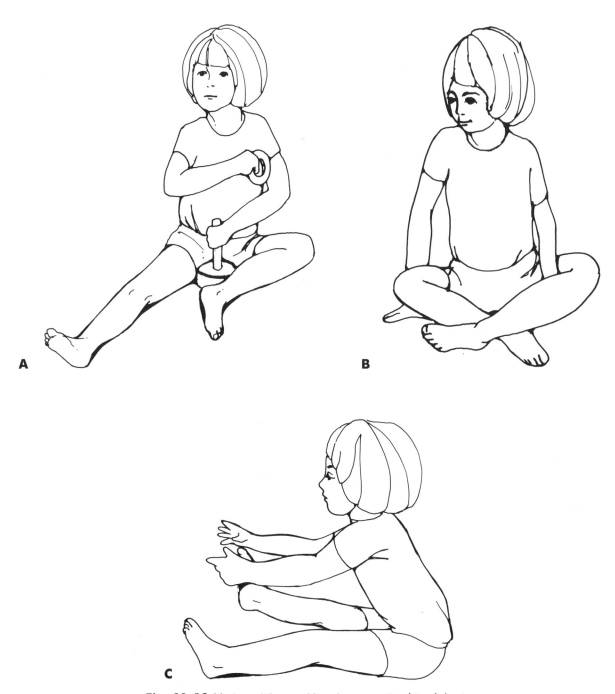

Fig. 21-13 Various sitting positions incorporating hip abduction.

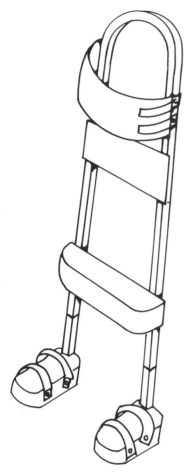

Fig. 21-14 Standing frame to ensure alignment of the lower extremities.

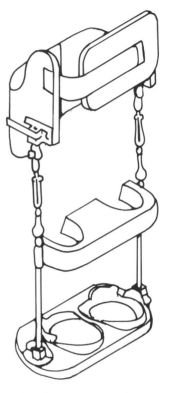

Fig. 21-15 Parapodium.

in the postoperative course, splints are usually only removed during therapy or bathing. Parents should be instructed in how to place and remove the splints and in appropriate skin care during the period of splinting. See details on cast and skin care above.

It is most important to maintain the newly acquired range of motion that results from the surgical procedure. As soon as the surgical site is healed, pool therapy or hydrotherapy can be a most effective modality to ensure range of motion in the presence of postoperative stiffness.

The period immediately after surgery can be extremely important in helping the cerebral palsied child to learn new patterns of posture and movement. Often previously dominant patterns of posture and movement are no longer available after myotomy or tenotomy of component muscles. Take full advantage of this opportunity to emphasize extension and abduction activities, particularly if they were difficult to attain preoperatively.

The child who undergoes osteotomy spends a longer period immobilized. Occasionally upright weight-bearing activities will be encouraged while the child is still in a cast. These are used by some surgeons to encourage bone healing. Stiffness after removal of the cast is a greater problem after osteotomy than after myotomy because of the duration of casting. Again, hydrotherapy should be used if possible to relax the child and encourage active movement through kicking and swimming about. If this is not possible, incorporate lower extremity movement activities into the child's bathing routine.

Have as a goal full range of movement within 1 week of cast removal. The longer it takes to achieve

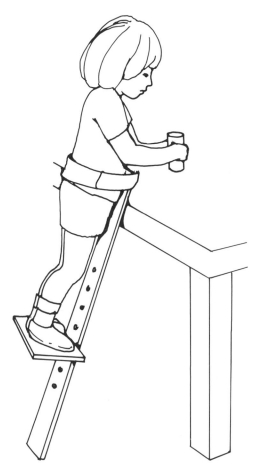

Fig. 21-16 Glenrosa prone board in use.

full movement after casting, the harder the process becomes.

SUGGESTED READINGS

Asher C: Postural Variations in Childhood. Butterworth, Boston, 1975

Bayley N: Manual of the Bayley Scales of Infant Development. The Psychological Corp., New York, 1969

Bernbeck R, Sinios A: Neuro-Orthopedic Screening in Infancy. Urban & Schwarzenberg, Baltimore, 1978

Cailliet R: Scoliosis. FA Davis, Philadelphia, 1975

Coleman SS: Congenital Dysplasia and Dislocation of the Hip. CV Mosby, St. Louis, 1978

Hensinger RN: Standards in Pediatric Orthopedics. Raven Press, New York, 1986

Lovell WW, Winter RB: Paediatric Orthopaedics. JB Lippincott, Philadelphia, 1978

MacEwen GD: The management of neuromuscular imbalance in the growing child. In Straub LR, Wilson PD (eds): Clinical Trends in Orthopaedics. Thieme, New York, 1982

Moe JH, Winter RB, Bradford D, Lonstein JE: Scoliosis and Other Spinal Deformities. WB Saunders, Philadelphia, 1978

Salter RB: Textbook of Disorders and Injuries of the Musculoskeletal System. 2nd Ed. Williams & Wilkins, Baltimore, 1983

Samilson RL: Orthopedic Aspects of Cerebral Palsy. Clinics in Developmental Medicine. Nos. 52/53. JB Lippincott, Philadelphia, 1975

Tachdjian MO: Pediatric Orthopedics. Vols. 1 and 2. WB Saunders, Philadelphia, 1972

Appendix 21-1
Length and Weight of Children*

These charts and tables were constructed using current body measurement data; they exploit the most recent advances in data analysis and computer technology. The data are derived either from studies done at the Fels Research Institute or from the health examination studies of the National Center for Health Statistics (NCHS). One set of charts for children from birth to 3 years is based on body measurements collected at the Fels Research Institute during 1929–1975. The set of charts for children 2 to 18 years of age is based on the NCHS data collected between 1963 and 1974.

---

* Graphs from Hamill PVV, Drizd PA, Johnson CL, Reed RB, Roche AF. National Center for Health Statistics (NCHS) growth curves for children, birth to eighteen years. Washington, D.C.; U.S. Government Printing Office, 1977; DHEW publication no. (PHS)78-1650.

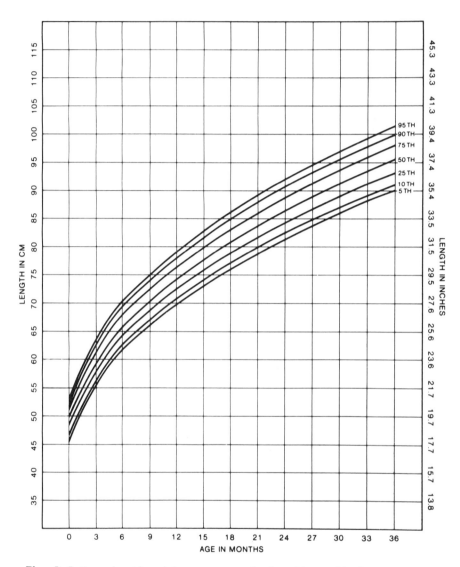

Fig. A-1 Recumbent length by age percentiles for girls aged birth to 36 months.

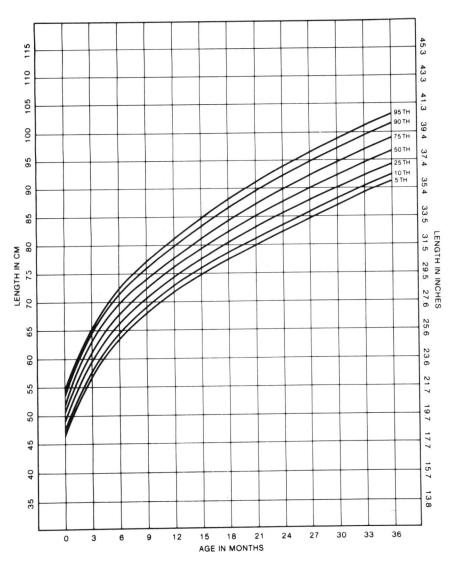

Fig. A-2 Recumbent length by age percentiles for boys aged birth to 36 months.

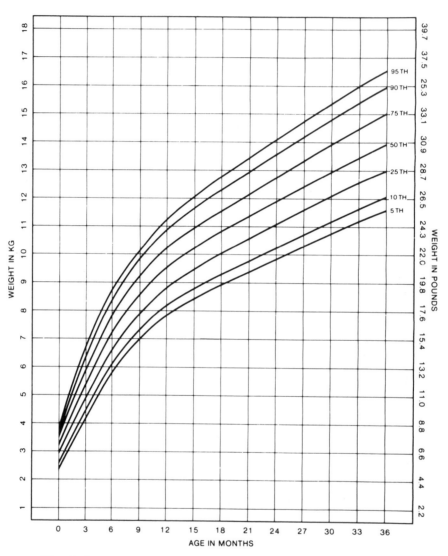

Fig. A-3 Weight by age percentiles for girls aged birth to 36 months.

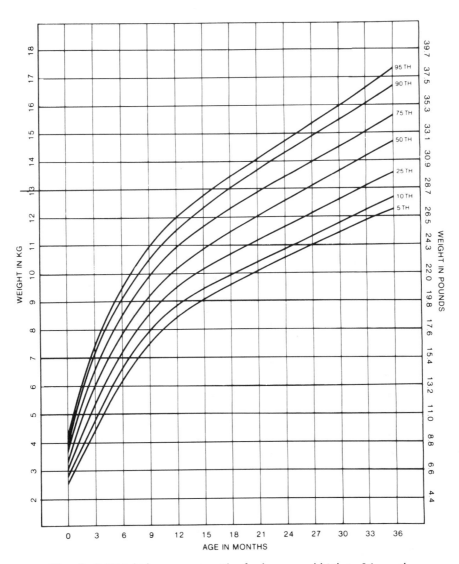

Fig. A-4 Weight by age percentiles for boys aged birth to 36 months.

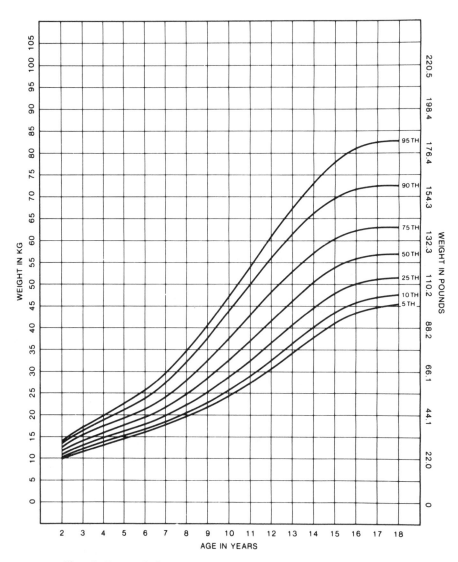

Fig. A-5 Weight by age percentiles for girls aged 2 to 18 years.

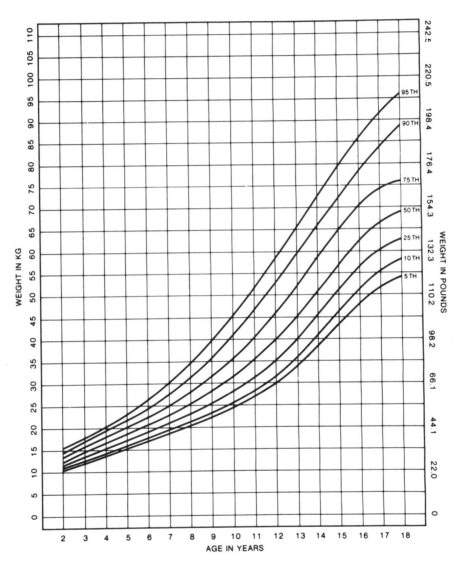

Fig. A-6 Weight by age percentiles for boys 2 to 18 years.

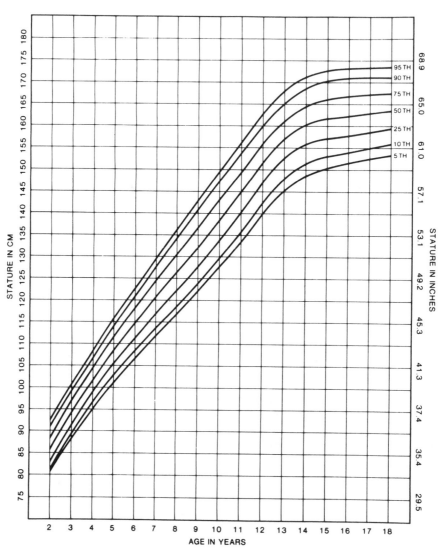

Fig. A-7 Stature by age percentiles for girls aged 2 to 18 years.

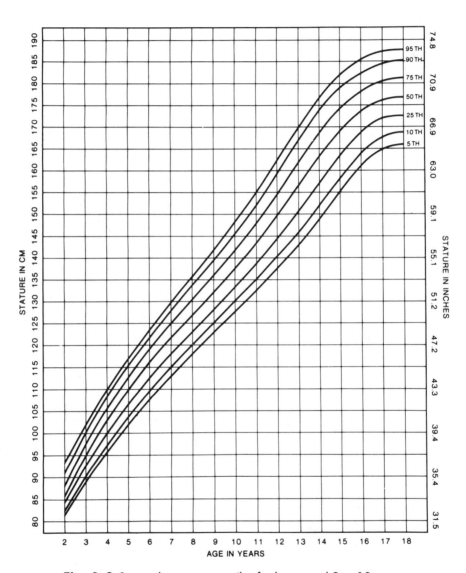

Fig. A-8 Stature by age percentiles for boys aged 2 to 18 years.

Table A-1 Sitting Height of Children by Race, Sex, and Age at Last Birthday[a,b]

Race, sex, and age	n	N	$\overline{X}$	s	$s_{\overline{x}}$	Percentile						
						5th	10th	25th	50th	75th	90th	95th
WHITE						In centimeters						
Boys												
6 years ------------------	489	1,787	65.0	2.68	0.13	60.4	61.4	63.2	65.1	66.7	68.5	69.7
7 years ------------------	551	1,781	67.2	2.74	0.15	63.0	64.0	65.4	67.2	68.9	70.8	71.8
8 years ------------------	537	1,739	69.5	2.94	0.12	65.1	65.7	67.6	69.6	71.5	73.3	74.3
9 years ------------------	525	1,730	71.6	3.15	0.19	66.4	67.4	69.6	71.6	73.7	75.6	76.7
10 years ----------------	509	1,692	73.3	3.07	0.20	68.3	69.5	71.4	73.3	75.4	77.3	78.7
11 years ----------------	542	1,662	75.6	3.10	0.13	70.6	71.5	73.5	75.5	77.7	79.6	80.7
Girls												
6 years ------------------	461	1,722	64.2	3.00	0.18	59.2	60.4	62.3	64.3	66.1	68.2	69.1
7 years ------------------	512	1,716	66.4	2.99	0.12	61.5	62.6	64.3	66.5	68.4	70.4	71.4
8 years ------------------	498	1,674	68.8	2.89	0.13	63.7	64.8	67.1	68.9	70.8	72.4	73.3
9 years ------------------	494	1,663	71.1	3.19	0.17	65.8	67.1	68.9	71.1	73.4	75.3	76.3
10 years ----------------	505	1,632	73.5	3.39	0.14	68.2	69.2	71.1	73.5	75.7	77.6	79.1
11 years ----------------	477	1,605	76.5	3.96	0.15	70.4	72.0	74.2	76.2	78.8	81.6	83.7
BLACK												
Boys												
6 years ------------------	84	289	63.2	2.48	0.35	59.2	59.7	61.4	63.2	64.8	66.5	68.1
7 years ------------------	79	286	65.6	2.58	0.29	61.6	62.3	63.5	65.6	67.5	69.1	70.1
8 years ------------------	79	279	67.8	2.81	0.29	63.5	64.3	66.2	67.5	69.4	71.8	72.7
9 years ------------------	74	269	69.3	3.69	0.40	63.7	64.5	66.7	68.6	71.7	74.5	75.8
10 years ----------------	65	264	70.9	3.54	0.33	64.8	66.1	68.3	70.6	73.2	75.4	77.5
11 years ----------------	83	255	73.4	3.36	0.37	67.8	68.7	71.4	73.6	74.8	77.5	79.3
Girls												
6 years ------------------	72	281	62.3	2.78	0.35	57.4	58.8	60.4	62.3	64.5	66.2	66.6
7 years ------------------	93	284	64.9	3.05	0.40	60.0	61.2	62.7	64.7	67.0	69.3	70.5
8 years ------------------	113	281	66.6	3.50	0.26	61.5	62.4	64.5	66.3	68.6	71.5	73.4
9 years ------------------	84	265	69.6	3.43	0.44	64.2	65.4	67.4	69.5	71.6	74.4	75.5
10 years ----------------	77	266	71.9	3.77	0.48	66.3	67.6	69.3	71.5	74.4	76.8	78.9
11 years ----------------	84	253	75.1	4.08	0.38	68.3	69.3	72.5	75.3	78.4	80.3	81.4

n = sample size; N = estimated number of children in population in thousands; $\overline{X}$ = mean; s = standard deviation; $s_{\overline{x}}$ = standard error of the mean.

[a] From Hamill PV, Johnston FE, Gram W. Height and weight of children, United States: height and weight measurements by age, sex, race, geographic region of children 6 to 11 years of age, United States 1963–65. National Center for Health Statistics, Series II, No. 104; Public Health Service Publication No. 1011, No. 104, U.S. Government Printing Office, Washington, D.C., 1970.

[b] Related Reference: Hamill PVV, Johnson FE, Lemeshow S. Body weight, stature and sitting height: White and Negro youths 12 to 17 years, United States. DHEW Publication No. (HRA) 74-1608, U.S. Government Printing Office, Washington, D.C., 1973.

Appendix 21-2
Passive Range of Hip Motion in Normal Children*

Table A-2 Range of Hip Motion in Normal Subjects

Age	Flexion Contracture (°)		"Frog Leg" Abduction (°)		Internal Rotation (°)		External Rotation (°)	
	Mean	Range	Mean	Range	Mean	Range	Mean	Range
Newborn[b]								
Male	28.0	20–75	76.7	50–90	60.8[a]	45–100[a]	87.5[a]	45–110[a]
Female	27.5	20–45	76.2	60–90	63.1[a]	35–90[a]	90.6[a]	60–110[a]
6 weeks[c]	19	6–32			24	16–36	48	26–73
3 months[c]	7	1–18			21	15–35	45	37–60
6 months[c]	7	−1–+16			21	15–42	46	34–61
4 years[d]					36		40	
9 years[d]					26		36	

[a] Internal and external rotation were determined with the hip flexed 90°.
[b] Normal ranges of hip motion in the newborn. Hass SS, Epps CH, Adams JP. Clin Orthop 1973; 91:114–18.
[c] Normal ranges of hip motion in infants—six weeks, three months, and six months of age. Coon V, Donato G, Houser C, Bleck EE. Clin Orthop 1975; 110:256–60.
[d] Femoral torsion and its relation to toeing in and toeing out. Crane L. J Bone Joint Surg (Am) 1959; 41:421–28. Note that these figures were estimated from a graph in Crane's paper.

* From Hensinger, RL: Standards in Pediatric Orthopaedics, p. 47. Raven Press, New York, 1986, with permission.

Appendix 21-3A
Developmental Chart for Routine Examination of Children*

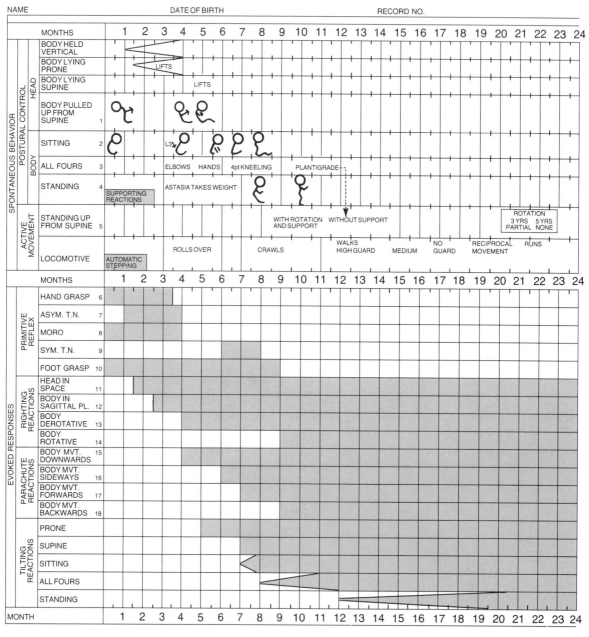

NAME   DATE OF BIRTH   RECORD NO.

Fig. A-9 The first letter of any word in the chart is aligned vertically with the age at which the phenomenon usually appears.

Divided into two sections, the upper section is a behavioristic scale modified from Koupernik (1954), and the lower section contains the primitive reactions and specific reactions. Entries in the chart are made by writing the chronological age in months below the functional finding indicated at the head of the columns. The chart was developed over a 5-year experience in regular weekly sessions in a children's clinic. (Koupernik C. *Developpement Psychomoteur du Premier Age*. Presses Universitaires, Paris, 1954.)

---

* From Milani-Comparetti A, Gidoni EA. Routine developmental examination in normal and retarded children. Dev Med Child Neurol 9:631–8, 1967, with permission.

(1) The figurines indicate that from birth until 4 months the head lags when gentle traction is applied to the arms of the supine child; at 4 months the head is maintained in alignment with the trunk as it is raised; at 5 months the child 'collaborates' with the examiner by flexing the head and exerting traction through the shoulders and elbows.

(2) L3 against the second figurine indicates that the progressive craniocaudal uncurving of the vertebral column has normally extended downwards to the level of the third lumbar segment at the age of 4 months.

(3) The words "elbows" and "hands" imply that at $3\frac{1}{2}$ months the normal infant extends the trunk by thrust through the elbows; at 5 months through the hands with extended elbows. These are considered to be the earliest phases of the adoption of the quadrupedal position. (4)

The *hatched area* (supporting reaction) is in fact a primitive reflex. These are assessed separately (*see* below), but it is convenient to record the supporting reactions in the examination of standing.

(5) Standing up without support is achieved in two different ways. The supine child rotates into the prone position, gets into four-foot kneeling, and then either climbs up using the hands as a support, or straightens the knees so that the plantigrade position is assumed, and from this position the trunk is lifted without support. This second alternative is recorded by putting the figure for the month on the arrow connecting "plantigrade" to "standing without support." The box is a convenience to extend the time covered by the chart. *N.B.* The conditions for performing tests in the bottom half of the chart are critical, because we are not so much interested in whether a particular reaction can be elicited, but rather in whether its presence under certain conditions and at a particular stage of development is interfering with the "funczione statica."

(6) Hand grasp is assessed by placing the child in the prone position and stimulating the palms by contact with the couch. The grasp reflex normally ceases to interfere with the supporting function of the arm at $3\frac{1}{2}$ months (*shading*).

(7) The asymmetric tonic neck reflex is assessed by placing the child supine and by rotating the head (without flexion). It is marked as positive if the elbow on the "occipital" side is more flexed than the elbow on the "chin" side.

(8) The Moro reflex is elicited by holding the child in a sitting position and tilting the trunk backwards. The effective stimulus is the falling back of the head when the examiner arrests the tilting movement at the shoulder level. The minimum positive reaction is a slight extention of the fingers. No parachute or tilting reactions usually exist until this minimal sign in the fingers has disappeared. The leg and foot response to this maneuver persists longer.

(9) The symmetric tonic neck reflex is assessed in the "all-fours" position. The presence of the S.T.N. at 6 months is indicated by flexion of the hips when the head is passively extended. The disappearance of the S.T.N. is seen when the child can lift the buttocks from the heels without flexing the head and upper limbs.

(10) Foot grasp is assessed with the child standing and by stimulating the sole of the foot by contact with the couch.

(11) We consider head-righting in space to be present when we see lifting of the head with the child in the prone position, or righting of the head when the vertically held child is tilted.

(12) The child is suspended prone with the upper abdomen on the examiner's hand. A positive reaction is indicated by extension of the head, trunk, and legs (first phase of the Landau reflex).

(13) The child is supine, and the examiner rotates the pelvis by using one flexed leg as a crank; alternatively he may rotate the flexed head. A positive reaction is indicated by "derotation" of the applied rotation, starting with flexion of the shoulder on the raised side. When this reaction appears the mother must be warned that the child should not be left alone lying on a bed because spontaneous rolling over is on the point of appearing.

(14) The child is placed supine and the normal 9 month infant tries to get out of this position and stand up by a sequence of movements ("chain reaction") starting with a flexion of the head and shoulder girdle. In cases where it is difficult to see this reaction on a couch in the clinic the mother may ask if, when waking up, the child immediately stands.

(15) The child is held vertically under the armpits and rapidly lowered; the normal reaction as seen in the lower limbs is extension, abduction, and external rotation. (*N.B.* Reaction in the upper limbs is impeded with this type of suspension.)

(16) The child is placed sitting and is pushed sideways on one shoulder with sufficient force to make it lose balance. The positive reaction is abduction of the opposite arm, with extension of the elbow, wrist, and fingers.

(17) The child is held with the trunk vertical and not inclined head-down as more usually described for testing the "sprungbereitschaft." In the vertical position the child is tilted forwards towards the couch. The arms project forwards with extended elbows, wrist, and fingers.

(18) The child is sitting and is pushed backwards. The full reaction is backward extension of both arms, but more frequently an element of trunk rotation comes in, and the reaction is seen in one arm only.

(19) The stimulus for all the tilting reactions is a slow tilt of the couch, either done smoothly, or in a series of small jerks. The examiner's attention is focused only on the reactive curving of the spine. Reactions in the limbs are ignored as it is difficult to separate the reaction to tilting from parachute reactions. With the "all-fours tilting reaction" the arrows should taper to 12 months and for the "standing tilting reaction" they should taper to 21 months.

Appendix 21-3B
Primitive Reflex Profile[a,b]

Asymmetrical Tonic Neck Reflex

Description   When the child is supine he may be seen to lie with head turned to one side with extension of the extremities on that side, and contralateral flexion of the extremities. This may also be noted in the sitting position. It is often described as the "fencer" position.

Technique   The child is placed supine. He is first observed for active head turning and subsequent extremity movement. If the reflex is not noted, the head is turned to each side for 5 seconds. This is repeated five times, to each side. If no movement is noted, the head turning is repeated and changes in tone are observed. This is then repeated with the child in a seated position.

Grading

0   Absent

1+   Tone changes in extremities with head rotation. On the chin side there is increased tone on flexion. On the occiput side there is increased tone on extension. Active head rotation on the child's part may yield slight movement of the extremities. Passive movement of the head does not yield movement of the extremities.

2+   Visible extension of extremities on the chin side and flexion of extremities on the occiput side. Movement is noted on both passive and active movement of the head. This is habituated on repeat trials. (This is seen in normal development of the reflex between 1 and 3 months of age.)

3+   Exaggerated quality with full extension of extremities on the chin side (180°) or full flexion of extremities on the occiput side (greater than or equal to 90° at the elbow). Some habituation is noted during the trials.

4+   Pathologic. Obligatory extension/flexion for more than 60 seconds.

---

[a] The basic distinction between the different scores was intended to reflect the following distinctions:
0   absent
1+   transient; elicited involuntarily by passive action of the infant, or noted only by change in tone
2+   elicited by voluntary active motion (physiologic)
3+   pronounced or sustained; more exaggerated than normally seen at chronologic age; not readily habituated
4+   obligatory; infant unable to break out of reflex for a minimum of 60 sec (pathologic).
[b] Capute, AJ: Primitive Reflex Profile. p. 24. University Park Press, Baltimore, 1978, with permission.

Symmetrical Tonic Neck Reflex

Description   On raising the head of a prone child, extensor tone increases in the arms and flexor tone increases in the legs; flexing the neck has the opposite effect with increased flexor tone in the arms and increased extensor tone in the legs.

Technique   The child is prone, suspended, sitting, or kneeling. Active neck extension/ flexion is sought through visual stimulus or command. Movement or tone change in extremities is assessed. If there is no active movement, the neck is passively extended/ flexed five times and movement/tone is assessed. The maneuver may have to be repeated in all positions.

Grading
- 0   Absent
- 1+   Mild, intermittent arm extension and leg flexion with neck extension; the reverse with neck flexion. Frequently only tone changes in the extremities with neck flexion/extension.
- 2+   Visible and consistent arm extension, or leg flexion with neck extension; the reverse is noted with flexion. (Physiologic appearance of reflex at 20 weeks.)
- 3+   Marked arm extension or leg flexion with neck extension, reverse with flexion. Not easily overcome by the child. Not readily habituated and present after five trials.
- 4+   Pathologic. Obligatory. Position remains after 60 seconds.

Tonic Labyrinthine Reflex

Description   The position/posture of the limbs changes with respect to the position of the head in space (orientation of labyrinths). Supine, the limbs extend or extensor tone increases. Prone, the limbs flex or flexor tone increases.

Technique   The child is observed supine. Support is then placed between the shoulders so that the head is extended to 45°. The position/tone of extremities as assessed. The child's head is then flexed to 45° with the back still supported, and finally he is asked to grasp in the midline. The child is then placed prone and position/tone is assessed.

Grading
- 0   Absent
- 1+   In the supine position, the shoulders are retracted and arms are lying in a "surrender" posture. There would be momentary shoulder retraction and leg extension when support is placed between the shoulders and the head is extended to 45°. When the child is made to flex his head, shoulder retraction is broken and the hands immediately come to the midline. In the prone position there may be momentary flexion noted at the hips.
- 2+   With his head in extension the child is not able to overcome shoulder retraction. His hands do not come to the midline when his head is flexed, but he can overcome this on command. Prone, some degree of flexion with increased flexor tone is noted.
- 3+   When the child's head is extended there is significant shoulder retraction and leg extension. He is unable to bring his hands together fully when asked to flex his head and his shoulders do not protract. In prone there may be considerable flexion.

4+   Obligatory severe extensor thrust or opisthotonus. The back is arched and the position is held for greater than 60 seconds.

Positive Support Reflex

Description   Upon stimulation of the hallucal area, cocontraction of opposing muscle groups occurs so as to fix the joints of the lower extremities in a position capable of supporting weight.

Technique   The child is suspended in the vertical position and the balls of the feet are brought in contact with the floor or surface for 60 seconds. The child is then bounced five times.

Grading
   0   Absent. No attempt at weight bearing.
   1+   The child does not maintain his weight for 60 seconds. He may land flat-footed with no discernible movement from heel to toe. The knees may be partially flexed without evidence of extension.
   2+   The child is able to support his weight for greater than 60 seconds. There is quick movement from plantar flexion to dorsiflexion. There is extremity extension with body support. Slight hip and knee flexion may be noted.
   3+   There is delayed movement from plantar flexion to dorsiflexion. The child remains in the equinus position. The knees may be hyperextended in a genu recurvatum position or there may be fixed and persistent knee flexion. The child seems to be standing on his toes.
   4+   The child remains on his toes in an equinus position. He is not able to move out of the position without circumducting the legs and stays in this position for greater than 60 seconds.

Derotational Righting Reflex

Description   The body turns to untwist itself in a segmental fashion when rotation is applied along the body axis.

Technique   The child is supine. Initially the head is rotated to turn the shoulders to midline and any rotation is observed. The legs are then rotated to turn the pelvis to midline and derotation is observed.

Grading
   0   Absent
   1+   The child does not roll over until midline is reached, but then completes the maneuver in a derotational (segmental) fashion. Movement occurs in a proximal to distal fashion when the shoulders are turned and in a distal to proximal fashion when the pelvis is turned.
   2+   The body follows the head in a derotational manner. The child rolls before the shoulders or the hips reach the midline, and essentially can roll over by himself. (This is the physiologic stage beginning at 4 to 6 months.)
   3+   The body follows in a nonderotational fashion. It may be noted that on rotating the legs the head will rotate before the trunk and upper extremities, or on rotating the head the legs will rotate before the arms.
   4+   The child will continue to roll in a nonderotational ("log rolling") manner and cannot inhibit the reflex. It is obligatory.

Moro Reflex

Description On sudden extension of the head there is rapid, symmetrical abduction and upward movement of the arms. The hands open and there is a gradual adduction and flexion of the arms in a clasping manner.

Technique The child is supine and the head is allowed to drop back suddenly on five trials.

Grading

0	Absent
1+	Minimal arm extension or abduction. There may be momentary flexion of the fingers.
2+	Full arm extension/abduction, then arm adduction with wrist flexion and finger extension. Habituates during trials (physiologic under 4 months).
3+	Back arches, minimal opisthotonus. Hyperextension of legs. Does not habituate.
4+	Shoulders retract, marked opisthotonus. Fingers are noted to be splayed during movement. Remains consistent during trials.

Galant Reflex

Description On stroking the back along the paravertebral area the child arches his trunk with concavity towards the stimulated side.

Technique The back is initially stroked with the dull side of a safety pin in the lumbar area and movement is noted. This is repeated five times. If there is no movement the sensory testing wheel is used five times to provide sharper yet consistent sensory input.

Grading

0	Absent
1+	Very mild and inconsistent incurvature.
2+	Persistent trunk incurvature (physiologic under 2 months).
3+	Exaggerated trunk incurvature with hips swinging to 45°. Not readily habituated.
4+	Persistent trunk incurvature and elevation of hips. No habituation on trials.

Appendix 21-4
Various Sensory Modalities Tested with Traditional Tests of Infant Reflexes

Touch
    Rooting reflex
    Galant's sign
    Flexor withdraw
    Righting reactions

Pain and Temperature
    Flexor withdraw

Touch/Pressure
    Palmar and plantar
    grasp reflexes
    Positive support reflex
    Automatic stepping
    Righting reactions

Proprioception
    Tendon reflexes
    Traction response
    Tonic neck reflex
    Righting reactions
    Tilting reactions

Vestibular System
    Semicircular canals
        Moro reaction
        Parachute reactions
        Tilting reactions
    Otoliths
        Righting reactions
        Tilting reactions

Section III

Cardiopulmonary Dysfunction

Edited by
Elizabeth J. Protas

22 Health Risk Appraisal

Robert Friberg

What is the role of the physical therapist in helping individuals in the community prevent cardiovascular disabilities? That physical therapists may assume a role in prevention is justified by the profession's body of knowledge and skills. Physical therapists possess the knowledge and skill to evaluate and treat musculoskeletal, neuromuscular, and cardiovascular disorders. To understand the pathological processes associated with each system, an understanding of the normal structure and function of that system is essential. To engage in the restorative process the physical therapist also understands and applies the principles of work physiology. In addition, a knowledge of the normal and abnormal responses to work also provides a basis for the practice of physical therapy.

The relationships between structure and function and their implications for those on the continuum from wellness to disease provide a model from which to identify an appropriate role. The role potential is multifaceted and can impact individuals along the continuum of wellness and disease. Specifically, it should include the cardiovascular system.

Physical therapy, by definition, is a further justification for accepting responsibility in the area of health risk appraisal of the cardiovascular system. To be involved in the arena of movement dysfunction, the physical therapist must focus attention on the prevention of dysfunction as well as the rehabilitation of dysfunction. Physical therapy provides opportunities for interaction with individuals in the context of prevention and rehabilitation of movement dysfunctions. Practically, it provides a forum to evaluate, plan, and implement physical therapy programs that are directly or indirectly related to the cardiovascular system.

The challenge for the physical therapist, then, is to assume responsibility for the prevention of movement dysfunction. An excellent tool to facilitate the adoption and implementation of this role is a health risk appraisal (HRA) instrument. This chapter will provide a basis for the selection and use of HRA instruments for the cardiovascular system. To provide a groundwork for the application of the HRA in physical therapy, information is provided about HRA types, uses, characteristics, and limitations. In addition, specific information about the HRA of the cardiovascular system is reviewed. Resources are also provided for future reference and use.

HEALTH RISK APPRAISAL

HRAs are techniques that provide a quantitative way of defining or describing the risk of death or certain diseases. These techniques are also known as health hazard appraisals or health risk assessments. They are predictions based on epidemiological data. To use some form of an HRA as part of a larger health promotion effort means that decisions must be made about which assessments to use and how the information fits the overall wellness or prevention program. General reasons for using HRAs include helping accomplish objectives of larger programs, providing a framework for presentation of health-related messages, increasing the awareness and concern about personal health, and increasing the personal motivation for change.

551

There are many choices of HRA instruments available for doing health risk assessment. Certain criteria should be considered when selecting the tool. They include the purpose; the nature of the population that will utilize the tool; overall goals of the wellness program; and the quality of the instrument.

All HRA instruments have basic characteristics. Each is primarily a data collection instrument intended to gather information about health habits, medical history, specific physiological measurements, and important social and demographic information. An HRA will also provide a summary profile that might include a score or ranking based on the responses, specific behavioral change recommendations, and resources, for instance, health promotion programs in the local area. The instrument itself must include appropriate types and numbers of questions about risk factors so that some type of risk calculation can be determined. The tool should also be characterized by an attractive format that is easy to read and understand.

By their very nature, health risk assessments have some limitations. A major limitation is that little empirical evidence exists regarding the relationship between individual mortality and HRA score. There is also evidence that suggests that the tool itself has little effect on individual health outcomes. However, the instrument can provide a positive influence. To gain this effect, it must be used in conjunction with a well-defined and integrated program.

APPLICATION TO PHYSICAL THERAPY

The current use of HRA by a wide variety of groups provides the profession of physical therapy a vehicle for capturing the awareness and attention of the public in the areas of movement dysfunction specifically associated with the cardiovascular system. Physical therapists are able to provide a service that may lead to increased levels of professional utilization by the public, in the contexts of wellness and prevention.

In addition to the potential for assuming responsibilities in the area of wellness and prevention, the opportunity for development and implementation of comprehensive client programs exists. All programs should contain an educational role and a direct role in the intervention of cardiovascular disorders. Physical therapists have the unique training to provide input to individuals in all phases of wellness or disease.

There are existing HRA models that will provide the basis for physical therapy involvement in cardiovascular health risk appraisal. The models are not inclusive or designed to meet the needs of physical therapists specifically. They are, however, appropriate for the role of increasing the knowledge and awareness of individuals. The physical therapist should not be limited by these approaches, but use them to pursue professional development. Physical therapy training provides a foundation in the etiological basis of cardiovascular pathology. This training can lead to the development of additional assessment tools to meet specific population or program needs.

CARDIOVASCULAR HEALTH RISK APPRAISAL

In 1980, 51 percent of all deaths in the United States were associated with cardiovascular disease. Coronary artery disease accounted for 56 percent of all cardiovascular disease. In other words, one of three deaths in the United States is attributable to coronary artery disease. Even more important are the numbers of individuals who have significant life style alterations owing to coronary artery disease. These individuals will suffer significant movement dysfunction.

Movement dysfunctions can be effectively evaluated and therapeutic intervention can be initiated by a physical therapist. This section reviews the risk factors associated with coronary heart disease. This review provides a basis for reviewing the implications of physical activity on associated risk factors. Finally, there is a discussion of practical ways to evaluate and implement the programs.

RISK FACTORS ASSOCIATED WITH CORONARY HEART DISEASE

There are numerous risk factors identified or suspected to cause cardiovascular disease. A comprehensive list of known or suspected risk factors would include age, sex, familial history, race, levels of serum cholesterol and triglyceride, level of systolic and diastolic blood pressure, cigarette smoking, impaired vasocompliance, obesity, abnormal glucose tolerance, diabetes, hyperuricemia, gout, hypothyroidism, sociopsychological stress, physical activity, and sedentary life. Various classification systems are available to organize all of these known and suspected risk factors. The risk factors can be organized by using four criteria in a two-by-two cell (Table 22-1). The cells on the horizontal axis represent primary and secondary (known and suspected) risk factors that are either unalterable or modifiable. The vertical cells represent risk factors that are of personal or socioenvironmental categories.

Primary risk factors are those that are empirically implicated to contribute to the development of atherosclerosis. Secondary risk factors are recognized for influencing cardiovascular disease but the specific weight or mechanisms of involvement need further research. Both primary and secondary risk factors can be altered through medical management or life style changes. There are also specific risk factors that can be classified as unalterable. Additionally, risk factors can be differentiated as personal or socioenvironmental. For example, hypertension can be classified, according to the scheme in Figure 22-1, in the cell representing both a personal and primary modifiable risk factor. Unalterable personal risk factors would include age, sex, race, and family history. Personal, secondary modifiable risk factors would be emotional stress, obesity, and sedentary life style. Emotional stress could also be classified as containing socioenvironmental and secondary modifiable characteristics.

It is generally accepted that the most powerful predictors for cardiovascular disease include age,

sex, level of blood pressure, level of serum cholesterol, cigarette smoking, and physical activities. Each of these predictors is described below.

Hypertension

Blood pressure, primarily arterial blood pressure, is one of the most powerful predictors of coronary heart disease. Both mortality and morbidity from coronary heart disease demonstrate a positive relationship with systolic and diastolic blood pressure. Studies have demonstrated that the risk of premature cardiovascular disease and death rises sharply with increased resting levels of both systolic and diastolic blood pressure. In addition, even within the "statistically normal" level of blood pressure, there are greater numbers of strokes and heart attacks among persons in the so-called high normal category than in persons with lower blood pressure. In the presence of other coronary heart disease risk factors, elevated blood pressure is a dangerous precursor to coronary heart disease.

Cigarette Smoking

Cigarette smoking is possibly the most significant and important risk associated with coronary heart disease.[1-3] It has been demonstrated that cigarette smoking accentuates the influence of the other coronary heart disease risk factors. Mortality is twice as high in the smoking group as in nonsmokers. However, once cigarette smoking habits stop, the risk (after a period of time) reverts to that of nonsmokers, although this period of time may be as long as several years. Cigarette smoking is, however, one factor that lends itself most readily to programs for prevention of coronary heart disease.

Table 22-1 Risk Factors Associated with Coronary Heart Disease

	Modifiable Factors		Unalterable
	Primary (Known)	Secondary (Suspected)	
Personal	Hypertension	Emotional Stress	Age
	Cigarette Smoking	Personality Type	Sex
	Diabetes	Obesity	Race
	Level of Serum Cholesterol and Triglyceride	Sedentary Life	Family History
Socioenvironmental		Emotional Stress	

Serum Lipids

Hyperlipidemia refers to elevation of serum cholesterol and triglycerides. As with blood pressure, there is no cutoff point in the distribution of serum cholesterol or triglycerides above which individuals are at risk or below which they are free from risk. In general, the higher the level, the greater the risk. Persons with diets high in saturated fats and cholesterol have elevated levels of serum cholesterol and increased incidence of cardiovascular disease.[4,5]

Obesity

It has been demonstrated that weight gain in middle age leads to increased risk of coronary heart disease.[6,7] It is theorized that weight gain influences other, more potent factors, such as elevated blood pressure and level of serum triglycerides. However, there is no current evidence that weight reduction alone will reduce the incidence of coronary heart disease, but weight reduction is one component for successful management of elevated blood pressure.

Family History

Those with a positive family history for heart disease are considered at risk. Positive family history is defined as a close relative (parent or grandparent) with coronary artery disease under 60 years of age. This is because the genetic factors associated with coronary heart disease are multifaceted. When individuals with a positive family history also have one or more other conventional risk factors, they are considered very vulnerable.

Stress and Behaviorial Patterns

There is some evidence to suggest that there is a positive relationship between how an individual responds to occupational or environmental stress and coronary heart disease. Because this varible is only one of many risk factors associated with the incidence of coronary heart disease, it must be evaluated in conjunction with all other variables to determine potential cardiovascular implications.[8]

Age and Sex

The risk of coronary heart disease increases with age for both sexes. This includes all races, although black males are more susceptible. There is an exponential rise of death rates with age. Because of increasing numbers of persons in middle age with coronary heart disease, coronary heart disease can no longer be considered a degenerative disease of the elderly.[1,2]

Physical Activity

Even though different opinions exist as to how much vigorous activity is appropriate, most research evidence suggests that it is a deterrent to coronary artery disease.[9-14] There is a strong inverse relationship between high energy output and fatal heart attack. Yet, empirical evidence also states that the potential benefits cannot be retained if physical activity is discontinued. Therefore, this association should be considered protective rather than selective.

The probable cause for activity being a deterrent to coronary heart disease is related to the effect it has on other risk factors. Consistent aerobic exercise has been shown to reduce resting and exercise blood pressure, to reduce the elevation of serum cholesterol and triglycerides, to improve glucose tolerance, to reduce sociopsychological stress, and to be an important factor in the reduction of obesity. Therefore, even though it is not a major direct link to the prevention of coronary heart disease, physical activity is probably the one single variable able to affect multiple other risk factors.

MECHANISMS FOR CARDIOVASCULAR HEALTH RISK APPRAISAL

Initial contact to screen individuals can occur in many different ways, for instance, shopping center health promotion booths, pre-employment screens, health fairs, preseason physicals for athletes, or your clinical facility. Regardless of the location or the intended goal of the health risk appraisal, certain information must be collected.

Once that information is collected, decisions can be made regarding the need for, types of, and levels of intervention. The following paragraphs provide more specific details regarding the probable nature of a series of decisions, the types of information that must be collected, and a brief overview of a sample protocol for cardiovascular health risk appraisal.

When health risks are assessed for cardiovascular disease, decisions regarding the role of physical therapy will be made. Although the role initially may not be to develop and monitor exercise programs, an equally valid role of educator can be adopted. Figure 22-1 provides a model that reflects the probable interaction with a client representing both high risk and limited risk for cardiovascular disease. The initial evaluation must contain specific information. The thoroughness with which all possible factors are evaluated will depend on the purpose of the screen, resources, etc. However, an initial decision must be made regarding risk level after the preliminary collection of data. Depending on the initial decision, there are several

paths leading ultimately to the development of an exercise program. Again, even for those patients at high risk, physical therapists may play a role in education or coordination during the intervening steps leading to the opportunity for exercise program development. Specific tasks for the physical therapist in this model obviously are related to the characteristics of your individual settings.

Figure 22-2 is a more detailed graphic representation that identifies information that should be collected in both the ideal and practical conditions. The ideal situation obviously reflects no limitation on your or your client's resources. The practical information, although lacking in thoroughness, will provide information to make the initial decision regarding high risk or limited risk. The decision to refer the patient for further medical evaluation because of high risk will be based on specific high-risk indicators. These include personal history of myocardial infarction; abnormal electrocardiogram; hypertension greater than 140/90; history of inactivity; obesity defined as greater than 22 percent for females and greater than 19

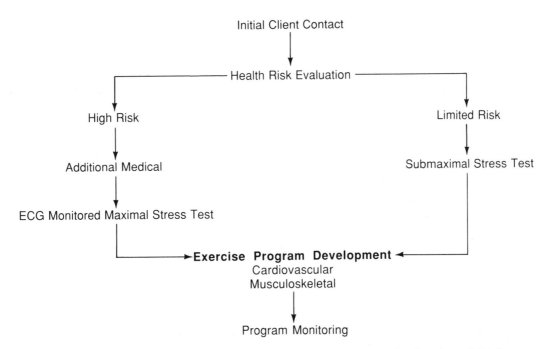

Fig. 22-1 Model for interaction with a client who may have a high risk or limited risk for cardiovascular disease.

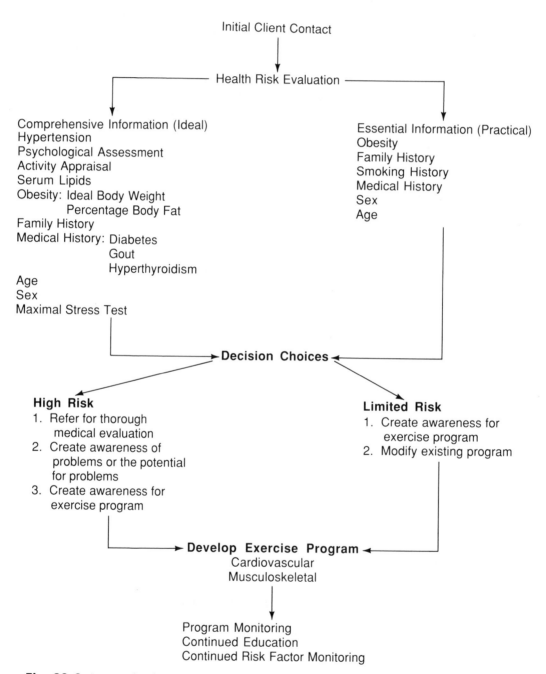

Fig. 22-2 A more detailed model for interaction with a client who is at risk for cardiovascular disease.

percent for males; hyperlipidemia with a cholesterol level greater than 200; triglyceride level greater than 150; glucose level greater than 100; family history of cardiovascular disease; history of smoking; history of tension or anxiety; diabetes; and age. If the client is positive for three or more of these risk factors, he should be referred for a more complete evaluation.

HEALTH RISK APPRAISAL PROTOCOL

There are a variety of ways to collect the initial information. The following paragraphs are brief descriptions of a protocol currently available that could be used.[15] The protocol is fairly comprehensive and reflects a thorough review of not only cardiovascular risk but some musculoskeletal function as well. It is an excellent example to use or modify to meet individual circumstances.

How the protocols are used is also described. The component parts represent the type of information that can be gathered and used for decision making. The information will provide an excellent basis for making the initial decision.

1. Record Sheet for *Level I Risk Assessment;* Record Sheet for *Level II Fitness Assessment; General Coronary Risk Profile; Health Factors Review;* and *Health Hazard Appraisal.* The information from each component is summarized on the Record Sheets for Level I Risk Assessment and Level II Fitness Assessment. This protocol provides a basis for cardiovascular and musculoskeletal assessment. The two can be used for an overall comprehensive HRA or individually for the specific system of interest.
2. The *Level I Risk Assessment* (Fig. 22-3) organizes information from other sources, several of which are written protocols reviewed in this chapter and various other physical measurements. The number of categories used on the Level I Risk Assessment in client evaluation is determined by program goals, resources, etc. The form used to organize and review data for Level I Risk Assessment provides a mechanism to identity primary and secondary risk factors

quickly. The format also facilitates the assessment of the client's progress over time.
3. The *General Coronary Risk Profile* (Fig. 22-4) provides information summarized on the Level I Risk Assessment. This evaluation tool consists of seven categories of forced choice answers. The categories represent the major risk factors for cardiovascular disease. Patients with "moderate" risk and above (>15 points) would be referred for further medical evaluation. The instrument is of value as a model even if the data regarding resting and exercise electrocardiograms are not available. Five important and powerful predictors are available to assist in decision making.
4. The *Health Factor Review* (Fig. 22-5) also provides information summarized on the Level I form. This instrument provides more general information about the overall physical and psychological health of an individual. There are specific questions that review cardiovascular risk factors, and those can be used for a variety of purposes.
5. The *Health Hazard Appraisal* (Fig. 22-6) evaluation forces the reviewer to select the most appropriate response for relevant variables in different categories to ultimately predict life expectancy. This information is also used on the Level I summary sheet. This specific protocol is excellent as a source for the collection of a variety of data useful in HRA in contexts other than cardiovascular. It can also be used as a model for the development of other protocols more appropriate to individual program goals.
6. The final part of this comprehensive model is the *Level II Fitness Assessment Summary* (Fig. 22-7) format. The major subcategories for this protocol reflect the importance of information regarding not only cardiovascular but musculoskeletal health risks. Flexibility and strength are important to evaluate owing to the ultimate goal of exercise program development.

The types of information, presentation-format, and potential uses of this set of protocols provide a way to initiate HRA. Modifications for individual

BASIC FITNESS APPRAISAL

NAME: _____ Activity interests/hobbies: _____

Family History of Disease: _____

Medical Precautions (personal): _____

Medications: _____

LEVEL I (Risk Assessment   DATE   DATE   DATE

Coronary Risk Profile Score _____

Health Factors Review X Score _____

Life Expectancy Score _____

Resting Heart Rate (radial/apical) _____

Blood Pressure (resting) _____

Pulmonary Function (residual volume) _____

Blood Chemistry (cholesterol) _____

    HDL/LDL Ratio _____

    Triglycerides _____

TEST

Body Fat Calipers _____

Skindex Method _____

Hydrostatic Weighing (Fat %/% Lean) _____

TEST

Postural Deformity–Neck _____

Postural Deformity–Trunk _____

Postural Deformity–Arms _____

Postural Deformity–Legs _____

STRESS

Stressors–Chemical _____

Stressors–Physical _____

Stressors–Social _____

Ability to Cope with Stress _____

NUTRITION

Nutritional Deficiencies _____

Further Medical Exam (tests needed) _____

Fig. 22-3 The Level I Risk Assessment form.

GENERAL CORONARY RISK PROFILE

CHECK THE APPROPRIATE BOX AND TOTAL SCORE

PERSONAL HISTORY OF HEART ATTACK

Points
- 0 ☐ None
- 2 ☐ Over 5 years ago
- 3 ☐ 2–5 years ago
- 5 ☐ 1–2 years ago*
- 8 ☐ 0–1 year ago*

TENSION-ANXIETY

Points
- 1 ☐ No tension, very relaxed
- 0 ☐ Slight tension
- 1 ☐ Moderate tension
- 2 ☐ High tension
- 1 ☐ Very tense, "high strung"

FAMILY HISTORY OF HEART ATTACK

Points
- 0 ☐ None
- 2 ☐ Yes, over 50 years
- 4 ☐ Yes, 50 years or under

RESTING ECG

Points
- 0 ☐ Normal (negative)
- 1 ☐ Equivocal (borderline)
- 3 ☐ Abnormal (positive)
- 2 ☐ Don't know

EXERCISE ECG

Points
- 0 ☐
- 4 ☐
- 8 ☐
- 2 ☐

SMOKING HABITS

Points
- 0 ☐ None
- 1 ☐ Pipe/cigar
- 1 ☐ Past only/Quit
- 2 ☐ 1–10 daily
- 3 ☐ 11–30 daily
- 4 ☐ 30 + daily

AGE FACTOR

- 0 ☐ Under 30 years
- 1 ☐ 30–39 years
- 2 ☐ 40–49
- 3 ☐ 50–59
- 4 ☐ 60 + years

ADD UP ALL POINTS (TOTAL) _____

RISK 0–4 very low; 5–14 low; *15–24 moderate; 25–34 high; 35 + very high

Fig. 22-4 The General Coronary Risk Profile form. (Modified from Cooper,[15] with permission.)

HEALTH FACTORS REVIEW

Please complete the questions below and bring it with you to the screening. Each question has a subjective ranking of 1–10. Circle the response or number closest to how you feel at this time in your life.

I am overweight or underweight?

1	2	3	4	5	6	7	8	9	10
Extremely over/under 50 + lbs.	Markedly over/under 40 + lbs.	Moderately over/under 20 + lbs.	Minimally overweight 10 + lbs. always	Average 6–10 lbs. overweight	Above average 1–5 lbs. overweight always	Subperfect 1–5 lbs. overweight sometimes	Perfect proper height always Women-22% fat Men-16% body fat	Sub Super Perfect 1–5 lbs. underweight sometimes Women-20% body fat Men-14% body fat	Super Perfect 1–5 lbs. underweight always Women-18% body fat Men-12% body fat

I am under stress at work?

1	2	3	4	5	6	7	8	9	10
Always. Can't handle it. Like walking a tight rope 300 ft. up in a cross wind 50 MPH and snowing	Always. Can handle it.	Most often	Often	Occasionally. Like walking a tight rope 30 ft. in the air. No wind, cool day (daily)		Periodically (3 x per week)			Hardly ever walking a tight rope on the ground; no wind; sunny day

Personal life stress is?

1	2	3	4	5	6	7	8	9	10
Like sitting in a bathtub with eight 2 year olds (severe stress)		High stress		Like watching TV and having your spouse talk with you at the same time (moderate stress)					Like sitting on a park bench on a sunny day just enjoying life quietly. (minimal stress)

My last dental checkup?									
1	2	3	4	5	6	7	8	9	10
No dentists for past 4 years	Within last 3 years	Within last 2 years	Within last 18 months	Within the last year	Within past 10 months	Within past 8 months	Within past 6 months	Within past 5 months	Within past 4 months

During the night I sleep?									
1	2	3	4	5	6	7	8	9	10
No time for sleep (less than 3 hours)	More than 12 hours sleep	Less than 5 hours sleep	More than 10 hours sleep	At least 5 hours sleep	At least 5½ hours sleep	At least 6 hours sleep	At least 6½ hours sleep	*	At least 7–8 hours per night

Presently I smoke?									
1	2	3	4	5	6	7	8	9	10
Like a chimney, 2 packs per day	At least 1½ packs	At least 1 pack		At least 10 per day	At least 8 per day	At least 6 per day	At least 4 per day	At least 2 per day	Nothing

With my current general health, I can									
1	2	3	4	5	6	7	8	9	10
Recognize people sometimes but can't hear them									Do anything superman or superwoman can do

Fig. 22-5 The Health Factor Review questionaire for patients. (Modified from Cooper,[15] with permission.)

561

HEALTH HAZARD APPRAISAL

I CORONARY HEART DISEASE (CHD) RISK FACTORS

Cholesterol and Triglycerides

CHOLESTEROL less than 160 HDL more than 70 TRIGYLCERIDES less than 60 +2	CHOLESTEROL 160–200 HDL 50–70 TRIGYLCERIDES 60–100 +1	CHOLESTEROL 200–240 HDL 40–50 TRIGYLERIDES 100–140 0	CHOLESTEROL 240–280 HDL 30–40 TRIGYLERIDES 140–180 −1	CHOLESTEROL more than 280 HDL lessthan 30 TRIGYLERIDES more than 180 mg% −3

Blood Pressure: Systolic/Diastolic

110 systolic +1	110–130 50–90 0	130–140 90–100 −2	140–170 100–110 −2	170 more than 110 −4

Smoking

Never used +1	Quit 0	Cigar, pipe, or close family member smokes −1	One pack of cigarettes daily −3	Two or more packs daily −5

Heredity

No family history of CHD +2	One close relative over 60 with CHD 0	Two close relatives over 60 with CHD −1	One close relative under 60 with CHD −2	Two or more close relatives under 60 with CHD −4

Body Weight (or fat)

5 lbs below desirable weight	−5 to +4 lbs desirable weight	5 to 20 lbs overweight	20 to 35 lbs overweight	35 lbs overweight
less than 10% fat— men; less than 16% fat—women +2	10–15% fat—men; 16–22% fat—women +1	15–20% fat—men; 22–30% fat—women 0	20–25% fat—men; 30–36% fat—women −2	25% fat—men; 35% fat—women −3

Sex

Female under 45 years 0	Female over 45 years −1	Male −1	Stocky male −2	Bald, stocky male −4

Stress

Phlegmatic, unhurried, generally happy +1	Ambitious, but generally relaxed 0	Sometimes hard driving, time conscious, competitive −1	Often hard driving, time conscious, competitive −2	Always hard driving, time conscious competitive −3

Fig. 22-6 The Health Hazard Appraisal form. (*Continues.*)

Physical Activity

Intensity—high duration—long 30 frequency—daily	Intermittent. 20–30 minutes, 3–5 times/wk	Moderate 10–20 minutes, 3–5 times/wk	Light. 10–20 minutes, 1–2 times/wk	Little or none
+3	+1	0	−1	−3

TOTAL: I (CHD) RISK FACTORS

II HEALTH HABITS (associated with good health and longevity)

Breakfast

Daily	Sometimes	None	Coffee	Coffee and donut
+1	0	−1	−2	−3

Regular Meals

3 or more	2 daily	Not regular	Fad diets	Starve and stuff
+1	0	−1	−2	−3

Body Weight: Smoking, Physical Activity (previously considered in Part I, CHD)

Sleep

7–8 hours	8–9 hours	6–7 hours	9 hours	under 6 hours
+1	0	0	−1	−2

Alcohol

None	Occasional social	1–2 drinks daily	2–6 drinks daily	6 drinks daily
+1	+1	0	−2	−4

TOTAL: II HEALTH HABITS

III MEDICAL

Medical Exam and Screening Tests (blood pressure, diabetes, glaucoma)

Regular tests, see doctor when necessary	Periodic medical exam and regular tests	Periodic medical exam	Sometimes get tests	No test or medical exams
+1	+1	0	0	−1

Heart

No history—self of family	Some history	Rheumatic fever as child, no murmur now	Rheumatic fever as child, have murmur	Have ECG abnormality and/or angina pectoris
+	0	−1	−2	−3

Fig. 22-6 (*Continued.*)

Lung (including penumonia, TB)

No problem	Some past problem	Mild asthma or bronchitis	Emphysema, severe asthma or bronchitis	Severe lumg problems
+ 1	0	− 1	− 2	− 3

Digestive Tract

No problem	Occasional diarrhea, loss of appetite	Frequent diarrhea or stomach upset	Ulcers, colitis, gallbladder or liver problems	Severe gastrointestinal disorders
	0	− 1	− 2	− 3

Diabetes

No problem or family history	Controlled hypoglycemia (low blood sugar)	Hypoglycemia and family history	Mild diabetes (diet and exercise)	Diabetes (insulin)
+ 1	0	− 1	− 2	− 3

Drugs

Seldom take	Minimal but regularly use aspirin or other drugs	Heavy use of aspirin or other drugs	Regular use of amphetamines, barbiturates or psychogenic drugs	Heavy use of amphetabarbiturates, or psychogenic drugs
+ 1	0	− 1	− 2	− 3

> TOTAL: III MEDICAL

IV SAFETY

Driving in Car

4000 miles per year, mostly local	4000–6000 miles, local and some highway	6000–8000 miles, local and highway	8000–10,000, highway and some local	10,000 miles, mostly highway
+ 1	0	0	− 1	− 2

Using Seat Belts

Always	Most of the time (75%)	On highway	Seldom (25%)	Never
+ 1	0	− 1	− 2	− 3

Risk Taking Behavior (motorcycle, skydive, mountain climb, fly small plane, etc.)

Some with careful preparation	Never	Occasionally	Often	Try anything for thrills
+ 1	0	− 1	− 1	− 2

> TOTAL: IV SAFETY

V PERSONAL

Diet

High complex carbohydrates and low refined sugar	Balanced, moderate fat and refined sugar	Balanced, typical fat and sugar	Fad diets	Starve and stuff
+ 1	0	− 1	− 2	− 3

Fig. 22-6 (*Continued.*)

Longevity

Grandparents lived past 90; parents past 80	Grandparents lived past 80; pastents past 70	Grandparents lived past 70; parents past 60	Few relatives lived past 60	Few relatives lived past 50
+2	+1	−1	−2	−3

Love and Marriage

Happily married	Married	Unmarried	Divorced	Extramarital relationship
+2	+1	−1	−2	−3

Education

Post graduate or master craftsman	College graduate or skilled craftsman	Some college or trade school	High school	Grade school
+1	+1	0	−1	−2

Job Satisfaction

Enjoy job, see results, room for advancement	Enjoy job, see some results, able to advance	Job OK, no results, no where to go	Dislike job	Hate job
+1	+1	0	−1	−2

Social

Have some close friends	Some friends	No good friends	Stuck with people I don't enjoy	No friends at all
+1	0	−1	−2	−3

Race

White or Oriental	Black or Hispanic	American Indian
0	−1	−2

TOTAL: V PERSONAL

VI PSYCHOLOGICAL

Outlook

Feel good about present and future	Satisfied	Unsure about present or future	Unhappy in present, don't look forward to future	Miserable, rather not get out of bed
+1	0	−1	−2	−3

Depression

No family history of depression	Some family history— I feel OK	Family history and I am mildly depressed	Sometimes feel life isn't worth living	Thoughts of suicide
+1	0	−1	−2	−3

Fig. 22-6 (*Continued.*)

Anxiety

Seldom anxious	Occasionally anxious	Often anxious	Always anxious	Everybody hates me
+1	0	−1	−2	−3

Relaxation

Relax or meditate daily	Relax often	Seldom relax	Usually tense	Always tense
+1	0	−1	−2	−3

TOTAL: VI PSYCHOLOGICAL

VII FOR WOMEN ONLY

Health Care

Regular breast and pap exam	Occasional breast pap exam	Never exam	Treated disorder	Untreated cancer
+1	0	−1	−2	−4

The Pill

Never used	Quit 5 years ago	Still use (under 30 years of age)	Use pill and smoke	Use pill, smoke (over 35 years of age)
+1	0	−1	−3	−5

TOTAL: VII FOR WOMEN ONLY

Complete the following pages and then fill in the boxes below.

I (CHD) Risk Factors ☐

II Health Habits ☐

III Medical ☐

IV Safety ☐

V Personal ☐

VI Psychological ☐

VII For Women Only ☐

LIFE EXPECTANCY

Nearest Age	Expectancy
30	74
35	74
40	75
45	76
50	76
55	77
60	78
65	80
70	82

total	life expectancy	longevity estimate	BASED ON CURRENT BEHAVIOR AND HEALTH HABITS
	+	=	

Fig. 22-6 (*Continued.*)

566

BASIC FITNESS APPRAISAL
(continued)

NAME: _____

LEVEL II (Risk Assessment   DATE   DATE   DATE

Age _____
Height _____
Weight _____
Fantasy Weight (subjective) _____
Ideal Weight (objective by formula) _____

Step Test Endurance _____
Bicycle Ergometer Endurance _____
1.5 Mile Run Endurance _____
   (or 12 minute test)

Sit/Reach Flexibility _____
Shoulder Elevation Flexibility _____

Grip Strength (lbs) _____
Sit-Up Strength (Reps/Minute) _____
Bench Press (lbs) _____
Hip Extension (lbs) _____
Orthotron Strength (flex) _____
Orthotron Strength (ext) _____
Standing Jump _____
Medicine Ball Throw _____

50-Yard Dash _____
Agility Drill _____
Hop/Step/Jump _____

Fig. 22-7 The Level II Fitness Assessment Summary form. (Modified from Cooper,[15] with permission.)

needs can easily be completed. The protocols provide a functional mechanism from which to develop measures that meet individual program expectations.

RESOURCES

Resources for the evaluation of cardiovascular health risk or physical therapy program development are available in a variety of forms. There are several excellent textbooks available that provide information essential in the evaluation of and

program planning for clients with cardiovascular disease.[16,17]

The American Heart Association is a valuable resource for information regarding not only evaluation and identification of cardiovascular disease but also guidelines for comprehensive program development. The American Heart Association publishes a specific tool for the assessment of cardiovascular disease called *RISKO*.[18] It is an excellent and easy-to-use tool for gaining the attention of groups regarding their risk for cardiovascular disease. In addition, the Aerobics Center in Dallas has developed comprehensive programs for not only screening, but also remediating people with suspected and known cardiovascular disease.[15]

REFERENCES

1. Acheson RW: The etiology of coronary disease. A review from the epidemiologic standpoint. Yale J Biol Med 35:143, 1962
2. Primary Prevention of Atherosclerotic Diseases. Report of the Intersociety Commission for Heart Disease Resources (abstract). Circulation 42:55, 1970
3. Epstein FH: Coronary heart disease epidemiology. In Stewart GT (ed): Trends in Epidemiology. Charles C Thomas, Springfield, IL, 1972
4. A Guide To and Treatment of Cardiovascular Disease. American Heart Association: Heart Book. EP Dutton, New York, 1980
5. Ross R: The genesis of atherosclerosis. In National Research Council: 1980 Issues and Current Studies. National Academy of Sciences, Washington, D.C., 1981
6. Rabkin SW, Mathewson FAL, Hsu PH: Relation of body weight to development of ischemic heart disease in a cohort of young North American men after a 26-year observation period; the Manitoba study. Am J Cardiol 39:452, 1977
7. Gordon T, Kannel WB: The effects of overweight on cardiovascular disease. Geriatrics 28:80, 1973
8. Friedman M, Rosenman RH: Type A behavior and your heart. Fawcett Publications, Greenwich, CT, 1974
9. Morris JN, Heady JA, Raffle PAB, et al.: Coronary heart disease and physical activity of work. Lancet 2:1053, 1111, 1953
10. Morris JN, Heady J, Raffle PAB: Physique of London busmen: the epidemiology of uniforms. Lancet 2:569, 1956
11. Froelicher VF: Does exercise conditioning delay progression of myocardial ischemia in coronary atherosclerotic disease? In Corday E, Brest A (eds): Controversy in Cardiology. Cardiovascular Clinic Series. Vol. 8. No. 1. FA Davis, Philadelphia, 1977
12. Zukel WJ, Lewis R, Enterline P, et al.: A short-term community study of the epidemiology of coronary heart disease. Am J Public Health 49:1630, 1959
13. Froelicher V, Battler A, McKirnan MD: Physical activity and coronary heart disease. Cardiology 65:153, 1980
14. Froelicher VF, Brown P: Exercise and coronary heart disease. J Cardiac Rehab 1:277, 1981
15. Cooper K: The Aerobics Program for Total Well-Being. M Evans, New York, 1982
16. Pollock ML, Wilmore JH, Fox SM: Exercise in Health and Disease: Evaluation and Prescription for Prevention and Rehabilitation. WB Saunders, Philadelphia, 1984
17. Amsterdam EA, Wilmore JH, DeMaria AN: Exercise in Cardiovascular Health and Disease. Yorke Medical Books, New York, 1977
18. American Heart Association: Heart Facts, 1983. American Heart Association, Dallas, 1982

23 Coronary Artery Disease and Medical Management

Peggy Blake Gleeson

Heart disease represents the leading cause of death in the United States; its mortality rate is twice that of cancer.[1] The incidence of heart pathology has been rising steadily as the age of our population increases; however, the young are no longer felt to be immune. Epstein[2] stated that heart disease "is no longer a 'degenerative' disease of the elderly," and it has been affecting younger individuals in recent years. The most common forms of heart pathology are coronary artery occlusion, and hypertensive heart disease.

CORONARY ARTERY OCCLUSION AND ATHEROSCLEROSIS

Coronary artery disease has become a wastebasket term for a number of pathological conditions, all of which result in an obstruction to the blood flowing though the coronary arteries. Atherosclerosis is the leading cause of coronary disease, accounting for 90 percent of all cases; other causes of coronary disease include thombosis, arteritis, chronic valvular disease, and a variety of infectious diseases.[3]

The atherogenic process begins with trauma to the intimal layer of the artery, caused by mechanical, chemical, or even epidemiological factors (Fig. 23-1). As a result of this trauma, platelet aggregation occurs and a prostaglandin, called thromboxane, is released that stimulates further aggregation. The thromboxane also acts as a vasoconstrictor. Concurrently, the injured layer

itself releases a chemical factor, known as prostacyclin, that opposes the constriction of the blood vessel by retarding platelet aggregation and by dilating the vessel. With minor or only sporadic injuries, the two factors, thromboxane and prostacyclin, equalize each other and healing occurs. With chronic injuries, the ability of the intima to heal itself is compromised. Along with further platelet aggregation, the thromboxane promotes the replication of arterial smooth muscle cells that migrate into the internal elastic lamina. This lamina is responsible for vessel compliance, and these migratory muscle cells constitute the primary cellular component of atherosclerotic plaque. The stability of the growing plaque is further enhanced by the elaboration of collagen and glycoprotein matrices. Excessive amounts of fat and low-density lipoproteins are stored within the cells forming the plaque.[3,4]

Normally, visible signs of sclerosis in the arterial wall do not become evident until nearly 70 percent of the lumen has become obstructed. The first signs that can be seen are a focal thickening of the intima and a "fatty streak," a smooth, yellow lesion composed of lipids. With maturity, this lesion becomes raised, incorporates more collagenous connective tissue, assumes a rigid, scarlike consistency, and may even form cholesterol crystals. Loss of local compliance is one obvious effect, but because the plaques grow with a relatively narrow neck and a weak vascular bed, they can easily break off, becoming thrombi, and block the lumen entirely.[1,3–5]

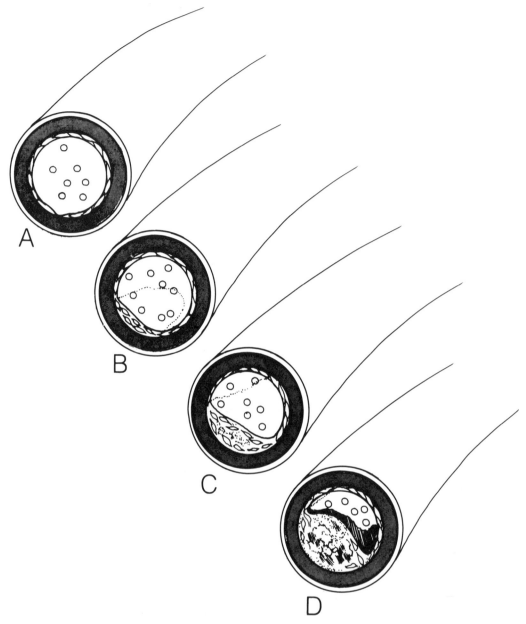

Fig. 23-1 The atherosclerotic process. **(A)** Injury to the arterial wall. **(B)** Lipoproteins invade smooth muscle cells in the intimal wall. **(C)** Fibrous plaque develops. **(D)** The final stage, calcification of the fibrous plaque.

Risk Factors of Atherosclerosis

Age

Age represents the greatest factor in the development of atheromas (plaques). Although there are marked variations in the extent of the disease, plaques have been found in the arteries of children. Kohn[4] stated that "probably all human beings show increasing atherosclerosis with increasing age." Plaques are almost always found in the arteries of young adults; atherosclerosis seems to be the culmination of a lifetime of minitraumas, rather than a few major incidents in an individual's later years.[5] Not only does the accumulation of injuries to the arteries become more evident with age, but a number of the risk factors for atherosclerosis, such as hypertension and elevated serum cholesterol, increase in either incidence or severity with age.

Sex

Although coronary heart disease represents the leading cause of death in women, they do seem to enjoy a relative immunity when compared with men.[6] Men are decidedly more at risk for atherosclerosis and the ischemia it produces. Women's advantage has been associated with every major risk factor.[7] The male and female sex hormones have been suggested as being responsible for the difference. Testosterone may in some way accelerate the development of the disease, whereas estrogen and progesterone may serve as a protective mechanism.[5] The relative immunity of women to coronary heart disease wanes with age, and seems to be lost completely upon menopause. Postmenopausal women are three times more likely to be at risk than are premenopausal women, and the younger the woman is at the time of menopause, the more striking this increase becomes.[7]

Obesity

Overweight must be considered a risk factor, primarily because of its effect on several other risk factors. Obesity is often associated with higher blood pressure, increased serum lipids, and a more sedentary, less active life-style. Furthermore, statistics indicate that the rate of mortality from coronary artery disease in the overweight individual is twice that of the same aged person of normal weight.[8]

Serum Lipids

Elevated serum lipids have long been associated with the development of clinically significant atherosclerosis.[4] The argument arises, however, when trying to determine the relationship between dietary cholesterol and serum cholesterol.

An excessive intake of dietary cholesterol and saturated fat prevails in industrialized countries, such as the United States, where coronary disease is a common cause of death. Roe,[9] among others, believes that hypercholesterolemia results from an excess intake of dietary cholesterol. People living in Southeast Asia, who consume small amounts of fat or cholesterol by American standards, have much lower plasma cholesterol levels.[10]

There are some researchers who dispute the relationship between dietary cholesterol and serum cholesterol. Controlling the ingestion of saturated fats may prove to be more effective in combatting atherosclerosis than limiting dietary cholesterol. Furthermore, regulating the types of food eaten may be less effective in lowering serum cholesterol than maintaining a normal body weight.

In considering the role of serum cholesterol in the development of coronary heart disease, a distinction must be made between the various groups of lipids. There are three major types: (1) high-density lipoproteins (HDL), (2) low-density lipoproteins (LDL), and (3) very low density lipoproteins (VLDL). Under normal circumstances, roughly 17 percent of the cholesterol in plasma from fasting individuals is located in HDL, 70 percent is in LDL, and 13 percent is in VLDL.[11] The concentrations of both HDL and LDL in the plasma are related to the risk of coronary disease; however, with HDL the correlation is a negative one, whereas the correlation is positive between heart disease and LDL. Men with coronary disease have been found to have depressed levels of HDL. Premenopausal women have concentrations of HDL that are 30 to 60 percent higher than those of their male counterparts; this seems to lend credence to the belief that an increase in HDL provides a type of immunity.[12]

Cigarette Smoking

Although the exact mechanism of the effect of smoking on heart disease is not completely understood, the fact that the two are closely related is clear. Shapiro et al.[13] found the incidence of coronary heart disease in men who smoked to be much higher than that in men who didn't smoke. Furthermore, the active nonsmokers had less than one-third the myocardial infarcts compared with the smokers. The risk of smoking is thought to be related primarily to the number of cigarettes smoked each day and may in fact not be related to the duration of the habit.[14] The risk of developing heart disease falls dramatically with termination of the cigarette habit.

Sedentary Life Style

Like obesity, the sedentary life style must also be considered a risk because of its effect on other risk factors. The sedentary individual is more likely to be overweight, to have higher serum cholesterol levels and higher blood pressure and to have fewer outlets for the emotional stresses of a fast-paced competitive world.

Several investigators have demonstrated a reduction in serum cholesterol or triglycerides or both with an increase in physical activity. However, this must be a regular, sustained increase to be effective. Holloszy[15] found that although an exercise program reduced serum triglycerides by 40 percent in middle-aged men, this effect lasted for only 2 days. For this reason, it is believed that only an on-going, continuous conditioning program will provide and maintain this reduction.

Hypertension

Although high blood pressure, or hypertension, is considered one of the primary risk factors in the development of coronary artery disease, it is a major topic in itself. In industrialized societies, the death rate from hypertension is assuredly age related; the rate and probability of dying from high blood pressure doubles at regular intervals with increasing age.[4] Merely because there is a high incidence of hypertension in the elderly, however, does not mean the increase in blood presure can be labeled normal. A substantial number of elderly individuals remain normotensive, and in nonindustrialized societies, many individuals demonstrate no significant correlation between an increase in blood pressure and increasing age.[7,16]

The incidence of hypertension greatly depends on what level is defined as abnormal. The World Health Organization defines hypertension as a supine systolic pressure of 160 mm Hg or greater, or a supine diastolic pressure of 95 mm Hg or greater. Although the diastolic pressure has gen-

erally been felt to be the major determinant of cardiovascular risk, it has become apparent that systolic pressure can be an important predictor variable.[17]

Coronary artery disease has been found to be a common sequela of hypertension. Edington and Edgerton[18] wrote that "at an advanced stage of the disease, it is hard to separate the vascular pathology and clinical manifestations due to the elevation of the blood pressure from those due to the basic atherosclerotic process."

Hypertension can have deleterious effects on both the heart and the arteries themselves (Fig. 23-2). The increase in workload that hypertension causes results in hypertrophy of the cardiac muscle; the left ventricle may double or even triple in weight. Because the coronary blood supply does not increase at an equal rate, a relative ischemia develops and the patient may experience angina. Not only does the increased pressure cause coronary sclerosis, but arteriosclerosis has been demonstrated in all areas of the body. Thrombosis and subsequent rupture of the blood vessels have very serious consequences if they develop in a cerebral vessel, causing hemorrhage and local tissue death, or in a renal blood vessel where kidney damage would ensue.[5]

Hypertension has been divided into two categories: primary, or essential; and secondary.

Essential Hypertension

Making up approximately 90 percent of all cases, essential hypertension is of unknown etiology. Both the kidneys and the adrenal cortex have a regulating effect on blood pressure and are

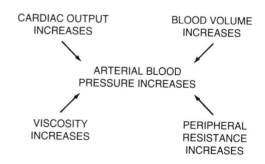

Fig. 23-2 Factors that affect arterial blood pressure.

thought to be involved in the development of this form of hypertension. Heredity seems to play a predominant role. Essential hypertension is characterized by a gradual onset and develops into a chronic condition of many years duration.[1]

Secondary Hypertension

Secondary hypertension can normally be linked with a specific lesion, such as chronic nephritis or an adrenal tumor. The hypertension that often results from the narrowing that occurs in the arteries of the aging population can also be included in this category; however, which is cause and which is effect remains unclear.[1]

PATHOLOGICAL CHANGES ASSOCIATED WITH ISCHEMIA

There are a number of ways in which the heart responds to the ischemia, or lack of blood, that results from coronary artery occlusion. When cardiac tissue is deprived of a sufficient amount of oxygen, the myocardial cells must shift from aerobic metabolism to anaerobic metabolism. Lactic acid, which is a by-product of anaerobic metabolism, accumulates in the tissues, causing a reduction of cellular pH. This resultant acidosis, together with the hypoxia, impairs left ventricular function. Because the contractions of the ventricle are no longer strong enough to completely empty the ventricle, pressure in the ventricle builds up; both blood pressure and heart rate become mildly elevated. The pain that is often experienced during the ischemic attack is termed angina and is characteristically felt as a radiating pressure in either the chest or left arm, although it has been experienced in other areas of the upper body as well. The exact cause of angina has not yet been determined; the accumulation of lactic acid or the mechanical stress that results from abnormal contractions are possible explanations.[19]

Typically, an ischemic attack will subside within minutes if the imbalance of oxygen is corrected. If the tissues do receive adequate oxygen, all of the above changes are reversible. However, if the ischemia is prolonged, an infarction occurs, and

irreversible cell damage and myocardial muscle death result.[19]

After a myocardial infarction (MI), the response of the cardiovascular system can be divided into three distinct stages.

Acute Stage

During the acute stage of an MI, there is a permanent loss of contractile function in the necrotic region (Fig. 23-3). The muscle appears cyanotic, and cellular edema as well as leukocytic infiltration can be noted within 24 hours. Cardiac output is reduced, and there is an increased systemic venous pressure. The cardiac output may still be sufficient to sustain life, but virtually no physical activity, even standing or sitting, can be tolerated. The stroke volume as well as the contractility of the ventricle are reduced. Fortunately, this phase is followed, within seconds in some cases, by the second stage, that of early compensation.[5,19,20]

Second Stage

During the second stage after an MI, the sympathetic nervous system becomes strongly stimulated and the parasympathetic nervous system is inhibited. This sympathetic response results in an increase in mean systemic blood pressure to almost 100 percent above normal; together these two occurrences are often able to raise the cardiac output to a normal level.[5] By the second or third day postinfarction, tissue degradation and removal of the necrotic fibers can be noted. Scar tissue, made of fibrous connective tissue, gradually re-

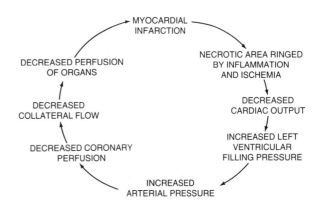

Fig. 23-3 The vicious cycle of myocardial infarctions.

places the damaged muscle. Scar formation begins around the third week postinfarction and is fairly strong by 6 weeks.[19]

Chronic Compensatory Stage

Chronic compensation is the final stage and is characterized by the retention of fluid. Renal function is directly affected by cardiac function, and in the presence of a drop in cardiac output, urinary output also falls. This reduction in renal output is a result of a reduction of glomerular pressure in the kidneys, and an increase in the secretion of aldosterone, which causes an additional amount of sodium to be absorbed by the renal tubules. Retention of fluid causes an increase in the venous return to the heart secondary to an increase in the pressure gradient of the blood flow.[5,20]

THERAPEUTIC DRUGS AND THEIR EFFECTS

There are a variety of medications that may be administered to the patient with coronary artery disease. A thorough understanding of how each medication affects the patient's response to exercise is crucial if the optimum benefits are to result from the rehabilitative efforts. The drugs most commonly used in the treatment of the patient with coronary disease are discussed, along with information on how these drugs may influence exercise response.[3,21–25]

Digitalis Series (Digitalis, Digoxin, Lanoxin)

Administered to treat congestive heart failure or atrial arrhythmias, this group of drugs increases contractility of the heart. Each heart beat is strengthened, resulting in a larger stroke volume and an increased cardiac output. Slowing of the heart occurs because of an increase in vagal tone. Ischemic ST changes may be accentuated, that is, there may be an increase in ST-segment depression either during or after exercise. People with normal coronary arteries may show exercise-induced ST-segment depression.

Cardiac Depressants (Lidocaine, Procainamide Hydrochloride, Quinidine)

Cardiac depressants control arrhythmias by preferentially depressing ectopic foci and by reducing excitability, conductivity, and automatic rhythmicity of the myocardium. Administered to treat both atrial and ventricular arrhythmias, including atrial premature beats, atrial flutter and fibrillation, paroxysmal tachycardia, and ventricular tachycardia, they can prevent ventricular fibrillation but cannot ordinarily be given in time to reverse it. (Electrical defibrillation is used for this purpose.)

Anticholinergics (Atropine)

Small doses of atropine slow the heart rate slightly and larger doses accelerate it markedly. There may be local vasodilation that causes flushing of the face, but blood pressure is normally not affected; however, the hypertension caused by cholinergic drugs can be prevented by administering an anticholinergic medication. These drugs are used to prevent or to counteract reflex bradycardia caused by excessive vagal tone, as in the carotid sinus syndrome and in certain types of heart block. There is often a loss of the patient's ability to sweat with these drugs, and this may affect heat elimination and, consequently, cause a decrease in exercise capacity.

Coronary Vasodilators (Nitroglycerine)

Coronary vasodilators primarily act on the smooth muscle walls of the heart. They are used to treat angina; by dilating the blood vessels, more blood and therefore more oxygen is able to reach the heart. In this manner, vasodilators may increase the patient's exercise tolerance.

Anticoagulants (Heparin, Dicumarol, Coumadin)

Anticoagulants are used to prolong the time required for the blood to coagulate by inactivating molecules of thrombin that may form. Heparin promotes the breakdown of newly formed clots by preventing blood platelets from sticking together, and also inactivates thromboplastin. Coumarin (sodium warfarin) and dicumarol lengthen the clotting time of the blood by competing with vitamin K for a place on the surface of an enzyme required for the synthesis of prothrombin and related clotting factors.

Diuretics (Diuril, Lasix, Aldactone)

In congestive heart failure, the blood flow may stimulate secretion of the adrenal cortical hormone aldosterone, a substance that acts on certain renal tubular cells to make them reabsorb sodium from the glomerular filtrate. This, in turn, stimulates the release of another hormone that aids in the reabsorption of water by the cells. A diuretic helps to break this cycle. Diuril (chlorothiazide) and Lasix (furosemide) remove sodium and chloride ions in equal amounts, and as a result, salt and water are removed from edematous tissues and excreted in the urine. Aldactone (spironolactone) acts by blocking the effects of the adrenal hormone on the cells of the kidney tubules.

Antihypertensives (Methyldopa, Reserpine, Aldomet)

Antihypertensive drugs are used primarily to treat mild-to-severe essential hypertension (about 90 percent of all cases of hypertension). However, they can also be used to control hypertension in the 10 percent of patients who have secondary hypertension. Antihypertensives act to reduce the number of nerve impulses passing out of the central nervous system and over sympathetic efferent pathways to the circulatory system. Some act directly on the vasomotor center; others act indirectly as a result of their primary peripheral effects. They also relax the blood vessels and bring about vasodilation by a depressant effect directly on the vascular smooth muscle walls.

Adrenergics-Vasopressors (Epinephrine, Dopamine Hydrochloride, Isoproterenol)

Adrenergics-vasopressors act by mimicking the actions of epinephrine or norepinephrine in the sympathetic nervous system on the receptor sites.

The three major types of receptors within the sympathetic nervous system are alpha, beta, and dopaminergic. Stimulation of the alpha receptors causes vasoconstriction; stimulation of the beta receptors will either increase the rate and force of myocardial contraction and the rate of atrioventricular node conduction, or produce bronchodilation and vasodilation of the blood vessels, depending on which beta receptors are stimulated. Stimulation of the dopaminergic receptors results in dilation of the splanchnic blood vessels.

Beta-Adrenergic Blocking Agents (Lopressor, Corgard, Propranolol Hydrochloride)

The beta-adrenergic blocking agents are used for a variety of conditions and include some of the medications listed in the categories already discussed. These drugs are administered in the treatment of hypertension, angina, cardiac arrhythmias, and hypertrophic subaortic stenosis. They have an affect on almost all of the parameters of the cardiovascular system. β-blockers, as they are often called, produce a decrease in heart rate, a reduction of cardiac output, a decrease in the resting stroke volume, a decrease in oxygen consumption, and an elevation of the left ventricular and diastolic blood pressures. These drugs are often used in long-term prophylaxis to prevent future MIs; by lessening the force of the heart's contraction, the heart does not have to work as hard. When patients who are taking a β-blocker participate in a cardiac rehabilitation program, their target heart rate must be lowered to compensate for the lowered maximal heart rate resulting from the effects of the drugs. These medications allow the patient with coronary heart disease to exercise longer and develop less ischemic ST-segment responses during exercise. They may cause false-negative responses for the exercise stress test. Because β-blockers may prevent the patient from reaching his maximal heart rate, a conventional endpoint to exercise, that of target heart rate, is impractical.

Calcium Blockers (Isoptin, Procardia, Adalat)

Relatively new in the treatment of cardiovascular disease, calcium blockers block the transport of calcium ions across the cell membrane in both the myocardium and vascular smooth muscle, preventing the heart from contracting too forcefully. Secondarily, calcium blockers act as a vasodilator, decreasing resistance to the flow of blood.

REFERENCES

1. Boyd W: An Introduction to the Study of Disease. p. 284. 6th Ed. Lea & Febiger, Philadelphia, 1971
2. Epstein FH: Coronary heart disease epidemiology. In Stewart GT (ed): Trends in Epidemiology. p. 181. Charles C Thomas, Springfield, IL. 1972
3. Kern LS, Gawlinski A: Stage managing coronary artery disease. Nursing 83 13(4):34, 1983
4. Kohn RR: Heart and cardiovascular system. p. 281. In Finch CE, Hayflick L (eds): Handbook of the Biology of Aging. Van Nostrand Reinhold, New York, 1977
5. Guyton AC: Textbook of Medical Physiology. pp. 316, 372, and 960. WB Saunders, Philadelphia, 1976
6. Kannel WB, Castelli WP: The Framingham study of coronary disease in women. Med Times 100:173, 1972
7. Kannel WB: Status of coronary heart disease risk factors. J Nutr Ed 10:10, 1978
8. Schottelius BA, Schottelius DD: Textbook of Physiology p. 1259. 17th Ed. CV Mosby, St. Louis, 1973
9. Roe DA: Clinical Nutrition for the Health Scientist. p. 9 CRC Press, Boca Raton, BL, 1979
10. Hodges RE: Nutrition in Medical Practice. p. 92. WB Saunders, Philadelphia, 1980
11. Lancet (editorial): July 2:131, 1976
12. Levy RI, Blum CB, Schaeffer EJ, p. 59 cited in Greten H (ed): Lipoprotein Metabolism. Berlin, 1976
13. Shapiro S, Weinblatt E, Frank CW, Sager R: Incidence of coronary heart disease in a population insured for medical care (HIP). Am J Public Health, suppl., 59:1, 1969
14. Hammond EC, cited in Kannel WB: Status of coronary heart disease risk factors. J Nutr Ed 10:10, 1978
15. Holloszy JO: Biochemical adaptations in muscle. Effects of exercise on mitochondrial oxygen uptake and respiratory enzyme activity in skeletal muscle. J Biol Chem 242:2278, 1967
16. Reed G, Anderson GR: Epidemiology and risk of hypertension in the elderly. Clin Ther special issue, 5:9, 1982
17. Shekelle RB, Ostfeld AM, Klawans HL, cited in Reed G, Anderson GR: Epidemiology and risk of hypertension in the elderly. Clin Ther special issue, 5:9, 1982
18. Edington DW, Edgerton VR: The Biology of Physical Activity. p. 473. Houghton Mifflin, Boston, 1975
19. Ford PJ: Cardiovascular pathophysiology. p. 390. In Price SA, Wilson LM (eds): Pathophysiology. 2nd Ed. McGraw-Hill, New York, 1978
20. Selkurt EE: Pathological physiology of the cardiovascular system. B. Congestive heart failure. p. 401. In Selkurt EE (ed): Physiology. 3rd Ed. Little, Brown, Boston, 1971
21. Brooks SM (ed): Nurses' Drug Reference. p. 230. Little, Brown, Boston, 1978
22. Ellestad MH: Stress Testing Principles and Practice. p. 251. FA Davis, Philadelphia, 1972
23. Govoni LE, Hayes JE: Drugs and Nursing Implications 27, 240. Merideth Publishing, New York, 1971
24. Grollman A: Pharmacology and Therapeutics Part 4, p. 460. Lea & Febiger, Philadelphia, 1962
25. Tjeng LH, Cardus D: Electrocardiogram monitoring during exercise and factors influencing its interpretation. p. 221. In Blocker WR, Cardus D (eds): Rehabilitation in Ischemic Heart Disease. SP Medical & Scientific Books, New York, 1983

24 Cardiac Rehabilitation during the Acute Phase of Recovery

Elizabeth J. Protas

Cardiac rehabilitation is primarily for individuals with coronary artery disease that results in myocardial infarction, angina pectoris, or cardiac surgery. The goal of the rehabilitative programs is to return the patient to a maximum level of function. Reaching this goal generally requires the efforts of multiple disciplines in working with the patient. Physicians, nurses, psychologists, exercise physiologists, and physical therapists all have a role to play in contributing to the patient's recovery. Cardiac rehabilitation is relatively new compared with some other areas of rehabilitation, having been a distinct health service area for only the last twenty years.

PURPOSE

The purpose of cardiac rehabilitation will change somewhat as the patient proceeds through a rehabilitative program. During the early stages, the emphasis is on patient education and determining whether or not the patient is sufficiently stable to resume ordinary daily activities. As recovery proceeds, the focus shifts to introducing longer-term behavioral changes. Life-style modifications such as smoking cessation, weight reduction, regular exercise, and stress reduction are encouraged for the patients and their families. Even though coronary artery disease is considered a progressive disease, rehabilitation is intended to ensure that the disease is managed and that the patient leads as high a quality of life as possible.

PHASES OF REHABILITATION

There are three distinct phases to cardiac rehabilitation, phases I, II, and III. This chapter describes exercise management associated with phase I for the patient with a myocardial infarction (MI). Chapter 25 discusses special concerns relating to the management of the patient after cardiac surgery. Chapter 26 discusses phase II and III outpatient cardiac rehabilitation programs.

Phase I

Phase I involves the acute stage of recovery and the associated period of hospitalization. The average length of hospital stay for an individual with an uncomplicated MI is 8 days, although this may vary in different regions of the country.[1,2] Complications, depending on their severity, can result in additional hospitalization.[3]

Patients should be observed for adverse signs and symptoms and complications during this period. Arrhythmias, congestive heart failure, and infarct extension can occur at this time. Close supervision of activities of daily living and ambulation ensure that the patient is not showing adverse signs to activity. Since patients frequently begin their rehabilitation program the second or third day after admission, a return to activity lessens the likelihood that the patient will become deconditioned during hospitalization.

An intense effort is also begun to educate the patient about the disease and factors that contribute to the progression of the disease. The patient frequently needs to know that a return to a normal life-style is not only possible after an MI, but quite common. Emphasis is placed on understanding and managing the disease.

Phase II

Phase II begins at the immediate postdischarge period and involves supervised exercise conditioning programs and continued efforts to assist the patient in life-style modification. Phase II programs are generally 8 to 12 weeks long; however, some programs may not begin until 2 to 6 weeks after discharge.[4] Patients are often given a home program to follow during the intervening weeks.

Phase III

Phase III is often referred to as community-based programs. After the patient successfully finishes phase II under medical supervision, he can be referred to an exercise and activity program such as those sponsored by the YMCA. The goals during this phase are to continue to improve functional and exercise capacity and to reinforce the changes that the patient has achieved.[5]

PHASE I—MYOCARDIAL INFARCTION

Symptoms

Awareness of a number of signs and symptoms that occur with an MI is important to the clinician who is supervising phase I activities. This information can be gathered by a careful chart review.

The symptom that most frequently brings patients to the emergency room is chest pain. The pain that accompanies an MI is a crushing, substernal chest pain that may persist for hours. Sweating, nausea, and severe anxiety occur with the chest pain. The pain may also radiate to the neck, back, jaw, shoulder, or down either arm. There are often no factors that precipitate the pain, and nitrate medications do not relieve the discomfort. Although these features seem quite specific, it is difficult to distinguish between MI pain and stable or unstable angina or even an anxiety attack. Since pain may be a complaint during rehabilitation, it is important to know some

characteristic differences.[6] Table 24-1 lists a comparison of the symptoms occurring with chest pain.

Electrocardiographic Changes

A number of characteristic changes occur on the electrocardiogram (ECG) after an MI.[7] A shift in the position of the ST segment is the first ECG change seen, and frequently the first to return to normal (Fig. 24-1). A depressed ST segment is common with angina pectoris, coronary insufficiency, subendocardial MI, digitalis toxicity, and during a positive graded exercise test (GXT). The ST-segment depression can be upsloping, horizontal, or downsloping. An elevated ST segment is seen with transmural and subepicardial MI, pericarditis, and, when persistent, ventricular aneurysm. Another change that occurs is an inverted T wave. This inversion will evolve during the first day or two after the MI and will revert to normal within a few days (Fig. 24-1). Finally, a Q wave appears. This change is permanent and will persist on the ECG as evidence of a previous MI (Fig. 24-1).

Where these changes appear in a twelve-lead ECG is useful in determining where the MI occurred. A chart review should provide information on the location of the infarct. If the patient is having an angina episode rather than an MI, the depressed ST segment will return to baseline quickly, and this change will not be associated with a Q wave.

Laboratory Findings

Laboratory tests will provide information on serum enzymes. There are three main enzymes that will show elevated levels when damage occurs in myocardial, liver, and skeletal muscle tissues. Elevation of serum enzymes caused by damaged myocardial cells can aid in the diagnosis of an MI.[6,7] Further analysis of isoenzymes provides patterns of elevation that are specific to one organ. Table 24-2 gives a description of the changes in these enzymes seen with an MI.

Differential Diagnosis

When the patient is first seen, he may have a decreased resting blood pressure and heart rate as a result of medications. If arrhythmias are

Table 24-1 Comparison of Chest Pain Symptoms

Symptom	Anxiety	Stable Angina	Unstable Angina	Myocardial Infarction
Duration	<1 min to several hours	Subsides gradually in 1 to 5 min	Subsides gradually, but lasts >4–5 min	May persist for hours
Radiation	None	Shoulder, neck, jaw, either or both arms, particularly the left, epigastrum	Similar to stable angina	Similar to stable angina as well as across chest to back
Quality	Sharp and stabbing or dull discomfort	Pressure or heavy discomfort, burning, choking, squeezing	Similar, but more intense	Crushing, accompanied by sweating, nausea, and anxiety
Preceding factors	Tiredness, emotion, often none	Exertion, stress, meals, smoking, cold weather, emotion	May occur at rest, often none	Often none
Pain relief	Lying down, sedation	Rest, sublingual nitrates relieve in 1–1.5 min	Incomplete or temporary relief	No relief with nitrates, narcotics for relief
ECG	Normal	Transient ST depression, which disappears with pain relief	Long-lasting ST depression and T wave inversion	T wave inversion, ST deviation, Q waves

present, these may be palpated as an irregular pulse. A fourth heart sound (S_4) can be auscultated. With the complication of congestive heart failure, the patient often displays tachycardia and hypotension with pulmonary rales and a third heart sound (S_3) on auscultation.[6,7]

An early task in the course of treatment is to determine whether the patient has experienced an MI or has angina pectoris. The diagnosis of an MI is generally made on the second day of hospitalization.

Arrhythmias and Arrhythmia Recognition

Normal Sinus Rhythm
Normal sinus rhythm is characterized by a resting rate of 60 to 80 beats/minute, a regular rhythm, and each wave equidistant from the next (e.g., each R wave is equidistant from the R waves on either side) (Fig. 24-2). Arrhythmias are deviations from this basic pattern, which is generated by the sinus node.

Atrial Arrhythmias
Atrial rhythms can be detected as variations in the P wave, which represents depolarization of the atrium. A premature atrial contraction (PAC) would occur earlier than expected and would have a P wave that is shaped differently than the sinus-generated P wave (Fig. 24-3). The P wave is shaped differently because the depolarization is stimulated from an ectopic area in the atrium. Atrial flutter represents multiple atrial firings before a ventricular depolarization. This is evident on the ECG tracing as multiple, equally shaped P waves and an irregular rhythm. Atrial fibrillation, on the other hand, is the firing of numerous ectopic areas in the atrium. This produces a wavy baseline with no distinct P waves between the QRS complexes, and an irregular rhythm (Fig. 24-4).

Nodal Rhythms
Nodal rhythms get their name from depolarizations that are stimulated by firing of the AV node. Since the AV node is situated between the atria

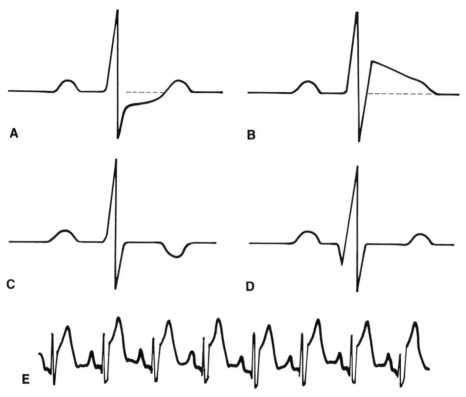

Fig. 24-1 Characteristic ECG changes in myocardial infarction. **(A)** Depressed ST segment. **(B)** Elevated ST segment. **(C)** Inverted T wave. **(D)** Q wave. **(E)** Rhythm strip demonstrating elevated ST segment and Q wave.

and ventricles in the heart's special conduction system, a beat stimulated by the AV node would not be preceded by a P wave. This firing would stimulate a ventricular depolarization, but not an atrial depolarization. Similar to atrial rhythms, a premature nodal beat would occur earlier than expected and an escape beat follows a pause. Neither beat would have a P wave, and each can be felt in the pulse as an irregular rhythm (Fig. 24-5).

Supraventricular Rhythms

Sometimes when the heart rate is rapid, it is difficult to distinguish between atrial and nodal beats. Rapid, irregular rhythms with regularly shaped QRS complexes are often referred to as supraventricular arrhythmias.

Ventricular Arrhythmias

Ventricular rhythms are beats that originate directly in ventricular muscle rather than being stimulated through the normal conduction system. These depolarizations appear on the ECG as un-

usually large, wide QRS complexes because they are being conducted through the muscle tissue (Fig. 24-6) and muscle is a slower conductor than the specialized conduction system.

Premature Ventricular Contractions. The ventricular contractions that are stimulated by ectopic ventricular depolarizations produce a poor cardiac output because of the slow coordination of the electrical with the mechanical contractile event. As a result, ventricular beats are difficult to palpate when taking the pulse and will feel like skipped beats. These can occur either prematurely, and are called premature ventricular contractions or PVCs, or as escape beats. PVCs can occur singly or in a variety of patterns.

1. Coupling. When PVCs fire in a regular pattern along with normal beats, this is called coupling. The coupling of the PVC can occur every second beat, known as bigeminy, every third beat (trigeminy), or every fourth beat (quadrigeminy) (Fig. 24-6).

Table 24-2 Enzymes in Myocardial Infarction

Enzyme	Normal Value	Elevation after MI	Peak	Return to Normal
CPK (Creatine phosphokinase) CPK-MD (isoenzyme for cardiac muscle)	Men: to 100 mU/ml Women: to 50 mU/ml	2–5 hours	First 24 hours 5–15 times normal	Day 2 to 3
SGOT (Serum glutamic oxaloacetic transaminase)	10–50 mU/ml	6–8 hours	24–48 hours 2–15 times normal	Day 4 to 8
LDH (lactic dehydrogenase) LDH1 (heart enzyme) LDH5 (liver enzyme)	Serum: 90–200 mU/ml Isoenzymes: LDH1: 20.0–34.0%	6–12 hours	48–72 hours 2–8 times normal	Day 7 to 10, may stay elevated for 10 days to 2 weeks
HBDH (hydroxybutyric dehydrogenase)	175–325 IU/L, indirect measure of cardiac LDH isoenzymes	12 hours	48–72 hours	1–3 weeks

Note: SGPT (serum glutamic pyruvic transaminase) will be elevated if enzyme elevation is due to liver rather than heart disease.

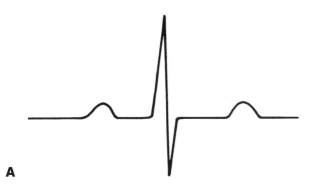

A

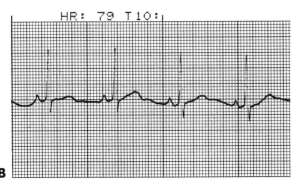

B

Fig. 24-2 Normal sinus rhythm. Each P–QRS–T complex looks the same with each wave equidistant. The rhythm is regular. **(A,B)**

2. Irregular PVCs. PVCs can also fire on an irregular basis. This can be felt as a very irregular pulse. PVCs emanating from a single, irritable ventricular area will have the same shape and appearance. PVCs that are occurring from multiple areas will have different shapes and appearances. Four or more PVCs in a row are termed ventricular tachycardia, since it is a fast ventricular rate (Fig. 24-7).

Some irregular PVCs are considered to be particularly dangerous because of their poor cardiac output.[7] These are:

A PVC that occurs more frequently than 1 in 10 beats
Three or more PVCs in a row
Ventricular tachycardia
Multifocal PVCs
PVC landing near a T wave

Several rapid and particularly malignant ventricular arrhythmias should also be mentioned.

1. Ventricular flutter. Ventricular flutter is a regular, rapid series (200 to 300/min) of ventricular depolarizations that looks like a sine wave pattern (Fig. 24-8). It is relatively

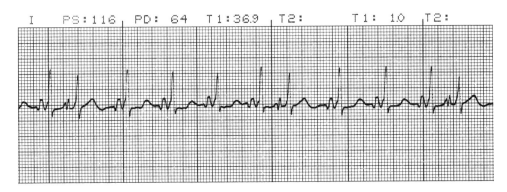

Fig. 24-3 Premature atrial contraction. The P–QRS–T complex is early with a different shaped P wave. The rhythm is irregular.

rare since it rapidly degenerates into a pattern of ventricular fibrillation.

2. Ventricular fibrillation. Ventricular fibrillation is extremely irregular with no discernable pattern. It is the result of multiple ectopic firings throughout the ventricles. There is no cardiac output and no pulse. This is a cardiac arrest and is a highly serious situation (Fig. 24-8).

Heart Blocks
Interference with a pulse conduction that occurs anywhere along the heart's conduction system is a heart block.

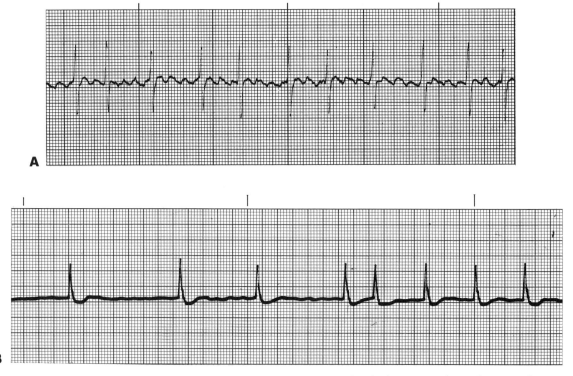

Fig. 24-4 (A) Atrial flutter. Multiple, similar P waves are seen. The rhythm is irregular with an atrial rate of 250–350/minute. **(B)** Atrial fibrillation. The baseline is wavy with no distinct P waves. The rhythm is irregular.

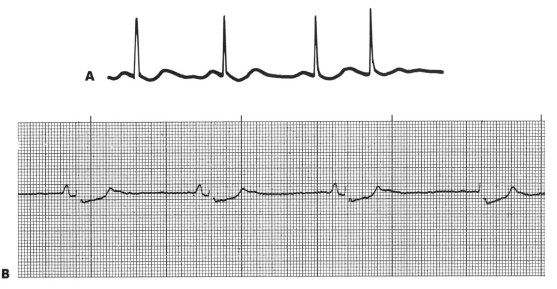

Fig. 24-5 (A) (AV) nodal premature. The QRS–T complex is early with no preceding P wave. The rhythm is irregular. This is rarely seen. **(B)** (AV) nodal escape beat. The QRS–T complex is preceded by a pause with no P wave present. The rhythm is irregular.

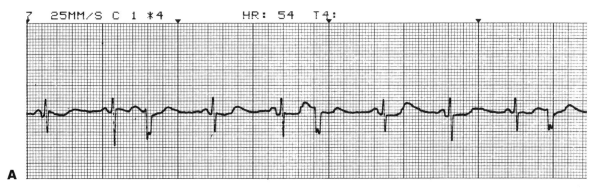

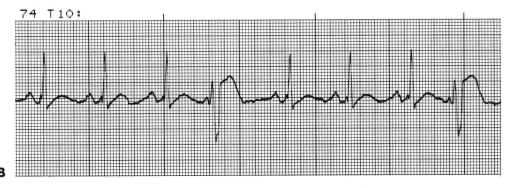

Fig. 24-6 (A) Premature ventricular contraction (PVC). The QRS complex is large and wide and occurs early. No P wave is present. **(B)** Quadrigeminy. A PVC occurs every fourth beat.

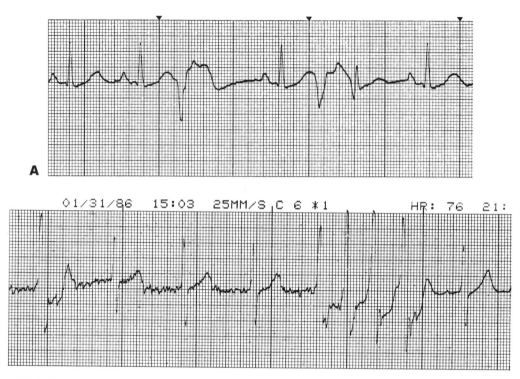

Fig. 24-7 (A) Multifocal premature ventricular contractions. The QRS complex is large and wide with different shaped PVCs. The rhythm is very irregular. (B) Ventricular tachycardia. PVCs occur four or more in a row. The rhythm is very irregular.

SA Block. A block at the sinus node, or SA block, results in a missed P-QRS-T cycle followed by a resumption of the sinus pattern (Fig. 24-9).

AV Blocks. An AV block slows the conduction of an impulse through the AV node. This will effect the P–R interval on the ECG. There are first, second, and third degree AV blocks.

1. First degree AV blocks. A first degree AV block will appear as a lengthened P–R interval (Fig. 24-9). This interval is normally less than 0.2 seconds long from the beginning of the P wave to the beginning of the upsweep of the R wave. On standard ECG recording paper, this would be the time covered in one large square.
2. Second degree AV blocks. There are several types of second degree AV blocks (Fig. 24-10). One type is seen in which there are multiple P waves to every QRS complex. Another pattern will display a progressively

lengthening P–R interval until finally a QRS complex is completely dropped. This is called a Mobitz I pattern. The other pattern, a Mobitz II pattern, will drop a QRS complex without a lengthened P–R interval.
3. Third degree AV blocks. A third degree block means that no impulses are passed through the AV node, which results in a slow rate. There is also no relationship between the atrial and ventricular patterns, that is, P waves are not related to the QRS complexes in any way (Fig. 24-11). A permanent pacemaker is generally implanted in instances of third degree heart block.

Bundle Branch Blocks. A bundle branch block is a slowing of conduction through either the right or left bundle branches of the ventricular portion of the conduction system. This slows the depolarization of one ventricle versus the other and shows as two R waves on the ECG (Fig. 24-11). In other

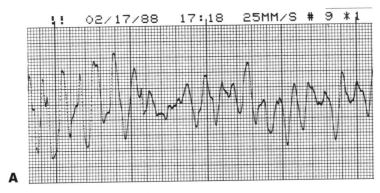

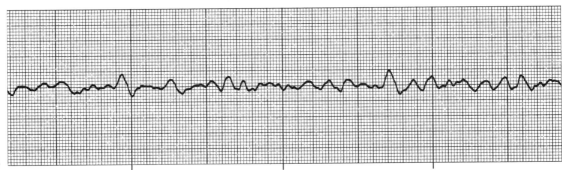

Fig. 24-8 (A) Ventricular flutter. The pattern is of a sine wave with a rate of 200–300/minute. **(B)** Ventricular fibrillation. No distinct waveforms are present, and the appearance is erratic. No pulse is present.

words, the ventricular depolarization is out of phase, and a wide QRS complex will also be evident.

Medications

Several medications have an influence on ECG patterns that the clinician should be able to identify. Many patients will be on β-blocking medications. These drugs will reduce the resting heart rate and blood pressure, as well as mute the heart rate response to exercise.[8] In other words, a lower heart rate and blood pressure will result from a standard exercise than if the patient were not on β-blocking drugs. Digitalis toxicity will cause an upsloping ST interval on the ECG (Fig. 24-12).[9]

PHASE I REHABILITATION PROGRAM

Most phase I programs use a combination of self-care, range-of-motion (ROM) exercises, ambulation, and other exercises such as cycle ergometry to enable the patient to progress from bedrest in intensive care to sufficient daily activity for discharge some 7 or 8 days later.[4,5,10–12] Careful monitoring and observation of the patient during these activities ensures that the patient is not experiencing any adverse reactions such as arrhythmias. Most activities used during this period are considered to be low intensity and are not intended to stress the patient as the myocardium heals.

Immediately Post-MI

The patient's self-care is frequently monitored by the nursing staff during the early days of hospitalization. The patient is generally allowed to perform his morning care and to feed himself if he is stable on the first day in the coronary care unit. By day 2 the patient is allowed to be up in the chair at bedside several times a day and to use the bedside commode. If the patient is progressing without incident, limited bathing and walking to

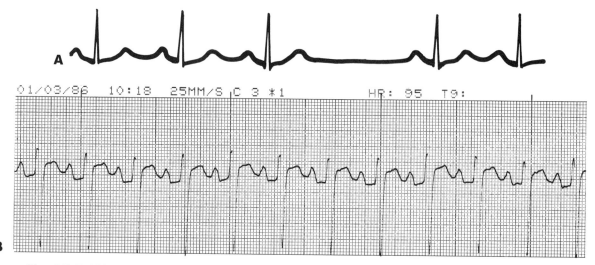

Fig. 24-9 (A) SA block. After a missing P–QRS–T complex, the sinus pattern resumes. This is rarely seen. **(B)** 1° AV block. The PR interval is greater than 0.2 seconds.

the bathroom and the chair in the room are encouraged. After the patient has been monitored once during the self-care activity, he will continue to perform the activity on his own. In an uncomplicated case, this can occur in the third or fourth day of hospitalization.

Some programs include ROM exercises during the first few days. These consist of supine or sitting, active ankle, knee, hip, and shoulder ROM activities. These activities are very low intensity and will enhance circulation, particularly in the lower extremities.[13] After the physical therapist ensures that the patient is not having adverse responses during the activities, the patient can continue these activities unsupervised.

Ambulation

Early ambulation during recovery from an MI has been found to be a safe, low-intensity exercise. For the uncomplicated patient, supervised, monitored ambulation can begin as early as day 4. The physical therapist generally uses the hallway outside of the patient's room to have enough distance for the patient to walk. The patient's ECG should be observed by using telemetry. The therapist should take the patient's blood pressure before and during the walk. The initial walks can be either according to distance, for example, 100 yards, or according to time, for instance, 3 to 5 minutes. The patient's responses to ambulation

can be used to assess whether the patient progress to increased time or distance. Most patients can be ambulating for as long as 15 to 30 minutes before discharge.[10] Ambulation is an activity that is very well tolerated by most patients during the acute recovery phase. This activity should produce an increase in heart rate of less than 10 beats from resting levels and only a slight increase of less than 10 mm HG in systolic blood pressure. Before discharge, patients should also be monitored while walking up and down a flight of stairs.

ROM Exercises

A number of programs also include in their phase I regimen a series of sitting and standing upper and lower extremity ROM exercises.[4] Although these exercises are primarily geared toward overall joint ROM, they can add variety and be a useful adjunct during recovery. These are also well tolerated by most patients and can be incorporated as a warm-up activity before ambulation.

Later Stage

Patients can be brought to the physical therapy department to exercise during the later stage of their phase I program. In this way, exercise with bicycle ergometers and treadmill walking can be introduced. This provides variety to the exercise program, and it is relatively easy to monitor the ECG while the patient is on either the bicycle or

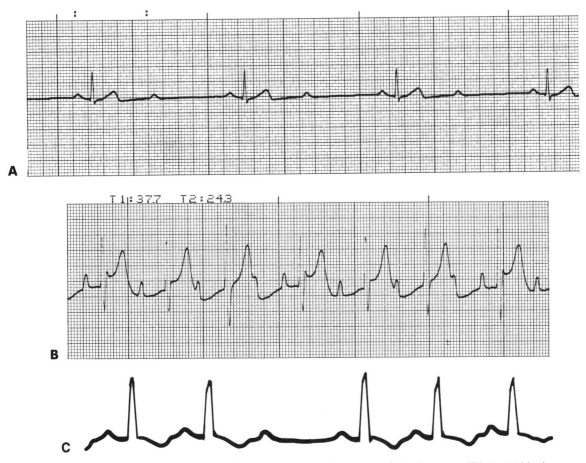

Fig. 24-10 (A) 2° AV block. For each QRS complex, there are multiple P waves. **(B)** 2° AV block—Mobitz I. The PR interval progressively lengthens until the QRS complex is dropped. **(C)** 2° AV block—Mobitz II. The PR interval is within normal limits, but the QRS complex is dropped. This is rarely seen.

treadmill (Fig. 24-13). An additional advantage to the use of either a bike or treadmill is that it is easier to standardize the energy costs of the exercise. For example, by controlling the speed and elevation of the treadmill, the metabolic equivalent (MET) level is known (Table 24-3). In a similar fashion, the approximate MET values for bicycle ergometer exercise can be established (Table 24-4).[14]

Precautions and Adverse Reactions to Exercise

Complications

Since patients are in the acute stage of recovery after an MI, many conditions can occur that will complicate the recovery process. In one study of 258 patients recovering from an MI, ventricular arrhythmias, supraventricular tachycardias, heart failure, and heart block were the most common complications. Table 24-5 lists that complications in order of occurrence seen in that patient series.[15] In contrast, the complications seen in patients who have undergone cardiac surgery are reported in Table 24-6.[16] Patients experiencing complications will generally be hospitalized longer and will be managed more cautiously during this stage.

Precautions associated with activity during this stage are related to common complications. Treatment can be deferred, or a decision may be made either to reduce the patient's activity or to stop the patient's progress as a result of some complications. The physical therapist should be aware of symptoms that occur at rest and their potential significance in making decisions about an individual patient's treatment (Table 24-7).

There are also signs of disproportionate re-

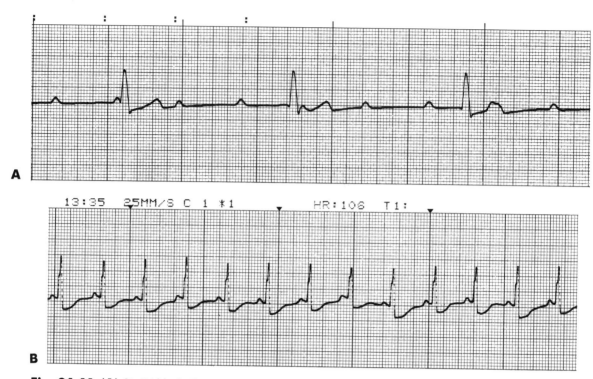

Fig. 24-11 (A) 3° AV block. The ventricular rate is slow with no relationship between P waves and QRS complexes. **(B)** Bundle branch block. The QRS complex is wide with two R peaks.

sponses to activity that may indicate problems. Since most activities and exercises that the patient engages in at this time are of low intensity, many programs suggest a heart rate limit of 120 beats/minute or an increase of less than 20 beats from the standing resting heart rate.[4,16] This is based on an average heart rate increase of less than 15 beats/minute in response to activities during the acute stage of recovery. A patient who has a higher heart rate response than this may have a poor ejection fraction and is compensating with a higher heart rate. It is not uncommon to note a resting heart rate of 120 beats/minute in a complicated patient; however, even a patient like this can be closely supervised during light activity. The inten-

sity and duration of activity are often kept very low in this instance. A decrease in heart rate of greater than 10 beats during exercise may indicate that the patient is experiencing a heart block with activity. A patient like this should be observed carefully with telemetered monitoring. The occurrence of significant arrhythmias during exercise is considered a reason to stop the activity and observe the patient. This is also true if the patient experiences chest pain, dyspnea, or an increased ST-

Fig. 24-12 Effect of digitalis on ST segment.

Table 24-3 Approximate MET Values for Treadmill Walking

| % Grade | MET Value[a] at the Following Speed (mph): | | | | | |
	1.7	2.0	2.5	3.0	3.4	3.75
0	2.3	2.5	2.9	3.3	3.6	3.9
2.5	2.9	3.2	3.8	4.3	4.8	5.2
5.0	3.5	3.9	4.6	5.4	5.9	6.5
7.5	4.1	4.6	5.5	6.4	7.1	7.8

(From American College of Sports Medicine,[14] with permission.)
[a] One MET = 3.5 ml/kg/min at rest.

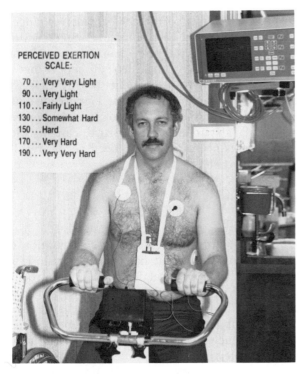

Fig. 24-13 Patient exercising on a bicycle ergometer while being monitored by telemetry.

segment displacement during exercise. A decrease in systolic blood pressure of greater than 20 mmHg may be associated with poor left ventricular function with exercise. Finally, if the patient is overly fatigued, feels faint, or demonstrates pallor or perspiration in response to the low-intensity activities, the activity should be stopped until the patient recovers.

Table 24-4 Approximate MET Values for Bicycle Ergometry

Body Weight (lbs)	(kg/min) (watts)	MET Value[a] with the Following Exercise Load:			
		300 50	450 75	600 100	750 125
110		5.1	6.9	8.6	10.3
132		4.3	5.7	7.1	8.6
154		3.7	4.9	6.1	7.3
176		3.2	4.3	5.4	6.4
198		2.9	3.8	4.8	5.7
220		2.6	3.4	4.3	5.1

(From American College of Sports Medicine,[14] with permission.)
[a] One MET = 3.5 ml/kg/min at rest.

Table 24-5 Complications with MI during Hospitalization[a]

Complication	% of Patients[b]
Ventricular arrhythmias	70
Supraventricular tachycardias	37
Heart failure	18
Heart block	14
Nonanginal chest discomfort	9
Cardiorespiratory arrest/resuscitation[c]	6
Extension reinfarction[c]	4
Thromboembolism[c]	2
Death[c]	1
Cardiac surgery[c]	2

(Percentages extrapolated from data from Sivarajan et al.[15])
[a] During the first 7 days of hospitalization.
[b] Percentage of 258 patients.
[c] During entire hospitalization.

LOW-LEVEL GRADED EXERCISE TEST

Before discharge, most patients undergo a low-level graded exercise test (LLGXT). A commonly used protocol for a treadmill test is shown in Table 24-8. The purpose of the test is to observe the patient under standardized and well-defined circumstances. Patients who are at high risk for subsequent cardiac events or who have poorly controlled arrhythmias or hypertension can be identified during the test.[17,18] The test can also be

Table 24-6 Complications Found in Postsurgical Patients

Complication	% of Patients (n = 521)
Ventricular arrhythmias	44
Superventricular arrhythmias	17
Multifocal PVCs	17
Incisional discomfort	14
Dizziness	14
Hypotension	8
Frequent PVCs	6
Couplets	5
Angina pectoris	4
Claudication	3
ST-segment change	2
Ventricular tachycardia	1
Hypertension	1

(From Dion et al.,[16] with permission.)

Table 24-7 Resting Symptoms and Associated Complications

Symptom	Potential Complication
Irregular pulse	Arrhythmia
Heart rate >120 beats/min	Supraventricular tachycardia or heart failure
Dyspnea	Heart failure
Heart rate <50 beats/min	Bradycardia associated with heart block, β-blocking medications
Chest pain	Infarction extension, angina, or nonanginal chest discomfort
Increased ST-segment displacement	Infarction extension
Systolic blood pressure <90 mm Hg	Heart failure, β-blocking medications

a basis for exercise prescription for the outpatient program, that is, a patient can be found to be without adverse signs and symptoms up to a particular heart rate.[4,19]

Predetermined endpoints for these tests are generally established. The most common endpoint is reaching a heart rate of 120 beats/minute. Other endpoints include the signs and symptoms of serious cardiac arrhythmias, chest pain, a systolic blood pressure that falls or fails to rise at least 10 mm Hg, fatigue, dizziness, or ataxia. A patient who completes the test can exercise to a heart rate of 120 beats/minute without adverse reactions. Patients with symptoms are advised to exercise at an intensity below the point at which the symptoms occurred. Antihypertensive and antiarrhythmia medications are usually reevaluated in these patients.

Patients who exhibit signs of ischemia during the LLGXT are considered to be at higher risk for subsequent and potentially fatal coronary

Table 24-8 Protocol for LLGXT

Speed (mph)	% Grade	Duration (min)
1.7	0	3
1.7	5	3
1.7	10	3
1.7	12	3

(From Schwartz et al.,[17] with permission.)

events.[17,18] Angina pectoris, ST-segment changes, and drops in systolic blood pressure suggest severe coronary artery disease or poor left ventricular function.[17,18,19] Irwin and Blessey[19] report that in a series of 134 post-MI patients during LLGXT, 22 percent experienced angina, 17 percent demonstrated ST-segment depression, and 10 percent had a fall in systolic blood pressure. Patients with these results need to be monitored very carefully during exercise.

HOME PROGRAM

Home programs are generally a continuation of the activities the patient has been performing in the hospital. The physical therapist should provide written instructions for the patient as well as review these verbally before the patient's discharge. Specific recommendations regarding exercise intensity, frequency, and duration should be included. For example, a series of standing upper and lower extremity ROM exercises can be used for a 5- to 10-minute warm-up before the patient takes a 20- to 30-minute walk. An additional 5-minute period of ROM can be a cool-down session after the walk.

The patient must be cautioned not to exercise if he is experiencing chest pain, feeling fatigued or not well, after meals, or in extremely hot or cold weather. If the patient can accurately take a pulse rate, he can be instructed to note the pulse during exercise and to exercise only up to a particular pulse level, often 120 beats/minute. The patient should be encouraged to contact the attending physician or the therapist with any questions or unusual symptoms. Patients tolerate this program routine well if the activities are performed once per day.

SUMMARY

An acute care cardiac rehabilitation program can provide a sound foundation from which to encourage the patient's recovery. The ability to perform low-level activities can indicate that the patient is safe to a resume normal daily routine without adverse consequences. The patient education that begins during this phase can reinforce more intensive efforts begun during an outpatient program. A knowledgeable physical therapist can guide the patient on the road to recovery in a safe and effective manner.

REFERENCES

1. List ND, Fronczak NE, Gottlieb SH, Baker RE: A cross-national study of differences in length of stay of patients with cardiac diagnoses. Medical Care 21:519, 1983
2. McNeer JF, Wagner GS, Ginsberg AS, et al.: Hospital discharge one week after myocardial infarction. N Engl J Med 288:1141, 1978
3. Madsen EB, Hougaard P, Gilpin E, et al.: The length of hospitalization after acute myocardial infarction. Circulation 68:9, 1983
4. Pollock ML, Pels AE, Foster C, Ward A: Exercise prescription for rehabilitation of the cardiac patient. p. 477. In Pollock ML, Schmidt DH (eds): Heart Disease and Rehabilitation. John Wiley & Sons, New York, 1986
5. Froelicher VF, Pollock ML (eds): Cardiac rehabilitation programs. The state of the art. J Cardiac Rehab 2:429, 1982
6. Conti CR, Griffith LSC, Ross RS: Thoracic pain and angina pectoris. p. 325. In Harvey AMH, Johns RJ, Owens AH, Ross RS (eds): The Principles and Practice of Medicine. Appleton-Century-Crofts, East Norwalk, CT, 1976
7. Young JB, Luchi RJ: Coronary heart disease. p. 516. In Kaye D, Rose LF (eds): Fundamentals of Internal Medicine. CV Mosby, St. Louis, 1983
8. Tesch PA, Kaiser P: Effects of beta-adrenergic blockade on O_2 uptake during submaximal and maximal exercise. J Appl Physiol 54:901, 1983
9. Dubin D: Rapid Interpretation of EKG's. Cover Publishing, Tampa, FL, 1975
10. Ice R: Program planning and implementation. In Irwin S, Tecklin J (eds): Cardiopulmonary Physical Therapy. CV Mosby, St. Louis, 1985
11. Graf RS: Rehabilitation during the acute and convalescent stages following myocardial infarction. p. 99. In Amundsen LR (ed): Cardiac Rehabilitation. Churchill Livingstone, New York, 1981
12. Pollock ML, Wilmore JH, Fox SM: Prescribing exercise for rehabilitation of the cardiac patient. p. 298. In Pollock ML, Wilmore JH, Fox SM (eds): Exercise in Health and Disease. WB Saunders, Philadelphia, 1984
13. Dehne PR, Protas EJ: Oxygen consumption and heart rate responses during five active exercises. Phys Ther 66:1215, 1986
14. American College of Sports Medicine: Guidelines for Graded Exercise Testing and Prescription. 3rd ed. Lea & Febiger, Philadelphia, 1986
15. Sivarajan ES, Bruce RA, Almes MJ, et al.: In-hospital exercise after myocardial infarction does not improve treadmill performance. N Engl J Med 305:357, 1981
16. Dion W, Grevenow P, Pollock ML, et al.: Medical problems and physiologic responses during supervised inpatient cardiac rehabilitation: the patient after coronary bypass surgery. Heart Lung 11:248, 1981
17. Schwartz KM, Turner JD, Sheffield LT, et al.: Limited exercise testing soon after myocardial infarction. Correlation with early coronary and left ventricular angiography. Ann Intern Med 94:727, 1981
18. Theroux GJ, Waters DD, Halpen C, et al.: Prognostic value of exercise testing soon after myocardial infarction. N Engl J Med 301:341, 1979
19. Irwin S, Blessey RL: Patient evaluation. In Irwin S, Tecklin JS (eds): Cardiopulmonary Physical Therapy. CV Mosby, St. Louis, 1985

25 Rehabilitation of the Postsurgical Cardiac Patient

Ann Winkel Fick
Viola Holloway

Physical therapy rehabilitation of the postsurgical cardiac patient often has a different focus than the later phases of cardiac rehabilitation. Patients may need physical assistance to return to their normal activities of daily living. This assistance is often needed for those patients who have had complications related to surgery, for elderly patients, or for those patients with multiple diagnoses. In this chapter, some of the common cardiac surgeries are briefly explained. General evaluation and treatment procedures are then described.

Aspects of cardiac transplantation will also be addressed. Since the development of cyclosporin A, this procedure has become a more common and acceptable treatment for patients with end-stage cardiac disease.[1] In this chapter, donor criteria, surgical procedures, drugs, rejection, infection, cardiac denervation, and treatment for cardiac transplant recipients are described.

CARDIAC SURGERY

Aortocoronary Bypass

A common type of revascularization procedure performed for an ischemic myocardium is the aortocoronary bypass (ACB), using the greater saphenous vein. During this procedure, a midline sternal incision is made and the sternum is opened, as the saphenous or other selected vein is being harvested (Fig. 25-1). To remove possible clots, the vein is irrigated and then put in a cold blood solution. The patient is then usually placed on cardiopulmonary bypass. The surgeon sews the graft (vein) at a point distal to the occlusion of the artery and then to the aorta (Fig. 25-2). Air is aspirated out of the vein to avoid introducing air into the coronary system. The patient is taken off cardiopulmonary bypass, chest tubes are inserted into the mediastinum, and temporary pacemaker wires are inserted into the right ventricle. The sternum is then wired closed.[2]

If the greater saphenous veins cannot be used or are not preferred, the left internal mammary artery can be used to bypass the left anterior descending coronary artery. According to Reul, the internal mammary artery is now the "conduit of choice by most surgeons."[3] Studies by Lytle and Campeau showed that the internal mammary artery grafts remained opened longer during the first 5 years postsurgery than the saphenous vein.[3]

Percutaneous Transluminal Coronary Angioplasty

Percutaneous transluminal coronary angioplasty (PTCA) is a procedure done under local anesthesia to open the blocked area of a coronary artery. In this procedure, a guiding catheter is placed through the skin, into the lumen of the femoral or brachial artery, and up to the left or right coronary artery. Another catheter, called a balloon catheter, is passed through the guiding catheter and into the narrowed area of the occluded coronary artery. The balloon is then inflated, causing the stenotic artery to dilate (Fig. 25-3). The goal of this procedure is to restore blood flow through this area of the artery.[4]

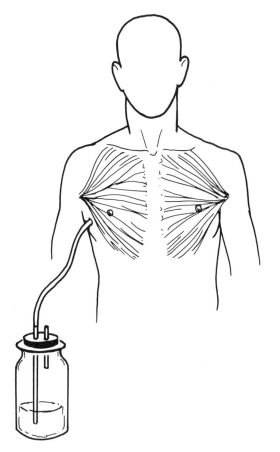

Fig. 25-1 An example of midline sternotomy with chest tubes in place.

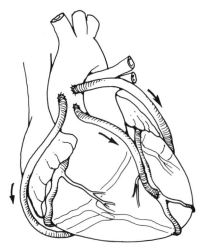

Fig. 25-2 A completed triple ACB graft to the right, left anterior descending, and obtuse marginal coronary arteries. The saphenous veins were used in this procedure.

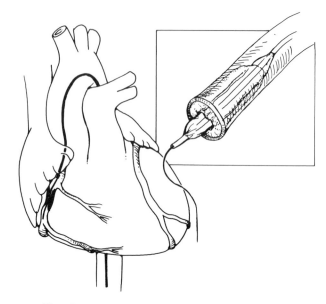

Fig. 25-3 Percutaneous transluminal coronary angioplasty before and during procedure.

Valve Replacements

For those patients with stenosis or regurgitant valves, valve replacement, usually of the aortic, mitral, or tricuspid valve, may be needed. The chest is opened and the patient is placed on cardiopulmonary bypass. A prosthesis is implanted after the diseased valve or leaflets are removed (Fig. 25-4). The chest is closed after cardiopulmonary bypass is removed.[5] Other common valve surgeries are annuloplasty for incompetent valves and commissurotomy for stenotic valves. Annuloplasty refers to plastic valve reconstruction, while

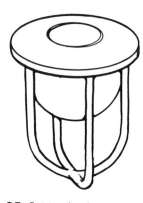

Fig. 25-4 Mitral valve replacement.

commissurotomy is surgical division, for example, division of the fibrous ring of the mitral valve.[6]

Pacemakers

Pacemakers can be implanted by the subxiphoid, transthoracic, or transvenous approach (Fig. 25-5). The transthoracic and subxiphoid procedures are done by epicardial lead placement. Epicardial placement means that the pacemaker leads are implanted on the outside surface of the heart. The subxiphoid method is preferred except when the heart is already exposed during cardiac surgery. During the transvenous endocardial approach, the electrodes are inserted into the left subclavian vein and then into the selected chamber of the heart. These leads are attached to the pulse generator, and the pacemaker is placed in the infraclavicular region.[7] A letter code system tells what part of the heart is paced, what heart chamber is sensed, and the type of response of the pacemaker. For example, a code of VVI says that the electrode is attached to the ventricle (V), and if the ventricle (V) is spontaneously stimulated to fire, the pacemaker stimulation is inhibited (I).[8] If the ventricle

is not stimulated, the pacemaker will fire (Fig. 25-6). Indications for pacemakers may include

1. Hypersensitive carotid sinus syndrome
2. Sick sinus syndrome
3. Tachycardia or bradycardia arrhythmias
4. Complete heart block
5. Stokes-Adams syndrome
6. Cardiac surgery

Precautions and possible problems of pacemakers may include

1. Temporary pacemaker wires should stay dry and be covered with something like a latex glove
2. Possible pacemaker generator failure, that is, sensing, pacing failure, or pacemaker battery depletion
3. Possible pacemaker-induced dysrhythmias
4. Possible right ventricular perforation
5. Possible diaphragmatic stimulation
6. Possible infection
7. Possible pacemaker function interference if diathermy is used or, especially with older pacemaker models, if the patient is in close contact with microwave ovens

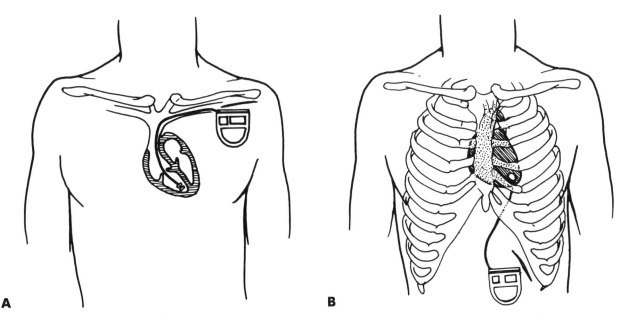

Fig. 25-5 Two examples of pacemaker implantation sites. **(A)** Endocardial or transvenous. **(B)** Epicardial.

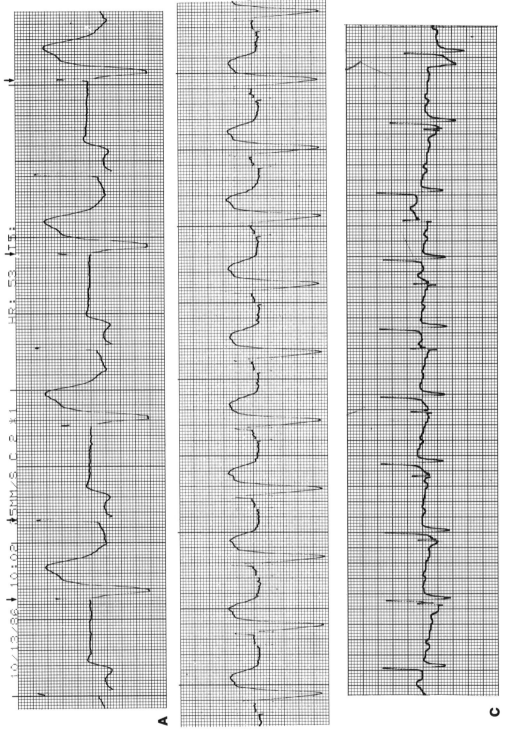

Fig. 25-6 Standard pacemaker ECG tracings. Notice the pacemaker spike before atrial and/or ventricular contraction. **(A)** Capturing ventricular pacemaker. **(B)** Capturing AV sequential pacemaker. There are two pacer spikes for each beat (one for the atrium and one for the ventricles) **(C)** Noncapturing pacemaker. In the noncapturing pacemaker tracing, the pacemaker spike is independent of atrial or ventricular electrical stimulation (spikes and QRS are not together).

8. Possible catheter dislodgement or displacement, especially after transvenous catheter pacement or temporary pacemaker placement. Check with the physician or hospital policy for these precautions. The patient's upper extremity (the side where the transvenous pacemaker was implanted) may be placed in a sling initially after surgery. Limited shoulder flexion, abduction, and extension as well as limited pushing and pulling activities may be advisable for up to 3 weeks.
9. Possible exercise intolerance may occur depending on the type of pacemaker or patient. The heart rate may be fixed. Be sure to monitor blood pressure and watch for possible electrocardiogram (ECG) abnormalities.[9,10]

Complications of Cardiac Surgery

Complications can occur with any invasive or surgical procedures. The following is a listing of some of the possible complications:

1. Respiratory failure or insufficiency
2. Cardiac arrest or myocardial infarction
3. Arrhythmias
4. Infection
5. Renal failure or insufficiency
6. Neurological deficits
7. Cerebral infarction or transcient ischemic attack
8. Pulmonary or peripheral embolus
9. Unstable sternum
10. Anemia

Chart Review

Before physical therapy rehabilitation is started, a review of the chart is necessary. Previous and recent history of cerebral vascular accidents, myocardial infarctions, surgeries, or other problems should be noted. Besides the normal information usually found in the chart such as mental status, the therapist treating postoperative cardiac patients should also note:

1. Heart catheterization and arteriogram, for the evaluation of valve and heart function[11] as well as which coronary arteries may be occluded
2. Nuclear cardiac imaging studies, for ejection fraction, "a measure of the pump function of the left or right ventricle,"[12] which is normally 50 percent at rest. Severe left ventricular dysfunction can produce an ejection fraction that is less than 30 percent.[13] Nuclear medicine studies can also assess whether the heart wall motion is normal, abnormal (bradykinetic, dyskinetic), or stationary (akinetic). Cardiovascular hemodynamics during exercise and any other tests may also be charted.
3. Baseline vital signs, including heart rate, blood pressure, respiratory rate, and temperature
4. ECG reports, for evaluation of arrhythmias
5. X-ray, for possible atelectasis or other cardiopulmonary problems
6. Laboratory reports. Look for hemoglobin (M = 13 to 16.5g/dl, F = 12 to 15 g/dl), potassium (3.6 to 5.5 mEq/L), blood glucose (70 to 110 mg/100 ml), prothrombin time results, recent blood gases, etc. Low hemoglobin values are not uncommon after surgery and may be a cause for a decrease in endurance.
7. Cardiac drugs. Certain drugs, such as β-blocking drugs, may lower the amount of increase in heart rate with exercise. Knowing the drug group and its effect on exercise may be necessary for better understanding of the patient's exercise response.
8. Home environment, including if the patient will live alone or with someone, how many steps there are to get into the house, etc. The therapist may need to question the patient if this information is not in the chart.

Evaluation

General Physical Therapy Evaluation

After reviewing the chart, general physical therapy evaluation is performed. The range of motion of the upper extremities should be determined without placing undue stress on the sternum, particularly in poststernotomy patients. When checking the range of motion of the upper and lower extremities, watch for possible:

1. Brachial plexus injury
2. Weakness of one side

3. Decreased range in the leg from which the saphenous vein was taken after coronary artery bypass surgery
4. Foot drop

Other parts of the evaluation can include:

1. Checking for edema
2. Checking for pain
3. Strength after a sternotomy—little to no resistance should be given to the upper extremities
4. Endurance
5. Bed mobility
6. Transfers
7. Posture
8. Self-care activities
9. Ambulation status
10. Vital signs at rest, with exercise, and with postural changes

Every patient should be evaluated and should progress individually, keeping in mind the patient's status and level of disability.

Vital Signs

Heart Rate

Evaluation of vital sign responses with exercise can be a significant part of early postoperative cardiac rehabilitation. Heart rate is one vital sign that should be taken before, during, and after exercise. Heart rate is obtained by palpating the radial pulse, auscultating the heart rate, or from an ECG tracing. The most accurate method is using an ECG tracing. This method also allows the therapist to check for significant arrhythmias. If an ECG machine is not available, the pulse should be described as regular, regular with ectopic beats, that is, an occasional missed or fast beat, or irregularly irregular, that is, no pattern to the rhythm.

Heart rate at rest is normally between 60 to 100 beats/minute. Excessive increases in heart rate with low-intensity exercise or resting heart rates above normal may be seen in cardiac patients with poor ventricular function, arrhythmias, low hemoglobin-hematocrit values, pulmonary dysfunction such as chronic obstructive pulmonary disease (COPD), bed rest and deconditioning, or fever.[14,15] Lower than normal resting heart rates and little increase in heart rate with exercise may be also

seen in patients with coronary artery disease. This response in patients with coronary artery disease is considered abnormal as long as the patient is not taking any medication that slows the heart rate.[14]

Blood Pressure

Blood pressure should be taken using the American Heart Association standards. The arm with the higher blood pressure reading should be used and these values should be recorded. The position of the patient and the time the blood pressure was taken, that is before, during, or after exercise, must also be noted. Proper cuff and bladder size are important since a bladder that is too narrow for a patient's forearm may give a higher blood pressure reading than the true value, while a cuff bladder that is too wide may give a lower blood pressure value. In other words, if the cuff is too small for the patient, the value may be higher than the true reading, and a cuff that is too big for the patient may give a lower reading than it should. Before taking the patient's blood pressure, the therapist should palpate the radial pulse to get an estimate of the systolic blood pressure value. Once the cuff is properly placed on the patient's forearm and the bladder is inflated, the blood pressure reading at the first radial pulse palpated during deflation is an estimate of systolic blood pressure. The blood pressure should then be auscultated. The bell of the stethoscope should be placed at the antecubital fossa. Deflation of the blood pressure cuff is to be done at 2 to 3 mmHg per second.[16]

Systolic Versus Diastolic Values. The first sound heard at rest in an adult patient is the systolic blood pressure. The diastolic blood pressure is recorded as the pressure at which the sounds disappear. During or after exercise and for children, the diastolic blood pressure values are recorded when the muffling sound occurs. These blood pressure values "should be read to the nearest 2 millimeter of mercury mark of the manometer scale."[17] Systolic blood pressure normally increases with increased exercise. A flat response or a decrease or inadequate rise in systolic blood pressure with increasing intensity of exercise is "indicative of inadequate pumping by the heart."[18] A drop of inadequate systolic blood pressure responses, according to Irwin, "should not be acted upon unless additional abnormalities are noted."[19] These abnormalities can include shortness of breath, angina, and significant ST-segment changes.[19]

Respiratory Rate

Respiratory rate, usually 10 to 20 ventilations per minute, is another important vital sign to monitor during exercise.[20] During low-intensity exercise, mainly tidal volume or "the volume of air entering or leaving the lung during a single breath" increases.[21] More air is inspired and expired without a needed increase in respiratory rate. With heavier levels of exercise, the tidal volume and the respiratory rate increased.[20-22] Shortness of breath is common in cardiac patients with severe disease.[14] Undue shortness of breath with any cardiac patient during exercise should be avoided.

Postsurgical Physical Therapy Treatment

Early after surgery, deep breathing and splinted coughing should be taught. Forced coughing should be avoided. Chest physical therapy of percussion, vibration, and postural drainage may also be needed to improve the patient's pulmonary status[23] (see Ch. 29).

Ambulation

Ambulation usually can begin with physician approval a few days after surgery. At this time, bed mobility, sitting, and transfer training can be started if not already initiated by the nursing staff. In initially getting the patient out of bed, vital signs during supine, sitting, and standing postures should be taken.

Exercise

During exercise and evaluation periods, listen to and observe the patient. Signs and symptoms of abnormal responses to exercise according to the American Heart Association include:

1. Flat or progressive decrease in systolic blood pressure
2. Bradycardia or excessive tachycardia
3. Significant arrhythmias
4. Angina

5. Undue shortness of breath
6. Dizziness
7. Confusion
8. Lower extremity claudication
9. Cyanosis
10. Pallor
11. Mottling of skin
12. Cold sweat
13. Ataxia
14. Glassy stare
15. Abnormal heart sounds

These can be related to cardiac ischemia, poor ventricular function, pulmonary disease, anemia, drugs, cardiac valvular disease, bed rest, and other causes. Contraindications to exercise according to the American Heart Association include:

1. Acute febrile illness
2. Uncontrolled, active chronic systemic disease
3. Anatomical abnormalities
4. Functional abnormalities such as third-degree heart block[15]

Exercise may aggravate these problems. Other factors to be considered before exercise include:

1. Drugs
2. Age
3. Weight
4. Level of fitness
5. Muscle strength
6. Orthopaedic problems
7. Cerebral dysfunction
8. Environmental temperature and other factors[15]

Bed Rest and the Critically Ill

For those patients who have been on bed rest for a prolonged period of time, an excessive increase in heart rate with exercise and postural hypotension can occur. Postural hypotension can generally be described as a decrease in systolic blood pressure of 10 to 20 mmHg or greater, or a resting systolic blood pressure lower than 90 mmHg.[25] For this problem, try getting the patient out of the bed slowly, have them exercise their legs before and during sitting or standing, and inquire about dizziness or lightheadedness of the patient. Muscle contractions help decrease venous pooling in the legs, thus decreasing the dizziness felt by the patient.[25] Supine range of motion exercises and sitting in a chair can help to prevent this problem.[15] When prolonged bed rest has occurred, continued efforts in remobilizing the patient should lessen these problems.

For those patients who have been seriously ill, the activity performed should be of low intensity. The activities may include deep breathing, bed mobility, proper bed positioning, dangling, transfer training, or self-care activities. A gradual increase in activity may eventually be appropriate. These activities help prevent problems that are associated with bed rest such as muscle weakness, pulmonary complications, and vascular thrombosis.[15]

Summary

In the acute stage after cardiac surgery, the basic goal should be to get the patient functional in activities of daily living. At the same time, it would be beneficial for the therapist to evaluate for the appropriateness of vital sign responses before, during, and after these activities. The therapist must keep in mind the patient's medical history, surgeries, and current problems to achieve optimal results from patient treatment. Before discharge, exercise guidelines and a low-intensity aerobic home program can be given to these patients. It must be stressed that later progression of the program should be under the direction of a qualified professional.

CARDIAC TRANSPLANTATION

Since the development of cyclosporin A, heart transplantation has become a more common and acceptable treatment for patients with end-stage cardiac disease. Cyclosporin A helps to reduce rejection of the transplanted heart, thus improving patient survival. Many centers are now performing cardiac transplantation because of cyclosporin A and other recent advances in cardiac transplantation.[1]

Criteria For Transplantation

Criteria for both the recipient and the donor must be met before cardiac transplantation is performed. The recipient must have a cardiac disa-

bility meeting the classification of the New York Heart Association functional class IV. Severe diabetes or serious medical conditions should not be present. For some heart transplant programs, an age limit of 50 years is set. At the Texas Heart Institute, there are no specific age requirements. Requirements of the donor include absence of heart disease, cardiac arrest, and active infection. The donor should be less than 35 years of age. A legal definition of brain death and family consent is required. There must be ABO blood-type compatibility, and the size of the donor must be similar to the size of the recipient.[26,27]

Surgical Procedure for Orthotopic Cardiac Transplantation

The surgical procedure can be performed after the previously described criteria have been met. After the donor's chest has been opened, the donor heart is stopped by a cardioplegic solution. Ample lengths of the aorta, pulmonary arteries, and superior vena cava are left during the excision of the heart. Once removed, the heart is kept in a saline slush solution at 4°C before transplantation. A median sternotomy is performed on the recipient and he is placed on cardiopulmonary bypass. The posterior shell of the right and left atria is still intact after the recipient's heart is removed. The recipient's sinoatrial node is spared. The two left atria are first sewn around the entire circumference. The two right atria are then anastomosed. Next, the pulmonary arteries and ascending aorta are connected (Fig. 25-7). Air is aspirated out of the donor heart chambers, and the heart is restarted.[1]

The recipient sinoatrial node is left intact during orthotopic heart transplantation to "avoid the need for difficult venous anastomoses."[28] Although it lacks a blood supply, the recipient sinus node ordinarily continues to function. It is believed that bronchial collaterals continue to supply the blood needed by the sinoatrial node. The sinoatrial node works by electrically stimulating the atrial remnants to contract. Two separate P waves may be seen on the ECG. One P wave seen is caused by the remaining recipient sinus node. The recipient P wave will fire independently of the donor P wave and QRST complex (Fig. 25-8). During exercise, anxiety, or other sympathetic stimulation, the rate

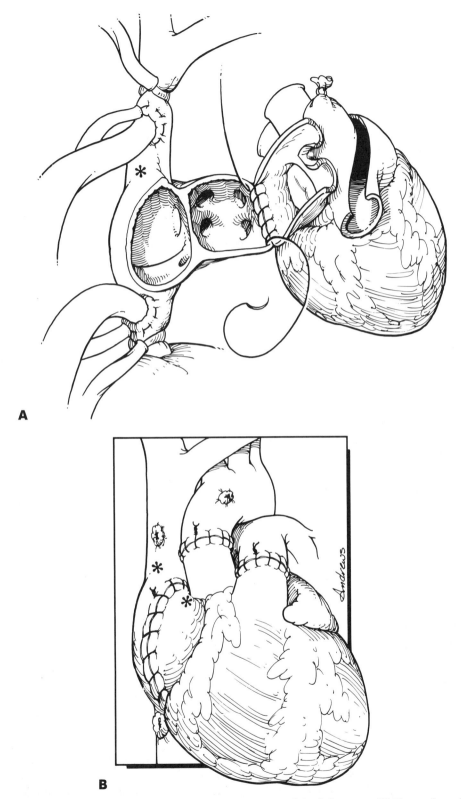

A

B

Fig. 25-7 (A) Implantation is initiated with anastomosis of the left atrium. **(B)** The end result of orthotopic heart transplantation. The asterisks (*) denote the two sinoatrial nodes. (Cooley DA (ed): Techniques in Cardiac Surgery. p. 370–371. 2nd ed. WB Saunders, Philadelphia, 1984.)

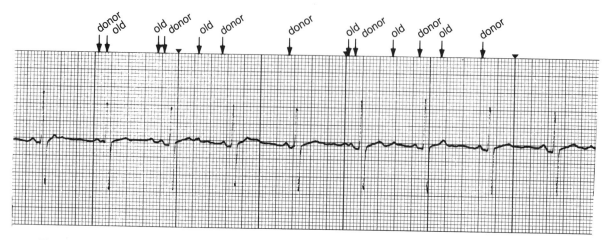

Fig. 25-8 An ECG tracing of an orthotopic heart transplant recipient. Two P waves can result. The recipient's own (old) sinoatrial node generates a P wave that cannot propagate beyond the suture-scar line of the anastomosis. The donor sinoatrial node generates a P wave that stimulates the ventricles to fire and produce the QRS complex.

of the innervated recipient P wave will increase according to increases in the intensity of sympathetic stimulation.[28] The donor sinus node has been denervated and therefore does not display the rapid rate change seen in the innervated heart.

Heterotopic Cardiac Transplantation

Heterotopic ("piggyback") heart transplantation is an alternative technique to the well-established orthotopic heart transplant. The operation consists of transplanting a donor heart into the right pleural cavity of the patient and connecting it to the patient's own heart. The two hearts are connected by sewing the two right atria and the two left atria together, making one right and one left atrium (Fig. 25-9). The ascending aortas are anastomosed, and the pulmonary artery trunks are connected with a Dacron tube graft. After the surgery is completed, the donor heart lies to the right side of the native heart with the left ventricle facing anteriorly and sits in front of the right lung in the right pleural cavity.[29,30]

Both hearts share in the venous return from the body. The donor heart generally has a greater cardiac output than the diseased native heart. Each heart is electrically stimulated by its own sinus node. The contraction of each heart is therefore independent of the other and two separate PQRST complexes are seen on ECG recordings[29,31] (Fig. 25-10).

Advantages of heterotopic cardiac transplantation over orthotopic cardiac transplantation have been described by Novitzky et al.[32] The native heart can assist the donor heart with cardiac output during its ischemic phase immediately postoperatively and during severe rejection episodes. If irreversible rejection occurs, the native heart is still present and potentially can sustain blood flow until a new donor is located. This procedure can be done despite high pulmonary vascular resistance. The hypertrophied right ventricle of the native heart can continue to maintain pulmonary circulation, whereas a normal right ventricle may not be able to meet this demand.[32,33] In urgent cases, heterotopic transplantation can be a valuable alternative when a smaller than optimal heart is the only available heart. Potential disadvantages include arrhythmias and angina of the native heart. Long-term anticoagulation therapy is also needed to help prevent emboli possibly caused by thrombus formation in the weakly contracting native left ventricle.[29]

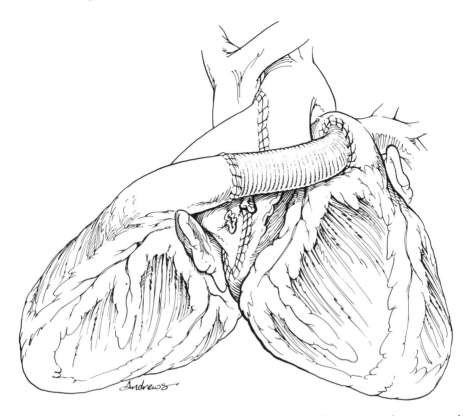

Fig. 25-9 An anterior view of heterotopic heart transplantation. The donor and recipient pulmonary arteries are connected with a Dacron tube graft. (Cooley DA (ed): Techniques in Cardiac Surgery. p. 373. 2nd ed. WB Saunders, Philadelphia, 1984.)

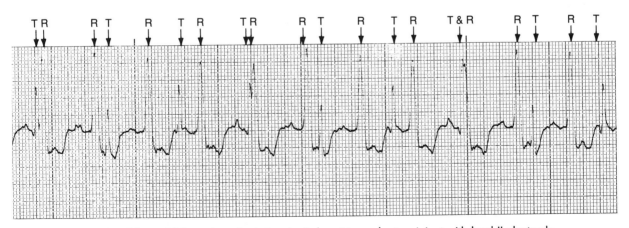

Fig. 25-10 An ECG tracing of a heterotopic heart transplant recipient with lead II electrode placement. T, the transplanted heart QRS complexes. R, the native heart QRS complexes.

Drugs Specific to Heart Transplantation

Cyclosporin A

Cyclosporin A, steroids, and antihypertensives are three of the drugs needed by patients after orthotopic heart transplantation. Cyclosporin A is an immunosuppressant used to help prevent rejection of the donor heart. It works by suppressing selective T lymphocytes, while the nonspecific immune system is spared.[1,34]

Antihypertensives

One common side effect of cyclosporin A treatment is hypertension. As a result, antihypertensive medication is needed to maintain the blood pressure at an acceptable level.[35]

Steroids

Steroids act as anti-inflammatory agents that help the body accept the donor heart. Although steroids assist in the acceptance of the new heart, these drugs, especially in high doses, impair the body's ability to fight infection. The use of masks and good hand-washing techniques and limited visitor exposure are therefore routine precautions for these patients. Steroids may also cause muscle weakness and joint pain, which can be reduced by moderate exercise.[35]

Rejection

Rejection is a common problem associated with heart transplantation. One or more rejection episodes are experienced by most patients. Arrhythmias, fever, shortness of breath, and increased resting blood pressure can be signs and symptoms of rejection. These signs and symptoms are nonspecific and do not always occur. For more reliable and accurate detection of rejection, frequent endomyocardial biopsies are performed.[35]

Endomyocardial biopsy is done in the cardiac catheterizaton laboratory. A cardiologist inserts a bioptome into the patient's femoral or jugular vein. The instrument is threaded through the body and into the right ventricle. Five to six small pieces of the right ventricle are taken and are examined by a pathologist. Moderate to severe grades of rejection are treated. Treatment consists of more im-

munosuppression drugs. The additional drugs are then quickly reduced on a daily basis until the rejection episode has subsided.[35]

Infection

Another problem after heart transplantation is infection. Infection is the major cause of death in cardiac transplant patients.[36] The patients are especially susceptible to infection when the dose of steroids is high. Measures are needed to decrease the likelihood of getting an infection at all times. Good hand washing by hospital personnel and patients is a must. Masks are worn by patients when they leave the room. Mask wearing is continued until the patient is on a maintenance steroid dose. Personnel may be asked to wear masks to limit the patient's exposure to common respiratory disease, since the pulmonary system is the most common site of infection.[35]

The Denervated Transplanted Heart

After cardiac transplantation, denervation of the autonomic nerves to the donor heart takes place. The direct autonomic stimulation is lost, but the indirect stimulation from the adrenal medullae is still intact. When an organ such as the heart is denervated, a phenomenon called denervation supersensitivity occurs. It has been found that after denervation the heart becomes overly sensitive to circulating catecholamines. Since the transplanted heart is denervated, the hormonal stimulation from the adrenal medullae will have a heightened impact on the heart.[37]

The denervated transplanted heart at rest generally has a higher than normal heart rate as a result of the removal of vagal stimulation to the donor sinus node. The heart rate in the cardiac transplant patient is not affected by the Valsalva maneuver or carotid sinus massage.[38] Normally these maneuvers reduce heart rate. No appreciable change occurs in the heart rate of cardiac transplant recipients when they move from supine to standing or receive the drug atropine (normally these actions would increase heart rate). Cardiac output, stroke volume, and respiratory rate remain within normal limits at rest in the transplanted heart. It is thought that cardiac output, although within the normal limits, may be slightly lower than that of an innervated heart.[38-41]

In healthy individuals during dynamic exercise, heart rate increases immediately and is mainly responsible for the increase in cardiac output. In the cardiac transplant recipient, the heart rate starts higher initially, increases gradually over time, and does not reach normal peak maximum heart rate values. Since the transplanted heart lacks sympathetic stimulation that normally increases heart rate, this atypical heart rate response is thought to be due to the circulating catecholamines.[40]

Stroke volume normally "remains virtually unchanged" until more strenuous exercise occurs.[42] Stroke volume is enhanced with exercise by an increase in venous return to the heart. An increase in venous return occurs through the pumping action of the exercising skeletal muscles, an increase in venous tone from sympathetic stimulation, and changes in intrathoracic and intra-abdominal pressure from increased respiration. The increase in venous return to the heart results in a greater stretch of the cardiac muscle. The stretched muscle fibers of the heart then contract harder, and an increase in stroke volume results. This is Starling's law of cardiac muscle mechanics. In the cardiac transplant recipient, since heart rate increases more slowly and gradually with exercise, stroke volume through Starling's law is thought to initially increase cardiac output. With higher-intensity exercise, a further increase in stroke volume occurs as a result of an increase of preload or end-diastolic volume (from increased venous return) and of the positive inotropic (cardiac muscle-strengthening) actions of the circulating catecholamines. This in turn causes a further increase in cardiac output.[41]

Cardiac output at peak exercise has been shown to be slightly less in cardiac transplant patients than in normal individuals. Oxygen consumption and physical work capacity also appear to be lower during exercise in this population. Peak exercise ventilation values were similar to those of the healthy population, but ventilation was higher in transplant patients during submaximal exercise.

The anaerobic threshold seems to occur sooner in the patient with a denervated heart. A higher postexercise buildup in lactic acid is also noted.

Perceived exertion levels in cardiac transplant patients seem to corroborate this. These findings could be related to medication or "subclinical rejection, as dogs with autotransplants are able to perform maximally."[41] Savin and co-workers have shown that physical work capacity does decrease with a significant rejection history.[40]

During the recovery period after exercise, the heart rate quickly returns to the resting level. In a denervated heart, it decreases more gradually as a result of the slow re-uptake of the circulating catecholamines (Fig. 25-11). Normally, stroke volume promptly begins to decrease after exercise because of reduced volume of blood in the ventricles before systole. In a denervated heart, stroke volume may not return to resting levels as soon as in the normal population. It is theorized that after exercise, the heart rate and stroke volume will take longer to return to resting values because of the transplanted heart's supersensitivity to circulating catecholamines. Since heart rate and stroke volume are decreasing after exercise, cardiac output is reduced. The respiratory rate returns to pre-exercise values or slightly higher than before exercise because of pre-exercise anticipation.[39,41]

With isometric exercise, a similar increase in systolic and diastolic blood pressure occurs in

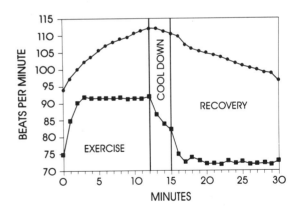

Fig. 25-11 An example of the differences in heart rate between the denervated transplanted heart (circles) and the healthy innervated heart (squares) during low-level exercise. Heart rate of the transplanted heart is higher at rest (from lack of vagal stimulation) and increases with exercise slower than normal. During the cool-down and recovery periods, the heart rate response of the transplanted heart is again a more gradual response than normal.

normal individuals and heart transplant patients. An increase in total peripheral resistance versus an increase in cardiac output is responsible for this increase. No significant increase in stroke volume occurs in normal persons or those with heart transplants. Heart rate reflexively increases in the normal population, while no change in heart rate is seen in the transplant group.[43,44]

In the heterotopic heart transplant patients, the donor heart responds as a denervated heart while the native heart responds as a diseased innervated heart. When this type of patient exercises, the donor and diseased hearts should be monitored separately. Arrhythmias and poor ventricular pumping of the diseased native heart are expected. With physician approval and absence of infection or of donor rejection, the arrhythmias of the native heart may be ignored and emphasis on donor function should be a priority. Shortness of breath may occur during exercise in these patients, especially because of the postoperative pulmonary problems these patients experience.

Chart Review

The review of the chart is similar to that of any patient after cardiac surgery. Previous and recent history should be noted. ECG reports, X-ray reports, drugs, baseline vital signs, and laboratory reports can give the therapist general information about the patient before treatment. The therapist should also look for cardiac biopsy results and white blood cell reports. If the patient is in moderate to severe rejection, the level of activity should be discussed with the transplant team. If the white blood cell count is lower than the normal range (4 $\times$ 10^3/μL), the patient may be more susceptible to infection. Anyone with a cold or other infection should not visit or treat the patient.

Evaluation

Evaluation of the heart transplant patient is generally like that of any cardiac patient, including:

1. Checking for edema
2. Checking for pain
3. Range of motion without undue stress on the sternum
4. Strength testing. This is especially important in this population since muscle atrophy from previous low exercise tolerance or bed rest may be seen. Again, after a sternotomy, little to no resistance should be given to the upper extremities. Watch for symmetry in strength.
5. Endurance
6. Bed mobility
7. Transfers
8. Posture
9. Self-care activities
10. Ambulation status
11. Vital signs. The response of the denervated heart must be kept in mind. Little to no increase in heart rate with low levels of exercise may be seen. According to Bexton et al., if the patient is taking a β-blocker, such as propranolol, the patient may have a lower exercise tolerance to maximal exercise. β-blockers combine with β-receptor sites, inhibiting the catecholamine response of the heart. During mild exercise those patients taking β-blockers should have a basically unchanged exercise tolerance since the circulating catecholamine influences with low-level exercise are small.[47]

Postsurgical Physical Therapy Treatment

Chest Physical Therapy

Postoperatively, heart transplant patients need to perform deep breathing and splinted coughing techniques as in other open heart surgery. (Forced coughing should be avoided in the immediate postoperative period.) Chest percussion and other chest physical therapy procedures may be needed to help clear the lungs, especially after heterotopic cardiac transplantation. In the latter patient, chest physical therapy is needed because the right lung collapses during this surgery[30] (see Ch. 29).

Exercises

Range of motion and strengthening exercises are important since these patients are often quite deconditioned before surgery. No undue stress can be placed on the sternum. The decision to use weights for upper extremity strengthening within the first few months after surgery should be jointly made by the physical therapist and physicians.

Dangling on the side of the bed, transfers to a chair, and ambulation exercises can usually be started within the first few days after surgery. During the early postoperative period, these patients are usually on high doses of steroids and other immunosuppressant drugs. Consequently, their activity may be restricted to their room or other areas. The patient may need to wear a face mask once outside of his room. Good postural techniques and back care should be stressed early in the program as a preventive measure. The back muscles may already be weakened or stressed from bed rest, and since these patients are usually on steroids, good posture is important. (Steroids can cause muscle weakness, joint pain, and possibly osteoporosis.) Some patients poststernotomy tend to sit and stand with an increased kyphosis, forward head, and rounded shoulders to flex their upper trunk and splint their sternum. Later in the program, usually after the sternum has healed, stretching of the anterior chest by scapular squeezes, chin tucks, and shoulder rolls can be started to encourage better posture.

Aerobic Exercise

The patient should be instructed in an aerobic exercise program as soon as it is appropriate. The exercise should be continuous and repetitive in nature. Walking and cycling are two of the best types of aerobic exercise for early post-transplant patients. As stated before, the denervated heart responds differently during exercise. In addition, for the heterotopic cardiac transplant recipient, there is a diseased heart and a transplanted heart. Therefore, Borg's[45] perceived exertion levels of "fairly light" to "somewhat hard" may be useful with exercise. (These subjective feelings normally correspond to a heart rate of 110 to 130 beats/minute.) Another effective and more objective measurement is the "dyspnea index" that is used by Stanford. The patient counts to 15 while exercising. If he breathes more than twice during the count of 15, he is probably exercising too hard.[46] Shortness of breath seems to be the most common limiting factor in heart transplant patients. Angina cannot be used as a limiting factor in the donor heart of the recipient, because no angina is felt after denervation. The exercise can

be started at any intensity and gradually increased to 20 to 30 minutes duration with a 3- to 5-minute warm-up and 3- to 5-minute cool-down period.

Low-Level Exercise

The exercise program may need to be less intense during times of moderate to severe cardiac rejection, significant infection, severe pancreatitis, or for other unusual problems. During these periods, the exercise intensity should be discussed with and determined by the transplant team.

Summary

Physical therapy treatment after heart transplantation is still fairly new to many physical therapists. To effectively treat a cardiac transplant patient, a good understanding is needed of the following:

1. Surgical procedures
2. Exercise response in the denervated heart
3. Transplant ECG interpretation
4. Immunosuppressant drugs
5. General transplant precautions and contraindications of exercise

With this information, an appropriate physical therapy plan for each patient can be formulated and carried out.

REFERENCES

1. Cooley D, Frazier O, Kahan B: Cardiac transplantation with the use of cyclosporin A for immunologic suppression. Tex Heart Inst J 9:247, 1982
2. Reul G: Revascularization of the ischemic myocardium. p. 223. In Cooley D (ed): Techniques in Cardiac Surgery. WB Saunders, Philadelphia, 1984
3. Reul G: Present status of the internal mammary artery as a coronary artery bypass conduit at the Texas Heart Institute. Tex Heart Inst J 12:211, 1985
4. Gruntzig A, Senning A, Siegenthaler W: Nonoperative dilatation of coronary artery stenosis. N Engl J Med 301:61, 1979
5. Cooley D: Mitral valve repair and replacement. p. 206. In Cooley D (ed): Techniques in Cardiac Surgery. WB Saunders, Philadelphia, 1984
6. Stedman T: Stedman's Medical Dictionary. pp. 83 and 303. Williams & Wilkins, Baltimore, 1976
7. Reul G: Implantation of permanent cardiac pacemaker. p. 75. In Cooley D (ed): Techniques in Cardiac Surgery. WB Saunders, Philadelphia, 1984

8. Cohen L, Goldberg K, Peck V (eds): Clinical Pocket Manual: Cardiovascular Care. p. 156. Springhouse Corp., Springhouse, PA, 1985

9. Andreoli K, Fowkes V, Zipes D: Artificial cardiac pacemakers. p. 258. In Comprehensive Cardiac Care. CV Mosby, St. Louis, 1979

10. Carveth S, Chameides L, Creed J: Invasive therapeutic techiques. p. 205. In McIntyre K, Lewis A (eds): Textbook of Advanced Cardiac Life Support. American Heart Association, Dallas, 1981

11. Andreoli K, Fowkes V, Zipes D: Assessment of patients with coronary artery disease. p. 58. In Comprehensive Cardiac Care. CV Mosby, St. Louis, 1979

12. Simoons M: Introduction to imaging of the heart: contrast angiography, digital angiography, nuclear imaging echocardiography. p. 5. In Simoons M, Reiber J (eds): Nuclear Imaging in Clinical Cardiology. Martinus Nijhoff Publishing, Boston, 1984

13. Iskandrian A: Nuclear Cardiac Imaging: Principles and Applications. p. 131. FA Davis, Philadelphia, 1987

14. Irwin S: Clinical manifestations and assessment of ischemic heart disease. J Am Phys Ther Assoc 65:1806, 1985

15. Kattus A, Brock L, Bruce R: Exercise Testing and Training of Individuals with Heart Disease or at High Risk for its Development: A Handbook for Physicians. pp. 20 and 40. American Heart Association, Dallas, 1975

16. Kirkendall W, Feinleib M, Freis E: Recommendations for Human Blood Pressure Determination by Sphygmomanometers. p. 1146A. American Heart Association Committee Report, Dallas, 1979

17. Kirkendall W, Feinleib M, Freis E: Recommendations for Human Blood Pressure Determination by Sphygmomanometers. p. 1150A. American Heart Association Committee Report, Dallas, 1979

18. Kattus A, Brock L, Bruce R: Exercise Testing and Training of Individuals with Heart Disease or at High Risk for its Development: A Handbook for Physicians. p. 14. American Heart Association, Dallas, 1975

19. Irwin S: Abnormal exercise physiology. In Irwin S, Tecklin J (eds): Cardiopulmonary Physical Therapy. p. 55. CV Mosby, St. Louis, 1985

20. Astrand P, Rodahl K: Textbook of Work Physiology. McGraw-Hill, New York, 1977

21. Stedman T: Stedman's Medical Dictionary. p. 1567. Williams & Wilkins, Baltimore, 1976

22. Irwin S: Abnormal exercise physiology. p. 59. In Irwin S, Tecklin J (eds): Cardiopulmonary Physical Therapy. CV Mosby, St. Louis, 1985

23. Kleinfeld M, Castle P: Physical therapy for patients with abdominal or thoracic surgery. p. 250. In Irwin S, Tecklin J (eds): Cardiopulmonary Physical Therapy. CV Mosby, St. Louis, 1985

24. Dion W, Grevenow P, Pollock M: Medical problems and physiologic responses during supervised inpatient cardiac rehabilitation: the patient after coronary artery bypass grafting. Heart Lung 11:248, 1982

25. Vander A, Sherman J, Luciano D: Human Physiology—The Mechanisms of Body Function. p. 277. McGraw-Hill, New York, 1975

26. Okereke O, Frazier O, Cooley D, et al.: Cardiac transplantation: current results at the Texas Heart Institute. Tex Heart Inst J 11:228, 1984

27. Copeland J, Salomon N, Mammana R: Cardiac transplantation, a two-year experience. Heart Transplant 1:67, 1981

28. Bexton R, Hellestrand K, Cory-Pearce R: Unusual atrial potentials in a cardiac transplant recipient. Possible synchronization between donor and recipient atria. J Electrocardiol 16:313, 1983

29. Frazier O, Okereke O, Cooley D: Heterotopic heart transplantation in three patients at the Texas Heart Institute. Tex Heart Inst J 12:221, 1985

30. Novitzky D, Cooper C, Barnard C: The surgical technique of heterotopic heart transplantation. Ann Thorac Surg 36:476, 1983

31. Melvin K, Pollick C, Hunt S: Cardiovascular physiology in a case of heterotopic cardiac transplantation. Am J Cardiol 49:1301, 1982

32. Novitzky D, Cooper C, Rose A: The value of recipient heart assistance during severe acute rejection following heterotopic cardiac transplantation. J Cardiovasc Surg 25:287, 1984

33. Cooper D, Lanza R: Heart Transplantation: The Present Status of Orthotopic and Heterotopic Heart Transplantation. p. 305. MTP Press, Lancaster, England, 1984

34. Kahan B: Cyclosporin A: a new advance in transplantation. Tex Heart Inst J 9:253–265, 1982

35. Chandler L: Cardiac Transplantation Patient Handbook. pp. 14–15, 9–12. Texas Heart Institute, Houston, 1987

36. Radovancevic B, Frazier O, Gentry L: Successful treatment of invasive aspergillosis in a heart transplant patient. Tex Heart Inst J 12:233, 1985

37. Guyton A: Structure and Function of the Nervous System. p. 223. WB Saunders, Philadelphia, 1976

38. Leachman R, Leatherman L, Rochell D: Physiologic behavior of the transplanted heart in six human recipients. Am J Cardiol 23:123, 1969

39. Hammond H, Froelicher V: Normal and abnormal heart rate responses to exercise. Prog Cardiovasc Dis 27:271, 1985

40. Savin W, Haskell W, Schroeder F: Cardiorespiratory responses of cardiac transplant patients to graded, symptom-limited exercise. Circulation 62:55, 1980

41. Cooper D, Lanza R: Heart Transplantation: The Present Status of Orthotopic and Heterotopic Transplantation. p. 148. MTP Press, Lancaster, England, 1984

42. Cooper D, Lanza R: Heart Transplantation: The Present Status of Orthotopic and Heterotopic Transplantation. p. 149. MTP Press, Lancaster, England, 1984

43. Haskell W, Savin W, Schroeder J: Cardiovascular responses to handgrip isometric exercise in patients following cardiac transplantation. Circ Res, suppl. 1, 48:156, 1981

44. Savin W, Alderman E, Haskell W: Left ventricular response to isometric exercise in patients with denervated and innervated hearts. Circulation 61:897, 1980

45. Borg G, Noble B: Perceived Exertion: In Wilmore J (ed): Exercise and Sport Sciences Reviews. New York, Academic Press, p. 138, 1974

46. Sadowsky H, Rohrkemper K, Quon S: Rehabilitation of Cardiac and Cardiopulmonary Recipients. Appendix I. An Introduction for Physical and Occupational Therapists. Stanford University, Stanford, CA, 1986

47. Bexton R, Milne J, Cory-Pearce R, English T, Camm A: Effect of beta blockade on exercise response after cardiac transplantation. British Heart J 49(6):584, 1983

26 Community-Based Cardiac Rehabilitation

Gary E. Adams

Heart disease is the leading cause of death in the United States, with an annual mortality exceeding .5 million adults and an annual morbidity of 1.5 million adults. The prevalence of affected adults is nearly 5 million, indicating that many adults survive a heart attack and resume a relatively normal life-style.

The estimated economic cost of cardiovascular disease in the United States is nearly one-fourth of the federal 1987 deficit at 64.4 billion dollars, a staggering figure that few citizens can comprehend. The cost does not relate so much to medical costs but rather to the loss of income produced by those who work and the loss of federal, state, and local tax dollars that provide important programs in our society.[1]

The patient recovering from a life-threatening event has many questions about his role in the community, family, and society. Am I going to live much longer? Will I be able to return to work and provide for my family? Will my employer believe that I can carry out my job? Will I be able to resume sexual activity? Will my diet become bland and unpalatable? These and many other clinical, vocational, social, recreational, and domestic issues confront the typical heart attack patient and his family.

The process of educating patients about what has happened to them should begin soon after admittance to the hospital, ideally within 2 days in an uncomplicated case of recovery.

The history of cardiac rehabilitation programs is relatively brief, dating back to approximately 1965 when a few curious cardiologists in different areas of the country began adding cardiac patients to existing adult exercise-centered fitness programs. From their experiences and reports in the literature, other programs followed, generally addressing the rehabilitation problem usually 3 months postmyocardial infarction.[2]

Even though the history of cardiac rehabilitation is brief, it is safe to say that traditionally the nomenclature used to describe programs was phase I, phase II, and phase III to describe in-hospital, early outpatient electrocardiogram (ECG) monitored, and unmonitored gymnasium setting exercise-centered programs respectively.[3] The system of describing programs by phases, while helpful in the past, has undergone much change over the last 15 years and is no longer appropriate. Many patients do very well after a cardiac event and return to the domestic and vocational setting soon after myocardial infarction or bypass surgery. Therefore, it is suggested that patients be described as either inpatient or outpatients.[4]

Community programs in cardiac rehabilitation can be found in rural and urban communities throughout the United States, Canada, and many European countries. Most began in the outpatient setting and can be divided into two large groups: monitored and nonmonitored, depending on the level of direct ECG surveillance employed. Regardless of the type of program, it should include provision for both inpatient and outpatient periods of the recovery and rehabilitation.

The propose of a rehabilitation plan is to identify and try to modify areas of behavior that are thought to contribute to the developmental process

611

of atherosclerosis (i.e., smoking; poor diet resulting in elevated cholesterol, triglycerides and glucose; hypertension; inactivity; obesity, and many other avoidable or manageable risk factors. The plan should include a variety of information sources and, whether the program is carried out by one person or several professionals, it should address the factors of risk through dietary, recreational, and psychological intervention techniques known to improve the patient's physiological and psychological well-being. The techniques used to teach patients and ultimately the community should try to draw upon the resources within the setting to help individuals who need help when their lives are interrupted. Social service agencies and non-profit agencies, such as the Heart Association and Department of Human Resources with its vast array of state and federally funded services, should be brought together with the specific professional services in medicine and counseling to create an atmosphere of community effort—an atmosphere of community-based cardiac rehabilitation.

Cardiac rehabilitation should ideally be thought of as an extension of physician services. It should be able to complement the physician's role in the patient care and increase the servalence component of a medical plan. A plan should be designed to react quickly to difficulties that may arrise concerning the patient's stability; adherence to diet, activity, and drug regimens; and compliance with this and other programs prescribed by the patient's physician. Most communities would be best served by establishing a network of community-based programs that consolidate the professional services and talents within a community rather than the duplication of services that now exist in most communities. By creating cooperative medical adversary boards that could include physician representation for all segments of the cardiology profession within a community, every patient could benefit from the resources available within the entire community rather than the limited resources usually available within a single clinical setting.

How patients respond to the multi-intervention cardiac rehabilitation program varies depending on several independent needs. Nevertheless, most individuals are physically capable of resuming the physical demands of vocational tasks some-

where between 5 and 10 weeks after discharge from the hospital. After a person returns to gainful employment, it is hard to maintain compliance to the set time schedule usually associated with a cardiac rehabilitation program. For this reason, as well as reasons associated with perceived wellness, that the principal effective time course of cardiac rehabilitation is approximately 10 to 12 weeks after the myocardial event. By that time, deitary, vocational, psychological, recreational, domestic, and medical intervention should be well stabilized with a provision for a maintenance program in the long-term follow-up of the patient.

The process of beginning a program is complex. Anyone interested in beginning a cardiac rehabilitation program should consult with an established program and contract with consultants who can provide the plans and materials necessary to operate a successful program. Membership in the recently, created American Association of Cardiovascular and Pulmonary Rehabilitation, P.O. Box 5177, Madison, Wisconsin 53705-0177 is recommended. Miller et al.[4] have recently described several considerations in beginning a program. They discuss types of community programs, program implementation, identification of patient potential, program development, and financial support. They have drawn upon the ongoing program development project that was started through the sponsorship of the North Carolina Department of Vocational Rehabilitation and The North Carolina Heart Association nearly 15 years ago.

To be called community-based, the program should feature multi-intervention, be tailored to the needs of the community in general (rural or urban), and be accessible to a large segment of the community's population.

THE UNIVERSITY MEDICAL CENTER CARDIAC REHABILITATION PROGRAM: A COMMUNITY-BASED APPROACH

The University Medical Center of Southern Nevada is a 400 bed tertiary care, teaching facility located in Las Vegas, Nevada. It serves as the teaching center for the University of Nevada School of Medicine Residency Program in Surgery, Obstetrics and Gynecology, Family Medicine, and

Internal Medicine. The Cardiac Rehabilitation Program is a part of the Division of Cardiology. An elective in cardiac rehabilitation was established in 1984 for third year residents in internal medicine that gives resident physicians an opportunity to participate in all aspects of the program including testing, education, vocational counseling, dietary, consultation and social services. The inpatient and outpatient programs are administered by the same staff, which allows for a more ideal progression from hospitalization to outpatient participation. Many aspects of outpatient services can be started while the patient is in the hospital. The current program has been operating for 11 years and has served approximately 500 new patients a year and 4,000 continuing patients in the last 5 years.

The information presented in this description of the program at University Medical Center was obtained by Janet Bezner Pfau who presented it to the graduate faculty at Texas Women's University.[5]

Staff

The program director is an exercise physiologist with a doctoral degree. In addition, the cardiac rehabilitation staff consists of three cardiac rehabilitation nurses, a Navada state vocational rehabilitation counselor, a registered dietician, and a Master's degree level cardiac rehabilitation 12-month intern appointment.

Patients in the hospital are exposed to other *disciplines* in the course of the rehabilitation, such as

1. Social services
3. Physical therapists
3. Nurses (Intensive Care and Intermediate Care Units)
4. Counseling—marriage and family therapists and psychiatrists
5. Psychological counselors—by referral when considered by the staff to be necessary

Immediately after discharge from intensive care, patients are introduced to the rehabilitation concept in the Coronary Intermediate Care Unit and thus became familiar with the team early on in their recovery process.

The Program: Inpatient Phase

The inpatient phase of the program begins in the step-down unit, the Cardiac Intermediate Care Unit (IMC), where patients are monitored continuously by telemetry. The unit nurses conduct most of the rehabilitation, including exercise and education.

The program was designed by the rehabilitation staff and is processed by a standing order system, according to diagnosis. The patient types commonly involved are postmyocardial infarction, aortocoronary bypass surgery, valve replacement, agina pectoris, and postangioplasty.

The program director, a clinical exercise physiologist, makes daily rounds with each patient to monitor progress and to answer any questions and maintains frequent communications with the head nurse of the IMC about patient responses to activities.

Daily rounds are also made by the medical director, residents in internal medicine, the head nurse, and graduate student interns make daily rounds to examine and discuss each patient relative to drug therapy, pathophysiology, ECG interpretation, and treatment options.

Progress through the inpatient rehabilitation program is documented in the patient's chart by the unit nurses and the rehabilitation staff. Patients are given extensive written information that they may take home with them. In addition, they receive one-on-one instructions and demonstrations about their specific diagnosis or program.

The exercise program is a progression from bed exercise to standing exercises to ambulation to stationary cycling. Heart rate, blood pressure, and electrocardiographic responses are recorded before, during, and after each activity and are documented daily on a flow sheet. In addition, a Holter monitor study is routinely performed before discharge at the cycling stage of the activity program.

The activity program is intended to offset the deleterious effects of bed rest on the cardiorespiratory system. It is intended to preserve the patient's original level of physical conditioning before the myocardial attack. It is not designed to significantly improve functional aerobic capacity. Patients do, however, gain confidence soon after a myocardial event and discover that they are not disabled. This is an important consideration because it is a basic belief of the program staff that early intervention prevents the onset on psychological disability that results in physical disability so often found in patients who receive little guidance after hospitalization.

Education includes information about the patient's diagnosis and/or procedure (i.e., cardiac catheter or coronary angioplasty), the atherosclerotic process, pulse taking, facts about aerobic exercise, dietary information, stress management, home exercise, and the return to previous activities, such as automobile driving, sexual activity, grocery shopping, etc. Patients are evaluated on their knowledge *retention* with a written test before discharge.

The final step before discharge, when ordered by a physician, is the discharge treadmill exercise evaluation. The evaluation serves as the basis for the outpatient exercise prescription and is also used to determine the patient's readiness for discharge. The exercise test protocol is presented in this section under Exercise Testing.

The program is carried out by nurses, who do most of the teaching, monitoring of exercise responses, and reporting to attending physicians. They work as members of a multi-intervention team. The program director has successfully used nurses in a program that also includes a component of exercise therapy because he feels that nurses spend more time with the patients and are better able to monitor the patient's status and report information to the many attending physicians.

The Program: Outpatient Phase

The first stage of the outpatient program is called the cardiac rehabilitation monitored (CRM) session and occurs during the first week postdischarge in the IMC unit. Patients are monitored by telemetry while they ride a stationary bicycle for up to 15 minutes at a comfortable speed and resistance. Vital signs are recorded at rest, every 5 minutes, and during a cool-down. The purpose of these sessions is to detect any problems the patient may have during exercise before participation in the outpatient program, where there are up to 50 patients exercising at once. This setup allows close

monitoring of the patient and recognition of dysrhythmias, undesirable heart-rate and blood pressure response, and complaints of angina or shortness of breath. Attendance at two CRM sessions is encouraged (usually Monday and Wednesday), and the patient is enrolled in the outpatient program.

The outpatient program, conducted at a local YMCA, is a 12-week program offered at 7:00 and 8:00 a.m., three days a week. Patients are charged $11.00 per session. Patients are oriented to the program at the first session and are given information about pulse taking, recording their own vital signs, the purpose of warm-up and stretching exercise for conditioning, and an overview of the program structure.

Patients are encouraged to monitor and record their vital signs independently, seeking assistance when necessary. Blood pressures are routinely taken by a staff member on Mondays and ECGs are performed on Wednesdays and whenever needed during the sessions as indicated by the patients' responses to exercise. Flow sheets are reviewed periodically by the staff for undesirable responses and the ECG strips are analyzed weekly and recorded.

The exercise session begins with a 10 to 15 minute warm-up period of floor exercises and stretching, led by a staff member. Patients then have the option of walking indoors or out, stationary bicycling, and in certain instances, to weight training and rowing. Clocks are conveniently located throughout the YMCA and the entire rehabilitation staff participates in the exercise sessions in order to be close at hand should any problems or questions arise. This setup allows for frequent interaction between patients and staff and is when much of the education and counseling occurs. Spouses or significant others are welcomed and usually accompany the patient during the first few weeks of the program. The session ends with an optional volleyball game, with modifed rules, and cool-down stretching.

Once a week, on Fridays, exercise is conducted in the teaching pool. Using the same format of warm-up, training, and cool-down, patients are led through a 40 to 50 minute water exercise routine, with frequent pulse monitoring. This session is very popular with the patients and is perceived as a positive addition to the program because it

1. Breaks up the monotony of walking/cycling
2. Decreases the stress of weight bearing
3. Allows for easier movement of the body in space (important for patients with other neurological or orthopaedic problems)
4. Creates a great social experience
5. Alleviates fear of water recreation
6. Allows patients to raise heart rates without perceiving that they are working as hard as they would be if they were out of water

Postsurgical patients whose incisions are not yet healed may either ride the bicycle or walk around the pool area where they can also be monitored by the staff from the water. After the initial 12-week period is over, patients are given the option to continue the program at the same cost per session or they can join the YMCA, which is more economical in the long run. Many patients do continue the program, and several have been faithful attenders for years.

Dropout in this phase of rehabilitation is mostly the result of financial constraints. Either the patient must return to work and cannot afford the time or they are just unable to afford the program itself. The vocational rehabilitation counselor, who is employed by the state, covers the cost for many patients who are not insured. Because a large number of patients are uninsured, the vocational rehabilitation involvement is a big plus for the program. Another probable reason for the low attrition rate is that the patients are scheduled for follow-up treadmill tests at 5 and 10 weeks, 6 months, and 1 year postdischarge. The treadmill tests may serve as motivation for some patients and they also allow the staff to keep track of patients for at least a full year after discharge.

The accessibility of the staff during the outpatient sessions at the YMCA enabled the patients to seek advice very easily. Additionally, the exercise leaders are very knowledgeable about proper and improper stretching techniques, and their routines are biomechanically sound.

Exercise Testing

A majority of the staff's time is spent administering exercise tests, which may total 20 to 30 a week.

Testing is performed in the hospital on the same floor as the CCU and IMC units, where it is easily accessible to inpatients and outpatients.

As previously mentioned, inpatients usually undergo discharge evaluation on the day they leave the hospital. The protocol is a modified Bruce test, termed a low-level test.[6] A 4-MET maximum is allowed for this test, which translates into 6 minutes of exercise. Patients are properly prepped by a nurse and monitored with a 12-lead ECG. Resting rhythm, blood pressure, and heart rate are recorded in supine, sitting, and standing positions. In addition hyperventilation values are obtained in supine and sitting positions. Hyperventilation serves to mimic the potential breathing pattern during the test and thus enables identification of any problems before exercise.

Once the test begins, blood pressure and ECGs are recorded at every stage of exercise by the nurse and the ECG technician, respectively. The director administers the testing procedures and monitors the patient's response to the graded exercise to determine the end point of the evaluation. Testing is terminated according to the criteria set by the American College of Sports Medicine (ACSM) in Guidelines for Exercise Testing and Prescription.[7]

Patients are continuously monitored for 7 minutes after the test, in a supine position, with vital signs taken at 1, 3, 5, and 7 minutes. The supine position is assumed immediately after exercise to increase the end diastolic filling pressure.

The evaluation is then interpreted by the physiologist, and a cardiologist classifies the patient according to the New York Heart Association (NYHA) functional class criteria (Table 26-1).[2] The results of the test are used to calculate a target heart rate for the patient to use to exercise in the outpatient program. The Karvonen method is used at 80 percent of the achieved maximum heart rate.

Table 26-1 NYHA Functional Classification System

Class	METS	Peak O$_2$ Consumption
I	7	22–60
II	5–6	≤21
III	3–4	≤16
IV	≤2	7

(From Naughton and Hellerstein,[2] with permission.)

Follow-up testing is scheduled for approximately 5 weeks after discharge and consists of symptom-limited tests using a modified Bruce protocol. The same criteria exist for stopping the test, but the patient is allowed to achieve as a level as can be tolerated rather than a maximum 4 METS as stipulated in the discharge test. It is not uncommon for patients to achieve 7 METS and above on this evaluation, thus placing them in the NYHA functional class I category.

In addition to ECG, heart rate, and blood pressure monitoring in the tests, patients breathe into a Beckman CO_2/O_2 analyzer, which calculates VO_2, METS, and the respiratory quotient. A computer printout at each minute of exercise is useful to determine when the patient is reaching maximum capacity (by an respiratory quotient approaching 1.0) and also to compare the calculated MET level with the predicted MET level at the test. These measured values are recorded and are later entered into the computer for research purposes (Table 26-2).

After each follow-up test, a new target heart rate is calculated, and the patient is counseled regarding progress made. The patient is given the opportunity to ask questions at this time and is encouraged to do so. If the patient is in the outpatient program the new target heart rate (THR) is implemented there. Exercise testing with all levels of cardiac patients is a safe and very useful tool necessary to determine readiness for discharge from the hospital and to calculate accurate exercise prescriptions. In addition, the results enable the vocational rehabilitation counselor to assess the level of work to which the patient can safely return, as well as to determine physical work capacity. Finally, sequential testing allows the patient to see positive and negative changes in responses, which is a significant motivational factor for most.

Cardiac Vocational Rehabilitation

One goal of a successful rehabilitation program should include the return of the patient to gainful employment. The methods by which that goal is met may be indirect, such as attempting to improve functional capacity to a level high enough to speculate on a patient's possibility of success.

In 1978 the regional director of Vocational Rehabilitation (VR) within the Nevada Department of Human Resources, was asked to consider assigning all VR cardiac clients in the Las Vegas community to one counselor and consider placing the VR counselor in an office within the hospital along with the rest of the cardiac rehabilitation staff. After 5 years, the program conducted a study to measure the effect of assigning a state-employed vocational rehabilitation counselor to a hospital-based cardiac rehabilitation program by comparing the cardiac rehabilitation "experimental" program and the State Department of Vocational Rehabilitation "Control" Program regarding their abilities to return cardiac patients to gainful employment.[8] The Cardiac Rehabilitation Program, as previously described, includes several staff members representing a variety of disciplines. Intervention begins in the hospital, usually within 2 to 3 days after the cardiac event and is continued without interruption throughout the rehabilitation process for approximately 12 weeks. All staff members, including the vocational rehabilitation counselor, participate in the in-hospital phase of the rehabilitation process.

The study period from 1979 to 1983 compared the state's approach versus the hospital's approach

Table 26-2 Treadmill Protocol

Stage	MPH	Grade (%)	METS	Minutes
	Discharge Protocol: Low Level Test			
I	1.7	0	2	1.00
II	1.7	5	3	2.00
III	1.7	10	4	3.00
Totals			4	6.00

Stage	MPH	Grade (%)	METS	Minutes
	Modified Bruce Protocol: Symptom-Limited Test			
I	1.7	0	2	1.00
II	1.7	5	3	2.00
III	1.7	10	4	3.00
IV	2.0	10	5	2.00
V	2.5	10	6	2.00
VI	2.5	12.5	7	2.00
VII	3.0	12.5	8	2.00
VIII	3.0	15.0	9	2.00
IX	3.4	15.0	10.5	2.00
X	3.4	17.0	12	2.00

in the following areas:

1. The number of clients served
2. The number of cardiac patients successfully returned to gainful employment
3. The cost of successful case closure (NOTE: A case was considered successfully closed if the patient returned to work and was still working 6 weeks after the start of employment)

Comparisons are now being prepared for the state representing the years 1984 through 1988. The data continue to support the following findings and conclusions.

Over the 5-year study period, the number of cardiac patients served by the hospital increased from 50 clients per year to 80 clients per year, but the rest of the state remained constant from year to year at approximately 150 clients per year. The total number of clients served by the state and hospital was 1,106.

The percentage of clients served to successful case closure during the first 4 years for the hospital was 33 percent versus 16 percent for the state, and in the fifth year, the hospital successfully closed 42 percent of its cases, whereas the state closed 9 percent of its cases.

The mean per client cost (in dollars) was approximately the same for the state and the hospital program for the first 4 years. The success rate of successful case closures was significantly different as previously stated. In 1982 and 1983, for example, the state successfully closed 12 percent and 9 percent of their cases, whereas the hospital program successfully closed 27 percent and 42 percent, respectively. Additionally, the number of cases closed unsuccessfully in 1982 and 1983 by the State was 52 percent of all cardiac cases each year, whereas the unsuccessful rate for the hospital was 24 percent in 1982 and only 8 percent in 1983. The average cost per patient to successful case closure by the state and by the hospital was $181.

The success of the Hospital "Experimental" Program was demonstrated to the State and it was allocated more money to expand client services to include

1. The cost of blood analysis
2. Memberships in the YMCA on an as-needed basis

3. Transportation costs to the program
4. Use of the Holter monitor during the initial phase of returning to work
5. A monitored exercise program during the first week after hospitalization to screen patients for rhythm abnormalities and exercise responses

Why was the hospital program more successful in returning people to gainful employment? First, the emphasis in the state program has always been assessment and retraining. The hospital program, by contrast, has principally emphasized early physical restoration after a cardiac event. The restoration of physical fitness within the first 12 weeks after a cardiac event has resulted in employers preserving jobs with the expectation that the employee will return to work in a reasonably short period of time.

Second, the hospital emphasizes an in-hospital early intervention approach where a counselor visits the patient in his hospital room and decides with the patient and cardiac rehabilitation staff to open a case during the hospital stay. Frank discussions with the rehabilitation staff about what to expect from the patient coupled with communicating with the employer and employee about what each can expect has relieved a great deal of stress associated with job security. The state program, by comparison, has not emphasized early intervention and is, therefore, usually included in the care of a patient after a substantial period of time has elapsed (usually greater than 3 months). By the time state vocational rehabilitation is called in to help, the patient is

1. Unemployed
2. Psychologically impaired
3. Without sick time and payments
4. Without vacation time
5. Without most or all insurance benefits

Early intervention can help avoid these vocational and personal catastrophic events.

Third, in 1978 with the cooperation of the State Regional Director of Vocational Rehabilitation, most of the cardiac cases in the Las Vegas community were consolidated and responsibility for them was given to one vocational rehabilitation counselor who occupied an office within the cluster of offices set aside in the hospital for cardiac rehabilitation. Most of the cases of interest to vocational rehabilitation were presented at the "Experimental Hospital Program" because it is a county facility that accepts patients with a need for financial support from the state and county agencies.

During the course of the study the state decreased funding in a dramatic fashion. The allocation of money within the agency has been made, on large part, on the basis of previous successful case closures. The state has demonstrated a low success rate (15 percent over the 5-year study, 12 percent in 1982, and 9 percent in 1983). Accordingly, the state cut funding for training in general, which severely affected the money available for cardiac intervention. Since retraining was the only intervention approach used by the state for cardiac patients, few cases were opened and few cases were successfully closed.

A study of the vocational rehabilitation counselor in the team approach to exercise-centered cardiac rehabilitation and their effect on returning cardiac patients back to work resulted in the following conclusions and recommendations:

1. Early intervention (usually within 1 week) increased the rate of patients returning to work.
2. Physical restoration during the first 12 weeks after a cardiac event improves the rate of patients returning to work.
3. Assigning a vocational rehabilitation counselor to the cardiac rehabilitation staff improves the rate of patients returning to work.
4. The consolidation of most of the vocational rehabilitation clients in a community to become the responsibility of an actively participating cardiac vocational rehabilitation counselor improves the rate at which patients to return to work.

The following recommendations were made:

1. Consolidate the cardiac cases in a community and assign those cases to a cardiac rehabilitation vocational specialist.
2. Emphasize the fact that vocational rehabilitation is a consumer of services and teach counselors how to buy services within a community.
3. Begin the vocational rehabilitation process early while the patient is still in the hospital setting.
4. Educate physicians, especially cardiologists, that early vocational counseling through vocational rehabilitation can increase the percentage of patients returning to gainful employment.
5. Emphasize physical restoration rather than retraining as a means by which to improve the number of patients gainfully employed after a cardiac event.
6. Commit state financial support to start up community-based multi-intervention cardiac rehabilitation programs in urban and moderately large rural areas to carry out the basic programs needed to implement these recommendations.

MONITORED EXERCISE IN CARDIAC REHABILITATION

The necessity of using continuous monitoring in cardiac rehabilitation is a controversial issue at this time. A number of programs adhere to the following advice:

> Direct observation, including continuous electrocardiographic monitoring, is recommended at the onset of an exercise program for those with diagnosed coronary artery disease. Intermittent monitoring, when participants are responsible for determining their own heart rate, is less effective in recognizing cardiac abnormalities and, therefore, is less safe.[3]

A key point is that recognition of cardiac abnormalities by itself will not improve patient safety unless there is a subsequent alteration in the mode of management of the patients. These issues have been confused in the literature. In an article entitled "Dysrhythmia Detection in Myocardial Revascularization Surgery Patients," the authors[9] note that "80% of the patients exhibited significant dysrhythmia" where significant dysrhythmias were defined as: (1) Premature ventricular contractions (PVCs) greater than 10 per minute, (2) multifocal

PVCs, (3) coupled PVCs, (4) ventricular tachycardia, and (5) supraventricular tachycardia.

Although the abstract statement implied that something had been modified in the medical management of the patient, the text of the paper states the following:

> The administration of cardiac medications was relatively unchanged throughout the study and the higher prevalence of dysrhythmia found during GXT II (66th week of training) and ambulatory monitoring II were not related to changes in medications.[9]
>
> The greatest number of significant dysrhythmia were detected during ambulatory electrocardiography at 8 weeks post-myocardial revascularization surgery. These significant dysrhythmias were, interestingly, not necessarily associated with physical activity.[9]

There is, in fact, little evidence to support the idea that monitoring that results in the detection of arrhythmia actually resulted in a change in the medical management of the patient when looked at with regard to (1) a change in training approach, (2) a change in training intensity, or (3) a change in medications. An abundance of evidence in both the literature and by history to demonstrate that cardiac arrest in cardiac patients participating in well-supervised nonmonitored cardiac rehabilitation programs is rare.[10–12]

A Study of Monitoring

The University Medical Center Cardiac Rehabilitation Program conducted a study to observe the incidence of ventricular arrhythmia during exercise in a group of diagnosed heart disease patients and to record alterations in the medical management resulting from electrocardiographic monitoring.[13,14]

The study period was 3 years. During that time, 300 consecutive patients were evaluated on a motor-driven treadmill 1 day before discharge at no more than a 4-MET load and then assigned a starting date to begin a monitored cycle ergometer exercise surveillance program.[15]

Each patient performed cycle ergometry for 3 days during the first week following discharge. The duration of the exercise was a continuous 15-minute ride per session. The intensity was approximately 85 percent of the highest heart rate achieved during the discharge treadmill evaluation.

Each patient was surveilled during the cycling program just described and then entered a YMCA-based, medically supervised program for approximately 11 weeks. There were two groups from within the 300 consecutive patients: 245 patients representing the no-arrhythmia group and 55 patients representing the arrhythmia group. No attempt was made to differentiate between complex and noncomplex arrhythmia or to label the arrhythmias as significant or nonsignificant. Patients were divided into one of the two groups on the basis of exhibiting one or more ventricular ectopic beats either at rest or in exercise during one of the three monitored exercise sessions.

During the discharge treadmill evaluation, the measured oxygen uptake was determined on 112 patients in the no-arrhythmia group and 33 patients in the arrhythmia group.

When compared to predicted MET values for speed and grade, our patients responded normally. The workload, however, represented a maximal effort for many and near maximal effort for most.

Respiratory exchange ratio values serve as a guideline in this functionally fair to poor group. When ratios exceeded .90 the onset of work intolerance closely followed. In the present study, the mean respiratory exchange ratio was .90 and .91 for the no-arrhythmia and arrhythmia groups respectively. The differences were not statistically significant.

The cycle training intensity was 15 to 18 miles per hour, zero resistant, which represented 84 and 89 percent of the highest heart rate at discharge for the no-arrhythmia and arrhythmia groups respectively.

The intensity presented as a mean percentage of the oxygen uptake at discharge was 71 and 73 percent for the no-arrhythmia and arrhythmia groups. The differences again were not significant.

Of the 300 patients who participated, 245 did not exhibit ventricular arrhythmias, but 55 patients did demonstrate some form of ventricular arrhythmia. Of the 245 patients who did not demonstrate arrhythmias while on exercise, 20 were on antiarrhythmic therapy and 225 were not. None of the patients in the arrhythmia group were on antiarrhythmic therapy throughout the study.

One hundred nine patients in the no-arrhythmia group and 17 in the arrhythmia group who entered the outpatient YMCA centered Cardiac Rehabilitation Program remained for at least 1 year. Arrhythmia recognition was monitored by the staff and patients by palpation and through the use of defibrillator paddles.

Arrhythmia was documented in 20 patients in the no-arrhythmia group and 11 individuals in the arrhythmia group. Two individuals, not previously on antiarrhythmia medication and from within the no-arrhythmia group were found to have frequent multifocal PVCs associated with dizziness that required medication; therefore, two patients received alterations in their medical management due to arrhythmia recognition during the study.

There were no cardiovascular accidents (cardiac arrest) in the supervised outpatient program during 1 year of follow-up.

There were two deaths during the course of the study. The subjects died while sleeping within 6 days after discharge and before entering the YMCA centered program. Both patients exhibited the following similarities:

1. Their treadmill electrocardiograms recorded no arrhythmias at rest and exercise and one bigeminal complex during 7 minutes of continuous monitoring during supine recovery.
2. Twenty-four-hour Holter studies revealed occasional PVCs, which did not increase with physical exertion.
3. ECG monitoring during cycling in the first week after discharge showed occasional PVCs at rest, less than 10 per minute and no arrhythmias in exercise.
4. The occasional PVCs at rest along with treadmill and Holter data were reported to the referring cardiologist resulting in no change in medications.

In summary, our group responded as expected for predicted values, worked to almost maximal levels as indicated by respiratory exchange ratio data, achieved peak heart rates of approximately 120 beats per minute, and worked at 70 percent of their demonstrated oxygen uptake and approximately 85 percent of the peak heart rate at discharge. The differences between the two groups were not statistically or physiologically significant. Therefore, a group of 300 consecutive patients worked at moderate to heavy workloads for 15-minute periods monitored during their first week after discharge and responded normally.

We concluded that (1) the incidents of ventricular arrhythmia after myocardial infarction or cardiac bypass surgery is low, (2) the detection of ventricular arrhythmia in cardiac rehabilitation programs rarely result in an alteration of the medical management of the patient, and (3) patients can safely exercise at relatively high loads soon after discharge from the hospital.

This study supports the concept that the indiscriminate use of long-term monitoring during exercise is probably not necessary in the prudent medical management of most patients.

Finally, to whose benefit does so much monitoring contribute? Serious questions still lie unanswered after almost a decade of common application. Where is the evidence that supports the "unsafe" label of nonmonitored programs found in the opening quote of this presentation and serves as a guideline to justify the widespread use of monitoring.

The knowledgable clinician should ask the following questions before adopting a strategy of continuous monitoring for cardiac rehabilitation.

1. How does monitoring benefit the patient medically?
2. How does monitoring bring about a change in the medical management of cardiac patients?
3. Does monitoring prevent cardiovascular accidents?

We await the carefully controlled study that will give us a clear understanding of the single most expensive issue now facing third-party providers who purchase cardiac rehabilitation services.

CONCLUSION

Cardiac rehabilitation is most often an exercise-centered approach to intervention medicine. It provides a vehicle by which assessment can lead to intervention methods intended to bring about desirable and perhaps some measurable changes. Here lies a dilemma in the profession. What changes do we report? What is important to report?

We have seen a variety of physiological parameters reported in the literature that leave us with the job of speculating about whether a patient is, in fact, able to resume a satisfactory life style. The ability to report how many patients returned to gainful employment probably tells us more about the effect of cardiac rehabilitation on reducing disability and handicap than the common methods of reporting the effects of rehabilitation in terms of a statistical association to morbidity and mortality.

Patients do need answers to their questions. The questions are not always the same for each patient and, therefore, several areas of preparedness within the program structure are important. It should be a model of multi-intervention, a patient-centered approach recognizing that most of the disability after a cardiac event is psychological and that much of the disability can be erased by allowing patients to discover in an exercise-centered setting that they are, in fact, not disabled. While the process of discovery within the patient unfolds, patients can and should examine identifiable factors within each area to determine if modification is recommended.

An attempt has been made to demonstrate the usefulness of multi-intervention. Perhaps one day, the model of multi-intervention will be recognized for its unique contribution in addressing the patient as a complex being in need of assessment and intervention in many areas. One day, we may look back and find it difficult to remember that this model of intervention was applied in such a limited way. When that day does arrive, in the not too distant future, the team approach to patient centered multi-intervention rehabilitation will be the practice of rehabilitation medicine.

REFERENCES

1. American Heart Association: Heart Facts. American Heart Association, Dallas, 1987
2. Naughton JP, Hellerstein HK: Exercise Testing and Exercise Training in Coronary Heart Disease. Academic Press, Orlando, FL, 1973
3. Wilson PK, Farkoy PS, Froelicher VF: Cardiac Rehabilitation, Adult Fitness, and Exercise Testing. Lea & Febiger, Philadelphia, 1981
4. Miller H, Ribisl P, Adams G, et al: Community programs of cardiac rehabilitation. p. 437. In Pollock ML, Schmidt DH (eds): Heart Disease and Rehabilitation. 2nd Ed. John Wiley & Sons, New York, 1986
5. Pfau JB: The University Medical Center of Southern Nevada Cardiac Rehabilitation Program Practicum Report. P.T. 5103. p. 1. Texas Women's University. Feb. 14, 1987
6. Adams GE, Marlon AM, Quinn EJ: O_2 uptake in cardiac patients during treadmill testing. CVP Feb/March, 1980
7. American College of Sports Medicine: Guidelines for Exercise Testing and Prescription. 3rd Ed. Lea & Febiger, Philadelphia, 1986
8. Kostelac JM, Adams GE, Marlon AM, et al: The vocational rehabilitation counselor in the team approach to exercise centered cardiac rehabilitation: Their effect on returning cardiac patients back to work. Med Sci Sports Exerc (abstract) 16:2, 1984
9. Dolatowski RP, Squires RW, Pollack M, et al: Dysrythmia detection in myocardial revascularization surgery patients. Med Sci Sports Exerc 15(4):281, 1983
10. Franklin B: The role of electrocardiographic monitoring in cardiac exercise programs. J Cardiovasc Rehabil 3(11):806, 1983
11. Haskell WL: Cardiovascular complications during exercise training of cardiac patients. Circulation 57(5):920, 1978
12. Van Camp S, Peterson R: Cardiovascular complications of outpatient cardiac rehabilitation programs. JAMA 256:1160, 1986
13. Adams GE, Allen P, Pokroy N, et al: The effects of an exercise centered multidisciplinary intervention program on the chronic renal failure patient. Abstracts of the Western Dialysis and Transplant Society. 11th Annual Meeting. Oct 24–26, 1980
14. Adams GE, Marlon AM, Quinn EJ, Kaufman JA: The incidence of ventricular arrythmia and alterations in medical management of cardiac patients resulting from electrocardiographic monitoring during exercise. Int J Sports Med 6(4):239, 1985
15. Muth JW, Adams GE, Kaufman JA, et al: Exercise centered cardiac rehabilitation: the effects of monitoring the ECG on the medical management of the exercise plan. Med Sci Sports Exerc (abstract no. 409) suppl., 18:S83, 1986

27 Pulmonary Pathology and Medical Management

Grace Moffat Minerbo

Pulmonary diseases are one of the ten leading causes of death, and bronchogenic carcinoma of the lungs is the leading cause of death from cancer in the United States.[1,2] Finally, whatever the primary disease, the immediate cause of death most often is lung disease: pulmonary edema, pulmonary embolism, or pneumonia.

The importance of the pulmonary system cannot be overstated. Lung disease in the United States is the fifth (pneumonia and influenza) and sixth (chronic obstructive pulmonary disease [COPD]) leading cause of death in males of all ages and is the fifth and eighth leading cause of death in females of all ages.[1] Pulmonary disease may have an effect on other body organs, while diseases in other body organs may have an effect on the lungs.

PATHOPHYSIOLOGY

Blood-Gas Exchange

The interface between air and blood in the lungs is approximately 0.2 μm thick (Fig. 27-1).[3] It is the only place where gases may be effectively exchanged. The alveolar membrane is composed of two types of epithelial cells. The epithelial cells involved in the gaseous exchange are the more numerous *type I* cells: flat squamous cells with long, thin cytoplasmic processes. The epithelial cells that secrete surfactant are the less numerous but larger *type II* cells. The surfactant reduces the surface tension of the tissue fluid lining the alveolar sacs, allowing air to inflate the alveolar sacs easily during inspiration. The lower surface tension of the alveolar tissue fluid during expiration allows the alveoli to become smaller but not collapse with each breath. Surfactant principally consists of lecithin with phospholipids. Inadequate surfactant levels in the fetal lung are determined by the low ratio of lecithin to sphingomyelin in the aminotic fluid.[4] The lower the ratio, the more immature the lung.

Pulmonary Function Tests

Pulmonary function tests are numerous, but the most common involve spirometry and arterial blood-gas analyses.[5] The most widely used pulmonary function tests (Fig. 27-2) evaluates ventilation, whereas arterial blood-gas analyses primarily evaluate perfusion. It is important to recognize, however, that these pulmonary function tests are rarely useful in making a specific diagnosis. The tests provide supportive data for the documentation of the physiological state of the respiratory system in disease and in health.

Ventilation-Perfusion Relationships

There are a number of mechanisms that contribute to bring air into the lungs so that exchange of gases can take place. The difference in air pressure between the alveoli in the cavity and the external environment (atmosphere) plays a vital role. Air moves in and out of the lungs because of pressure gradients established. The mechanical function of moving air in and out of the lungs is known as ventilation. Perfusion refers to the blood flow in the capillaries. When the ventilation-perfusion ratio of the lungs is matched, lung function is normal. Mismatching of ventilation with perfusion leads to arterial *hypoxemia*, secondary *erythrocytosis*, and *cor pulmonale* with congestive heart failure.[6]

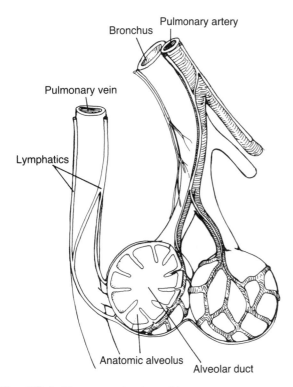

Fig. 27-1 Diagrammatic view of lung structures. A, alveolus; AD, alveolar duct; RB, respiratory bronchiole; TB, terminal bronchiole.

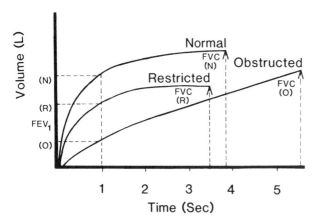

Fig. 27-2 Pulmonary function tests. A diagrammatic view of the relationship between forced vital capacity (FVC) and forced expiratory volume in 1 second (FEV$_1$) in normal individuals (N) and in individuals with either obstructed (O) or restricted (R) lung disease. (From Rothstein JM [ed]: Measurement in Physical Therapy. p. 232. Churchill Livingstone, New York, 1985, with permission.)

Blood-Gas Analysis

Standard values obtained from blood-gas analyses of normal arterial blood are shown in Table 27-1. There are several general rules for evaluating arterial blood-gas values. First, as the bicarbonate ions (HCO$_3^-$) increase in the blood, the pH of the blood increases, resulting in alkaline serum. As the arterial carbon dioxide (PaCO$_2$) increases, the pH of the blood decreases, resulting in acidic serum. For every increase of 1 mmHg of the PaCO$_2$, the pH decreases by 0.0075 (acidic serum). For every decrease of 1 mmHg of the PaCO$_2$, the pH increases by 0.0075 (alkaline serum).

$$\uparrow HCO_3^- \rightarrow \ \uparrow pH \ (\text{alkaline})$$

$$\uparrow PaCO_2 \rightarrow \ \downarrow pH \ (\text{acidic})$$

Acid-Base Balance

Fluid and electrolyte balances are maintained in healthy individuals. Electrolyte imbalances usually occur secondary to other diseases (e.g., ketoacidosis in diabetes mellitus) or as secondary complications of drug therapy in the medical management of a disease. The normal pH of arterial blood is 7.40 ± 0.04, producing a normal pH range of 7.36 to 7.44 (Table 27-1) (Fig. 27-3A). When the blood pH drops below the normal range, the patient is said to be in *acidosis* (acidic pH is less than 7.36). Conversely, when the blood pH increases above the normal range, the patient is said to be in *alkalosis* (alkaline pH is greater than 7.44). Neither acidosis nor alkalosis is compatible with life. The blood pH imbalance, also known as the acid-base imbalance, must be corrected. Normally, the kidneys regulate blood levels of HCO$_3^-$ while the lungs regulate blood levels of CO$_2$, preventing

Table 27-1 Standard Arterial (Normal) Blood-Gas Values

Function	Normal Values
Hematocrit	40–45%
pH	7.40 ± 0.04 (7.36–7.44)
PaCO$_2$	40 ± 4 mmHg
PaO$_2$	80 mmHg
HCO$_3^-$	24 (23–27 mEq/L)
O$_2$ saturation	95%

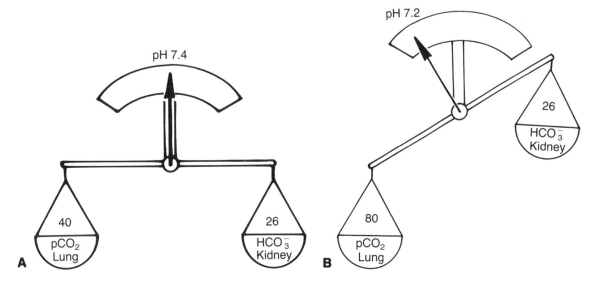

Fig. 27-3. (**A**) Normal blood-gas values. The lungs function to maintain normal PCO_2 levels between 40 and 44 mmHg. The kidneys function to maintain normal HCO_3^- levels between 23 and 27 mEq/L. (**B**) Uncompensated respiratory acidosis. When serum PCO_2 levels increase and the serum O_2 levels decrease, the pH decreases, resulting in serum acidosis. Since the lung is responsible for the increase in PCO_2, this type of acidosis is known as respiratory acidosis.

acidosis and alkalosis from occurring. Acidosis and alkalosis have a metabolic or respiratory origin.[7,8]

Uncompensated Respiratory Acidosis

Pulmonary CO_2 retention results in *uncompensated respiratory acidosis* (Fig. 27-3B) in which the pH of the blood is lowered to acidic levels. This is accomplished by poor ventilation that induces *hypercapnea* and *hypoxia*, leading to respiratory acidosis—the cardinal signs of respiratory failure. There are several pathophysiological conditions that may result in the production of respiratory acidosis. Alveolar hypoventilation occurs in respiratory acidosis owing to muscle weakness induced by diseases such as poliomyelitis, muscular dystrophy, or hypothyroidism or may be drug induced, for example, by sedatives, morphine, or anesthesia. COPD (emphysema and chronic bronchitis) causes hypoxemia because of regional hypoventilation resulting from obstructive lesions in the airways. In emphysema, loss of septal walls further contributes to this condition. In respiratory acidosis, patients normally develop compensatory mecha-

nisms to reverse the low levels of O_2 and high levels of CO_2 in the blood.

Compensated Respiratory Acidosis

Compensated respiratory acidosis allows the pH of the blood to return to its normal neutral value of 7.4 (Fig. 27-4). The kidney attempts to lower CO_2 blood levels by forming more HCO_3^- and excreting more H^+ ions (Figure 27-4). However, it takes several days for the kidneys to compensate for respiratory acidosis. The increased $PaCO_2$ depresses the respiratory center of the medulla. Hypoxia stimulates the respiratory centers of the carotid and aortic bodies to increase breathing. Therefore, if the patient is administered O_2 while in respiratory acidosis, then the respiratory centers will be deprived of the remaining stimulus for breathing, which could lead to CO_2 narcosis and death. Hence, O_2 therapy is *not* recommended for treatment of respiratory acidosis. The treatment for respiratory acidosis is improved ventilation through intubation and mechanical ventilation in acute respiratory failure.

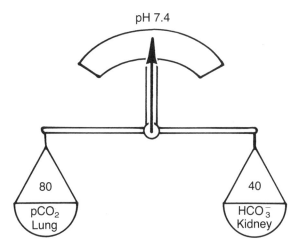

Fig. 27-4 Compensated respiratory acidosis. To compensate for respiratory acidosis, the kidneys increase the serum levels of HCO_3^-. It takes several days for the kidneys to compensate for respiratory acidosis.

Respiratory Alkalosis

Hyperventilation causes *respiratory alkalosis* with an increase in the pH of the blood (Fig. 27-5). Through stimulation of the respiratory center, the lungs blow off more CO_2 than normal, thereby

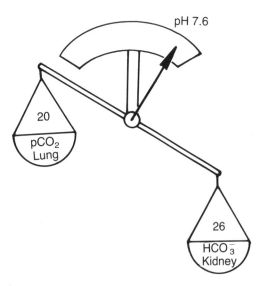

Fig. 27-5 Uncompensated respiratory alkalosis. When serum PCO_2 levels decrease, the serum pH increases, resulting in serum alkalosis. Since the lung is responsible for the increase in PCO_2, this type of alkalosis is known as respiratory alkalosis.

decreasing serum CO_2 levels and increasing the pH to alkaline levels. There are many factors that cause hyperventilation and thus respiratory alkalosis. Hyperventilation is common with anxiety, hysteria, some pulmonary diseases (e.g., asthma and emphysema), and drug use. One of the most common drugs known to induce respiratory alkalosis shortly after a drug overdose is taken is aspirin. Later, as more aspirin is absorbed into the blood, metabolic acidosis occurs. To compensate for the decrease in serum CO_2, carbonic anhydrase in the lungs then breaks down more carbonic acid (H_2CO_3) to replenish the CO_2 lost by hyperventilation. The kidney compensates by excretion of the HCO_3^- along with K^- and Na^+ ions, which in turn may lead to hypokalemia and dehydration. The simplest method to treat hyperventilation is to put a bag over the patient's head and have the patient rapidly inhale and exhale air to increase CO_2 levels in the blood and thereby decrease pH to the normal range.

Pulmonary Edema

It is important to prevent pulmonary hypertension because it can lead to pulmonary edema. When this occurs, fluid seeps out of the capillaries, accumulating in the interstitial tissue of the lung and then in the alveolar sacs. Pulmonary edema interferes with gaseous exchange by interfering with the diffusion pathway between the alveolus and the capillary. Pulmonary edema is a common complication of congestive heart disease, pneumonia, and many other lung disorders. It occurs when the normal mean pulmonary hydrostatic blood pressure of 15 mmHg exceeds the normal colloidal osmotic pressure of the blood of 25 mmHg.

Blood Hydrostatic Pressure (Normal = 15 mmHg)

> Colloidal Osmotic Pressure (Normal

= 25 mmHg) = Pulmonary Edema

Acute pulmonary edema occurs with extravascular fluids accumulate in the interstitial tissue and alveolar air sacs of the lungs. It is a grave emergency that is fatal if not promptly treated. Pulmonary edema results from an increase in the pressure of the blood flowing through the pulmonary vessels secondary to left heart failure. Left heart failure leads to an increase in pulmonary venous blood pressure, followed by an increase in pulmonary capillary blood pressure that in turn makes the thin capillary walls of the lungs more permeable. Fluids leave the lung capillaries, primarily because of the increase in hydrostatic pressure of the blood, to fill the interstitial spaces of the lung. If pulmonary pressure continues to remain high, then interstitial fluid seeps out of the lung parenchyma to enter the alveolar air spaces, causing pulmonary edema. If pulmonary pressure continues to increase, pulmonary hypertension occurs, eventually resulting in right heart failure.[9]

Cor Pulmonale

When pulmonary artery pressures are higher than the pumping capacity of the right ventricle, the right ventricle dilates in its effort to maintain stroke volume. Cor pulmonale develops in response to right heart failure in which right ventricular enlargement occurs in response to pulmonary hypertension. Left heart failure can also increase blood pressure in the pulmonary vasculature but is excluded in the definition of cor pulmonale. In the United States, COPD is the most common cause of cor pulmonale.

Right heart failure results in venous congestion, peripheral edema, ascites, and Na^+ and H_2O retention. Systemic veins become distended. In particular, the increase in the jugular venous pressure is highly visible to the trained eye. Hypertrophy of the liver then follows in right heart failure.

Pulmonary Hypertension

Pulmonary hypertension is present when the pulmonary artery blood pressure rises higher than normal in response to cardiac output.[10] The etiology of pulmonary hypertension is diverse. Pulmonary artery blood pressure may increase by several mechanisms:

1. Lung vasoconstriction resulting from acidosis or hypoxia.
2. Loss of blood vessels resulting from lung diseases, for example, emphysema.
3. Obstruction of blood vessels of the lungs by thrombi, emboli, and parasites.
4. Increase in pulmonary venous pressure caused by left ventricular heart failure.

The most common cause of pulmonary hypertension is pulmonary artery vasoconstriction secondary to hypoxia and acidosis. The lung vasculature is unique in that acidosis and hypoxia induce vasoconstriction in the pulmonary arteries. Arteries in the remainder of the body do not respond in a similar manner to hypoxia and acidosis.

Pulmonary Thromboemboli (Pulmonary Emboli)

Blood clots or thrombi can form in any part of the cardiovascular system, but the most common site is in the deep veins of the lower extremities where approximately 90 percent of the thrombi form. The second most common site of origin of venous thrombi is the right heart.

When the thrombus is dislodged from its site of origin, either as a single entity or as fragmented parts, and is carried by the blood to other parts of the body where it lodges in a blood vessel causing its obstruction, it is known as an embolism. An embolism most commonly is derived from a thrombus, therefore, it is known as a thromboembolus. If the thromboembolus is lodged in a blood vessel in the lung, it is known as a pulmonary thromboembolus. Pulmonary emboli are primarily derived from venous thrombi.[4]

Some patients who develop pulmonary emboli whether in or out of the hospital die suddenly. However, approximately 80 percent of thrombi that form resolve spontaneously through the fibrinolytic system without medical intervention. The populations most susceptible to pulmonary embolus formation are immobilized, bedridden patients and postoperative patients in whom venous stasis is prevalent.

To a lesser extent, emboli may be produced by droplets of fat after fractures of the diaphysis of long bones, which allow fatty bone marrow to enter the blood. Amniotic fluid during childbirth may become an embolus in the maternal circulation. Eighty-five to 90 percent of these patients die during childbirth. In caisson disease (the bends), deep sea divers develop gas emboli if they ascend to the surface too rapidly. Nearly all myocardial infarctions result from thrombi or emboli occluding the coronary arteries of the heart, usually in conjunction with atherosclerosis.

Atelectasis

Atelectasis, the mechanical collapse of the lung, lobes, or lobules, occurs by several mechanisms (Fig. 27-6):[11]

1. *Congenital.* The lung is in its unexpanded state before birth and remains so after birth.
2. *Pneumothorax.* When air enters the pleural cavity either by an external wound (trauma) or by a tear in the lung, the lung collapses. This is known as pneumothorax or air in the thoracic cavity. In pneumothorax, the mediastinum is pulled toward the normal lung.
3. *Obstruction.* When the smaller air passageway becomes completely obstructed (e.g., by a mucous plug, tumor, peanut or popcorn, etc.), air trapping occurs, leading to the collapse of the affected lung. Resorption of the air induces atelectasis in focal areas. In obstructive atelectasis, the mediastinum is pulled toward the side of the collapsed lung.
4. *Compression.* Atelectasis may be caused by the accumulation of fluids or a tumor in the pleural cavity that in turn compresses the adjacent lung. In compressive atelectasis, the mediastinum is pulled toward the normal lung.

Emphysema

Emphysema is the permanent over-expansion of the distal air spaces of the lungs accompanied by the breakdown of the septal walls of the lung (Fig. 27-7). The alveoli lose their ability to recoil with respiration, resulting in expiratory airflow resistance. Most commonly, emphysema is due to cigarette smoking or inhalation of polluted urban air.[11]

Emphysema is the opposite of atelectasis. When atelectasis occurs in a lobe(s) of the lung or in the

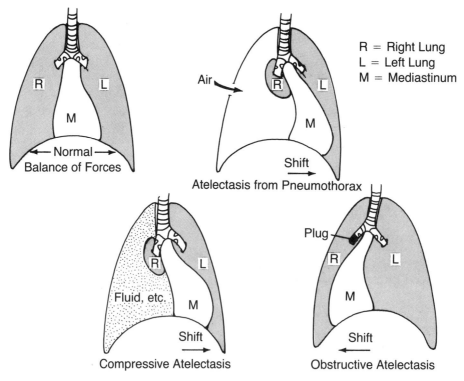

Fig. 27-6 Diagram of mechanism of atelectasis. In atelectasis from pneumothorax, the mediastinum is pulled toward the normal side of the lungs. In compressive atelectasis, the mediastinum is pulled toward the normal side of the lung. In obstructive atelectasis, the mediastinum is pulled toward the side of the atelectasis.

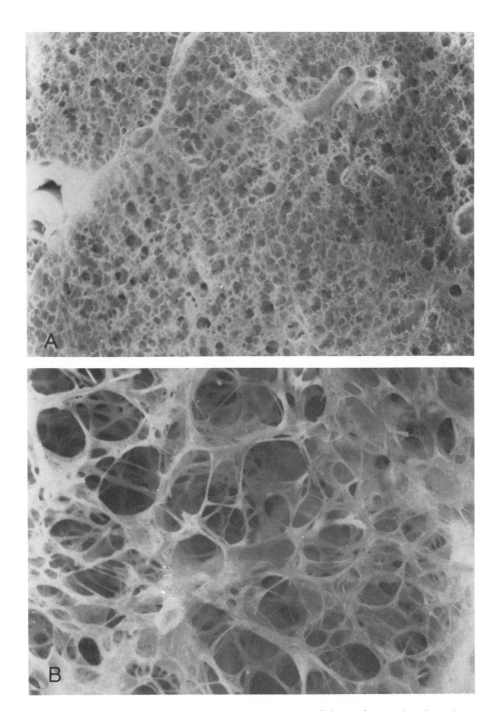

Fig. 27-7 Normal and emphysematous lungs. Appearance of slices of normal and emphysematous lungs. (**A**) Normal; (**B**) panlobular emphysema reveals the broken alveolar walls resulting in the expanded air spaces. (From West,[11] with permission.)

right or left lung, the affected lobe(s) or lung is made smaller as a result of its mechanical collapse. The normal lung will overinflate to expand to fill the space. Thus, emphysema may be compensatory to atelectasis, to fibrosis in which the lung shrinks owing to connective tissue deposition, or to surgical ablation of the lung. Emphysema also may occur secondary to an enlargement of the chest cavity.

Partial obstruction of the air passageways is another method by which emphysema may occur. With inspiration, air enters the alveolar sacs. With expiration, the lack of elastic recoil prevents most of the air from leaving, resulting in the over-expansion of the alveolar sacs. The obstructing substance may be a mucous plug, for example. Smooth muscle spasms in the distal bronchioles narrow the lumen of the bronchioles, as in asthma. Fibrosis of the bronchioles reduces lumen size. The narrower the bronchiole, the greater the air trapping in the lungs.[12]

PATHOLOGY

Emphysema

The destruction of the lung accompanied by the loss of elasticity of the alveolar sacs by smoking and inhalation of polluted air is the most common cause of emphysema.[4,10] Pathologically, there are two different types of emphysema: centrilobular and panlobular. In centrilobular emphysema, the respiratory bronchioles predominantly are dilated, while the alveolar sacs are spared. Consequently, the central portion of the lung lobules dilates, while the peripheral alveolar sacs remain relatively normal. This common form of emphysema is associated with smoking and inhalation of polluted air (Fig. 27-8). In panlobular emphysema, dilatation of the alveolar sacs becomes prominent (Fig. 27-8). However, dilatation occurs throughout the acinus, that is, alveolar sacs, alveolar ducts, and respiratory bronchioles are dilated. Consequently, in panlobular emphysema, all portions of the lung lobules are involved, producing a diffuse emphysema. Panlobular emphysema is an autosomal recessive hereditary disease resulting from a deficiency of α-1-antitrypsin enzyme.

Patients with severe emphysema are known as "pink puffers" because they have a pink complexion and hyperventilate. These patients maintain a relatively normal O_2 saturation through hyperventilation and thus do not become hypoxic, thereby retaining a pink complexion; they are puffing because of hyperventilation. This compensatory action allows the body to match ventilation with perfusion. Both centrilobular and panlobular emphysema are asymptomatic until the disease is well advanced.

Chronic Bronchitis

Chronic bronchitis is produced by the chronic inflammation of the lung bronchioles and usually the bronchi as well.[12] The inflammatory response results in excess mucus secretions. The airway passages are compromised further by the swelling or edematous condition of their mucosal lining. Thus, in chronic bronchitis, obstruction of the air passages results from inflammation and edema of the walls in addition to excess mucus production. The main symptom of chronic bronchitis is a chronic or recurrent productive cough. To be classified as having chronic bronchitis, the patient must have the cough a minimum of 3 months per year for at least two successive years. However, other causes of a productive cough must be ruled out, for example, pulmonary infection, neoplasms, and heart disease. Chronic bronchitis commonly precedes and accompanies centrilobular emphysema.

Patients with chronic bronchitis are known as "blue bloaters" because they are cyanotic and edematous. The airway passages are significantly narrowed, resulting in a striking mismatch of ventilation and perfusion. This leads to arterial hypoxemia, hypercapnia, respiratory acidosis, and secondary erythrocytosis including airway infections and obesity.

The term COPD is applied to patients who have emphysema (centrilobular or panlobular) or chronic bronchitis or both simultaneously. The mechanism of airway obstruction differs between these two COPDs, but the results are the same: chronic obstruction of the air passageways. In emphysema, the lung parenchyma is partly de-

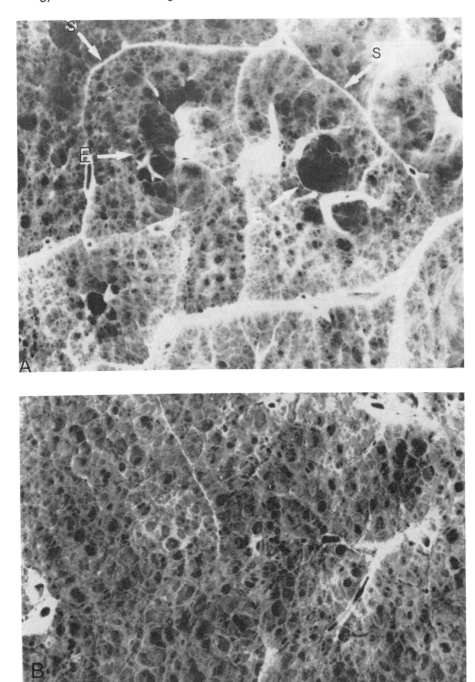

Fig. 27-8 Centriacinar (centrilobular) and panacinar (panlobular) emphysema. Appearance of lung slices in centrilobular (**A**) and panlobular (**B**) emphysema. Each photograph is magnified five times. Barium was injected into the arteries, which are consequently seen as dense white areas. Emphysematous (E) areas are seen adjacent to the blood vessels in centrilobular emphysema (**A**). In panlobular emphysema (**B**), there is diffuse involvement of the lung since the alveoli and alveolar ducts are primarily involved. The septal (S) wall is seen. (From Robbins and Kumar,[4] with permission.)

stroyed outside the air passageways, significantly reducing radial traction and causing the airways to narrow. In chronic bronchitis, the airways are obstructed by excessive mucus secretions, bronchospasms, and the inflammatory thickening of the mucosal membrane lining the air passageways.

Bronchiectasis

Bronchiectasis is a congenital or acquired disorder of the bronchi in which the elastic and muscle tissues of the bronchial walls are destroyed by recurrent infection or inflammation resulting in the permanent dilatation of the bronchial walls.[13] Cystic fibrosis accounts for approximately 50 percent of the cases of bronchiectasis. Foul-smelling purulent sputum in excess of normal quantities is the hallmark of this disease.

Asthma

Asthma is an allergic sensitivity disorder of the bronchial airways in which there are intermittent attacks of dyspnea and wheezing caused by the sudden narrowing of the bronchial airways upon exposure to multiple allergens.[10] Several factors play a role in the pathogenesis of the disease, such as the hypersensitivity of the airways to a given substance, for example, ragweed pollen, and the release of mediators that induce bronchoconstriction and excess secretion of highly viscid mucus contributing to the obstruction of air flow. The major chemical mediators of asthma include histamine, slow-reacting substance of anaphylaxis, eosinophilic chemotactic factor A, bradykinins, and prostaglandins.

Normally, the trachea and bronchial tree widen and lengthen with inspiration, increasing the area of the air passageways allowing air to enter the lungs. Expiration normally is passive by elastic recoil. In an acute asthmatic attack, the bronchial air passageways narrow suddenly in the presence of the allergen. With inspiration, air enters the lungs even though the bronchial air passageways are narrow. In expiration, the trapped alveolar air passively and slowly moves up through partially obstructed airways, producing the prolonged wheezing sounds. Wheezing with expiration is accompanied by feelings of tightness in the chest,

dyspnea, and a cough. Airflow is decreased on pulmonary function tests. Complete or partial reversibility of obstructed airways occurs with the use of bronchodilators.

The underlying cause of asthma is the decrease in diameter of the lumen of the bronchotracheal tree produced by the contraction of its smooth muscle, edema of the bronchial wall, and viscid mucus production. This results in a negative effect on almost all pulmonary functions. There is an increase in airway resistance; a decrease in forced expiratory volumes of air; a loss of elastic recoil of the alveolar sacs; mismatched ventilation-perfusion ratios; and increased breathing rates.

Cystic Fibrosis

Cystic fibrosis is an autosomal recessive hereditary disorder of the exocrine glands.[4] Almost all exocrine glands are affected, especially sweat glands and mucous glands. The sweat contains abnormally high levels of Na^+ and Cl^- ions and the abnormal mucus is highly viscid. The mucus obstructs the glands and ducts in various organs, especially the lungs. Obstruction of the ducts of the exocrine glands results in the eventual destruction of the glands and the organ involved.

Bronchogenic Carcinoma

The leading cause of death in the United States is heart disease, but the second leading cause of death is cancer. Until recently, lung cancer was the primary cause of cancer deaths in men, whereas women died primarily of breast cancer. In 1985, the mortality rates for lung and breast cancer in women in the United States equalized.[2] If the trend of increasing incidence of smoking continues among women, it is expected that the next census will reveal that lung cancer indeed is the chief cause of cancer deaths in both men and women in the United States. Bronchogenic carcinoma in nonsmokers is rare.

Bronchogenic carcinoma of the lung accounts for 90 to 95 percent of all lung neoplasms. Smoking cigarettes is closely linked with this aggressive, malignant tumor, whose prognosis is very poor. The 5-year survival rate without treatment is 8 percent. Since smoking is the prime cause of the disease, it is therefore a preventable disease.

Bronchogenic carcinoma arises from the mucosal layer of the bronchial tree. It is the most common intrathoracic malignancy.[4] It may present as an unresolved pneumonia, atelectasis, or pleurisy. Metastasis to other organs frequently produces initial symptoms. The adrenal glands, liver, brain, and bones are the primary sites for metastasis of this malignant neoplasm. Of the four cell types of bronchogenic carcinoma, squamous cell carcinoma is the most common, accounting for 30 to 60 percent of the cases (Fig. 27-9).

Approximately 25 percent of bronchogenic carcinomas are asymptomatic. The most common nonspecific manifestations of the disease are cough, dyspnea, and chest pain, frequently accompanied by a sudden, inexplicable weight loss. Biopsy of adjacent lymph nodes for pathological evaluation reveals the presence or absence of me-

tastasis of the bronchogenic carcinoma. If metastasis has occurred, usually confirmed by screening tests (e.g., bone scan), then there is no treatment except palliation. If metastasis of the tumor has not occurred, then surgical excision of the affected lung is the treatment. As with most malignant neoplasms, the earlier the diagnosis, the better the chance of survival.

Tuberculosis

At the beginning of the 20th century, tuberculosis was the leading cause of death in the United States. The incidence of the disease decreased dramatically along with the decrease in mortality rates during the 20th century.

Tuberculosis is caused by the bacterium *Mycobacterium tuberculosis*, which usually involves the lungs but may involve any other organ in the body. When all the organs of the body are infected, the

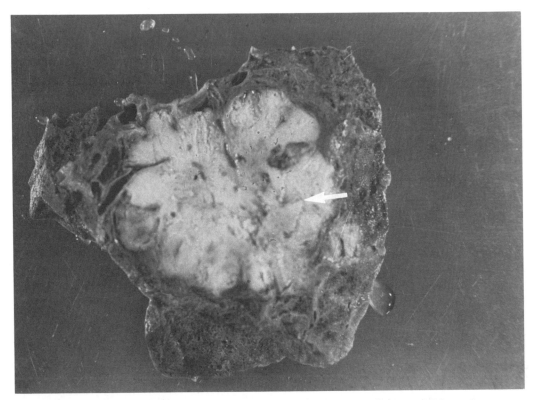

Fig. 27-9 Bronchogenic carcinoma of the lungs. The malignant tumor (white area) is a primary tumor (arrow) invading the adjacent lung tissue. The neoplasm was observed to have invaded the thoracic cavity as well as the pericardial sac of the heart.

disease is known as miliary tuberculosis. Widespread distribution of the tubercle bacilli occurs when the organisms massively invade the bloodstream and lymphatics.

The organism is transmitted person-to-person by droplet infection. The infected individual with active tuberculosis transmits the tubercle bacillus usually when coughing or sneezing. Droplets containing the microorganism are sprayed into the air. When a susceptible individual inhales the particles, the lungs become infected with the tubercle bacillus. Granuloma formation results when the body builds a wall of connective tissue around the infectious organisms, rendering the organisms viable but dormant for many years. The granuloma in tuberculosis is known as a tubercle. It is said to be a caseous granuloma when the core of the granuloma undergoes necrosis, producing a grossly visible soft, white, cheesy interior upon sectioning. When the defense mechanisms of the immune system are compromised, reactivation of the tubercle bacillus occurs, and the individual develops active tuberculosis. Most cases of tuberculosis in adults are due to reactivation of the disease rather than to a recent infection.

Tuberculosis may be considered to be a primary or secondary disease. Primary tuberculosis occurs in a previously unexposed and thus nonsensitized individual, usually a child infected with the tubercle bacillus. Secondary tuberculosis usually occurs in an adult with reactivation of a primary infection or reinfection of a sensitized host. In both primary and secondary tuberculosis, tubercles form by a granulomatous inflammatory reaction and granulomas in both diseases eventually become calcified. Primary tuberculosis usually develops subpleurally, either just above or below the interlobular fissure found between the upper and lower lobes of the lung. Secondary tuberculosis usually develops in the apices of one or both upper lobes of the lung. Cavitation of the tubercles or granuloma of tuberculosis is the hallmark of secondary tuberculosis.[4]

Pneumoconiosis and Fungal Diseases

When foreign matter enters the lungs, pneumoconioses may develop, usually resulting in pulmonary fibrosis. Anthracosis develops when coal dust enters the lungs, producing a black lung

grossly. Coal miners typically develop "black lung" disease. If asbestos fibers enter the lung, they produce not only a pneumoconiosis but lung cancer—mesotheliomas, primarily. Mesotheliomas are tumors arising from the pleural membranes of the thoracic cavity. There are many other contaminants of the air such as silica dust derived from sand and beryllium that form pneumoconioses.[4]

Fungal spores inhaled into the lung also can produce pulmonary diseases such as aspergillosis and histoplasmosis.

Pneumonia

Inflammation of the lungs is known as pneumonia. Many different types of microorganisms can cause pneumonia by invading the lung through inhalation of contaminated air, aspiration of oropharyngeal secretions, and hematogenous spread. These microorganisms usually are bacteria, viruses, or mycoplasmas but may also be other organisms such as fungi and protozoans. Foreign matter such as beryllium may also produce pneumonia when inhaled. Aspiration pneumonia may occur when vomitus is inhaled. Lipid pneumonia may occur with aspiration of oils. Ionizing radiation may also induce pneumonia.

There are two basic pathological patterns revealed when pneumonia develops.[4] The most common pattern occurs when fluid, an inflammatory exudate, fills the alveolar sacs in response to the presence of bacterial infections. When the fluid replaces the air in the affected part of the lung, an airless, solid-appearing mass of tissue results. This process is known as consolidation. The heavier lung now sinks when immersed in water, whereas a normal, air-ladened lung would float. The second pathological pattern to develop in pneumonia occurs less frequently, when the inflammatory exudate fills the spaces within the walls or septa of the lungs. This is known as interstitial pneumonia. It is usually due to the presence of viruses or mycoplasmas in the lungs. Two main types of pneumonia exist: lobar pneumonia and bronchopneumonia.

Lobar Pneumonia

When an entire lobe or major part of it is infected with an organism, this is known as lobar pneumonia. Approximately 90 percent of these cases are caused by the virulent bacterium pneumoncoccus. The infection usually occurs in otherwise healthy individuals.

The sudden onset of lobar pneumonia is characterized by shaking chills, fever, chest pain, and cough with a rusty sputum. Radiographs show lobar infiltration. Pneumococci are found in the sputum and blood upon bacteriological culture. If the pneumonia is not treated with antibiotics, there is a 20 to 40 percent mortality rate.

Bronchopneumonia

In bronchopneumonia, foci of infection are located around terminal bronchioles scattered throughout several lobes of the lungs. Areas of consolidation appear around these bronchioles. Bronchopneumonia usually occurs as a complication of surgery, anesthesia, trauma, aspiration, or even secondary to chronic pulmonary disease such as emphysema. It is usually due to opportunistic infections by organisms encountered in the body that are not pathogenic normally. In the compromised patient in whom the defense mechanisms of the host are impaired, the immune system cannot cope with these normally nonpathogenic microorganisms. This results in the opportunistic organisms causing disease; in this case, bronchogenic pneumonia. Consequently, bronchopneumonia is a type of mixed bacterial pneumonia in contrast to lobar pneumonia, which is due to one type of pathogenic organism at any given time.

Opportunistic Organisms

Cytomegalic Inclusion Disease

Approximately 70 percent of healthy adults have evidence of exposure to cytomegalovirus (CMV) but do not have cytomegalic inclusion disease (CID).[4,10] In 10 to 25 percent of healthy individuals, CMV may be cultured from the salivary glands, and it may be cultured from the cervix of 10 percent of healthy women, as well as from 1 percent of all newborns.

CMV may be transmitted by blood transfusions; intrauterine fetal infections when the mother is healthy but harbors the virus, or if the mother has the disease; during birth with maternal genital infection; infected organ transplants; respiratory droplet infection; and as a venereal disease. The virus has been isolated from both semen and vaginal fluids.

In an immunocompetent individual, CMV infection rarely results in clinical disease. However, in immunosuppressed individuals, CMV usually causes a severe opportunistic pneumonia. Interestingly, CMV infection also can result in immunosuppression that in turn increases the possibility for other opportunistic organisms to become pathogens, for example, *Pneumocystis carinii*.

CMV produces disease in many organs of the body in immunosuppressed individuals, but the most important infections are in the lungs and liver. The intranuclear virus is in the herpes family (human herpesvirus type 5) and forms intranuclear (viral) inclusion bodies in all infected cells (Fig. 27-10). Pneumonitis occurs frequently in the lungs and is accompanied by severe hypoxia. Radiographs reveal diffuse interstitial infiltrates or well-defined nodular lesions. Intracranial periventricular calcifications seen in radiographs of the skull or brain are highly suggestive of CID (Figs. 27-11 and 27-12). Aspiration biopsy of the lungs reveals interstitial pneumonitis with hyaline membrane formation (Fig. 27-13). "Owl-eye" cells may be seen in infected renal tissue or in urine from infected individuals (Fig. 27-10). The infected cells lining the renal tubules are enlarged, and the intranuclear CMV is seen in the nuclei of these cells as dense, homogeneous, basophilic, intranuclear inclusions (Fig. 27-10). There is a halo around the intranuclear inclusion body that forms a clear zone between the inclusion body and the nuclear membrane.

Pneumocystis carinii Pneumonia

Pneumonia may be caused by the opportunistic microorganism *Pneumocystis carinii* in individuals who are taking immunosuppressive drugs for the management of organ transplants and cancer, or in individuals whose immune system is defective owing to disease, such as in the acquired immune deficiency syndrome (AIDS), or owing to agenesis of the immune system in utero (congenital).[4,14]

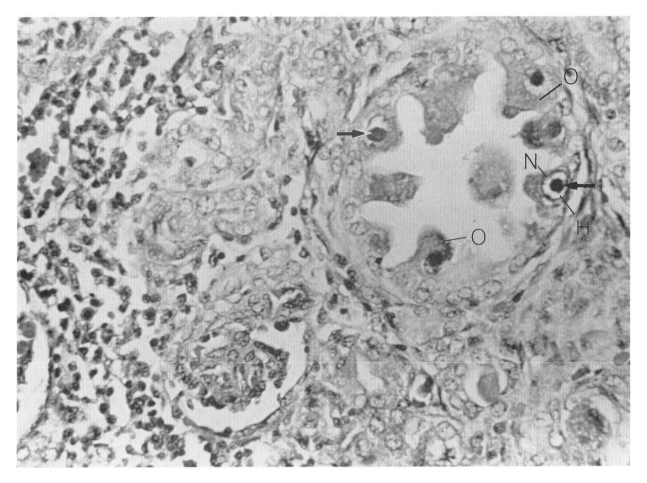

Fig. 27-10 Kidney with CMV infection (light microscopy). Owl-eye cells (O) seen in renal tubule in CMV infection in patient with AIDS. Viral inclusion bodies can be seen in the cell nuclei (arrows). There is a halo (H) effect produced by a space that develops between the viral inclusion bodies in the nucleus and the nuclear membrane (N). The infected owl-eye cells are about to be extruded into the urine. (From MEDCOM, Inc., 12601 Industry St., Garden Grove, California, with permission.)

P. carinii is a protozoan with intracellular and extracellular stages residing in the pulmonary alveoli (Fig. 27-14). It is found in most rodents and dogs. Its mode of transmission is unknown. When an individual's immune system is suppressed because of drugs or disease, this opportunistic organism is activated in the lungs, causing *P. carinii* pneumonia (PCP). Its complete life cycle usually occurs in the lungs (cysts, sporozoites, and trophozoites). It has been found that animals treated with immunosuppressive drugs or corticosteroids also develop PCP. However, it has not been determined whether or not rodents and dogs are vectors of PCP. In humans, almost all individuals with PCP also harbor CMV.

The disease is diagnosed by lung aspirate biopsy revealing an eosinophilic foamy or honeycomblike exudate in the alveolar spaces (Figs. 27-15 and 27-16). Through light microscopy, *P. carinii* is found enmeshed within the alveolar exudate, occurring singularly or in clusters of two to eight (Fig. 27-14). Radiographs reveal several clinical stages of the disease; the most readily identifiable stage shows the perihilar infiltration of the lung in early PCP (Fig. 27-17) compared to that of advanced PCP (Fig. 27-18).

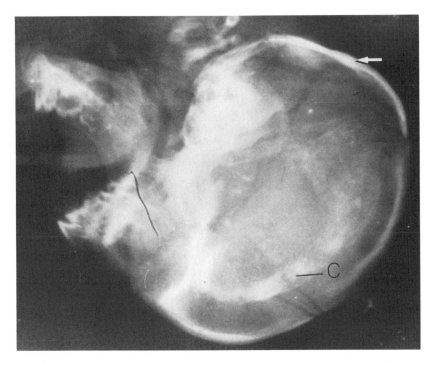

Fig. 27-11 Radiograph of skull of child with CMV infection. Intracranial periventricular calcifications (C) can be seen through the skull (arrow). (From MEDCOM by permission.)

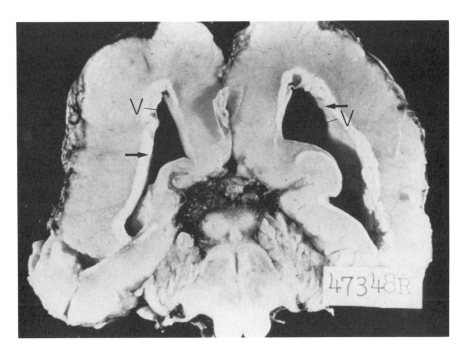

Fig. 27-12 Section of adult brain from CMV-infected AIDS patient. Periventricular calcification (arrows) is seen around the dilated ventricles (V). (From MEDCOM by permission.)

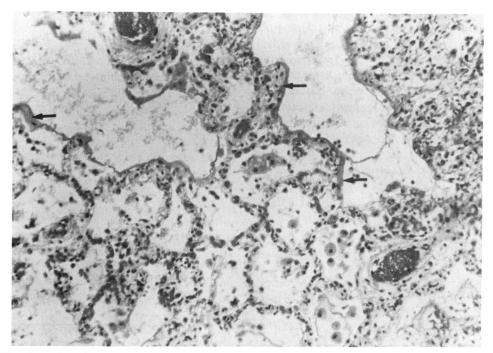

Fig. 27-13 Light microscopy view of lung with CMV infection. Interstitial pneumonitis is seen with hyaline membrane formation (arrows). (From MEDCOM by permission.)

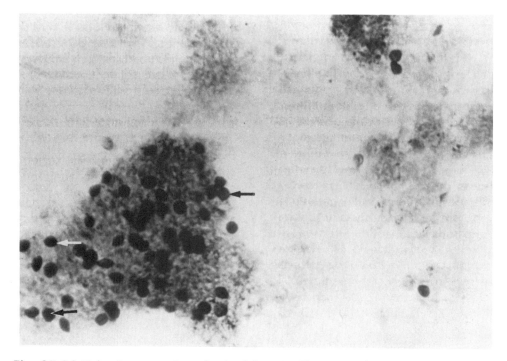

Fig. 27-14 Light microscopy view of stained *P. carinii*. These stained protozoans (arrows) are enmeshed within the lung exudate of an AIDS patient with PCP. (From MEDCOM by permission.)

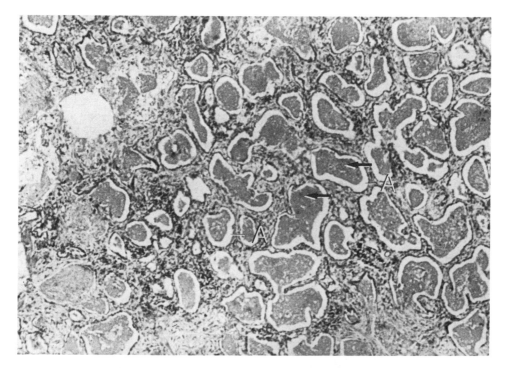

Fig. 27-15 Light microscopy view (low power) of PCP-infected lung. Foamy or honeycomblike exudate (arrows) are found in many of the alveoli (A). (From MEDCOM by permission.)

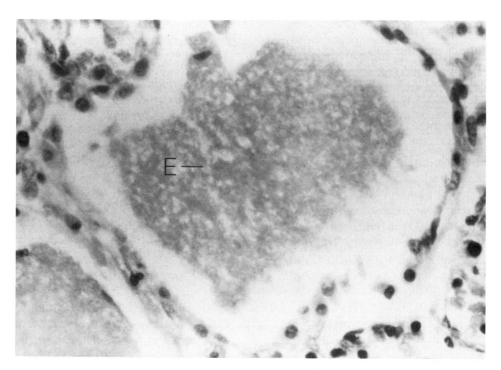

Fig. 27-16 Light microscopy view (high power) of PCP-infected lung. The foamy nature of the exudate (E) is visible. *P. carinii* cells, not specifically stained, are vaguely seen in the exudate. (From MEDCOM by permission.)

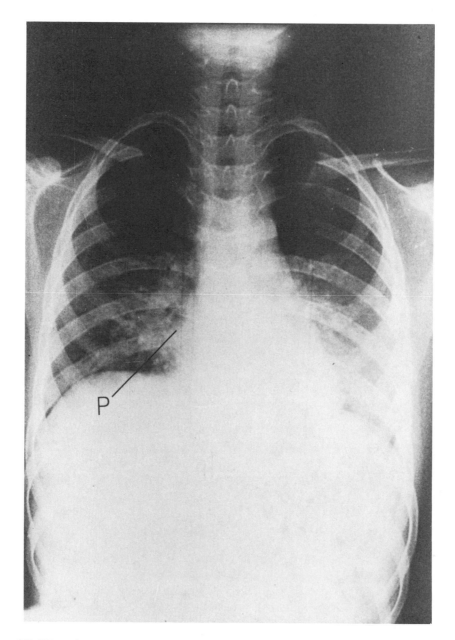

Fig. 27-17 Radiograph of lungs Infected with *P. carinii* in AIDS patient. Note the perihilar (P) involvement of the lungs in early PCP. (From MEDCOM by permission.)

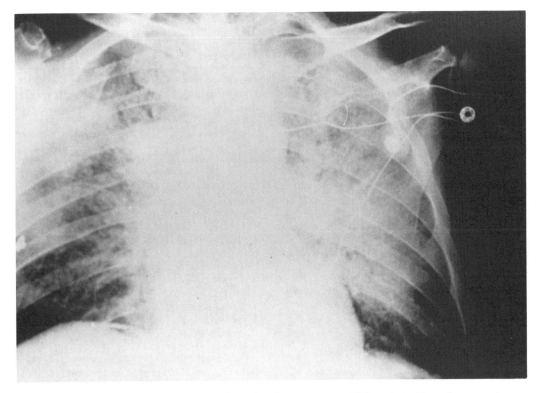

Fig. 27-18 Radiograph of lungs infected with *P. carinii* in AIDS patient. Note the extensive involvement of the lungs in PCP with advanced disease. (From MEDCOM by permission.)

MEDICAL MANAGEMENT

Opportunistic Infections

Cytomegalic Inclusion Disease

CMV infection may be diagnosed by viral culture from blood, urine, or other secretions and tissues. Observation of giant cell formation in the urine in the presence of owl-eye cells and the presence of rising titers of CMV complement-fixing antibodies in the blood also are diagnostic (Fig. 27-10). There is no cure for any viral disease including CID. Palliative treatment with appropriate drugs is used to control pain, fever, and convulsions.[14]

P. carinii Pneumonia

P. carinii can be diagnosed by light microscopy when stained (Fig. 27-14) from sputum, bronchial washings, bronchial brushings, and tracheal aspirates. The treatment of choice is trimethoprim and sulfamethazole. If the patient cannot tolerate the toxic side effects of these drugs, then pentamidine may be administered.[14,15]

Emphysema

The signs and symptoms of emphysema are nonspecific (Tables 2 and 3). The diagnosis of emphysema is made by pathological examination of the involved tissue demonstrating enlarged air spaces and the loss of alveolar tissue. The patient presents clinically with exertional dyspnea that progressively worsens with time and is accompanied by a minimal cough. The patient usually has a history of smoking. Radiographs reveal the diaphragm to be flat and the thoracic cavity to be enlarged, especially in the anteroposterior dimensions. These physical changes expand the area of the thoracic cavity to accommodate the expanded overinflated lungs. Auscultation of the chest reveals diminished breath sounds, rhonchi, and pro-

Table 27-2 Nonspecific Manifestations of Pulmonary Disease

Manifestation	Description	Associated Diseases
Cough	Most common symptom.	Heart disease, otitis media
Dyspnea	Difficulty breathing Dyspnea at rest with acute respiratory illnesses.	Heart disease
	Exertional dyspnea with impaired ventilation.	Angina (coronary heart disease)
Expectoration	Excessive sputum production with acute and chronic respiratory diseases.	Infections
Wheezing	High-pitched sound produced with asthma during expiration.	Pneumonia
Chest pain	Associated with lung disease, especially pleurisy.	Heart disease
Hemoptysis	Bloody sputum. Associated with bonchopulmonary diseases such as bonchitis, tuberculosis, bronchiectasis, and carcinoma of the lung.	Ruptured thoracic aneurysms
Cyanosis	Blue skin color caused by hypoxia associated with anemia, emphysema, etc.	Congenital heart disease
Polycythemia	Increase in total mass of erythrocytes. Compensatory response to chronic anoxia.	High altitudes

Table 27-3 Clinical Distinctions between Emphysema and Chronic Bronchitis

Emphysema	Chronic Bronchitis
Onset about 60 years	Onset about 50 years
Cough mild or absent	Cough severe, continuous, progressive
Mucus whitish, mucoid production sparse	Mucus yellow-greenish, mucopurulent, production excessive
Dyspnea chronic, severe and progressive	Dyspnea sporatic, mild
Weight loss	Weight gain
Cyanosis absent	Cyanosis present
Hypoxia absent or mild	Hypoxia moderate to severe
Hypercapnia absent	Hypercapnia mild to severe
Compensated: hyperventilation (pink puffers)	Noncompensated (blue bloaters)
Edema absent	Edema present
Hyperinflation of lungs	Absent
Chest diameter (anteroposterior) increased	Normal
Breath sounds decreased	Breath sounds increased (rhonchi)
Respiratory acidosis absent	Respiratory acidosis present

longed respiratory expiration accompanied by tachypnea. The lack of elastic recoil of the affected lungs makes it very difficult to exhale air, causing reduced air flow rates.

Therapy includes bronchodilator drugs such as aminophylline, a theophylline derivative, accompanied by bronchopulmonary drainage. The bronchodilators relieve the bronchospasm characteristically associated with this type of COPD. Postural drainage techniques then are applied by the physical therapist. Cessation of smoking is of paramount importance. Oxygen consumption during exercise is determined to assess the degree of lung impairment. Corticosteroids represent the second line of defense in the treatment of emphysema, but are used only if the bronchodilators and postural drainage are not effective. Steroids (prednisone, 30 mg once per day) may be effective in treating emphysema, but they are frequently without benefit. The long-term use of steroids beyond 2 to 4 weeks should be discontinued if there is no objective improvement. The complications associated with long-term use of glucocorticosteroids include adrenal gland atrophy with adrenal suppression, osteoporosis, edema, hyperglycemia, and an increased susceptibility to infections owing to depression of the immune system.[10,15]

Since hypoxemia is more deleterious than hypercapnea, oxygen therapy may be administered even though there is fear of suppressing ventilatory drive. Continuous oxygen therapy is indicated if arterial hypoxia persists in conjunction with cor pulmonale. Cor pulmonale is treated with dietary salt restrictions and diuretics.

If upper airway tract infections occur, antibiotic therapy should be initiated. Preferably, the offending organism should be identified by sputum culture. However, it is common to administer broad-spectrum antibiotics such as tetracycline or ampicillin for 7 to 10 days to combat infection.

Chronic Bronchitis

The onset of chronic bronchitis is due to irreversible bronchial obstruction and reversible bronchospasm. Excessive production of viscid mucus by the hypertrophied mucous glands in the large bronchi accompanied by chronic inflammation in the small airways are distinguishing characteristics (Table 27-3). Chronic bronchitis is diagnosed clinically by the presence of a productive cough with excess sputum production for at least 3 months a year for two consecutive years. Hypoxemia and hypercapnea result from the chronic alveolar hypoventilation (Table 27-3). The etiology of the disease is unknown. Chronic bronchitis, like emphysema, is associated with cigarette smoking, air pollution, airway infection, and allergies. The treatment is the same as that of emphysema, namely, bronchodilators, postural drainage by physical therapists, oxygen, corticosteroids, and antibiotics.

Cystic Fibrosis

The diagnosis of cystic fibrosis is suspected when a child or young adult presents with a history of chronic lung disease. Bronchitis, bronchopneumonia, bronchiectasis, and lung abscesses are common respiratory diseases afflicting this population and resulting in recurrent hospitalization. Nearly all patients develop chronic, progressive respira-

tory diseases that are the common cause of death and morbidity in cystic fibrosis patients.

Pancreatic dysfunction occurs in 85 percent of the patients. Growth failure and nutritional deficits result from pancreatic insufficiency. Pancreatic insufficiency also leads to fat and protein malabsorption. Diabetes mellitus results from insulin deficiency and recurrent pancreatitis. However, it must be emphasized that cystic fibrosis is a multisystem disorder adversely affecting all body systems.

Diagnosis of this genetic disease is determined by the pilocarpine iontophoresis test (sweat test).[15,16] Sodium and chloride ions are elevated in the sweat of patients with cystic fibrosis. The patient is diagnosed as having cystic fibrosis when the sweat test reveals concentrations of these ions above 80 meq/L on two separate tests administered on two consecutive days.

Treatment of this chronic progressive disease is palliative. Therapy consists of antibiotics for secondary pulmonary infections, bronchodilators to relieve bronchospasms, and postural drainage with chest percussion to clear the upper respiratory airways of the excessive mucus. Psychotherapy and genetic and occupational counseling also are critical. There is no cure for this disease. About one-half of the children with cystic fibrosis die before the age of 20 years.

Bronchiectasis

Cystic fibrosis accounts for approximately 50 percent of the patients who develop bronchiectasis. As a rule, drug therapy consists of antibiotics and inhaled bronchodilators. Physical therapists play a major role in providing postural drainage, chest percussion, and exercise. If the respiratory infection does not respond well to the antibiotic therapy, then surgical resection is indicated. Surgery also is indicated for massive hemoptysis.

Asthma

The symptoms and signs of asthma are intermittent periods of wheezing, coughing, dyspnea, and feelings of tightness in the chest. The characteristic wheezing sound occurs with expiration only. Prolonged expiration and diffuse wheezing are detected with chest auscultation. Pulmonary function tests reveal a limitation of airflow in the pulmonary airways. Bronchodilators readily open the airways by reversing the bronchoconstriction.

Laboratory findings consist of a slightly increased total white blood count with an increased number of eosinophils. It is normal for the eosinophil count to rise in allergies and parasitic infections. However, no single laboratory test for asthma is diagnostic. Chest x-rays reveal hyperinflation. Pulmonary function tests reveal the degree of airway obstruction.

Asthma is treated through three routes.[15–17] First, O_2 is provided until arterial blood-gas analysis indicates normal O_2 saturation. Second, postural drainage and deep coughing help to remove the obstructions from the airways thereby mobilizing the secretions. Adequate fluid replacement may be necessary to combat dehydration. Third, bronchodilators such as theophylline are provided to eliminate bronchospasms, thereby opening the airways.

Bronchogenic Carcinoma

Early diagnosis of cancer through screening is important. Obtaining a cure depends on localizing the primary lesion *before* metastasis has occurred, followed by surgical excision of the tumor. Chest x-rays screen for lung cancer in conjunction with light microscopy observation of cancer cells obtained from the diseased lung tissue.

Depending on the stage of the disease when diagnosed, bronchogenic carcinoma presents with variable findings. The clinical findings depend on the type of primary cancer, its metastases, and secondary physical effects of the tumor on other organ systems related to space-occupying lesions, as well as the development of paraneoplastic syndromes. These syndromes are complicated and poorly understood. Extrapulmonary organ dysfunctions occur in this syndrome but are not directly related to the primary tumor or its metastases. For example, gynecomastia is associated with large cell lung cancer.[17]

Persistent cough, dyspnea, hemoptysis, and unaccountable weight loss accompanied by chest pain generally characterize symptomatic lung cancer that is advanced and not resectable. Early lung cancer is asymptomatic. It can be diagnosed by cytological examination of the sputum. Chest x-

rays are nonspecific but helpful. The only definitive diagnosis requires cytological observation of cancer cells in sputum, pleural fluids, or lung tissue biopsy specimens. Only if lung cancer is detected early before metastasis can the surgeon remove the primary tumor and truly cure the disease. Fine-needle aspiration biopsies and exfoliative cytopathological studies are the least invasive techniques used to obtain tissue from the malignant tumor.

The majority of lung cancers belong to one of four major cell types.[4] These are malignant tumors of the epithelial tissue of the airways of the lung: squamous cell carcinoma, to 25–30 percent; adenocarcinoma, 30 to 35 percent; small cell carcinoma (oat cell), 20 to 25 percent; and large cell (anaplastic) carcinoma, 10 to 15 percent. Cigarette smoke and industrial carcinogens in the air are the most common cause of lung cancer. Primary malignant tumor of the lung in nonsmokers is rare.

After the pathologist makes the diagnosis of a specific cell type of bronchogenic carcinoma, the malignant tumor is graded and staged to determine treatment and prognosis. Malignant tissue is graded by determining the degree of cell differentiation and the mitotic index generally. The staging of cancer depends on the size of the primary lesion, its extent of spread to regional lymph nodes, and the presence or absence of metastases. The overall 5-year survival rate for all types and stages of bronchogenic carcinoma is approximately 10 percent.

Malignant neoplasms including bronchogenic carcinoma disseminate to other parts of the body by invading a body cavity such as the thorax, thereby seeding pleural surfaces, and by hematogenous and lymphatic spread to other body organs. Bronchogenic carcinoma metastasizes to the lymph nodes (70 to 80 percent), liver (30 to 40 percent), bone (20 to 40 percent), and brain (15 to 20 percent).

The primary treatments for lung cancer are surgery, chemotherapy, and radiation therapy. Surgery is the treatment of choice for lung cancer diagnosed early. Unfortunately, only about 25 percent of patients with lung cancer present with only a primary tumor; most have secondary metastases. The current combination chemotherapeutic treatment of choice for some bronchogenic carcinomas is cyclophosphamide, doxorubicin, methotrexate, and lomustine. Combination chemotherapeutic drugs may result in tumor regression, but the median survival time generally is not prolonged. Radiation therapy is applied as a palliative agent to relieve some symptoms, for example, to reduce the size of a tumor that is compressing the esophagus or the heart.[15,16]

Pulmonary Tuberculosis

Although tuberculosis is declining in Europe and North America, it continues to be an important cause of death in third-world countries. The disease most frequently affects the elderly, urban dwellers, and minority groups. Hispanic, Haitian, and Southeast Asian immigrants usually have case rates as high as those of the third-world country of their origin. With extensive immigration to the United States, especially in the post-Vietnam era, tuberculosis frequently is being seen in microepidemics centered around these families. Therefore, in some hospitals, interestingly, the number of tuberculosis cases in the wards may be increasing.

It is important for health care workers to determine whether or not they have been exposed to the tubercle bacillus prior to working. Health care workers generally are requested to have a chest x-ray and to take the tine tuberculin test to determine prior exposure to the tubercle bacillus. The tine test involves four tines or prongs, 2 mm long, attached to a handle; the tines are coated with tuberculin and pressed into the outer layer of the skin of the forearm. The skin is checked for the presence of an induration or swelling 48 to 72 hours later. If the induration around the puncture wounds is 2 mm or more in diameter, the test is considered positive. This is a screening test that is convenient and inexpensive but has decreased specificity. Individuals with positive tine tests should be given the intracutaneous tuberculin purified protein derivative test. A positive tuberculin test results when the area of induration is at least 5 mm in diameter by 48 hours. A positive reaction indicates previous or present contact and infection with tuberculosis. The positive reaction does not indicate whether the disease is currently active or inactive. Most health care workers at the beginning of their careers have a negative tuberculin test. Regular screening allows the time when a negative tuberculin test changes to positive to be observed, thereby revealing the individual as being recently infected and requiring drug therapy.[15,16]

The signs and symptoms of tuberculosis are fatigue, anorexia, low-grade fever, and night sweats. A cough accompanies these symptoms that at the onset is dry but then becomes productive with increasing quantities of sputum released. The sputum eventually becomes purulent and often bloody. Occasionally the disease is asymptomatic.

Definitive diagnosis of the disease can be made if *M. tuberculosis* grows in a culture of the sputum or bronchial washings. The microorganisms are stained with an acid-fast dye for light microscopy detection. Demonstration of acid-fast bacilli alone does not confirm the diagnosis since there are other species of mycobacteria that are not tuberculous. Radiographs provide clinical support of the diagnosis by revealing the presence of fibrocavities, nodules, and pulmonary infiltrates located in the apical or posterior segments of the upper lobes or the superior segments of the lower lobes.

The modern treatment of tuberculosis depends on multiple drug therapy. Single drug therapy protocols are not utilized in order to prevent the formation of drug-resistant mycobacteria. Lengthy periods of drug therapy also are important because of the slow turnover time and the long inactive periods of the mycobacteria. Treatment protocols are the same for pulmonary and miliary tuberculosis.

The basic drug regimen for treatment of tuberculosis consists of isoniazid and rifampin administered for 9 months. After sputum cultures are negative for *M. tuberculosis*, it is mandatory that the patient continue medication for 6 months. If drug resistance or patient intolerance develops toward either drug, then a third drug such as ethambutol or streptomycin should be used. If isonazid cannot be used, it is usually replaced by ethambutol; rifampin and ethambutol should be used for 18 months. If rifampin cannot be used, isoniazid plus ethambutol or streptomycin should be administered for 18 months.

Chemoprophylaxis is an important component of drug therapy of tuberculosis. It is the treatment of choice for individuals who are newly infected with the tubercle bacillus but do not have active disease, usually identified by conversion of tuberculin skin test results from negative to positive. These individuals with minimum infection should follow the chemoprophylaxis regimen of isoniazid therapy for 12 months. Chemoprophylaxis is a type of therapy for tuberculosis that utilizes only one drug, isoniazid, the drug of choice for treatment of any organ infected with *M. tuberculosis*. The following groups should be administered isoniazid for a year as chemoprophylaxis:

1. Newly infected individuals whose tuberculosis skin test turned positive in 2 years.
2. Household members and close contacts of people with active tuberculosis.
3. Individuals with positive tuberculin skin tests and positive radiograph findings suggestive of tuberculosis but without positive bacteriological evidence of disease.
4. Individuals with positive tuberculin skin test reactions with high risk factors of reactivated tuberculosis, for example, patients taking immunosuppressant drugs or cortisone and patients having diabetes mellitus or marasmus or undergoing hemodialysis.
5. Individuals under 35 years of age with positive tuberculin skin tests and no risk factors.

Pneumonia

Chest x-rays provide evidence to support the clinical suspicion of pneumonia by revealing consolidation and patchy infiltrates of single or several lobes of the lung or involvement of the whole lung. However, the diagnosis depends on culturing the organism from sputum, blood, and pleural fluid. The pathogen may be identified by examining Gram-stained smears of the cultured organism by light microscopy. The antimicrobial therapy used depends on the results of the drug sensitivity tests.

PHARMACOLOGICAL AGENTS

Bronchodilators

Methylxanthines

The methylxanthines are important sources of the bronchodilators known as theophylline, theobrom-

ine, and caffeine, which are derived from tea, cocoa, and coffee, respectively.[18] Theophylline is an important therapeutic agent in the treatment of asthma and in the management of chronic bronchitis and cystic fibrosis. The methylxanthines in vitro can be shown to inhibit the breakdown of the enzyme phosphodiesterase, which hydrolyzes cyclic nucleotides, thereby increasing the cellular concentration of cyclic adenosine monophosphate (cAMP). This would explain the smooth muscle relaxation and cardiac stimulation seen after administration of methylxanthines. These agents also inhibit the release of histamine by the mast cells, which is useful in the treatment of asthma. Of the methylxanthines, theophylline is the most effective bronchodilator.

Adrenergic Agents

Epinephrine

Epinephrine is an effective, rapidly acting bronchodilator. Its action is initiated 15 minutes after subcutaneous injection or inhalation, and its effect lasts 60 to 90 minutes. Tachycardia, dysrhythmias, and angina are serious side effects of the drug owing to the stimulation of both β_1 and β_2 receptors. Only β_2 receptors relax the smooth muscles lining the airways, producing bronchodilatation. The β_1 receptors affect the heart adversely by increasing cardiac stimulation. Therefore, epinephrine should only be used if theophylline is not effective.

Ephedrine

The bronchodilatation drug ephedrine has a longer duration and a much lower potency compared with epinephrine. It was one of the first drugs to be used to treat asthma.

Isoproterenol

Isoproterenol is a potent bronchodilator that acts within 5 minutes and is effective for 60 to 90 minutes. It is usually administered as an aerosol for the treatment of asthma. Adverse cardiac effects may occur with the use of high doses.

Muscarinic Antagonist (Atropine)

Atropine derived from the leaves of the datura plant is used to treat asthma by acting as a antimuscarinic agent. Muscarinic antagonists such as atropine effectively relax airway smooth muscles

Table 27-4 Antituberculosis Drugs: Actions and Complications

Drug	Actions	Complications
Isoniazid	Bacteriocidal to intracellular and extracellular mycobacteria. (Administration of vitamin B_6 [pyridoxine] prevents neuritis.)	Peripheral neuritis Hepatitis
Rifampin	Bacteriocidal (colors urine orange).	Hepatitis Discolors contact lenses Inhibits the effect of oral contraceptives.
Ethambutol	Bacteriostatic to both intracellular and extracellular mycobacteria.	Optic neuritis (reversible)
Streptomycin	Bacteriocidal to extracellular organisms.	Nephrotoxicity Destruction of the eighth cranial nerve

and decrease the secretion of mucus that occurs in response to vagal stimulation.

Chromolyn

Chromolyn is an effective prophylactic agent that prevents bronchoconstriction induced by exercise or aspirin. It also prevents bronchospasm induction by air pollutants. The effectiveness of this drug depends on preventing calcium transport across the mast cell membrane.

Corticosteroids (Prednisone)

It is believed that corticosteroids may decrease airway obstruction by decreasing inflammation or by enhancing the effects of β-adrenergic agonists. However, the dangerous side effects of long-term use of the drugs described earlier in this chapter necessitate short-term use of steroids as the drugs of last resort.

Drug Therapy of Tuberculosis

The actions and complications or toxicity of the antituberculosis drugs are presented in Table 27-4.

Drug Therapy of Bronchogenic Carcinoma

The actions and acute and delayed complications of the drugs utilized in the treatment of carcinoma of the lung are presented in Table 27-5.

Table 27-5 Drug Therapy of Bronchogenic Carcinoma: Actions and Complications

Drug	Actions	Complications Acute	Complications Delayed
Cyclophosphamide	Alkylating agent	Nausea Vomiting	Alopecia Hemorrhagic cystitis
Doxorubicin (Adriamycin)	Natural product	Nausea Colors urine red	Cardiotoxicity Alopecia Bone marrow depression
Methotrexate	Antimetabolite	None	Bone marrow depression Gastrointestinal tract ulcerations Leukopenia Thrombocytopenia
Lomustine	Alkylating agent	Nausea Vomiting	Leukopenia Thrombocytopenia

Table 27-6 Antimicrobial Therapy for Pneumonia: Common Microorganisms, Choice Drug Therapy, and Disease Complications

Common Microorganisms	Choice Antibiotic	Complications of Diseases
Streptococcus pneumoniae (pneumococcus)	Penicillin G	Bacteremia Endocarditis Meningitis Pericarditis
Haemophilus influenza	Ampicillin	Empyema Endocarditis
Staphylococcus aureus	Nafcillin	Empyema
Mycoplasma pneumoniae	Erythromycin	Skin rashes Hemolytic anemia Myringitis
Legionella species	Erythromycin	Endocarditis Pericarditis Empyema

Drug Therapy of Pneumonia

Some common microbes that cause pneumonia, the preferred therapeutic antibiotic administered, and the complications of the disease are presented in Table 27-6.

REFERENCES

1. Vital Statistics of the United States, 1981. U.S. Department of Health and Human Services, 1981
2. Silverberg E: Cancer Statistics, 1985. American Cancer Society, New York. Reprinted from Ca-A Cancer Journal for Clinicians, Vol. 35, No. 1, 1985
3. Ham A, Cormack D: Histology. JB Lippincott, Philadelphia, 1979
4. Robbins SL, Kumar V: Basic Pathology. WB Saunders, Philadelphia, 1987
5. Protas EJ: Pulmonary function testing. In Rothstein JM (ed): Measurement in Physical Therapy. Churchill Livingstone, New York, 1985
6. West JB: Disturbances of respiratory function. In Braunwald E, Isselbacher KJ et al. (ed): Harrison's Principles of Internal Medicine. 11th Ed. Vol. II. McGraw-Hill, New York, 1987
7. Levinsky NG: Acidosis and alkalosis. In Braunwald E, Isselbacher KJ et al. (eds): Harrison's Principles of Internal Medicine. 11th Ed. Vol. I. McGraw-Hill, New York, 1987
8. Narins RG, Emmett M: Simple and mixed acid-based disorders: a practical approach. Medicine 59:161, 1980
9. Staub NC: The pathophysiology of pulmonary edema. Hum Pathol I:419, 1970
10. Fishman MC, Hoffman AR et al.: Medicine. 2nd Ed. JB Lippincott, Philadelphia, 1985
11. West JB: Pulmonary Pathophysiology: The Essentials. Williams & Wilkins, Baltimore, 1982
12. Fishman AP: The spectrum of chronic obstructive disease of the airways. In Fishman AP (ed): Pulmonary Diseases and Disorders. 2nd Ed. McGraw-Hill, New York, 1987
13. Murray JF: Bronchiectasis and broncholithiasis. In Braunwald E, Isselbacher KJ et al. (eds): Harrison's Principles of Internal Medicine. 11th Ed. Vol. II. McGraw-Hill, New York, 1987
14. Lopez C, Fitzgerald PA et al.: Deficiency of interferon-alpha generating capacity is associated with susceptibility to opportunistic infections in patients with AIDS. In Selikoff I et al. (eds): Acquired Immune Deficiency Syndrome. Ann NY Acad Sci 437:39, 1984
15. Stauffer JL, Carbone JE: Pulmonary Diseases. In Krupp MA et al. (eds): Current Medical Diagnosis and Treatment 1986. Lange Medical Publications, Los Altos, 1986
16. Schroeder SA, Krupp MA, Tierney LM (eds): Current Medical Diagnosis and Treatment 1988. Lange Medical Publications, Los Altos, 1988
17. Braunwald E, Isselbacher KJ et al. (eds): Harrison's Principles of Internal Medicine. 11th Ed. McGraw-Hill, New York, 1987
18. Katzung BG (ed): Basic and Clinical Pharmacology. Lange Medical Publications, Los Altos, 1982

28 Acute Pulmonary Management: Respiratory Care Devices

L. Gail Robinson

The purpose of this chapter is to acquaint the physical therapist or physical therapist assistant with some frequently utilized respiratory care apparatus. The information presented serves as a foundation for evaluating and treating individuals who require respiratory care devices. These devices may be found in any patient care setting and are associated with a variety of cardiopulmonary dysfunctions the physical therapist encounters.

THE SETTING

The most common setting is the acute care hospital, and specifically the intensive care unit (ICU). The ICU environment may be somewhat foreign to the physical therapist. The physical therapist with minimal acute care experience may experience anxiety when called to provide services in the ICU. This environment is also stressful for the patient and family members. The various tubes, lines, and monitoring equipment are a serious challenge to work around. Once the physical therapist obtains confidence with handling the acute care monitoring equipment, this equipment can provide objective data on the patient's status and response to the intervention by the physical therapist.

The majority of devices presented here are associated with the adult population, but when appropriate, specifics are referred to for the neonate, infant, and child. The settings in which these devices appear are quite diverse. When pos-

sible, examples and specific considerations are presented for the physical therapy department, outpatient, home health, or other nonacute intensive care setting. Finally, an important role for physical therapists as health care providers is to educate and support the patient and family, and exercising this role is of extreme value when handling equipment during physical therapy intervention in any setting.

AIRWAYS

Figure 28-1A diagrams the upper airway anatomy. Airway obstruction is life threatening and should be avoided whenever possible. In the unconscious, spontaneously breathing adult, the tongue is associated with the most common cause of airway obstruction—soft tissue obstruction. Cardiopulmonary resuscitation (CPR) teaches the head-tilt/chin-lift maneuver to open the airway and establish breathlessness.[1] Figure 28-1B depicts the maneuver for opening the airway. Airway obstruction may also be due to a foreign body creating a partial or complete obstruction. In the child, foreign body obstruction is the common cause of airway obstruction. The Heimlich maneuver, as taught in CPR, allows us to manage foreign body airway obstruction in children and adults.[1] When laryngeal spasm causes an obstruction, advanced life support techniques are performed by individuals appropriately trained in these procedures.[1]

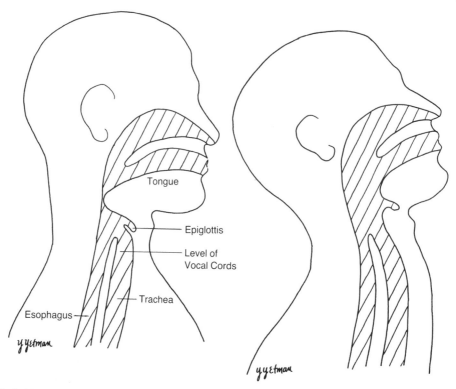

Fig. 28-1 Upper airway anatomy. **(A)** Tongue (soft tissue) obstructing the airway. **(B)** Result of head tilt/chin lift manuever—the airway is opened.

Pharyngeal Airways

In the context of this chapter the term "pharyngeal airways" is used to describe airway devices designed for short-term use (Fig. 28-2). Their purpose is to assist in maintaining a patent airway. The oropharyngeal airway (Fig. 28-2A) is inserted along the tongue until the teeth limit the insertion. This airway extends from the lips to the pharynx and conforms to the curvature of the palate.[2] These airways are usually rigid, and if it is positioned correctly using the correct size, the patient is able to breath around the device. It is designed to enable a suction catheter to easily pass along the side and into the laryngopharynx. This pharyngeal airway may induce gag reflex; therefore, it is better suited for the comatose patient. Once consciousness is regained, the device is frequently removed, since it is no longer needed to maintain a patent airway and can provoke vomiting and laryngospasms.

The nasopharyngeal airway, also called the nasal trumpet (Fig. 28-2B), is a device for insertion through one of the nares. It follows the posterior wall curvature of the nasopharynx and oropharynx. Distally, it is positioned at the base of the tongue, allowing the tongue to separate from the

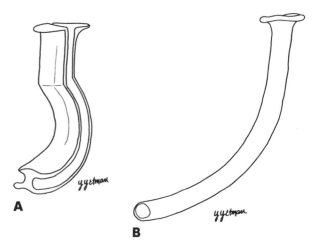

Fig. 28-2 Pharyngeal airways. **(A)** Oropharyngeal airway. **(B)** Nasopharyngeal airway.

posterior pharyngeal wall.[3] Extending from the nostril to the pharynx, it is usually constructed out of soft rubber material and is funnel shaped. The diameter size varies. A safety pin should be attached transversely through the nasal end to prevent slippage into the nose.[2,3] An advantage of the nasopharyngeal airway is that it does not ellicit the gag reflex as much as the oropharyngeal airway. Therefore, the semicomatose and awake patient will usually tolerate this airway better than the oropharyngeal airway. There can be minor trauma to the nasal area when the airway is inserted. Some clinicians recommend changing the nasopharyngeal airway daily from one naris to the other to decrease airway irritation and necrosis in the airway caused from tube pressure.[3] Oxygen humidification is recommended when the patient has a nasopharyngeal airway. Adequate suctioning is possible through the airway, but may increase airway resistance. Figures 28-3 and 28-4 depict the placement of the pharyngeal airways in a patient.

Artificial Airway

An artificial airway is "a tube inserted into the trachea that bypasses the upper airway and laryngeal structures as integral parts of the total airway."[3] Insertion of the tube is considered an invasive procedure, resulting in the establishment of an endotracheal tube (Fig. 28-5) or a tracheostomy tube.

An endotracheal tube can be inserted by either the oral or nasal route (Figs. 28-6 and 28-7). The instrument specifically developed for intubation of the trachea with an endotracheal tube is a laryngoscope; however, an esophageal obturator is sometimes utilized for establishing an airway in a CPR emergency.[3] "Intubation" is the term associated with the actual procedure of establishing an artificial airway with either an endotracheal tube (oral or nasal route) or a tracheostomy tube. "Intubation" is not synonymous with ventilator or oxygen therapy. The term used to refer to removal of the artificial airway is "extubation." The common indications for intubation, either by the endotracheal or tracheostomy tube, are divided into four categories:[3]

1. Relief of soft tissue and laryngeal obstruction.
2. Protection of the lower airway from aspiration

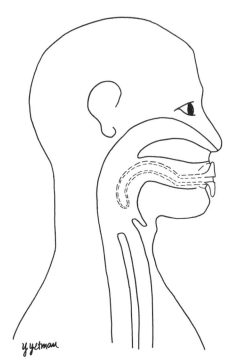

Fig. 28-3 Oropharyngeal airway.

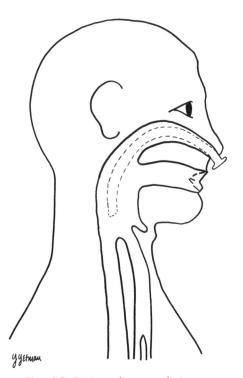

Fig. 28-4 Nasopharyngeal airway.

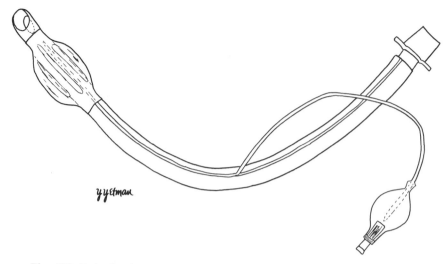

Fig. 28-5 Artificial airway specifically referred to as an endotracheal tube.

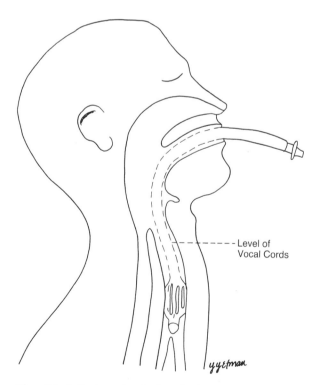

Fig. 28-6 Endotracheal tube. Oral route (orotracheal tube).

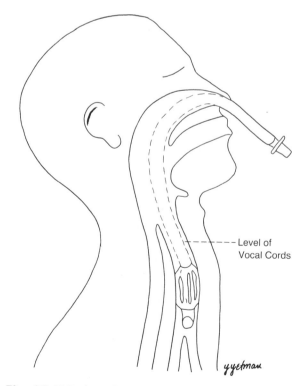

Fig. 28-7 Endotracheal tube. Nasal route (nasotracheal tube).

when the airway protective reflexes are not intact.

3. Facilitation of the removal of pulmonary secretions by tracheal suctioning.
4. Facilitation of prolonged artificial ventilation.

Extubation is indicated when the cause factor(s) for placement is not present.[3] This implies that the patient can independently maintain a patent airway without an assistive device, does not have an airway obstruction, does not require assistance with ventilation, and has the ability to swallow, cough, and maintain adequate pulmonary hygiene.

The hazards of any type of artificial airway are associated with the actual establishment of the airway, the type of airway utilized, and the ongoing care of the airway. Complications may occur during the intubation procedure, be created by pathological or mechanical problems after intubation, occur during the extubation procedure, or occur after extubation.[4]

The risk of complications is less significant than the original danger indicating the need to establish an airway. The complications are reduced with proper maintenance and airway care. Upper airway complications include sinusitis, pressure necrosis of the alsa nasi area, and otitis media.[3]

During the evaluation and treatment of patients with an artificial airway, the physical therapist should consider each of the following problems:

1. An artificial airway bypasses the body's normal defense mechanisms that prevent the lower airway from becoming contaminated with bacteria. This situation may result in bacterial contamination of the tracheobronchial tree. Therefore, evaluation of the airway secretions and provision of appropriate facilitatory and clearance techniques would be appropriate for these patients.
2. The cough or "clearance" mechanism is impaired since the vocal cords cannot approximate when an endotracheal tube is in place. The patient will need assistance in expelling secretions or require suctioning of the airway.
3. The patient is not able to speak. This communication handicap creates stress and anxiety for the patient, family, the physical therapist. Mechanisms for effective

communication should be considered to facilitate treatment and assist the patient to cope with the device.

4. An artificial airway creates a loss of personal and environmental control. Respect for the patient's dignity and consideration for his feelings are critical components of the treatment program.[3]

Endotracheal Tubes

Nasotracheal tubes are usually more suited for longer-term intubation than are oral tubes. However, the usual duration for endotracheal tube intubation is 3 days. After 72 hours, if more prolonged intubation is indicated, a tracheostomy tube is considered.

Swallowing is possible when the endotracheal tube is placed via the nasal route. While not all nutrients are provided orally the psychological benefits of swallowing liquids are significant to the critically ill patient. Drinking is difficult to perform and is *not* appropriate for *all* patients with nasotracheal tubes.[3] Caution should be given to the position, posture, appropriateness, and stability of the patient before initiating this activity.

Tracheostomy

The tracheostomy tube requires a surgical procedure for placement (Fig. 28-8). Using this particular airway has an advantage over the endotracheal tube since it does not enter the upper airway, allows the patient to swallow and eat solid food, is easier to stabilize, makes it easier to suction tracheobronchial secretions, and creates less airway resistance. Overall, this airway is better tolerated by the patient.[3] Complications from the tracheostomy may occur during the surgical procedure, and pathological or mechanical problems may occur after surgery or after extubation.[4]

Laryngeal and tracheal (lower airway) complications of artificial airways are important to consider when assessing the intubated patient. Complications may include sore throat, hoarseness, glottic or subglottic edema, ulceration of tracheal mucosa, vocal cord ulceration, granuloma and polyp, vocal cord paralysis, laryngotracheal web, and tracheal stenosis.[3]

Tracheostomy tubes can be "cuffed" or "un-

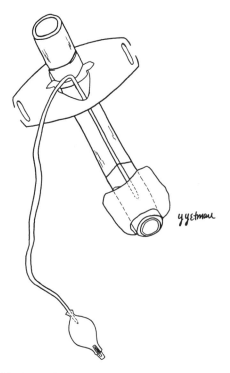

Fig. 28-8 Artificial airway—cuffed tracheostomy tube.

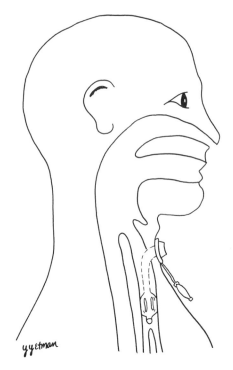

Fig. 28-9 Artificial airway—adult cuffed tracheostomy tube.

cuffed" (Figs. 28-9 and 28-10). It is important to note the appropriate management of the cuff in the total care of the patient who has an artificial airway.[3] Neonatal and pediatric artificial airways have one design feature distinguishing them from adult airways—none have cuffs. The care and considerations for these devices are similar to those of the adult population.

The complications described above may occur with either tube (endotracheal or tracheostomy) whether cuffed or uncuffed. Appropriate support and guarding of the device and airway is critical when treating patients. Pulling on the tube causes trauma to the airway.

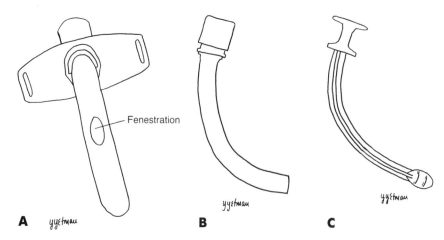

Fenestration

A   **B**   **C**

Fig. 28-10 Artificial airway. **(A)** Uncuffed fenestrated tracheostomy tube. **(B)** Inner cannula without fenestration. **(C)** Obturator.

A fenestrated tracheostomy tube has a "window" cut out of the posterior wall of the outer cannula (Fig. 28-10). This window allows the patient to breathe around and through the fenestration without requiring the actual removal of the artificial airway. This surgical procedure requires removal of the inner cannula, deflation of the cuff; and covering or plugging the opening of the outer cannula. This allows the clinician to evaluate the patient's ability to ventilate or "breathe," to clear secretions, and to protect his airway. The patient can also vocalize sounds in this manner. A variety of these fenestrated tubes are available. It is critical that they fit the patient appropriately. This device is not intended for long-term use, although special "talking tracheostomy tubes" are available for more extended use.[3]

"Tracheal buttons" are designed to keep the channel between the skin and trachea patent. They are utilized when the patient is extubated, but a potential for re-establishment of the airway exists. The stoma can be maintained open, and suctioning is permitted through the button. These devices are available for indefinite use.[3] Given adequate skin integrity, appropriate nutritional status, and good hygiene of the site, a tracheostomy stoma will usually seal within 48 hours of tracheostomy tube or button removal.[3]

Physical Therapy Intervention

Physical therapy management of the airway device and considerations of treatment are of great importance in *any* setting. Upon identifying the specific airway and its purpose, the physical therapist should evaluate the patient's pulmonary status and any indications for airway clearance techniques. It is important to consider how to support the tube and protect the anatomical airway when turning, exercising, or gait training the patient with an artificial airway. An airway (pharyngeal or artificial) assists in the management of the patient's anatomical airway. The overall goal of these devices is to keep the patient's airway patent. They provide a pathway for easily suctioning tracheobronchial secretions. These devices cannot ensure ventilation, respiration, adequate clearance, or oxygenation but provide a pathway for these functions. Complications can be minimized and some can be prevented; problems of communication and body image can be addressed.

OXYGEN THERAPY

Oxygen (O_2), a colorless, odorless, tasteless, highly combustible gas, is vital for maintaining cellular life in the atmosphere.[2,3] "Room air" is composed of 78.08 percent nitrogen, 20.95 percent oxygen, and other trace gases.[2,3,5] There is approximately 16 percent oxygen in the air we exhale.

"Supplemental oxygen" is commercial oxygen that is manufactured by fractional distillation. Manufactured oxygen is encountered in the following systems: liquid; concentrators; and cylinders. Supplemental oxygen or "oxygen therapy" is prescribed when the patient requires greater than 21 percent or more than atmospheric oxygen.

Therapeutic oxygen is extremely beneficial when utilized appropriately. Clinical goals that can be achieved through correct oxygen utilization are treatment and prevention of hypoxemia; decreased ventilatory work of breathing; and decreased myocardial work.[3,5]

Hypoxemia

The primary indication for oxygen is the treatment or prevention of hypoxemia. Supplemental oxygen does not reverse any underlying airspace abnormalities. Hypoxemia is the decrease in oxygen content of arterial blood (PaO_2). Normal ranges for PaO_2 are 80 to 90 mmHg and are obtained by a direct arterial blood measurement. This extremely important measurement is closely related to the oxygen saturation of hemoglobin (O_2SAT). O_2SAT can also be measured indirectly with an oximeter.[2–4,6]

Hypoxia

Hypoxia reflects a decrease of oxygen at the tissue level. It is related to but distinctly different from hypoxemia. Hypoxia is a "condition in which the metabolic demands of the tissues for oxygen exceed the ability of the lungs and circulatory system to supply it."[3]

A critical diagnostic and monitoring tool for patients utilizing oxygen therapy is the direct arterial blood-gas measurement. Whenever evaluating or treating patients receiving oxygen continuously or intermittently and patients with cardiopulmonary dysfunction not utilizing supplemental oxygen, it is essential for the clinician to assess for signs and symptoms of hypoxia. The clinician should first identify the type of hypoxia-associated factor(s). Four distinct types of hypoxia that are factors that lead to the clinical entities that require supplemental oxygen are:[2,4,5]

1. Hypoxic hypoxia (hypoxemia hypoxia).
2. Circulatory hypoxia (ischemia hypoxia).
3. Histotoxic hypoxia.
4. Anemic Hypoxia.

The clinician may assess changes in circulation, respiration, and central nervous system function that indicate hypoxia. Signs and symptoms will vary depending on the type of hypoxia.

Circulatory signs include:

1. Cyanosis. It is important to note that there are two different types, central and peripheral. It is difficult clinically to detect cyanosis, and it is not always considered a reliable index of hypoxia.
2. Acute hypertension with tachycardia.
3. Hypotension with bradycardia. It is important to note that this response is frequently seen in the decompensated individual (e.g., elderly patients; patients with known cardiopulmonary dysfunction).
4. Cardiac dysrhythmias.

Respiratory signs include:

1. Tachypnea.
2. Dyspnea. It is important to note that the sensation of shortness of breath does not always indicate hypoxia.

Central nervous system (CNS) symptoms include responses that are similar to alcohol intoxication or a hypoglycemic reaction in a diabetic, such as restlessness, agitation, disorientation, loss of judgement, confusion, paranoia, dizziness, drowsiness, headache, and nausea.

In addition to these signs and symptoms, the neonate may have a decreased rectal temperature.[2,4,5]

Complications

Hazards or complications of oxygen therapy include:[2,6,7]

1. Combustion. Oxygen increases the rate at which objects burn.
2. Respiratory depression or hypoventilation, especially in the patient who depends on the hypoxic drive to stimulate his ventilatory drive (chronic obstructive pulmonary disease).
3. Absorption atelectasis, alveolar collapse. "Airlessness" occurs with administration of 100 percent O_2.
4. Oxygen toxicity. Prolonged administration of high oxygen concentrations can affect the pulmonary system, CNS, retina, hematopoietic system, and endocrine organs.
5. In newborns and children, bronchopulmonary dysplasia and retrolental fibroplasia are associated with oxygen therapy.[4]

Oxygen therapy is considered potentially harmful when it is utilized inconsistently, inappropriately, and with poor monitoring and evaluation of the patient.

Delivery Systems/Oxygen Administration Devices

As previously mentioned, supplemental oxygen is provided by one of three delivery systems—(liquid, concentrators, and cylinders. Several variables are involved when choosing a particular system; therefore, in a variety of settings and patient populations, different systems may be encountered. Concerns of complications associated with oxygen therapy apply to *any* system.

Supplemental oxygen from one of the three delivery systems is administered to the patient by a variety of devices. It is important to understand that any of these administrative devices may be utilized with any system. Some of the numerous oxygen administration devices that are available commercially are depicted in Figures 28-11 to 28-14. Figure 28-15 depicts an oxygen conservation device to improve the efficiency of oxygen delivery. In addition to oxygen therapy, patients may receive humidity therapy, aerosolized medications, or any combination of these three, via these administration devices. Two categories or methods of classifying dry oxygen administration are (1) a low-flow system or variable performance device (e.g., cannula, mask); (2) a high-flow system or fixed performance device (e.g., venturi).

These systems are defined in terms of gas flow of the apparatus, *not* the oxygen flow rate through

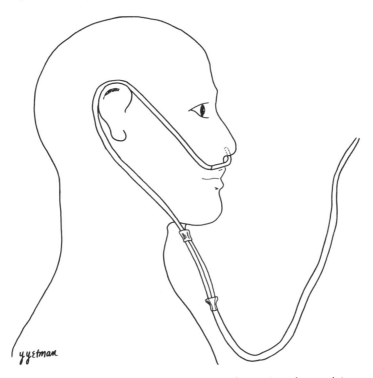

Fig. 28-11 Oxygen administration device (nasal cannula).

Oxygen
Delivery
System

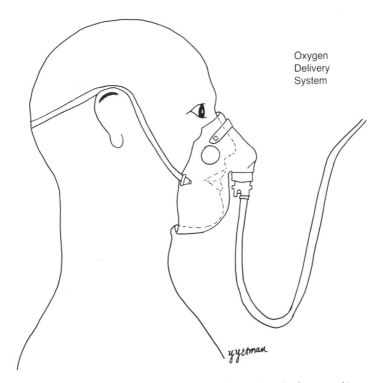

Fig. 28-12 Oxygen administration device (simple face mask).

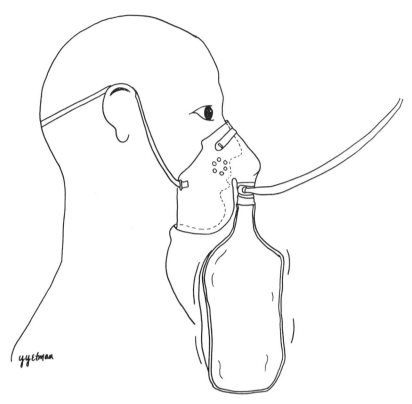

Fig. 28-13 Oxygen administration device. Rebreathing face mask can be partial or non-rebreathing depending on the specific set up utilized when high concentrations of O_2 delivery are required.

the device.[3,6] Liter flow refers to the number of liters of oxygen provided per minute (L/min). The fraction of inspired oxygen (FIO_2) is clinically defined as the "measurable or calculable concentration of oxygen delivered to the patient and indicates the percentage of oxygen present.[3]

Table 28-1 Guidelines to Estimate FIO_2 Comparing Oxygen Administration Devices

Apparatus	100% Oxygen Flow Rate (L/min)	FIO_2 (%)
Nasal cannula	1–6	0.25–0.45
Simple mask	6–15	0.35–0.65
Aerosol facemask or aerosol tracheostomy mask	6–15	0.40–0.70
Partial rebreathing mask	Flow rate so reservoir bag remains inflated	0.60–0.80
Nonbreathing mask	Flow rate so reservoir bag remains inflated	0.85–0.95

Guidelines for estimating FIO_2 with oxygen flow utilizing oxygen administration devices are provided in Table 28-1. These are estimates of oxygen delivered into the respiratory system. It is critical to understand that differences between individuals occur owing to variances in their tidal volume (V_T), breathing rate or frequency (f), minute volume, and pattern of ventilation.[3] The percentage of estimated supplemental oxygen delivered does not ensure "respiration." It is important, that the clinician performs an appropriate cardiopulmonary physical therapy evaluation on individuals receiving oxygen and assesses the effectiveness of the supplemental therapy. Key points in the evaluation and treatment of individuals requiring oxygen therapy include the following:

1. Recall that supplemental oxygen is a prescribed drug.
2. Obtain a baseline cardiopulmonary evaluation (especially noting vital signs and ventilatory pattern).

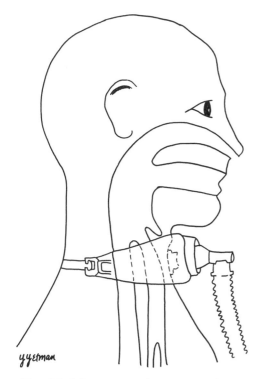

Fig. 28-14 Oxygen administration device (tracheostomy collar).

3. Monitor and record appropriate evaluative data during and after treatment.
4. Obtain oxygenation status directly by complete arterial blood-gas measurement, or indirectly with an oximeter for the percent O_2 saturation measurement.
5. Monitor patient for signs and symptoms of hypoxemia/hypoxia.
6. Evaluate the oxygen administrative device including correct flow (liters per minute or the FIO_2), appropriate fit, flexibility and mobility during treatment.
7. Evaluate oxygen delivery system including length of lines or cords, needed electrical outlet, portability, weight of portable unit, and leakage; and consider the mobility of the system given the patient's status.

VENTILATORS VERSUS RESPIRATORS

This section discusses assistive devices that support breathing. Terminology and concepts related to this equipment are important to clarify. Terms such as "artificial ventilator," "mechanical support," "mechanical ventilation," and "respirator" tend to be used interchangeably in the clinical setting. Terminology related to respiratory support devices can be confusing and at times seem contradictory. *Ventilation* is the process of supplying air (gas) to the pulmonary system for the actual gas exchange, or *respiration*, to occur at the alveolar level. Gas exchange occurs by simple diffusion of gas molecules along a gradient of differences in the partial pressure of the gas.

Definition

Machines provide for the movement of gases into and out of the pulmonary system. Ventilation does not ensure respiration; therefore, ventilators are not respirators.[3] A patient may receive artificial ventilation by various methods or devices. The most common manual breathing is mouth-to-mouth "rescue breathing" as performed in CPR.[1] Several types of masks are now available for mouth-to-mask rescue breathing. These are rec-

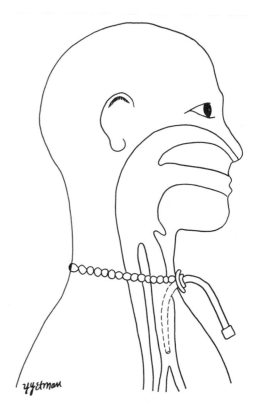

Fig. 28-15 Oxygen administration device (transtracheal oxygen conservation system).

ommended when working in areas with a high risk of infection. Rescue breathing can also be performed by using a manual resuscitator device, such as an AMBU (air-mask-bag-unit) or Laerdal bag. The purpose of a bag (manual resuscitator) is to manually apply positive pressure to the airway.[8] It is recommended that these bags be available for use in departments and clinics. They have an attachment so oxygen can be delivered along with the positive pressure. A variety of bags are manufactured, and they all function essentially in the same manner. It is important to recall that rescue breathing is performed at 12 breaths per minute or one every 5 seconds.[1] The patient is "bagged" at this rate with a smooth even rhythm. The "bagging" technique is also described below (see Suctioning, below).

Ventilators are found in *all* settings, not just an ICU. These settings include, but are not limited to, home, school, community, work, cars, outpatient clinics, rehabilitation centers, extended care facilities, standard hospital rooms, and physical therapy departments. Ventilators exist in a variety of sizes and shapes to better adapt to these settings. For purposes of this discussion, ventilators will be classified into two types: negative pressure and positive pressure.

Negative-Pressure Ventilators

Negative-pressure ventilators apply alternating or intermittent subatmospheric pressure to the patient's trunk or entire body. These machines are often thought of as large and cumbersome. Examples of negative-pressure ventilators include the iron lung, cuirass ventilator, rocking devices or bed, pneumobelt, and "raincoat."[2] These external ventilators do not require an artificial airway (intubation). Clinically, they are associated with individuals who have "normal" lungs, but who have difficulty, breathing. Patients with certain neuromuscular dysfunctions (diseases) may require this type of ventilatory support at night or intermittently. Evaluation and research on various negative-pressure devices may encourage the broader utilization of these ventilators with other individuals who have lung disease.

Positive-Pressure Ventilators

Positive-pressure ventilators apply supra-atmospheric pressure into the patient's airway by an endotracheal or tracheostomy tube.[2] These are the machines most commonly referred to as ventilators. They also come in various shapes and sizes, and their portability enables their use in any setting. These positive-pressure machines are further subdivided by describing their mechanism of ending or limiting inspiration and initiating expiration.[5]

Discussion of positive-pressure ventilators can be complex when listing the brands and describing the variety of models. A new generation of mechanical ventilators that were introduced in this decade has changed some approaches to ventilatory support. For example, microprocessor-controlled units are highly sophisticated, complex machines; however, the basic guidelines for assessing the patient are the same as those used with the older machines.

Considering all the equipment associated with the acute care environment, ventilators are typically viewed as the most intimidating. The acute care clinician may seek out opportunities to work around the machines; however, adjustments and fear reduction are necessary steps in the orientation and educational process to these machines.

Use of the Ventilator

In Figures 28-5 to 28-7 the patient requires an artificial airway (endotracheal tube). The endotracheal tube could be attached to a ventilator or to a source of oxygen or humidity (T-piece), or to any combination of these. When a patient is intubated, typically a mechanical ventilation is required. In the process of "weaning," or discontinuing ventilatory support, patients may be required to breathe or ventilate on their own, but will continue to utilize an artificial airway. The artificial airway ensures patency, but patients breathe on their own; and respiration is assessed by arterial blood-gas values (see Airways, above). The physical therapist has an important role in the treatment of ventilated patients and in their weaning process. In the evaluation and treatment of patients utilizing *any* type of mechanical assistance in *any* environment the following key points are suggested for review.

Evaluation of the Ventilator

1. What is the type and purpose of the ventilatory assistance?

2. How many breaths does the ventilator deliver (number per minute)?
3. Are the breaths in a predicted rhythmical pattern at a set rate?
4. Are the breaths intermittent?
5. What is the volume of air the ventilator is delivering?
6. Where are the alarms?
7. What is the length of the tubing connected to the individual?
8. How mobile is the unit and the connecting tubing?
9. Review chart data that indicate the prescribed ventilatory setting, mode, oxygen concentration, and any aerosolized medications.
10. What additional monitoring equipment is available to assist in evaluating the patient's response, for example, electrocardiograph, continuous heart rate, blood pressure readings, oximetry, etc.

Evaluations of the Patient

1. Note indications that airway suctioning is needed before continuing with the evaluation process.
2. Determine whether airway clearance and suctioning techniques are priority treatments at this time.
3. Identify which artificial airway the patient has attached to the ventilator.
4. Assess the patient's work of breathing, including:
   frequency of ventilation or respiratory rate.
   which muscle(s) is assisting the patient's ventilatory efforts.
   the effectiveness of the muscle(s) (strength or fatigue).
   the volume of air being ventilated.
   the overall "pattern of ventilation"—compare the patient's breathing pattern with the ventilator setting.
5. Determine the patient's functional and mobility status.

SUCTIONING

Tracheal aspiration or airway suctioning of tracheobronchial secretions largely depends on the effectiveness of the patient's cough and his ability to adequately clear the airway.[3] In the spontaneously breathing patient, effective mobilization and clearance of secretions is an important evaluation measure for the physical therapist. Tracheobronchial secretion aspiration is indicated for *all* patients who are intubated either with an endotracheal tube or a tracheostomy tube. Patients with these artificial airways are unable to cough effectively and thus expel their tracheal secretions.[3,5]

Clinically, physical therapy treatment for assistive cough techniques and secretion mobilization and clearance are commonly performed to minimize or even omit the airway suctioning procedure in the spontaneously breathing patient (see Ch. 00). When the suctioning procedure is necessary, physical therapy treatment modalities are utilized with the intubated patient to promote optimum clearing of the airway. It is important to consider the need of airway suctioning with either the spontaneously breathing or intubated patient once any facilitory techniques are performed and *before* any position changes occur. Frequency of suctioning is increased when the patient has copious secretions.[3] However, complications can occur with any amount of suctioning. It is critical for the physical therapist to evaluate and monitor the patient's medical status, to understand the indications for suctioning in the individual, and to be competent in the suctioning technique or procedure.

Hypoxemia, cardiac dysrhythmias, hypotension, and lung collapse are all complications associated with airway aspiration.[3,5] Hazards of an incorrect suctioning procedure include ulceration of the tracheal mucosa.[5]

Competent performance of the suctioning procedure can only be achieved in the clinical setting under the supervision of a clinician skilled in all aspects of tracheobronchial aspiration. Thus, the potential for complications can be minimized and the hazards of suctioning can be avoided.

Portable equipment is availble for the clinic or home settings since patients with impaired airway clearance will often be seen in these settings. Appropriate suctioning equipment and supplies should be in stock if treating patients with known dysfunction associated with airway clearance or if potential clearance problems exist.

Airway suctioning is critical to the total care of the patient with airway clearance dysfunction; however, it is not considered a pleasant procedure to execute. Potential hazards exist when one facilitates the mobilization of secretions and does not provide the appropriate skill of airway aspiration as necessary, and waiting for suctioning at a later time by someone else is not a recommended policy. Any clinician who supervises or performs treatment for patients with impaired airway clearance should be prepared to competently provide appropriate suctioning techniques. The outcome of an effective suctioning procedure should include improved ventilation-perfusion, improved oxygenation, decreased work of breathing, and improved clearance with decreased trauma.

Airway Suctioning Technique

The following key points are suggested for review with the appropriate protocol for suctioning.

Prepare the Patient

1. Provide a clear explanation of the procedure.
2. Provide support throughout the procedure, re-explaining and informing the patient of the steps. (This is an appropriate practice even when treating infants and unconscious individuals.)
3. Position the patient.
4. Evaluate and monitor the patient before, during, and after the procedure including auscultation and palpation.

Prepare the Equipment

1. Evaluate suctioning device for appropriate vacuum level:
   100 to 120 mmHg recommended for adults.
   60 to 80 mmHg recommended for infants.
2. Ensure availability of supplemental oxygen.
3. Have available:
   Appropriate size sterile suction catheter.
   Pair of sterile gloves (wear a glove on each hand). (Suction kits are available that include sterile gloves, catheters, and a container for sterile saline.)
   Sterile saline.
   Sterile lubrication gel, if indicated.

Prepare the Clinician

1. Wash hands using the correct procedure before and after suctioning.
2. Maintain medical asepsis throughout the procedure, that is, clean technique utilizing sterile gloves, catheter, and saline and preventing contamination of this equipment.

3. Evaluate patient for signs and symptoms of retained secretions and the clearance of these secretions.
4. Evaluate patient for potential complications.
5. Observe monitoring equipment if available.

The Procedure

During the actual suctioning procedure, a catheter is slowly and gently inserted into the airway with no suction applied. Once an obstruction is felt (carina), the catheter is slightly pulled back, and a vacuum is applied during this withdrawal. Rotation of the catheter and intermittently applied suction is recommended during the procedure. The duration of applied vacuum should be no longer than 10 to 15 seconds. Preoxygenation, postoxygenation, and appropriate rest periods are suggested for the patient.[3,5,9]

A slightly different procedure has been suggested for endotracheal suctioning of the neonate. The key points when performing suctioning with neonates include the following:

1. Utilization of a transcutaneous oxygen monitor to evaluate oxygenation status.
2. For bagging, attach bag to a pressure manometer to evaluate safe levels.
3. Limit duration of suctioning to 5 to 10 seconds.
4. Observe caution with hyperoxygenation while hyperventilating to minimize hyperoxia and hypoxia.
5. Set vacuum level of suction machine between 60 and 80 mm Hg.[9]

The bagging procedure is controversial and should be performed with caution. However, the procedure is sometimes utilized for the following reasons:[3,5,9]

1. To deliver an "extra" breath and preoxygenate the individual before airway suctioning.
2. To maintain a degree of positive end expiratory pressure.
3. To evaluate the lung compliance.
4. To facilitate tracheal lavage.

SUMMARY

This chapter provides information on devices associated with acute care, specifically respiratory care. The ICU environment and equipment is often viewed as intimidating, even offensive, to some clinicians. However, this setting can serve as a positive learning experience. Physical therapy interventions conducted in this environment are directed toward goals of promoting and restoring function and relieving or minimizing discomfort.

The acuity level of patients across all practice settings is rising, and they require skills for physical therapy interventions. Given that prevention and reduction of dysfunction is a key focus of early intervention, the acuity level of the patient and the amount of monitoring and supportive equipment should not retard or stop this critical role of

physical therapy. The physical therapist's role and contribution to the critically ill patient in the non-ICU environment is significant. Patients with primary or secondary cardiopulmonary dysfunction may require a variety of respiratory care devices. Equipment alone should not limit physical therapy treatment. Appropriately utilized equipment may actually enhance treatment outcomes. Table 28-2 is provided as a guideline when encountering medical equipment and monitoring apparatus. The ability to handle these devices is necessary in any setting or situation.

ACKNOWLEDGMENT

I acknowledge Yvonne Yetman for the drawings depicted in this chapter.

REFERENCES

1. Journal of the American Medical Association. Standards and Guidelines for Cardiopulmonary Resuscitation and Emergency Cardiac Care. Vol. 255. No. 21. American Medical Association, Chicago, 1986
2. Morrison ML: Respiratory Intensive Care Nursing. 2nd Ed. Little, Brown, Boston, 1979
3. Shapiro BA, Harrison RA, Kacmarek RM, Cane RD: Clinical Application of Respiratory Care. 3rd Ed. Year Book Medical Publishers, Chicago, 1985
4. Burgess WR, Chernick V: Respiratory Therapy in Newborn Infants and Children. 2nd Ed. Thieme, New York, 1986
5. Frownfelter D: Chest Physical Therapy and Pulmonary Rehabilitation. 2nd Ed. Year Book Medical Publishers, Chicago, 1987
6. Kofke WA, Levy JH: Postoperative Critical Care Procedures of the Massachusetts General Hospital. Little, Brown, Boston, 1986
7. Burton GG, Gee GN, Hodgkin JE: Respiratory Care. JB Lippincott, Philadelphia, 1977
8. McPherson SP, Spearman CB: Respiratory Therapy Equipment. 3rd Ed. CV Mosby, Princeton, NJ, 1985
9. Irwin S, Tecklin JS: Cardiopulmonary Physical Therapy. Vol. 1. CV Mosby, St. Louis, 1985

SUGGESTED READINGS

Cherniack RM, Cherniack L, Nalmark A: Respiration in Health and Disease. 2nd Ed. WB Saunders, Philadelphia, 1972

Guyton AC: Textbook of Medical Physiology. 4th Ed. WB Saunders, Philadelphia, 1971

Hislop HJ, Sanger JO: Chest Disorders in Children. American Physical Therapy Association, New York, 1968

Table 28-2 Guideline for Equipment Review

1. Identify equipment	Name and define the device(s); what is its purpose?
2. Identify the dysfunction that requires this equipment	Why is this patient using the device?
3. Identify how this dysfunction affects treatment	What are the signs, symptoms, and will they be altered by treatment?
4. Evaluate the equipment	Assess the device(s): Is it portable? Is it operating correctly?
5. Create a plan of action	What support or guarding is needed? Will assistance of another person or other piece of equipment be necessary? What precautions are necessary? What objective information is available to record?
6. Conduct the evaluation-treatment	Perform the physical therapy plan of care considering the plan identified in Step 5.
7. Evaluate the physical therapy treatment and how the equipment was handled	What should be done the same way during the next treatment? What should be done differently and how? Did the equipment assist in objectively measuring the patient's response to treatment?
8. Re-evaluate the equipment	Reassess the device(s): Is it operating correctly?

Lister MJ (ed): Physical Therapy. Journal of the American Physical Therapy Association. American Physical Therapy Association, Washington, 1982

MacKenzie CF (ed): Chest Physiotherapy in the Intensive Care Unit. Williams & Wilkins, Baltimore, 1981

McArdle WD, Katch FI, Katch VL: Exercise Physiology, Energy, Nutrition, and Human Performance. 2nd Ed. Lea & Febiger, Philadelphia, 1986

Nunn JF: Applied Respiratory Physiology. Butterworth, London, 1969

Petty T: Ambulatory Oxygen. Thieme, New York, 1983

Pollock ML, Wilmore JH, Fox SM, III: Exercise in Health and Disease. WB Saunders, Philadelphia, 1984

Rushmer RF: Cardiovascular Dynamics. 4th Ed. WB Saunders, Philadelphia, 1976

Shapiro BA: Clinical Application of Blood Gases. Year Book Medical Publishers, Chicago, 1973

Stephens GJ: Pathophysiology for Health Practitioners. MacMillan, New York, 1980

West JB: Respiratory Physiology—The Essentials. 3rd Ed. Williams & Wilkins, Baltimore, 1985

West JB: Pulmonary Pathophysiology—The Essentials. Williams & Wilkins, Baltimore, 1977

29 Pulmonary Physical Therapy

Elizabeth J. Protas

Pulmonary physical therapy encompasses a number of interventions used by the physical therapist to improve the respiratory and functional status of the patient with pulmonary disease or dysfunction. There is considerable variety in these interventions that reflects the variations encountered in the patient population. These problems run the gamut from postoperative atelectasis to the older adult with emphysema. This chapter provides an overview concerning pulmonary physical therapy techniques.

INDICATIONS

Secretion Retention

Secretion retention is the most common indication for pulmonary physical therapy. The retention of secretions can occur in the postoperative patient, in the patient with chronic obstructive pulmonary disease (COPD), or in the neurologically injured patient with poor control of the respiratory muscles. For whatever reason, the patient is having difficulty clearing these secretions from the lung.

Poor Pulmonary Function Values

Decreased forced vital capacities and flow volume loops suggest that respiration is not adequate to meet the body's needs during activity and exercise. Reduced pulmonary function is often associated with chronic pulmonary diseases.

Changes in Arterial Blood-Gases

Reduced arterial oxygenation and carbon dioxide retention are often seen when there is insufficient gas exchange between the pulmonary alevoli and the arterioles. Anything that would increase the effective width of the alveolar walls, such as secretions or edema, will decrease the gas exchange that occurs.

Decreased Cardiopulmonary Function

Decreased cardiopulmonary function can be the result of anesthesia during and pain after surgery, or it can occur as a result of chronic pulmonary disease. This can be manifested by poor pulmonary function and arterial blood-gas values as well as a tendency to retain secretions.

Decreased Activity Tolerance with or without Supplemental Oxygen

One of the most common complaints from patients with pulmonary disorders is the inability to tolerate ordinary activities of daily living. Shortness of breath during even moderate activities is often the first symptom that a patient demonstrates.

Decreased Respiratory Muscle Strength and Endurance

Changes in respiratory muscle strength and endurance can mean the loss of extremely important compensatory abilities. Decreases are especially notable in patients who are on ventilators.

665

Poor Posture

Abnormalities of the chest wall as well as adaptations to chronic respiratory distress can compromise the pulmonary system. Likewise, loss of range of movement in the chest wall can impinge on pulmonary function.

Abnormal Breathing Patterns

Changes in breathing patterns can result in an increase in the cost of the work of breathing. That is, more than a usual portion of the body's energy is required to maintain breathing.

Generalized Muscle Deconditioning.

Associated with many chronic illnesses is a vicious cycle of reduced activity that leads to decreased muscle strength and endurance. The reduced general endurance will also infringe on the patient's functional status.

GOALS OF PULMONARY PHYSICAL THERAPY

Increase Secretion Clearance

Improved effectiveness of the patient's ability to remove secretions and maintain the lung free of secretions is an important outcome for pulmonary physical therapy.

Improve Pulmonary Function

Significant improvements in pulmonary function have been documented after secretion clearance from the lung.[1] For patients with COPD, however, extensive pathological changes in the lung are irreversible and do not allow substantial changes in pulmonary function.

Improve Arterial Blood-Gas Values

Increases in the partial pressure of arterial oxygen (PaO_2) and decreases in elevated arterial carbon dioxide values have also been seen with secretion clearance.[1] Supervised breathing exercises and incentive spirometry have been credited with reversing atelectasis and thus improving blood-gas values in postoperative patients.

Enhance Cardiopulmonary Function

Enhancement of cardiopulmonary function may be a more generalized goal that relates to both pathology and the patient deconditioning that occurs with illness. Pulmonary physical therapy techniques are aimed at improving the patient's overall functional status.

Improve Physical Work Capacity

The physical work capacity (PWC) is the maximal level at which the patient can exercise. PWC is also referred to as the aerobic capacity and is frequently measured as the maximum oxygen uptake.[2] Individuals with pulmonary disease are often limited by dypsnea experienced during activities. An exercise program aimed at increasing activity tolerance will result in greater exercise efficiency and endurance.[3]

Enhance Respiratory Muscle Strength and Endurance

Exercises that are specifically designed to increase either respiratory muscle strength or endurance have been evaluated. Significant improvements in these functions have been reported.[4–8]

Improve Postural Alignment and Mobility

The goal is to encourage the assumption of a more normal posture, since many of these patients will tend to adopt a posture that has excessive tension in the respiratory accessory muscles and the appearance of a stressful position (Fig. 29-1). Likewise, decreased activity can lead to losses in range of motion of the upper extremities and thorax.

Establish Improved Breathing Patterns

There are several approaches to establish improved breathing patterns. Encouraging patients to breath deeply is important in fully aerating the lung and preventing atelectasis. Several authors also advocate breathing retraining to change a patient's breathing pattern.[9,10] An example would be the emphasis on lengthening the exhalation time.

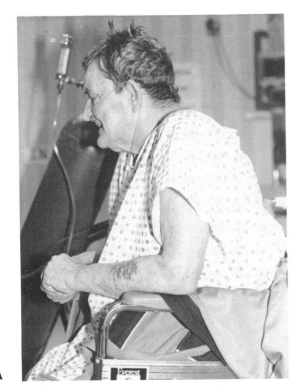

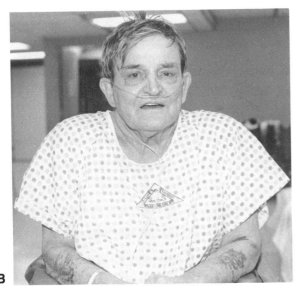

Fig. 29-1 (A,B) Posture of the patient with chronic obstructive lung disease.

Enhance General Muscle Performance

Improving muscle strength can improve the patient's tolerance for demanding activities such as lifting. Many patients will experience dypsnea when trying to lift heavy objects.

INITIAL PATIENT EVALUATION

Primary Diagnosis

Establishing a patient's primary diagnosis can be a difficult task, particularly in patients with chronic pulmonary illnesses. The following guidelines may be useful for the physical therapist when determining the patient's primary diagnosis:

1. The most straightforward situation is one in which the patient's primary medical complaint is the same as the admitting diagnosis. For example, the primary diagnosis is COPD with the admitting diagnosis an exacerbation of the COPD.
2. If a patient has a history of multiple medical problems and has been admitted for one of those problems, the primary diagnosis for the admission is that problem. For example, the patient has a history of coronary artery disease, diabetes mellitus, and hypertension. He is admitted for coronary artery bypass surgery secondary to coronary artery disease. His primary diagnosis is coronary artery disease.
3. A patient who has a history of multiple medical complaints, but is admitted for a new complaint, should be considered to have the primary diagnoses of the multiple medical problems. For example, the patient has a history of COPD, congestive heart failure, and hypertension, but is admitted for gastrointestinal tract bleeding. The primary diagnoses are COPD, congestive heart failure, and hypertension.

History

Note all pertinent information that could assist in the management of a patient. The following would be key points to examine:

1. Any *past medical history*, especially that which relates to pulmonary status, should be noted. For example, the patient with acquired immune deficiency syndrome (AIDS) who has a history of *Pneumocystis carinii* pneumonia is susceptible to the development of this pneumonia again.
2. Pertinent *past surgical history* can provide information about complications a patient experienced with surgery or anesthesia.
3. *Socioeconomic history* will provide information on life-style characteristics such as smoking, alcohol or substance abuse, living conditions, family and occupational history. Table 29-1 is a list of the most common pulmonary diseases that are associated with occupational exposure to noxious agents.[11]

Contraindications and Precautions

Many conditions can exist that would preclude certain pulmonary physical therapy techniques. For example, vibration and shaking of the chest is contraindicated with rib fractures. Likewise, some situations would require that precautions be taken during pulmonary physical therapy. For example,

Table 29-1. Pulmonary Diseases Associated with Occupational Exposure to Noxious Agents

Pulmonary Disease	Noxious Agent or Condition
Pulmonary fibrosis	Asbestosis (asbestos exposure) Silicosis (hard rock mining) Pneumoconiosis (coal dust exposure)
Pulmonary infiltrates of immunological origin	Farmer's lung (allergic alveolitis from animal and vegetable material) Beryllium disease (nuclear reactors, x-ray tubes, aviation)
Obstructive airway disease	Occupational asthma (induced by occupational inhalant) Byssinosis (cotton or flax dust in textile industry)
Toxic injury	Irritant gases (e.g., ammonia, chlorine, hydrogen chloride)
Cancer	Asbestosis Exposure to arsenic, chromates, and/or nickel

care must be taken when using percussion on a patient who has osteoporosis. The most common problems are presented in Table 29-2.

Table 29-2. Conditions Requiring Precautions in Relation to Pulmonary Physical Therapy

Technique	Condition Requiring Precautions
Percussion	Flail chest or surgical incision instability Rib fractures or lesions Bone disorders (e.g., osteoporosis, Paget's disease, metastatic bone lesions) Hemoptysis Bleeding disorders, hemorrhage, anticoagulant drugs, decreased blood platelets, petichiae Severe pain Fresh burns, skin grafts, or open wounds Incision sites with chest or heart surgery Unstable cardiac conditions (e.g., uncontrolled dysrhythmias) Acute tuberculosis without chest secretions Pneumothorax Fragile, elderly person Subcutaneous emphysema Recent spinal fusion
Trendelenberg position	Systemic and pulmonary hypertension Acute neurological problems (craniotomy, cerebral aneurysm, increased intracranial pressure, coma, recent cerebral vascular accident) Shortness of breath Unstable cardiac conditions Recent meals or tube feedings Unstable fluid balance (congestive heart failure, pulmonary edema, ascites, renal dialysis) Esophageal procedures Recent face and neck surgery
Shaking	Rib fracture, flail chest, or incisional instability Degenerative or metastatic bone disorders Hemoptysis Unstable cardiac conditions Severe pain Gastrointestinal distress

Vital Signs

Note any changes in vital signs that may influence treatment, for example, changes in the respiratory rate that occur during activity or when the patient is anxious. Any chronic dysrhythmias that occur during activity should be noted. The current status of the patient's vital signs should also be documented.

Laboratory Test Results

Admissions for patients with pulmonary complaints are generally associated with a battery of diagnostic procedures. Information such as increased white blood cells or decreased platelets can indicate an infection or a reduced immunological system. If a patient is on supplemental oxygen when blood gases are drawn, the therapist needs to know the fraction of oxygen in the inspired air (FIO_2) to make decisions concerning appropriate supplemental oxygen values during treatment.

Medication

The medications that the patient is taking can provide information on the stability of the patient's condition, as well as other related conditions that impinge on the patient. Bronchodilators, mucolytic agents, antibiotics, and steroids are commonly used in patients with pulmonary disorders.[12] Cardiac medications such as antiarrhythmic agents, cardiac stimulants, and vasopressors are often prescribed. Table 29-3 lists some of the most common medications in each of these categories.

Respiratory Therapy

A number of respiratory therapy situations will provide knowledge about the patient. The therapist should identify the mode of ventilation (spontaneous breathing or intubated with mechanical ventilation), the administration of supplemental oxygen as well as the FIO_2, the use of bronchodilator or aerosol therapy, and the use of incentive spirometry. The frequency with which a patient is receiving respiratory therapy modalities can assist the physical therapist in scheduling pulmonary treatments at optimal times, such as after the administration of bronchodilator medications.

Table 29-3. Common Medications in Patients with Pulmonary Diseases

Type of Medication	Examples
Antiarrhythmia drugs	Dilantin (phenytoin), Inderal (propranolol), Pronestyl (procainamide), quinidine, Xylocaine (lidocaine)
Antibiotics	Chloromycetin, erythromycin, gentamicin, Keflin (cephalothin), Mandol (cefamandole), tetracycline, tobramycin
Bronchodilators	Alupent (metaproterenol), aminophylline, Bronkosol (isoetharine), Cheledyl, Isuprel (isoproterenol), Metaprel (metaproterenol), Tedral, Vaponefrin (racepinephrine)
Cardiac stimulants	Atropine, calcium, digoxin, epinephrine, Isuprel
Mucolytic agents	Mucomyst (acetylcysteine)
Steroids	Decadron (dexamethasone), prednisone, Solu-Medrol (methylprednisolone)
Vasopressors	Dopamine, epinephrine, Levophed (norepinephrine), Nipride (nitroprusside), nitroglycerine

Patient Observation

The patient's general physical appearance, posture, color (cyanosis, pallor, flush), clubbing of the digits, condition of the skin, jugular vein distension, and the existence of extremity edema will provide information on how chronic and involved the patient's condition has been. A patient who has chronically experienced poor arterial oxygenation will exhibit facial signs of stress and a protective posture and often has hypertrophied sternocleidomastoid muscles. Jugular vein distension and edema are associated with congestive heart failure.

Chest Configuration

Postural abnormalities and asymmetries frequently occur in patients with pulmonary disease. Common chest problems and their definitions appear in Table 29-4. Deviations from normal postural alignment can further compromise lung function.

Table 29-4. Postural Abnormalities in Pulmonary Patients

Abnormality	Description
Kyphosis	Increased anterior-to-posterior curvature of the thoracic spine
Scoliosis	Lateral curvature in the vertebral column
Kyphoscoliosis	Combination of increased anterior-to-posterior and lateral curvature that can restrict lung volumes
Barrel chest	Ribs are fixed in a more elevated position that increases anteroposterior diameter and flattens the diaphragm
Pectus carinatum	Referred to as pigeon breast because there is an anterior displacement of the middle portion of the sternum and ribs
Pectus excavatum	Referred to as funnel breast since there is a depression of the lower one-third of the sternum and ribs

Breathing Patterns

The therapist should note the areas of the chest wall being used during breathing. The chest should expand symmetrically. Decreased unilateral expansion suggests that poor ventilation is occurring in some areas of the lung. This is commonly seen in patients after surgery when the patient will reduce chest expansion because of pain. Since the diaphragm is the primary muscle of respiration, an estimate of diaphragmatic movement should be established. This can be done by placing the thumbs on either side of the costosternal angle when the patient is supine, and asking the patient to take a deep breath. With normal diaphragmatic excursion, the therapist's thumbs will be moved apart and slightly upward.[10] Diaphragmatic movement is often limited in the patient who is barrel chested or has COPD or both, after chest or abdominal surgery, or after high cervical spinal cord injuries. Another common variation in chest expansion is shallow, apical breathing. This pattern is most often associated with pain and obstructive lung disease.

Breathing rate abnormalities are frequently ob-

served. Tachypnea is a fast, shallow rate associated with respiratory distress, whereas hyperpnea is an increased rate and depth of breathing. A decreased, regular rate of breathing is called bradypnea, and a total absence of breathing is apnea.

Abnormalities in the rhythm of breathing should be noted during the patient evaluation. Table 29-5 lists common rhythm abnormalities and their definitions. Additional observations should include minimal, moderate, or maximal use of accessory musculature, whether or not the patient is splinting painful areas, and the occurrence of nasal flaring.

Table 29-5. Breathing Rhythm Abnormalities

Name	Description
Dyspnea	Difficult or labored breathing that can occur at rest, spontaneously without exertion, or with exertion. When seen with ankle edema, dyspnea is indicative of right heart failure.
Orthopnea	Breathing difficulty when reclining that is often described as the one-, two-, or three-pillow orthopnea for the number of pillows required for comfortable breathing. Suggests left heart failure.
Obstructive	Prolonged expiration secondary to airway obstruction.
Parodoxical	General term referring to variation of normal breathing patterns.
Cheyne-Stokes	Progressive hyperpnea, alternating with periods of apnea.
Biot's	Abrupt, irregular onset of hyperpnea, alternating regularly with periods of apnea.
Kussmaul's	Panting, labored breathing characterized by increased rate and depth.
Apneustic	Prolonged, gasping inspiration, followed by short, inefficient expiration. Often seen in patients with asthma.
Pursed-lip	Slow inspiration followed by slow passive expiration through pursed lips.
Sighing	Breathing punctuated by frequent sighs.

Auscultation and Palpation

Breath sounds will provide additional information on how well the lung is being ventilated. The different areas of the lung may be auscultated as shown in Figure 29-2. Breath sounds can be described as normal (a slight rustling sound during inspiration and the first part of expiration), decreased, absent, or bronchial (heard normally over the manubrium as a hollow, loud, high-pitched sound). Decreased breath sounds can occur in situations such as a pneumothorax, severe emphysema, pleural effusion, pleural thickening, and early stages of lobar pneumonia. Bronchial breath sounds are abnormal when heard over lung tissue, and indicative of consolidation or compression of lung tissue secondary to increased pleural fluid.[13]

Abnormal or *adventitious breath sounds* can be classified as rales, rhonchi or wheezes, and pleural rubs.[14] Rales consist of short, discontinuous crackling or bubbling sounds that can be heard during inspiration or expiration or both. These sounds are often associated with the sudden opening of previously closed airways.[10] Rales that can be heard during both inspiration and expiration suggest fluid in the larger airways such as fluid occurring with pulmonary edema. Rhonchi or wheezes are loud, gurgling, rumbling, continuous sounds caused by air passing through airways that are obstructed by secretions, swelling, bronchospasm,

or tumors. Rhonchi are most commonly heard during exhalation and often represent diffuse airway obstruction. Most people are familiar with the audible wheezes heard in an individual during a bronchial asthma attack. Pleural rubs are creaking, dry, leathery sounds heard throughout inspiration and expiration, although they are often more audible during inspiration. Rubs denote pleural inflammation and subsequent loss of lubrication.

Voice sounds generated during auscultation can also be evaluated as normal, decreased, or increased. Whispered pectoriloquy is an increased transmission of a whisper indicative of consolidation of lung tissue or collapsed tissue such as with atelectasis. Bronchophony is exaggerated vocal resonance heard over a bronchus and suggests solidification such as that which might occur with a tumor or when pleural effusion compresses lung tissue. Egophony is a change of a vocalized "e" to an "a" sound heard through the stethoscope. This change is useful in distinguishing between consolidation and pleural effusion. Egophony is associated with and heard directly over an effusion.

By palpating the chest wall, the physical therapist can confirm information about areas of consolidation or hyperinflation detected through auscultation. Vibrations that can be palpated on the chest wall and are produced by speech or secretions are referred to as *tactile fremitus*. These vibrations can

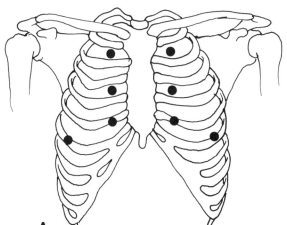

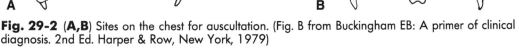

Fig. 29-2 (A,B) Sites on the chest for auscultation. (Fig. B from Buckingham EB: A primer of clinical diagnosis. 2nd Ed. Harper & Row, New York, 1979)

be increased, decreased, or rhonchal. Since sound is transmitted better through solid objects or fluids than through air, increased fremitus will take place with consolidation or compression of lung tissue. For example, atelectasis or pulmonary edema would increase the vibration felt when the patient repeatedly voices the number "99," whereas a pneumothorax will result in decreased tactile fremitus. Rhonchal fremitus is increased vibrations produced by an obstructed bronchus. The obstruction can be secondary to secretions, a tumor, bronchiectasis, or bronchitis in the large airways. The apical, anterior, lateral, and posterior chest wall should be palpated bilaterally for the therapist to determine whether there is an asymmetrical difference in the chest vibrations.

PULMONARY PHYSICAL THERAPY PROCEDURES

Postural Drainage

Postural drainage, as the name implies, is a method of positioning a patient so that gravity will assist in draining secretions from a particular lung area. The positioning used is illustrated in Figure 29-3. The positions used in a treatment will depend on the results of the initial patient evaluation. For example, if a patient has rales over the right middle lobe and radiographic evidence of atelectasis in that area, the patient would be positioned three-fourths supine with the foot of the bed elevated 14 inches. The time advocated for maintaining each postural drainage position varies in the literature. Both Frownfelter[15] and Humberstone[10] suggest a 20-minute period for each drainage position, although Humberstone notes that when postural drainage is combined with percussion and vibration, each position may be maintained as little as 2 minutes.[10] Mackenzie,[1] on the other hand, recommends that treatment be continued as long as sputum is produced and until auscultatory evidence of secretion clearance is produced when treating the patient in intensive care with an acute lung pathology. He suggests that, using these criteria, the duration of therapy may vary from 15 minutes to 2 hours. It is recommended that the physical therapist select an objective endpoint for each individual patient, rather than using a predetermined treatment time.

Postural drainage is indicated any time there are secretions to be cleared from the lung. Breath sounds and radiographic evidence are key indicators of the need for these positioning techniques, as well as which areas are in need of draining. As indicated in Table 29-2, the major precaution associated with postural drainage has to do with the head down or Trendelenburg position. There are a number of circumstances in which this position is not advisable or will be poorly tolerated by the patient. Under these conditions, a modified position is used and the postural drainage will be combined with percussion and vibration to achieve the same results.

Percussion

Percussion is the technique used in which cupped hands are alternately and rhythmically applied to the chest wall. The purpose of percussion is to dislodge secretions mechanically so that, together with postural drainage, they may be moved up the bronchial tree and removed by coughing or suctioning.

Percussion should be applied over the chest wall where evidence of secretion retention exists. The technique should be comfortable to the patient and not produce erythema on the skin. The spinous processes of the vertebrae are avoided during percussion to avoid patient discomfort.

The amount of time percussion is continued over an area may also vary from 3 to 5 minutes[15] to several hours.[1] Periods of percussion may also be interrupted by the patient's coughing. The coughing will help to remove any mobilized secretions. Percussion may also trigger a period of bronchospasm in the patient. This may require the patient to discontinue the treatment for a short period, and for percussion to be resumed after a bronchodilator is administered.

Crane[16] suggests modifications of percussion that can be used in infants and small children. These involve using only three fingers or the thenar or hypothenar surfaces of the palm to apply percussion to a small child (Fig. 29-4).

Precautions associated with percussion are noted in Table 29-2. Ciesla[17] has recently reported that percussion can be used with proper precautions even in the presence of rib fractures and soft tissue injury such as burns without increasing the problems associated with these injuries. Precautions that are observed in these instance are avoiding percussing directly over a fracture and using sterile coverings over burn areas.

Vibration

Vibration, as the name implies, is quite literally a vibration applied by the physical therapist to the chest wall during a patient's exhalation. Generally, the patient is asked to take a deep breath, hold the breath for a few seconds, and finally exhale while the therapist applies vibration. This is repeated for five or six deep breaths. The benefits of this technique in conjunction with postural drainage and percussion primarily seem to be to expand atelectic areas and enhance secretion mobilization. A patient who is unable to inhale deeply may be assisted with intermittent positive pressure breathing (IPPB) or by using an AMBU bag on a patient who has an artificial airway.[15] This will encourage optimal chest expansion along with moving secretions.

Shaking

Shaking or rib springing is a more forceful version of vibration. Shaking is begun at peak inspiration and continued throughout expiration. Since shaking is a more vigorous technique, more precautions are observed when using this technique on a patient. In general, the patient should have a flexible rib cage with no instability or degenerative bone disease (Table 29-2).

Breath Control Techniques

An inefficient and abnormal breathing pattern is often seen in the patient with pulmonary disease. Likewise, the pain accompanying thoracic and abdominal surgery can restrict chest expansion. Breath control techniques fall into two general categories: (1) deep breathing and (2) breath retraining.

Deep breathing is used to encourage full lung expansion. The patient is taught to place a hand on the abdomen to feel the stomach rise during inspiration and fall during exhalation. The patient may also be taught to place the hands on the lower ribs to encourage ventilation in the lower lung regions. This is referred to as lateral-costal breathing. This deep breathing can be incorporated with vibration and postural drainage. Incentive spirometers are another device to promote lung expansion.

Breath retraining is often a more complicated process because the physical therapist attempts to change an established breathing pattern. The most common of these retraining maneuvers is pursed-lip breathing. The patient is taught to exhale through pursed lips to increase the pressure within the lung and prevent early collapse of small airways. Pursed-lip breathing is meant to lessen trapping of air in the lung of a patient with chronic obstructive lung disease. Some patients will use this technique spontaneously. Another technique is to emphasize the role of the diaphragm during breathing. Diaphragmatic breathing teaches the patient to allow full descension of the diaphragm during inspiration and passive relaxation of the diaphragm during exhalation. The patient becomes aware of the proper movement by resting a hand on the abdomen while breathing quietly in the supine position. The patient is then encouraged to practice diaphragmatic breathing in different positions, such as sitting, standing, and walking. These measures are used to ensure the carryover of the procedure during ordinary activities of daily living. Diaphragmatic breathing can be combined with another technique, an attempt to lengthen exhalation. The patient is encouraged to develop a pattern of exhalation time that is at least twice as long as inhalation. This is most important for patients with obstructive airway disease.

The physical therapist must carefully evaluate the benefits of changing breathing patterns. A study by Willeput et al.[18] suggests that imposing breathing patterns on patients with chronic obstructive lung disease may lessen ventilation, increase paradoxical chest wall movements, and increase the work of breathing. The physical therapist should keep in mind that the spontaneous breathing pattern adopted by the patient may be optimal for a particular patient and disability.

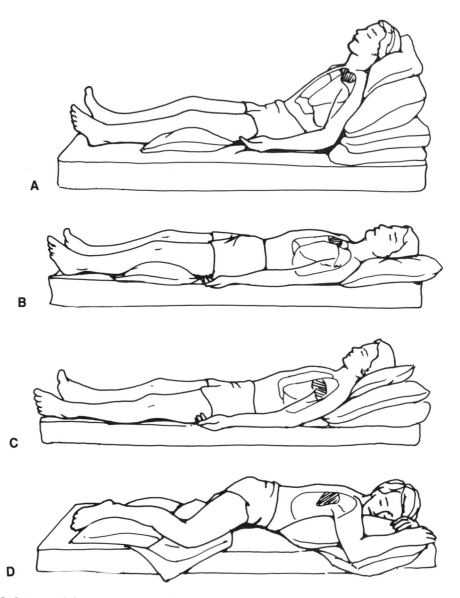

Fig. 29-3 Postural drainage positions. (**A**) Both upper lobes—apical segments. (**B**) Right upper lobe—anterior segment. (**C**) Left upper lobe—anterior segment. (**D**) Right upper lobe—posterior segment. (**E**) Left upper lobe—posterior segment. (**F**) Left upper lobe—posterior segment (alternate position). (**G**) Right middle lobe. (*Figure continues.*)

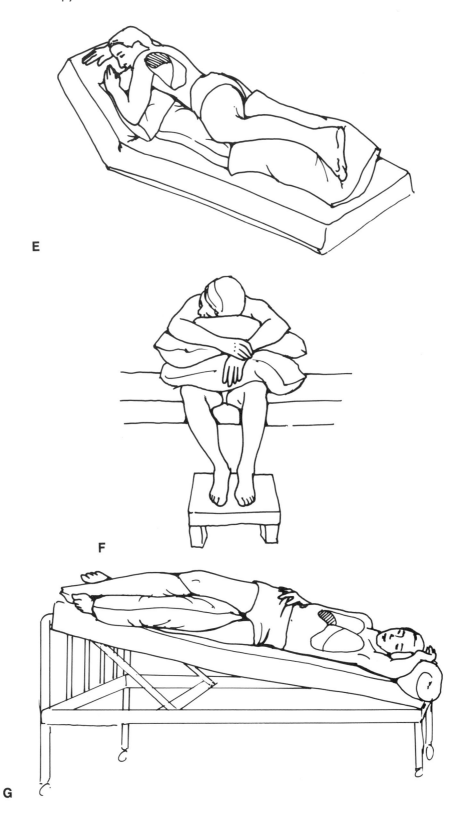

E

F

G

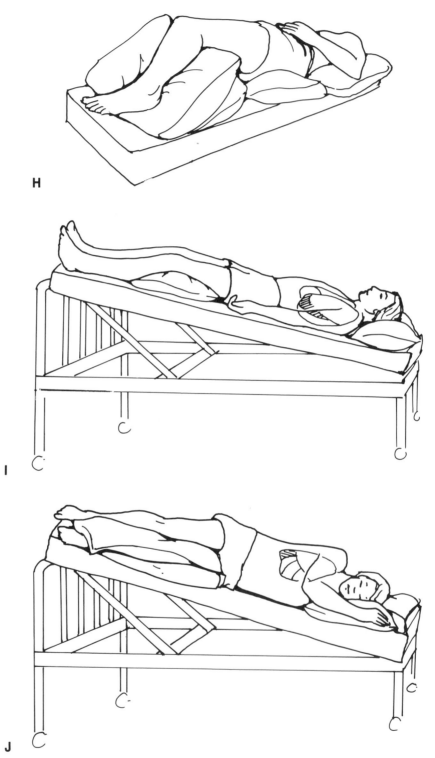

Fig. 29-3 (*Continued*). (**H**) Lingula (posterior view). (**I**) Both lower lobes—anterior segments. (**J**) Right lower lobe—lateral segment. (*Figure continues.*)

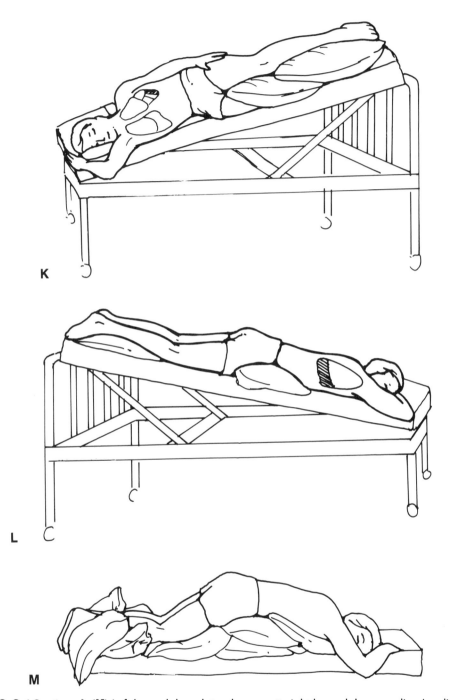

Fig. 29-3 (*Continued*). (**K**) Left lower lobe—lateral segment; right lower lobe—cardiac (medial) segment. (**L**) Both lower lobes—posterior segments. Note pillows under hips and knees, none under head. (**M**) Both lower lobes—posterior segments (shown using telephone books or pillows for home use).

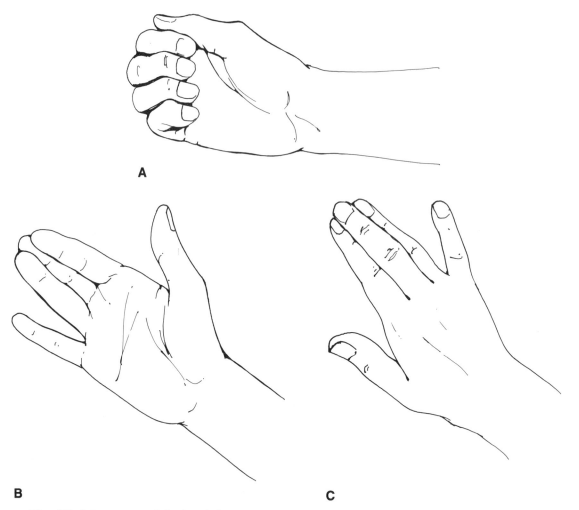

A

B   **C**

Fig. 29-4 Positioning of the hands for percussion of neonates or small children. (**A**) The position for using thenar or hypothenar surfaces; (**B,C**) the positions for using the fingers, in percussion.

Endurance Exercise Training

Repeated bouts of illness associated with some chronic pulmonary conditions frequently leave the patient deconditioned as a result of restricted activity. An exercise conditioning program can be selected for a patient to reverse some of the deconditioning associated with the illness.

The parameters of the exercise program should be determined after a standard graded exercise test (GXT). Several protocols are available that require the patient to walk on a treadmill while the elevation of the treadmill is increased by a few percent every 2 to 3 minutes beginning with level walking.[19] An example of one common testing protocol, a modified Balke-Ware protocol, is shown in Table 29-6.[20] If a bicycle ergometer is used, the resistance can be increased by 25 watts

Table 29-6. Modified Balke-Ware Exercise Testing Protocol

Time (min)	Speed (mph)	Elevation (%)
3	2	0
3	2	5
3	2	10
3	2	15
3	2	20
3	2	25

every 3 minutes. The physical therapist should monitor and record the electrocardiogram (ECG), heart rate, and blood pressure during the exercise test. The patient's arterial oxygen saturation can be monitored cutaneously by using a device such as a transcutaneous oxygen monitor (Figs. 29-5 and 29-6). Arterial oxygen saturation should remain stable during exercise, while the heart rate and blood pressure increase with increasing exercise.

The patient should continue increasing levels of exercise until there are indications that he has reached a maximum level of exercise. The age-predicted maximum heart rate, or 220 − age, is often used to define maximum, or the heart rate at which some significant signs and symptoms occur. Common significant signs and symptoms are:

1. Subjective (signs of hypoxia)
    Severe dyspnea
    Cyanosis
    Extreme fatigue
    Faintness or dizziness
    Chest pain
    Jugular vein distension
    Muscle cramps
2. Objective
    Decreased arterial oxygen saturation by
        oximetry

Sudden onset of pallor or extreme
    diaphoresis
Ventricular dysrhythmias
    More than six premature ventricular
        contractions (PVCs) per minute
    Bigeminy (PVC every other beat)
    Paired PVCs
    PVC falling near the T wave
ST-segment depression greater than 1 mm
Bradycardia
Blood pressure irregularities
    Systolic pressure over 215 mmHg
    Decreased systolic pressure with
        increasing exercise
    Increase in diastolic pressure of 20
        mmHg above resting or over 100
        mmHg
Mental confusion, apprehension

When the test is ended, the patient should be given a brief period of level, slow walking (1 mile/hour on the treadmill) or slow, unresisted pedaling on the bike to cool down after the test. In this way the patient will avoid feeling dizzy or faint after the exercise.

A number of patients will experience arterial oxygen desaturation during the exercise test. If desaturation occurs in the patient who is breathing room air, (1) have the patient rest after the exercise, (2) give the patient 1 liter of oxygen for 5

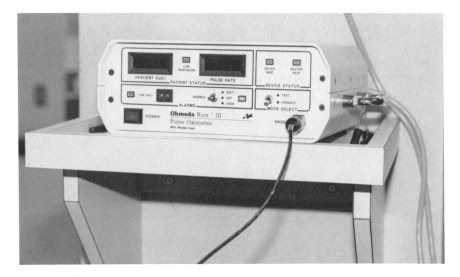

Fig. 29-5 Transcutaneous oxygen monitor.

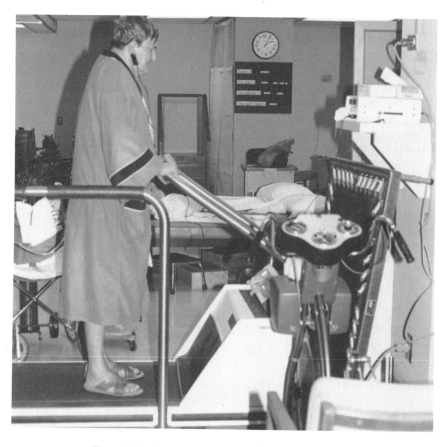

Fig. 29-6 Patient exercising with oxygen monitor.

minutes by nasal cannula, and (3) repeat the test. This procedure may be repeated with a flow rate of 2 or 3 liters of oxygen if the patient continues to experience desaturation with exercise. For a patient who is desaturating during exercise, the physical therapist should recommend to the attending physician a prescription for oxygen during exercise.

For patients who are already receiving supplemental oxygen, the physical therapist should document the arterial blood gases before exercise. If the patient desaturates on the usual flow of supplemental oxygen, then the patient should rest, the oxygen flow should be increased by 1 liter, and the exercise test should be repeated.

The highest heart rate achieved during the GXT is considered the patient's maximum heart rate or, if appropriate, the symptom-limited heart rate. This value is used to establish an exercise prescrip-

tion for the patient. A range of exercise intensities based on the heart rates can be established for the patient's exercise program. For example, if a patient experiences dyspnea during the test at a heart rate of 130 beats/minute, and began with a resting heart rate of 80 beats/minute the exercise heart rate can be determined as follows:[19]

Maximum heart rate	130
− Resting heart rate	− 80
Heart rate reserve	50
× 60–80%	× 60–80%
Heart rate range	30–45
+ Resting heart rate	+ 80
Target heart rate ranges	110–125

An exercise conditioning program could be prescribed for this patient that produced a heart rate of between 110 and 125 beats/minute. This should be an intensity below a point at which the patient experiences dyspnea.

The mode that is selected for the exercise should be something that the patient will continue and enjoys. A simple walking program often has the most functional carryover and is easy for most patients to perform on a regular basis; however, any form of exercise within the proper intensity can be planned. A rowing-type exercise can be most useful for enhancing the endurance of the upper extremity and truck musculature.

The duration of an exercise session should be at least 20 minutes, excluding a 3- to 5-minute warm-up and cool-down period, to enhance the patient's general endurance. These sessions should be planned at a time during the day when the patient is least fatigued and has not eaten a recent meal.

A frequency of three times per week is sufficiently regular so that it becomes a habit pattern for the patient without requiring the patient to exercise daily. This is a manageable schedule for most patients. Of course, some severely involved pulmonary patients who can only exercise at a low intensity may have to exercise more frequently to achieve any benefits.

The patient can progress in an exercise program if the target heart rates are no longer reached during the exercise. A seriously debilitated patient may require 8 weeks or more of an exercise program before requiring a progression.

In summary, an exercise program designed to enhance a patient's exercise endurance should have several elements defined by the physical therapist. Those elements include (1) the heart rate intensity, (2) the mode of exercise, (3) the duration of an exercise session, and (4) the frequency of the sessions.

Exercise for the Ventilator-Dependent Patient

An additional application of a general exercise program is for the patient who is ventilator dependent. Serious deconditioning is associated with the patient who is placed on a ventilator. To counter these deconditioning effects, ambulation is advocated for the ventilator-dependent patient.[1] Although little research data exist to document the outcomes of ambulation in ventilator patients, one study suggests that ambulation in place will positively influence ventilator weaning criteria and in a small sample of patients led to rapid ventilator weaning.[21]

Respiratory Muscle Training

Respiratory muscles, like skeletal muscles, will respond to the functional demands placed on them. Activities that are specifically designed to enhance endurance will result in extended endurance, whereas activities that require strength will tend to produce greater strength. The literature suggests that both the strength and endurance of the respiratory musculature can change as a result of specific exercise programs.[4,5,22] Respiratory muscle strength training is similar to isometric training for extremity muscles in that the individual works to produce maximum static inspiratory and expiratory pressures against a closed airway. Respiratory muscle endurance training targets the ability to sustain ventilation over a prolonged period. Leith and Bradley[5] had their subjects perform high levels of ventilation for 12 to 15 minutes. These subjects continued several repetitions of these bouts for 45- to 60-minute training sessions 5 days per week. Although this is a demanding training schedule, Leith and Bradley were able to demonstrate an improvement in the maximum voluntary ventilation in individuals with COPD.[5]

General Muscle Performance Training

Another well-defined consequence of chronic illnesses is the generalized muscle atrophy that accompanies inactivity. Most patients with chronic respiratory problems will require exercises aimed at the hypertrophy of disused musculature. Particular emphasis should be given to the upper extremity muscles if the patient experiences shortness of breath during lifting or similar activities. A program of light weight training performed twice per week can provide an outcome of improved muscle strength.

Relaxation and Energy Conservation

Many patients will require guidance in how to respond when their respiratory capacity is challenged by overexertion. Frownfelter[9] recommends that patients be taught a relaxation scheme such as biofeedback or hypnosis. For similar reasons, Humberstone[10] advocates teaching patients a forward leaning posture to assist respiratory muscle stabilization and reduce the work of breathing. Humberstone further suggests that a careful analysis of functional tasks may enhance energy conservation for the patient.[10] For example, if a patient becomes dyspnic while showering, the use of a shower chair could reduce the dyspnea experienced by the patient.

Postural Exercise

The goal of postural exercise is to maintain normal postural alignment and upper extremity and trunk mobility. The patient should be encouraged to assume correct sitting and standing postures. The physical therapist should also teach the patient activities that will promote trunk extension, as well as a full range of scapular and shoulder movements. With careful planning, the patient can combine these activities into general muscle conditioning exercises to minimize the time required for exercise.

PATIENT COMPLIANCE

Finally, the physical therapist should incorporate several strategies to ensure that the patient will adopt the program that the therapist is recommending. Most of the treatments discussed require substantial cooperation and behavioral changes from the patient. Several components of a program that would improve patient compliance are the following:

1. Involve the patient in the planning and selection of activities.
2. Demonstrate all exercises.
3. Write explicit directions on each activity, including frequency, duration, and any special directions.
4. Supervise the patient's program until correct performance of all exercises is ensured.

5. Whenever possible, have the patient working with a group of patients with similar problems. Group exercises promote greater compliance.
6. Observe the patient on a regular basis to answer any questions and encourage continued participation. This may have to be a phone call, but this does help to ensure patient cooperation.

REFERENCES

1. MacKenzie CF, Ciesla N, Imle PC, Klemic N: Chest physiotherapy in the intensive care unit. Williams & Wilkins, Baltimore, 1981
2. Astrand PO, Rodahl K: Textbook of Work Physiology. McGraw-Hill, New York, 1986
3. Sinclair DJM, Ingram CG: Controlled trial of supervised exercise training in chronic bronchitis. Br Med J 280:519, 1980
4. Keens TG, Inese RB, Krastins IR et al.: Ventilatory muscle endurance training in normal subjects and patients with cystic fibrosis. Am Rev Respir Dis 116:853, 1977
5. Leith DE, Bradley M: Ventilatory muscle strength and endurance training. J Appl Physiol 41:508, 1976
6. Rothman JG: Effects of respiratory exercises on the vital capacity and forced expiratory volume in children with cerebral palsy. Phys Ther 58:421, 1978
7. Shaffer TH, Wolson MR, Bhutani VK: Respiratory muscle function, assessment and training. Phys Ther 61:1711, 1981
8. Sobush DC, Dunning M: Providing resistive breathing exercise to the inspiratory muscles using the PFLEX (tm) device. Phys Ther 66:542, 1986
9. Frownfelter D: Breathing exercise and retraining, chest mobilization exercises. In Frownfelter D (ed): Chest Physical Therapy and Pulmonary Rehabilitation. Year Book Medical Publishers, Chicago, 1978
10. Humberstone N: Respiratory treatment. In Irwin S, Tecklin JS (ed): Cardiopulmonary Physical Therapy. CV Mosby, St. Louis, 1985
11. Murphy DMF: Environmental (occupational) lung disease. In Kaye D, Rose LF (ed): Fundamentals of Internal Medicine. CV Mosby, St. Louis, 1983
12. Siegel PD, Barch F: Chronic bronchitis and emphysema. In Kaye D, Rose LF (ed): Fundamentals of Internal Medicine. CV Mosby, St. Louis, 1983
13. Kuna ST, Levine S: Respiratory diagnostic procedures. In Kaye D, Rose LF (ed): Fundamentals of Internal Medicine. CV Mosby, St. Louis, 1983
14. American College of Chest Physicians-American Thoracic Society, Joint Committee on Pulmonary Nomenclature: Pulmonary terms and symbols. Chest 67:583, 1975
15. Frownfelter D: Percussion and vibration. In Frown-

felter D (ed): Chest Physical Therapy and Pulmonary Rehabilitation. Year Book Medical Publishers, Chicago, 1978

16. Crane L: Physical therapy for the neonate with respiratory disease. In Irwin S, Tecklin JS (ed): Cardiopulmonary Physical Therapy. CV Mosby, St. Louis, 1985

17. Ciesla N: The incidence of extrapleural hematoma with postural drainage and percussion. Phys Ther 66:492, 1987

18. Willeput R, Vachauclez JP, Lenders D, et al.: Thoracoabdominal motion during chest physiotherapy in patients affected by chronic obstructive lung disease. Respiration 44:204, 1983

19. Pollock M, Wilmore J, Fox S: Exercise in Health and Disease. JB Lippincott, New York, 1985

20. Froelicher VF: Exercise testing and training. Year Book Medical Publishers, Chicago, 1983

21. Fremstad R, Protas EJ: The effect of ambulation on ventilator weaning criteria. Cardiopulmonary Q, Winter, 1985 (abstract)

22. Gross D, Ladd HW, Riley EJ et al.: The effect of training on the strength and endurance of the diaphragm in quadriplegia. Am J Med 68:27, 1980

30 Cardiopulmonary Complications in AIDS Patients

Mary Lou Galantino

Human immunodeficiency virus (HIV), which is related to acquired immune deficiency syndrome (AIDS), is transmitted by sexual contact or parenterally via blood or blood products. There is no evidence of transmission of HIV or the AIDS-related retrovirus by respiratory means or casual contact with individuals infected with this virus. The transmission pattern of HIV is similar to that of hepatitis B virus. The risk groups include males with homosexual contact, female sexual partners of bisexual males, drug abusers, persons with multiple sexual partners, children born to mothers who are infected with HIV, intravenous drug abusers, and people who have received frequent blood transfusions or blood products. Since the screening of blood donors for HIV antibody and the heat treatment of blood products, transfusions of blood and blood products have a markedly diminished risk. Some AIDS patients have other infections that can additionally be transmitted to healthy individuals (such as hepatitis B, cytomegalovirus [CMV], Epstein-Barr virus [EBV], tuberculosis, salmonellosis, and cryptosporidiosis).[1]

GENERAL GUIDELINES

In the health care setting, there is a risk of exposure to a number of infectious diseases by being exposed to blood or body fluids. The hepatitis virus and the AIDS-related virus (HIV) may be carried in the blood of individuals who appear healthy or individuals who are sick but have not yet been fully diagnosed. All exposures to blood or body fluids from any individual should be considered potentially dangerous, and appropriate precautions should be taken. The control precautions outlined here will help prevent the transmissions of any blood-borne or body fluid-borne infection. In situations in which considerable contact with blood or body fluids is expected, such as deliveries, surgeries, and endoscopies, precautions should be used for all patients (i.e., gowns, goggles, and masks according to contact expected). All patients with blood-borne viruses may not be identified at the time of a procedure; therefore, precautions are indicated for all anticipated blood exposure from any patient.

DIAGNOSIS AND INITIATION OF INFECTION PRECAUTIONS

Identification of patients requiring isolation measures should be made by physicians caring for the patients and the head nurse or charge nurse on each hospital unit. The following instances warrent AIDS precautions.

Documented AIDS

The group with documented AIDS includes patients with Kaposi's sarcoma, *Pneumocystis carinii* pneumonia, and other opportunistic infections not associated with other underlying disease or therapy.

Possible AIDS

Patients with possible AIDS are from a high-risk group (such as homosexual males, hemophiliacs, and intravenous drug users) who exhibit symptoms such as unexplained fever, unexplained pulmonary symptoms or infiltrates, skin lesions that are highly suggestive of Kaposi's sarcoma (Fig. 30-1), and systemic illness characterized by fever, weight loss, adenopathy, muscle wasting, unusual perspiration, thrush, and diarrhea.

Patients Being Followed for AIDS-Related Problems

There is no indication for isolation of members of high-risk groups without symptoms suggestive of AIDS. AIDS precautions are not necessary for

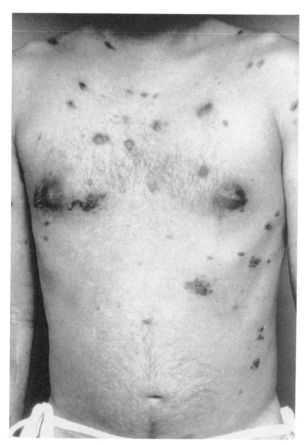

Fig. 30-1 Skin lesions associated with Kaposi's Sarcoma, an AIDS-related condition.

asymptomatic persons with antibody to HIV who do not fit into the documented AIDS or possible AIDS categories. However, these individuals may have virus in their blood, and general precautions for handling blood and other body fluids for *all* hospitalized patients should be followed. These precautions include careful hand washing after any contact with body fluids, extreme care in avoidance of puncture by used needles, no recapping of needles, and use of a puncture-resistant needle box for disposal of all sharp instruments.

PRECAUTIONS FOR AIDS

1. A private room is designated for some patients according to diagnosis, doctor's order, or request. This is to protect the patient from inffections to which he may be susceptible and to protect other immunocompromised patients. A private room is indicated for patients who are too ill to use good hygiene, such as those with profuse diarrhea, fecal incontinence, or altered behavior secondary to central nervous system infections.
2. Hand washing before and after direct care is important to protect the immunocompromised patient as well as the employee.
3. Needle disposal in puncture-resistant containers without breaking or recapping the needle should be done in the room or as close as possible to the area of use. This is to protect nursing and housekeeping staff. Needle recapping and disposal are frequent causes of needle sticks.
4. Gowns are not needed unless gross contamination of the uniform is expected, such as in cases in which direct contact between the uniform and draining wounds is expected or during bronchoscopy when splatter can occur. If unexpected contamination of the uniform occurs, washing in a home washer with detergent is adequate for decontamination.
5. Masks are not needed for patients with AIDS; however, a coughing patient with an undiagnosed pulmonary condition should be on mask precautions. Since tuberculosis (TB)

is a cause of pulmonary disease in a small percentage of cases, masks worn by the staff are a prudent precaution until TB is ruled out. There is no evidence that the AIDS virus is spread through the respiratory tract.[1]

6. Protective eyewear consisting of goggles, glasses, etc., should be worn when splatter and suctioning of blood is expected (e.g., surgeries, endoscopies including bronchoscopies, deliveries).

7. Double-plastic laundry bags are needed if the patient has draining wounds or is incontinent.

8. Dietary isolation trays are not needed. Dietary trays may be served, removed, and sanitized in the same manner as other patient trays.

9. Patients may use showers and tubs. Shower floors (both for AIDS patients and for others) should be decontaminated daily with 1:10 dilution of 5.25 percent sodium hypochlorite (household bleach) by the housekeeping department. Tubs used by infected patients (AIDS and others) should be cleaned first and then decontaminated with sodium hypochlorite (a 1:10 dilution of bleach).

10. All blood specimens from all patients whether known to be infected with AIDS or not should be handled with caution. All specimens from AIDS patients must be identified with "precautions" labels, placed in Ziploc bags, and sealed for transport to prevent spills from broken tubes. Laboratory slips should also be labeled and attached to the outside of the bag.

11. Spills of blood and other body secretions should be cleaned up promptly. Large spills should be cleaned by a gloved employee with paper towels. The towels should then be placed in an infectious waste container. A diluted 5.25 percent sodium hypochlorite solution should be used to disinfect the area. To protect employees from noxious fumes, sodium hypochlorite should not be placed directly on large amounts of protein matter (urine, stool, blood, sputum, etc.). A 1:10 dilution of bleach may be order for physical therapy and nursing units from the pharmacy or housekeeping departments.

12. Laboratory procedures should be adopted to prevent the formation of aerosols. Biological safety cabinets (class I or II) and other primary containment devices (e.g., centrifuge safety cups) are advised whenever procedures are conducted that have a high potential for creating aerosols or infectious droplets. Other standard laboratory safety practices should be followed.[2]

13. Equipment decontamination should be appropriate to the equipment involved. Respiratory therapy ventilator tubing should be decontaminated with ethylene oxide or pasteurization. Any instrument that has been in direct contact with blood or other secretions should be thoroughly washed and sterilized or exposed to a high-level disinfectant before re-use. Lensed equipment should be thoroughly cleaned and then sterilized or exposed to a high-level disinfectant (such as ethylene oxide or alkaline glutaraldehyde) for 45 minutes. Ideally, each patient should have his own disposable razor. If electric razors are used, they should be dismantled and the heads washed thoroughly with soap and water and then wiped with 70 percent alcohol or alcohol-Zephiran (benzalkonium) between patients. Such precautions should always be used, regardless of whether the patients have AIDS or hepatitis B. Other equipment such as electrocardiogram or electroencephalogram electrodes which contact nonbroken skin require only washing with detergent and water before re-use. Decontamination of other equipment such as thermometers, tonometers, laryngoscopes, and spirometers should be handled by routine procedures.

14. Clinitron and kinetic beds may be used for AIDS or suspected AIDS patients to prevent skin breakdown. Decontamination of Clinitron or kinetic beds will be done by the supplier.

15. Pregnant health care workers are not known to be at greater risk of contracting HIV infections than other health care workers who are not pregnant; however, if a woman develops HIV infection during pregnancy, the risks are increased for the infant, who may contact the virus through perinatal transmission. Consequently, pregnant health

care workers should be especially familiar with precautions for preventing HIV transmission.

PRECAUTIONS FOR OTHER DISEASES THAT MAY BE SEEN IN AIDS PATIENTS

Cytomegalovirus

Many AIDS patients are excreting CMV through their stools and urine. Good hygiene has been shown to prevent acquisition of CMV. Therefore, hand washing is very important after any contact with patient body fluid. Although some patients have CMV in their lungs, it is not known whether CMV can be transmitted through the respiratory tract.

Pregnant women should be aware that the CMV virus may cause birth defects. Consequently, pregnant women should be extremely cautious in the care of any patient, since not all patients who excrete this virus have been identified as carriers.

When a patient with an undiagnosed pulmonary process is coughing and has sustained close contact with others, masks should be worn by the patient when outside of an isolation room. Masks should also be worn by others exposed to the patient when the patient is not wearing a mask. These precautions should be followed until medical clearance is obtained.

Until a patient's respiratory illness is diagnosed, others need to be protected from diseases spread through the respiratory tract. Immunocompetent persons need protection from *Mycobacterium tuberculosis*. Immunocompromised persons need protection from *Mycobacterium avium* and *Pneumocystis carinii*.

Opportunistic and Other Infections

The patient with AIDS constantly faces the threat of acquiring opportunistic infections. To decrease the danger to the hospitalized AIDS patient, infection control procedures must be meticulously

Table 30-1 Summary of Important Recommendations and Work Restrictions for Personnel with Infectious Diseases

Disease or Problem	Relieve from Direct Patient Contact	Partial Work Restriction	Duration
Conjunctivitis	Yes		Until discharge ceases
CMV	No		
Diarrhea			
Acute stage (diarrhea with other symptoms)	Yes		Until symptoms resolve and *Salmonella* is ruled out
Convalescent stage (*Salmonella* [nontyphoidal])	No	Should not care for high-risk patients	Until stool is free of organism on two consecutive cultures not less than 24 hours apart
Other enteric pathogens	No		
Enteroviral infections	No	Should not care for infants	Until symptoms resolve
Group A streptococcal disease	Yes		Until 24 hours after adequate treatment is started
Hepatitis, viral			
Hepatitis A	Yes		Until 7 days after onset of jaundice
Hepatitis B			
Acute	No	Personnel should wear gloves for procedures involving trauma to tissues or contact with mucous membrane or broken skin	Until antigenemia resolves
Chronic antigenemia	No	Same as acute illness	Until antigenemia resolves
Non-A, non-B	No	Same as hepatitis B	Period of infectivity has not been determined

(continued)

Table 30-1 (*continued*)

Disease or Problem	Relieve from Direct Patient Contact	Partial Work Restriction	Duration
Herpes simplex			
Genital	No		
Hands (herpetic whitlow)	Yes	Note: Not known whether gloves prevent transmission	Until lesions heal
Orofacial	No	Personnel should not care for high-risk patients	Until lesions heal
Measles			
Active	Yes		Until 7 days after rash appears
Postexposure (susceptible personnel)	Yes		From 5–21 days after exposure or 7th day after rash appears
Mumps[a]			
Active	Yes		Until 9 days after onset of parotitis
Postexposure	Yes		From 12–26 days after exposure and/or 5 days after onset of symptoms
Pertussis			
Active	Yes		From beginning of catarrhal stage through 3rd week after onset of paroxysms, or until 7 days after start of effective therapy
Postexposure (asymptomatic personnel)	No		
Postexposure (symptomatic personnel)	Yes		Same as active pertussis
Rubella			
Active	Yes		Until 5 days after rash appears
Postexposure (susceptible personnel)	Yes		From 7–21 days after exposure or 5 days after rash appears
Scabies	Yes		Until treated
Staphylococcus aureus (skin lesions)	Yes		Until lesions have resolved
Upper respiratory infections (high-risk patients)	Yes	Personnel with upper respiratory infections should not care for high-risk patients	Until acute symptoms resolve
Varicella (chickenpox)			
Active	Yes		Until all lesions dry and crust
Postexposure	Yes		From 10–21 days after exposure or, if varicella occurs, until all lesions dry and crust
Zoster (shingles)			
Active	No	Appropriate barrier desirable; personnel should not take care of high-risk patients	Until lesions dry and crust
Postexposure	Yes		From 10–21 days after exposure or, if varicella occurs, until all lesions dry and crust

[a] Mumps vaccine may be offered to susceptible personnel. When given after exposure, mumps vaccine may not provide protection. However, if exposure did not result in infection, immunizing exposed personnel should protect against subsequent infection. Neither mumps immunoglobulin nor immune serum globulin (USG) is of established value in postexposure prophylaxis. Transmission of mumps among personnel and patients has not been a major problem in patients in hospitals in the United States, probably due to multiple factors, including high levels of natural and vaccine-induced immunity.

(Institute for Immunological Disorders: Manual of Infection Control, Houston, Texas 1986.)

followed. Hand washing before and after contact with the patient as well as strict adherence to aseptic techniques during invasive procedures and the management of indwelling lines and catheters are essential. In general, invasive procedures should be limited as much as possible for the protection of the AIDS patient.

The patient and the family should be taught how to assess an infection. The patient should be observed daily for signs and symptoms of infection including fever, chills, shortness of breath, cough, dysuria, inflammation of the skin or oral mucosa, diarrhea, and a deterioration of the mental status. The family should be encouraged to maintain a clean and clutter-free environment. Supplies should not be stockpiled in the patient's room.

The patient should be taught the importance of personal cleanliness and should be reminded to wash his hands before eating and after coughing, sneezing, or going to the bathroom. If the patient is confined to bed, hand-washing supplies should be provided. The patient should bathe or shower daily and should rinse thoroughly to remove soap. Teeth should be brushed twice daily with a soft toothbrush.

Precautions Related to Infections in the Health Care Worker

Although there is no evidence that health care workers who are infected with the HIV virus have transmitted infection to patients, a risk of transmission could exist in certain situations. Personnel who exhibit any of the clinical features described in the AIDS spectrum should be counseled to exercise precautions in an effort to minimize the risk of infecting others.

Table 30-1 provides a summary of important recommendations and work restrictions for personnel with various infectious diseases. The importance of protecting the patients from such infections cannot be overemphasized.

HELPING THE PATIENT COPE WITH ISOLATION

If a patient is in isolation, special measures must be taken to help him maintain a sense of connection with the hospital staff and the outside world. Emphasize that the isolation is temporary and will

be limited to the hospital stay. Reassure the patient that he is not "dirty." Encourage visits by the patient's family and friends. Acknowledge the visitors' fears of contracting AIDS, but reassure them that the disease cannot be transmitted through casual contact. Urge the patient to keep in touch with the outside world through television, radio, newspapers, and letters. Discuss current events with him. Brighten the hospital room with cards and pictures.

COMMON PULMONARY AND CARDIAC COMPLICATIONS

Pneumocystis carinii Pneumonia

More than 60 percent of patients with AIDS develop Pneumocystis carinii pneumonia (PCP), and 30 to 85 percent of these patients develop recurrent PCP within 12 months.[3-8] The pathology shows a predominant diffuse alveolopathy. By the time that clinical symptoms appear, numerous organisms fill the alveoli, and the condition in the lung is characterized by mononuclear cell infiltration of the alveolar septums. Interstitial fibrosis is rare but may be a sequela of PCP.

The clinical features of PCP include tachypnea, cough, fever, hypoxemia and increased alveolar-capillary oxygen gradient, respiratory acidosis, and bilateral diffuse alveolar disease. Patients with severe pulmonary involvement may have diffuse lymphadenopathy. Dry rales may be auscultated, but indications of consolidation are not generally observed.

Several tests may contribute to the diagnosis of PCP. Radiographic studies demonstrate bilateral pulmonary infiltrates that originate in the hilar regions and eventually extend peripherally to create a solid granular appearance (Fig. 30-2). Pulmonary function tests show reductions in total lung capacity and vital capacity, reduced single breath diffusing capacity for carbon monoxide, and increased expiratory flow rates. The analysis of induced sputum, bronchoscopy, open lung biopsies (rarely performed), and gallium lung scans can also contribute to the diagnosis.

Pulmonary physical therapy is indicated for the patient with PCP, as are general mobility activities as a means to encourage the gradual improvement of the patient's endurance.[9] Drug intervention

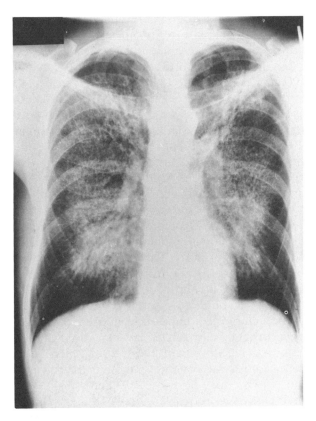

Fig. 30-2 Radiograph demonstrating the solid granular appearance of bilateral pulmonary infiltrates within the lungs.

includes oral trimethoprim-sulfamethoxazole or intravenous pentamidine. These drugs are considered equally effective in bringing about recovery in 75 percent of the cases. These drugs are also associated with a 50 percent incidence of significant toxicity and a failure rate of about 25 percent.[10–14] Inhaled pentamidine may be effective and less toxic therapy for mild PCP.[15] Larger and more controlled studies are needed to further establish drug recommendations.

Tuberculosis

Pulmonary TB in patients with HIV infection cannot be easily distinguished from other infections simply on the basis of radiographic and clinical findings. Chest radiographs frequently re-semble the pattern of primary TB (i.e., hilar or mediastinal adenopathy with or without noncavitating pulmonary infiltrates, located with approximately equal frequency in upper and lower lung fields).[16]

Chemotherapy should be initiated whenever acid-fast bacilli are found in a specimen. Patients with TB and HIV infection respond relatively well to standard anti-TB drugs.[17] These include isoniazid, rifampin, and either ethambutol hydrochloride or pyrazinamide. The appropriate duration of therapy may need to be longer than the standard duration of 9 months.[18] Despite the immunosuppressed state of patients with AIDS, the chest radiographic abnormalities related to TB clear within months of beginning anti-TB drug therapy.

Mycobacterium avium-intracellulare

Several reports have indicated that *Mycobacterium avium-intracellulare* (MAI) is common patients with AIDS and HIV.[19–25] Among all patients with AIDS, the most frequently isolated cause of infection is *Mycobacterium avium* complex. *Mycobacterium tuberculosis* is more common in intravenous drug users and Haitians. Extrapulmonary disease and noncavitary, nonapical pulmonary TB are also frequently seen.[26]

In contrast to primary pulmonary TB, sputum cultures for MAI are frequently positive, whereas pleural effusions are infrequent and tend to be small. Extrathoracic TB is very common.[27,28] Patients may present with a coexisting pulmonary infection.

Treatment of disseminated disease resulting from MAI includes several experimental drugs, ansamycin and clofazimine. After therapy, patients should be followed closely. Mycobacteriological examinations should be repeated if clinically indicated.

Pneumonia and Cytomegalovirus

CMV is associated with severe pneumonia in immunocompromised individuals. CMV may be associated with hemorrhagic exudative alveolar inflammatory response that includes cytotoxic suppressor T-lymphocytes.[18] In the lungs, CMV lesions represent a range from focal to diffuse pneumonitis with numerous characteristic intranuclear and intracytoplasmic inclusion cells.[29] Treatment with gancidozia (DHPG) and chest physical therapy is indicated to clear the lungs and enhance lung capacity.

Cardiac Complications

Physical therapists should be aware of this pathogenic process to ensure proper evaluation and treatment of the patient with AIDS-related complex (ARC). Cardiac disease secondary to multiple causes can be expected to complicate the clinical course of these patients. Although a more accurate estimation of the incidence of myocardial disease must await further study, emphasis on the importance of thorough cardiac evaluation is recommended.

The reported clinical manifestions of the cardiac involvement in AIDS have been limited to focal metastatic involvement of the heart by Kaposi's sarcoma.[30,31] Other cardiac complications have been associated with other disease processes. Unusual manifestations of TB have been noted in a study by Suderam et al.[17] The pericardium was involved, causing acute cardiac tamponade in one patient who subsequently had a chronic TB draining sinus despite several months of anti-TB chemotherapy.

Three cases were reported that demonstrated myocardial compromise secondary to dilated cardiomyopathy resulting from AIDS. In each case, recurrent opportunistic infection had been present for over 6 months before a rapidly progressing cardiac illness became evident 4 to 8 weeks before death.[32] Both cell-mediated and humoral immunity have been postulated to have an important pathogenic role in the occurrence and progression of viral cardiomyopathic processes.[33]

INTENSIVE CARE PATIENTS

Patients with AIDS who require mechanical ventilation present a special problem because of the potential for considerable environmental contamination from blood and oral secretions. Airborne pathogens may be disseminated in the expired air from the ventilator. Ventilator exhaust, when possible, should be vented outside, and if not, a filter should be placed in the expired gas line. Ideally, patients in an intensive care unit (ICU) should be cared for in a private room and have a private nurse. All health care professionals should be gowned and masked and use protective eyewear when necessary to prevent conjunctival contamination.

In a study conducted at San Francisco General Hospital, 82 patients with AIDS were admitted to the ICU between March, 1981, and December, 1985. Of these patients, 69 percent died in the hospital, as did 87 percent of the patients who required mechanical ventilation because of PCP and respiratory failure.[34] Since the time of the study at San Francisco General Hospital, the number of ICU admissions has considerably declined, despite the increasing number of AIDS patients admitted to hospitals. This decrease was not explained by a reduction in the number of patients with PCP or by an improvement in their treatment. A survey of physicians at San Francisco General Hospital indicated that physicians are aware of the poor prognosis of AIDS patients with PCP and respiratory failure and believe that mechanical ventilation is infrequently indicated for this condition. Also, they have become increasingly likely to discuss issues of resuscitation with their patients with AIDS. Consequently, a change in physician attitudes, more effective patient counseling, and the increased availability of hospital- and community-based support services that provide alternatives to terminal intensive care are contributing to fewer ICU admissions overall.

PULMONARY PHYSICAL THERAPY

Purpose

The purpose of implementing chest physical therapy is to assist the AIDS patient with an abnormal or ineffective airway and to drain secretions from the peripheral airways to the trachea so they can be removed by coughing or suctioning. In addition, improvement in effective coughing and expansion of the atelectatic areas in the lungs are also considerations for chest physical therapy.

Procedures

1. Review chart for orders, clinical data, and chest radiograph report and identify opportunistic or pulmonary infection of patient.

2. Wash hands and explain procedure to the patient. If you are wearing a face mask, you may want to also discuss this with the patient.
3. Do breath sounds assessment to identify area to be drained.
4. Properly position patient and proceed with percussion and vibration.
5. Patient should be instructed to relax and take slow deep breaths using diaphragmatic, pursed-lip breathing.
6. Do a series of procedures including postural drainage, clapping, and vibration of each area to be drained.
7. At the end of each procedure encourage deep breathing and coughing exercises. Dispose of used tissues in blood and body secretions labeled bag.
8. Assess the effectiveness of these procedures with chest auscultations.
9. Incorporate incentive spirometry into the program and post-treatment breathing regime.

Precautions

1. Use proper body mechanics.
2. Avoid chest physical therapy 1 to 2 hours after meals. Stop continuous enteral feeding 30 minutes to 1 hour before treatment.
3. If not contraindicated, encourage a high fluid intake program for these patients; however, patients should be discouraged from taking large quantities of fluid just before and during treatment.
4. Be overly cautious on the cachetic, debilitated patient. Deviation from proper techniques can cause fractures of the ribs, or hemoptysis can occur.
5. Use of masks and gloves is indicated for the physical therapist when working with patients on respiratory or reverse isolation. This includes patients with untreated TB or MAI.

CASE STUDY

J.F. is a 42-year-old patient with HIV infection who was admitted with a history of diarrhea and progressive mental deterioration (central nervous system encephalopathy).

Significant Past Medical History

Patient had been on ribavirin and azidothymidine (AZT, or Retrovir). J.F. also had an episode of severe herpes zoster that was well controlled by Retrovir.

Hospital Course

Patient was admitted October 23, 1987, with a temperature of 103°F and blood pressure of 120/80. Blood cultures were obtained, and intravenous fluids were administered. Do Not Resusitate (DNR) status was discussed with the patient's family at the patient's request.

10-23-87: Chest radiograph revealed atelectasis of the right lower lobe and complete collapse of the medial basal segment of the right lower lobe. The left lung was clear.
Antibiotics were started (Primaxin [Imipenem-Cilastatin Sodium, MSD] and Flagyl [metronidazole]).
Respiratory therapy consult was ordered. Pulmonary physical therapy was initiated.
Minimal dilation of the intracerebral ventricular system was noted with a computed axial tomograhy (CAT) scan of the brain; however, the dilation was increased since January 6, 1987. Minimal cerebral atrophy was noted.
10-26-87: A cardiology consult and echocardiogram were requested, and a diagnosis of congestive heart failure with pulmonary edema was given. The electrocardiogram demonstrated sinus trachycardia. Intravenous hyperalimentation (IVH) was halted, and support hose was placed on patient.

A Review of Pulmonary Physical Therapy

10-23-87: Orders were received and evaluation was performed. Respiratory rate (RR) was regular with no shortness of breath. Pulmonary physical therapy was administered in left side-lying position. The physical therapist taught breathing exercises to J.F., which included deep diaphragmatic, pursed-lip breathing. Incentive spirometry was introduced.

10-24-87: Bilateral breath sounds were auscultated, and no shortness of breath was noted. Pulmonary physical theray was continued twice a day.

10-25-87: Bilateral breath sounds were decreased. Pulmonary therapy was continued.

10-26-87: Auscultation of the lungs revealed continuous audible rales. The chest radiograph worsened, showing mild cardiomegaly. J.F. expressed minimal subjective relief from difficulty in breathing despite increased urine output from Lasix (furosemide). Supplemental oxygen at 3 liters was added to the regime, and pulmonary physical therapy was continued.

10-27-87: Bilateral breath sounds were decreased throughout the chest. Pulmonary physical therapy resulted in decreased auscultation of rales in the right lower lobe.

10-28-87: Chest radiograph now improved. Effusion diminished. Pulmonary physical therapy continued.

10-29-87: Atelectasis resolved. J.F.'s overall status improved. Breathing exercises reinforced.

This case study demonstrates the progression to more serious respiratory complications during the course of pulmonary physical therapy. A number of conditions could have contributed to the development of congestive heart failure. These include fluid overload; complications resulting from atelectasis with resultant congestive heart failure; staphylococcus associated with endocarditis (J.F. had blood cultures that were positive for staphylococcus); possible HIV-related myocardiopathy.

CONCLUDING REMARKS

The major focus of physical therapy in the treatment of AIDS patients with cardiopulmonary complications warrents careful evaluation and management in relation to pulmonary physical therapy. Moreover, a concerted look at one's fears when treating this patient population is highly recommended. Physical therapists are presented with many challenges in dealing with these patients; however, physical therapy can clearly enhance the quality of life in the AIDS patient.

ACKNOWLEDGMENT

The author acknowledges Eva Sanchez, administrative assistant, for manuscript support in editing and typing.

REFERENCES

1. Centers for Disease Control: Recommendations for prevention of HIV transmissions in health-care settings. MMWR 36, suppl. 25:2S, 1987
2. Centers for Disease Control: Laboratory safety practices. MMWR 31:577, 1982
3. Centers for Disease Control: Acquired immunodeficiency syndrome (AIDS), update—United States. MMWR 32:309, 1983
4. Hollander H, Golden J, Stulbarg M: Recurrent AIDS-related *Pneumocystis carinii* pneumonia (PCP): frequency, outcome and prevention. In: Program and Abstracts of the International Conference on AIDS, Paris. L'Association pour la Recherche sur les deficits Immunitares Viro-Induits. 51:7, 1986
5. Hardy D, Wolf PK, Gottlieb MS, et al.: Fansidar prophylaxis for *Pneumocystis carinii* pneumonia (PCP). p. 25. In: Abstracts from the International Conference on the Acquired Immunodeficiency Syndrome, Philadelphia, American College of Physicians, 1985
6. Fauci AS, Macher AM, Longo DL, et al.: NIH conference, acquired immunodeficiency syndrome: epidemiologic, clinical, immunologic and therapeutic considerations. Ann Intern Med 100:92, 1984
7. Kovacs JA, Hiemenz MD, Macher AM, et al.: *Pneumocystis carinii* pneumonia: a comparison between patients with immunodeficiency syndrome and patients with other immunodeficiencies. Ann Intern Med 100:663, 1984
8. Centers for Disease Control: Update: acquired immunodeficiency syndrome, United States, MMWR 35:757, 765, 1986
9. Small C, Harris C, Friedland G, Klein R: The treatment of *Pneumocystis carinii* pneumonia in the acquired immunodeficiency syndrome. Arch Intern Med 145:837, 1985
10. Jaffe HS, Abrams DI, Amann J, et al.: Complications of cotrimoxazole treatment of AIDS-associated *Pneumocystis carinii* pneumonia in homosexual men. Lancet 2:1109, 1983
11. Gordin FM, Simon GL, Wofsy CB, Mills J: Adverse reactions to trimethoprim-sulfamethoxazole in patients with acquired immunodeficiency syndrome. Ann Intern Med 100:495, 1984
12. Haverkos HW: Assessment of therapy of *Pneumocystis carinii* pneumonia. Am J Med 76:501, 1984
13. Wharton M, Coleman DL, Fitz G, et al.: Prospective randomized trail of trimethoprim-sulfamethoxazole versus pentamidine for *Pneumocystis carinii* pneu-

monia in the acquired immunodeficiency syndrome. Am Rev Respir Dis 129:188A, 1984

14. Leoung GS, Mills J, Hopewell PC, et al.: Dapsone trimethoprim for *Pneumocystis carinii* pneumonia in the acquired immunodeficiency syndrome. Ann Intern Med 105:45, 1986

15. Conte J, Hollander H, Golden J: Inhaled or reduced-dose intravenous pentamidine for *Pneumocystis carinii* pneumonia. Ann Intern Med 107:495, 1987

16. Weber AL, Bird KT, Janower ML: Primary tuberculosis in childhood with particular emphasis on the changes affecting tracheobronchial tree. AJR 103:123, 1968

17. Suderam G, McDonald R, Maniatis T, et al.: Tuberculosis as a manifestation of the acquired immunodeficiency syndrome (AIDS). JAMA 256:362, 1986

18. American Thoracic Society: Treatment of tuberculosis and other mycobacterial diseases. Am Rev Respir Dis 127:790, 1983

19. Cohen RJ, Samoszuk MK, Busch D, Lagios M: Occult infections with *M. intracellulare* in bone-marrow biopsy specimens from patients with AIDS. N Engl J Med 308:1475, 1983

20. Wong B, Edwards FF, Kiehn TE, et al.: Continuous high-grade *Mycobacterium avium-intracellulare* bacteremia in patients with the acquired immunodeficiency syndrome. Am J Med 78:35, 1985

21. Pitchenik AE, Cole C, Russell BW, et al.: Tuberculosis, atypical mycobacteriosis and the acquired immunodeficiency syndrome among Haitian and non-Haitian patients in South Florida. Ann Intern Med 101:641, 1984

22. Macher AM, Kovacs JA, Gill V, et al.: Bacteremia due to *Mycobacterium avium-intracellulare* in the acquired immunodeficiency syndrome. Ann Intern Med 99:782, 1983

23. Zakowski P, Fligiel S, Berlin GW, Johnson L, Jr.: Disseminated *Mycobacterium avium-intracellulare* infection in homosexual men dying of acquired immunodeficiency. JAMA 248:2980, 1982

24. Greene JB, Sidhu GS, Lewis S, et al.: *Mycobacterium avium-intracellulare:* a cause of disseminated life-threatening infection in homosexuals and drug abusers. Ann Intern Med 97:539, 1982

25. Chan J, McKitrick JC, Klein RS: *Mycobacterium gordonac* in the acquired immunodeficiency syndrome. Ann Intern Med 101:400, 1984

26. Centers for Disease Control: Diagnosis and management of the mycobacterium infection and disease in persons with human immunodeficiency virus infection. Ann Intern Med 106:254, 1987

27. Fraser RG, Pare JAP: Diagnosis of diseases of the chest. Vol 2. p. 731. WB Saunders, Philadelphia, 1979

28. Stead WW, Kerby GR, Schleuter DP, Jordahl CW: The clinical spectrum of primary tuberculosis in adults: confusion with reinfection in the pathogenesis of chronic tuberculosis. Ann Intern Med 68:731, 1968

29. Benyesh-Melnick M: Cytomegaloviruses. p. 701. In Lennette EH, Schmidt NJ (eds): Diagnostic Procedures for Viral and Rickettsial Infections. Public Health Association, New York, 1969

30. Silver MA, Macher AM, Reichert CM, et al.: Cardiac involvement by Kaposi's sarcoma in acquired immune deficiency syndrome (AIDS). Am J Cardiol 53:983, 1984

31. Autran B, Gorin T, Leibowitch M, et al.: AIDS in Haitian women with cardiac Kaposi's sarcoma and Whipple's disease. Lancet 1:767, 1983

32. Cohen I, Anderson D, Virmani R, et al.: Congestive cardiomyopathy in association with the acquired immunodeficency syndrome. N Eng J Med 315:628, 1986

33. Woodruff JF: Viral myocarditis: a review. Am J Pathol 101:427, 1980

34. Wachter R, Luce J, Turner J, et al.: Intensive care of patients with the acquired immunodeficiency syndrome. Am Rev Respir Dis 134:189, 1986

31 Evaluation and Treatment of the High-Risk Infant

Carolyn M. Oddo

Medical technology in the treatment of neonates has improved dramatically in the past several years. Approximately 250,000 high-risk infants are spending time in one of this country's specialized neonatal intensive care units (NICUs) each year. Pediatric physical therapists are vital health care team members who can bring their expertise and knowledge of neonatal development into the NICU early on in the management of these high-risk infants. Early detection of problems and intervention by physical therapy can greatly enhance the neonate's developmental outcome and facilitate the mother-infant bonding process.

WHO IS A "HIGH-RISK" INFANT?

Infants are classified as "high risk" if they have the potential to acquire developmental disabilities during childhood as a result of events that occurred prenatally, perinatally, or postnatally. Premature and low-birthweight (LBW) infants are two major categories of high-risk infants. The normal gestational period for a full-term pregnancy is 38 to 42 weeks. A premature infant has a gestational period of less than 38 weeks. Accordingly, a post-term infant has a gestational period of greater than 42 weeks. Gestational age can be defined as the time, in weeks, from the first day of the mother's last menstrual period until the infant is born. Once assignment of gestational age is made,

an assessment of the infant's birthweight must be made to determine whether the infant's size is appropriate for his gestational age. Any infant with a birthweight of 2,500 g or less is considered to be LBW regardless of the cause and without regard to the duration of gestation. The classification of LBW became necessary when it was realized that not all neonates weighing 2,500 g or less were premature. Infants born with a birthweight of less than 1,500 g are considered very low birthweight (VLBW).[1]

Knowing the infant's birthweight in relationship to the gestational age gives the medical care giver a better indication of the intrauterine growth and development. A LBW is expected for a premature infant; however, a LBW for a full-term infant can indicate some form of prenatal deprivation. The infant's height, weight, and head circumference are charted on standardized growth charts for determination of his percentiles for each gestational age. Infants between the 10th and 90th percentiles are considered appropriate for gestational age (AGA). Infants with parameters above the 90th percentile are considered large for gestational age (LGA), and those with parameters below the 10th percentile are small for gestational age (SGA).

Infants are considered high risk when one or more of the risk factors listed in Table 31-1 are present in their medical history. Infants in these groups would benefit from a screening for developmental disabilities.

Table 31-1 Risk Factors for Developmental Disabilities

Birthweight of 1,500 g or less
Ill neonates <2,500 g
Genetic or chromosomal abnormalities
Gestational age of 32 weeks or less
Hydrocephalus
Infants born to maternal drug or alcohol abusers
Intracranial or intraventricular hemorrhage
Microcephalus
Musculoskeletal or orthopedic abnormalities
Neurological impairments (cerebral palsy, meningitis, head trauma, spinal cord injuries)
Seizures
Sepsis
Small for gestational age
Term infants with anoxic insults before, during, or after delivery (birth asphyxia, meconium aspiration, fetal distress syndrome)
TORCH infections (toxoplasmosis, rubella, cytomegalovirus, herpes virus, syphilis)
Trauma

EVALUATION OF THE HIGH-RISK INFANT

History

Before handling the infant, the physical therapist should read the patient's medical chart to obtain a complete history as well as an awareness of any precautions that should be taken in caring for the infant. Important factors worth noting from the patient's history are diagnosis, date of birth, gestational age, birthweight, and medical complications. This information will assist in calculating the corrected age of those infants that are premature. The corrected age is used for up to 2 years of age when assessing development against standardized developmental assessment tools. Use of corrected age provides the infant with additional time to achieve developmental milestones appropriate for chronological age. The formula to calculate corrected age is as follows:

Corrected Age = Number of weeks from the date of birth − the number of weeks premature

Apgar Score

The Apgar score is an informative numerical evaluation of the newborn's physical status at 1 and 5 minutes after birth. Values from zero to two are given to the following parameters of the newborn:

Heart rate
Respiratory effort
Muscle tone
Reflex irritability
Color

A value of zero will be assigned for the absence of a response in that parameter, and a score of two is given when the best response possible is made. The sum of all ratings makes up the Apgar score, which is usually written as $X^1X_A{}^5$ (X = the score at 1 minute and X_A = the score at 5 minutes). A perfect score is 10. A score of six or less indicates that the newborn may have suffered some type of intrauterine distress. Interpretation of the usefulness of the Apgar score as a predictor of outcome has been varied. One generally accepted concept is that the 1-minute score is a reflection of the severity of the intrauterine distress and the 5-minute score is more predictive of morbidity and mortality.[2]

Delivery History

A description of the delivery history may include factors such as type of labor, type of delivery, complications of delivery, presentation of infant, etc. The mother's pregnancy history can be summarized in one of two ways. The most commonly seen method is recorded in the medical chart as $G_X P_{X_1} Ab_{X_2}$. Gravida (G_X) is the number of times the mother has been pregnant. Para (P_{X_1}) is the number of previous pregnancies that have gone to the period of viability (approximately 20 weeks of gestation). Abortion (Ab_{X_2}) is the number of births before the stage of viability.

Obstetrical History

A new methodology that summarizes the obstetrical history of the mother is presented as four digits separated by dashes.[3]

$$X - X_1 - X_2 - X_3$$

The first digit (X) refers to the number of full-term infants the mother has delivered. The second digit (X_1) refers to the number of premature infants born to the mother. The third digit (X_2) refers to the number of abortions. The fourth digit (X_3) refers to the number of children now alive.

Aside from the above numerical data from the infant's medical record, mention of the home and family situation will aid the physical therapist in getting the total picture of the child's disposition. Once the history is reviewed, the evaluation process can begin.

General Inspection

Before actually placing hands on the infant, the physical therapist should use visual observation skills to evaluate the effects that gravity has on muscle tone and positioning. Improper positioning can lead to positional deformities or skin breakdown. Visual observation can tell the physical therapist a lot about the infant's spontaneous movement before manually testing for responses. Identification of all tubes, intravenous lines, and monitors should be made at the onset of the evaluation so appropriate precautions can be taken to avoid injury to the infant.

The observer will also want to know the infant's general state of alertness at the start of the examination and how well the infant responds to changes in his environment. One method to determine the infant's response to changes in his environment is to make note of his state pre-examination, during examination, and postexamination.

Neonatal States

Quiet-alert. In the quiet-alert state the infant is able to orient to sound and locate and fix on objects.

Active-awake. Minimal fixation or visual tracking is observed, and movements of the trunk and extremities are seen.

Crying. The infant displays a high activity level and it is difficult to get him to attend to any stimulation.

Quiet-sleep. Regular breathing is apparent, the infant's eyes are closed, and little active movement is noted.

Active sleep state. The infant is in rapid eye movement (REM) sleep and slight active movement and sucking are observed.

During the general inspection and observation stage, and all throughout the evaluation, the physical therapist should document the infant's state in response to different stimuli as well as his ability to soothe and console himself by bringing his hands to his mouth or changing position.

BABY HANDLING

The physical therapist should now handle the infant and, if possible, swaddle him and hold him in her lap. Begin by softly talking to the infant and observe his ability to adapt to the change in his environment as he goes from the transition of pre-examination to during-examination state. Figure 31-1 illustrates one possible position for the therapist and infant to begin their evaluation.

This is a good time to perform informal visual and auditory testing on the infant. Observe for

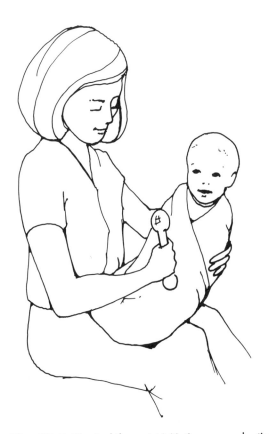

Fig. 31-1 Physical therapist initiating an evaluation.

fixing and tracking responses by holding a bright red object a few inches from the infant's face and slowly moving it to the left and right and then up and down. Auditory responses such as turning toward sounds, startling, or making a facial movement are observed as a result of ringing a bell near the right and left ears. Care must be taken not to talk to the infant when testing for visual responses and not to show the infant the toy used to test hearing to ensure accuracy in the testing procedure.

Any absent or asymmetrical responses in the visual or auditory testing should be documented in the patient's record and reported to the infant's physician so that formal testing can be considered.

DEVELOPMENTAL DIFFERENCES BETWEEN FULL-TERM AND PREMATURE INFANTS

The resting posture of a full-term infant is very different from that of a premature infant. A healthy, full-term infant will display the following resting posture: head turned toward the right or left, shoulders abducted and externally rotated, wrists held in midposition with fingers in flexion, hips flexed, and feet maintained in dorsiflexion. Generalized flexion is seen as a result of intra-uterine positioning. Muscular hypertonia is present in both the upper and lower extremities, and as they are pulled down during testing, they spring back into flexion when they are released. Active movements are seen as flexion or extension at all joints simultaneously.

Scarf Sign

The scarf sign is commonly used to assess the muscle tone of the newborn. It is performed by holding the infant by the wrist and attempting to bring the elbow past the midline when the infant is supine. The full-term infant resists this maneuver. The premature infant does not resist and allows the elbow to be moved to the opposite shoulder. Figure 31-2 illustrates this maneuver.

Heel-to-Ear Maneuver

Another commonly used test to evaluate the newborn's muscle tone and degree of flexibility is the heel-to-ear maneuver. Testing is done by placing the newborn supine on a table with his pelvis flat and gently lifting the legs in an attempt to touch the head with the feet. This maneuver is impossible with a full-term infant. The leg of the premature infant is so flexible that the foot can easily be raised to touch the ear. Figure 31-3 illustrates this test.

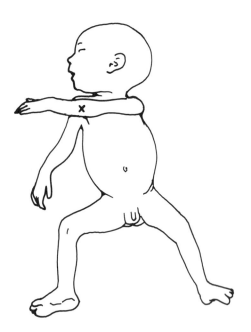

Fig. 31-2 Scarf sign.

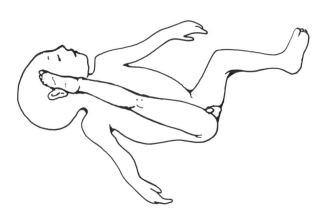

Fig. 31-3 Heel-to-ear maneuver.

Primitive Reflexes

The primitive reflexes are fully developed and symmetrical in the full-term infant. They are called primitive reflexes because they begin to appear before birth in utero and are controlled at the brain stem and spinal cord levels of central nervous system maturation. Primitive reflexes are integrated into voluntary movement during the first 4 to 6 months of life as the cortex matures and develops.

Important factors to note when testing the infant for primitive reflexes are not only their presence and appropriate integration, but the quality of their presence and any signs of asymmetry. Absence of or poor quality of performance of reflexes can be reflective of a neurologically depressed or weak infant. Any asymmetry in response of the reflex testing may indicate findings such as a hemiparesis, facial palsy, or Erb's palsy depending on the location and nature of the reflex. There are many different standardized reflex testing tools available to therapists that list not only acceptable integration periods for the reflexes, but also the procedures to perform them.

Muscle Tone

Babies born at 28 weeks gestation display generalized hypotonia with extension of all extremities in the resting position. They are born with a thick coating of white vernix that covers their body. When this coating is washed off, the infant's red translucent skin is exposed with tiny veins seen below the surface. Fetal hair, called lanugo, covers the infant's body. The infant at this stage in his development lacks skin creases on the soles of the feet, ear cartilage, and breast buds. The primitive reflexes are beginning to appear. The rooting reflex is becoming more consistent and organized at the corners of the mouth. The palmar grasp reflex is present in the finger flexors and beginning to spread to the muscles of the forearm. Extension of the upper extremity has been added to the Moro reflex, but abduction and bringing the hands to midline are still lacking.

The premature infant born at 32 weeks gestation has a complete rooting reflex and a firm grasp reflex of the fingers. The 32-week-gestation infant shows accelerated steps in fetal development. The

components of the Moro reflex and the primary stepping reflex are becoming more complete at this stage. An increase in muscle tone is now present in the thighs and trunk, and more active movement is seen as generalized movements of the whole body. The arms are still held in extension.

At 35 weeks of gestation, the hypertonia has progressed to the upper extremities. The characteristic "frog-leg" positioning of the lower extremities is seen while in the supine position. Infants born at 37 weeks gestation present much like a full-term infant. All extremities are held in loose flexion. The primitive reflexes are more consistent and organized. An increase in muscle tone is now seen in the cervical region, and all that remains for the development of normal muscle tone is the balance between the flexors and extensors of the neck and the differences between the upper and lower extremities.

It is important to note that the muscle tone of the premature infant who has reached 40 weeks gestation is not the same as that of the full-term newborn. Muscle tone in the infant develops caudocephally. The full-term infant displays a newborn posture of flexion of the trunk and extremities because his muscle tone was developed in utero and was influenced by the restriction of space in the uterus. Active movement and extension of the trunk and extremities is developed by the newborn soon after birth as his body is exposed to the effects of gravity and the presence of the primitive reflexes. Premature infants, on the other hand, are not restricted in utero because they are smaller in size and are born with much less muscle tone and flexion of the trunk and extremities.

TREATMENT OF HIGH-RISK INFANTS

Before initiation of evaluation and treatment, all patients should have a referral from a physician. Once this is obtained, an initial evaluation is performed and a treatment program is specifically designed to meet the unique needs of the particular neonate.

The criteria for physical therapy intervention in the NICU and other high-risk nurseries varies from facility to facility. One major criterion for

Table 31-2 Indications for Physical Therapy Referral

Feeding difficulties
Abnormal neurological examination (hypertonia, scissoring, clonus, hypotonia)
Obligatory or absent primitive reflexes
Abnormal positioning (frog-leg positioning of the lower extremities, torticollis, retracted shoulders and extended arms, etc.)
Potential for decreased range of motion or joint contractures
Neurologically depressed infants
Asymmetrical use of the extremities

direct intervention in terms of developmental stimulation is that the patient be medically stable. If the patient is not medically stable or on mechanical ventilation, the physical therapist's intervention in the NICU may be limited to providing a positioning program and "crib" stimulation. In some settings, physical therapists provide chest physical therapy to this population and become more involved with the "acutely ill" infants who have respiratory involvement. Some of the most common indications warranting a physical therapy referral are listed in Table 31-2. NICU personnel should receive inservice training on a regular basis on the indications warranting a physical therapy referral. If the physicians are geared toward observing for potential problem areas instead of referring by diagnosis, then the facility can strive for appropriate coverage of the nursery by physical therapists.

Short-term and long-term goals for the treatment of the high-risk infants are:

To develop normal movement patterns
To prevent positional deformities
To prevent contractures
To promote an environment for mother-infant bonding
To establish correct handling of the infant
To attain developmental milestones appropriate for age level

Treatment times for neonates will be shorter than for most patients seen by physical therapists and will be dictated by the neonate. During the treatment session, the physical therapist must be astutely aware of the neonate's signs of overstimulation or fatigue. These signs might include an increase in respiratory rate, yawning, spitting up, burping, cyanosis, or covering the face with the hands. These infants have very immature central nervous systems and overload easily; therefore, if an infant displays a sign of overstimulation, it is best to place him back in his incubator and follow up later with another treatment session.

TREATMENT TECHNIQUES

Developmental Stimulation

Developmental stimulation to promote visual and auditory responses can begin by decorating the infant's incubator with crib toys and mobiles. Premature infants have a short field of vision (approximately 6 to 10 inches) and respond well to people's faces and sharp, contrasting designs. Pictures of people's faces from magazines or hand-drawn faces and designs with contrasting shapes in black and white are most effective when placed on the wall of the incubator and moved regularly to provide the infant with a variety of visual experiences. Musical toys that play soft, soothing songs are beneficial to have in or near the incubator to calm the infant and to help him tune out some of the common nursery noises such as the constant hum of alarms. Figure 31-4 illustrates some examples of crib stimulation.

Swaddling

Swaddling is a technique that can be used by physical therapists and other health care workers to help the infant organize his response to his new environment. The infant has difficulty controlling his head, arms, and legs against gravity, and this makes it difficult for him to concentrate on an activity; thus, he becomes "disorganized" and frustrated. By swaddling the infant with only his head exposed, the physical therapist or parent can introduce age-appropriate developmental toys to him and work on visual and auditory stimulation. As the infant becomes proficient with only his head exposed, the physical therapist can expose one hand and begin working on hand-to-mouth or grasping techniques. This sequence can be continued until the neonate can handle having all his extremities exposed to the environment. Infants find comfort sleeping in the swaddled posi-

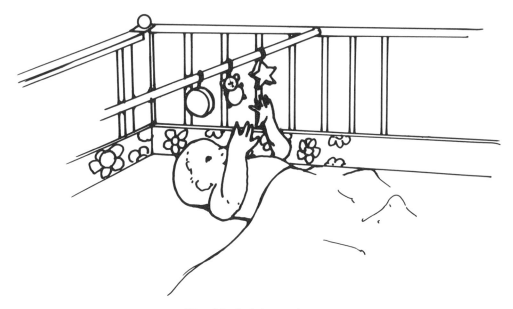

Fig. 31-4 Crib stimulation.

tion because it provides neutral warmth and a simulation of their mother's womb, which they were deprived of for a period of time by being born prematurely. Swaddling also aids the neonate in maintaining his body temperature while being fed or treated outside of the incubator.

Swaddling is an especially beneficial technique for infants going through drug withdrawal from maternal drug abuse. These infants are very jittery and irritable and need the swaddling to calm them and help them to organize their central nervous system in their new environment. Figure 31-5 illustrates the technique for swaddling an infant.

Being rocked back and forth in a rocking chair is another treatment technique that provides the swaddled infant with a calming and soothing effect. Many NICUs are equipped with rocking chairs that can be utilized by physical therapists in their treatment programs.

POSITIONING PROGRAMS

Proper positioning of the neonate plays an important role in the prevention of abnormal postures and contractures that later could produce stumbling blocks in his development. A positioning program should be developed specifically for the infant based on the results and findings of his initial evaluation. For the positioning program to be effective and followed consistently, it is recommended that the physical therapist write out and illustrate the program and display it on the infant's incubator so that the care givers and parents can follow it. In addition, the physical therapist may want to demonstrate the program to the care givers and the parents to ensure that it is carried out correctly. Below are some examples of general guidelines for an effective positioning program.

Prone

The prone position is probably the most favorable position for these neonates because it promotes flexion of the extremities. When the infant is supine, all movements become very difficult because they are largely performed against gravity. Often the infant is so weak that he does not have the strength to move his extremities, and he will lose interest in reacting to his environment. By lying prone, the infants tend to keep their extremities close to their bodies, which will help them "organize" better toward their environment. Care must be taken to see that the infant's head is turned toward the right and left equally to prevent

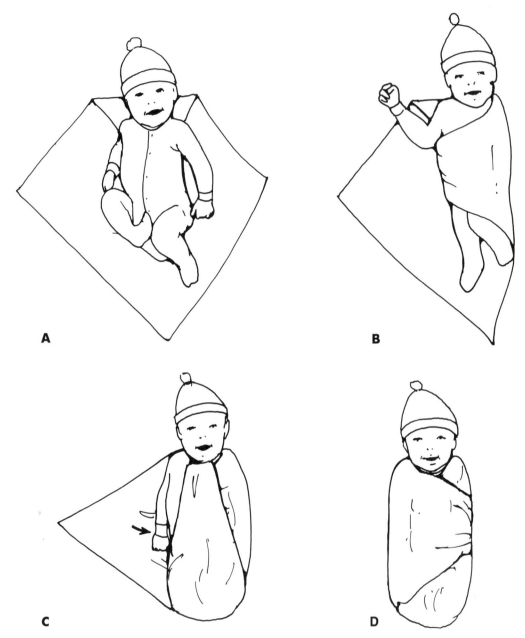

Fig. 31-5 (A,B,C, and **D)** The technique for swaddling an infant.

positional deformities such as a torticollis. If the lower extremities are markedly abducted while the infant is lying prone, the physical therapist can gently bring them up under the hips and secure them there with a blanket or towel rolls. The prone position also encourages hand-to-mouth activity and lifting the head up off the bed.

Supine

When the infant is supine, it is important to encourage the head to the midline position to prevent the asymmetrical tonic neck reflex from becoming obligatory as this will interfere with bringing the hands to the midline and grasping in the future. The next area of concern would be the possibility of retracted and abducted shoulders, which would again interfere with bringing the hands to the midline. The lower extremities frequently are abducted or in the frog-leg position. If this is not prevented, it could cause marked external rotation of the legs that could later interfere with crawling and ambulation. The supine position provides the infant with the optimal environment for social interaction and encourages active movement of all extremities. Generalized flexion of the neonate needs to be encouraged

whilie he is lying supine. Figure 31-6 provides some examples of how towel rolls can be used to help encourage the desired flexion.

Side Lying

Towel rolls can also be used to help position the neonate in side lying. The neonate should lie equally on the right and left sides to prevent any asymmetries from developing. Benefits of side lying include encouraging the hands to move to the midline, improving visual awareness of the hands, and adduction of the lower extremities. The side-lying position is optimal for discouraging the frog-leg position. Figure 31-7 illustrates an example of the use of towel rolls in the side-lying position.

Range of Motion/Splinting

Premature infants are rarely born with contractures, but occasionally the full-term infant with neurological problems develops contractures secondary to spasticity in the hands and feet. The upper extremity will present with shoulder internal rotation, flexion of the elbow, pronation of the forearm, wrist flexion, and finger flexion with

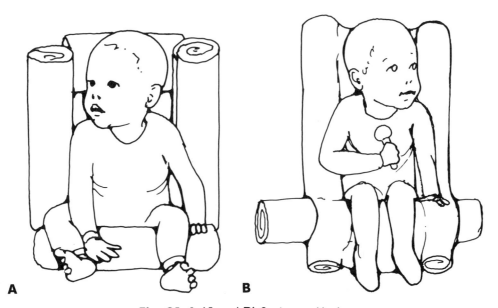

A　　　　　　　　　　　　　　　　**B**

Fig. 31-6 (A and **B)** Supine positioning.

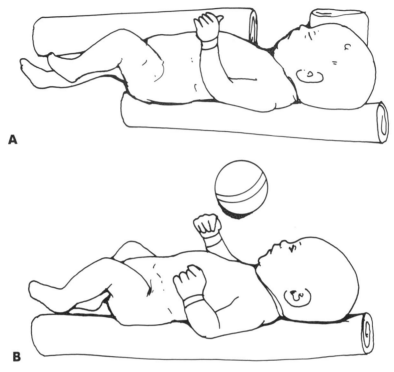

Fig. 31-7 (A and **B)** Side-lying positioning.

cortical thumbing. If the infant has decreased active movement and is unable to break out of this pattern, it may be necessary to fit him with a resting hand splint and provide passive range of motion exercises to prevent contractures and the overstretching of the extensor muscles of the wrist. If the forearm and wrist are in a neutral position and the only abnormality noted is the presence of a cortical thumb, then the splint of choice would be a cortical thumb splint.

Plantar flexed positioning of the feet without active movement at the joint encourages the potential for contracture development. Conservative management for the prevention of contractures may include passive range of motion exercises and splinting. Splinting techniques for the foot are numerous, and some possible alternatives include the construction of a splint to encourage neutral positioning of the foot, the application of a miniature foot board, taping the foot, or positioning with towel rolls. If the infant's foot is large enough and the degree of involvement is minimal, the wearing of a soft baby high-top shoe or booties may provide the support needed to maintain full range of motion.

Parent Education

Vital to the success of any physical therapy intervention program is the education of the parents about the purposes and specific techniques of their infant's individualized treatment program. Physical therapists should make an effort to meet with parents at the infant's bedside and demonstrate handling and positioning techniques to them. Parents should also be taught swaddling techniques and developmental stimulation activities appropriate for their infant's age level. Parents should be given time to practice these techniques in the presence of the physical therapist as this will help them build their confidence and allow them to ask questions. Return demonstration of the exercises and handling techniques by parents should be evaluated by the physical therapist to identify areas in which additional instruction or time to practice is needed. Having these exercises written in the form of a home program will aid the parents in remembering exactly how the program should be performed. Remember that the parents are bombarded by many different health care providers and often find it difficult to remember everything that is told to them. The purposes of good inter-action in the nursery between the physical therapist and the parents include providing emotional support, promoting mother-infant bonding, and paving the way for a smooth transition and compliance in the outpatient follow-up setting.

FOLLOW-UP CARE

Once early detection and identification of infants that are at risk of delays in their development is made, it is essential that they are referred to an outpatient follow-up clinic. The first year in the life of a high-risk infant can be filled with numerous medical appointments with a large number of health care providers. The follow-up clinic can serve as an important bridge between the gap of medical care givers and the patients, which can be tremendous for the families of the high-risk infant. Continuity of patient care can be strived for by having the follow-up clinic serve many functions and staffing it with consistent health care providers. Familiarity with the system and the health care providers can greatly enhance compliance with home programs and follow-up appointments. Appointments to the follow-up clinic can be made in conjunction with actual physical therapy appointments if deemed necessary as a result of the infant's initial evaluation. Infants should be seen in the follow-up clinic at 6 weeks, 3 months, 6 months, 9 months, and 12 months corrected age. The frequency of appointments after 1 year can be decided on by the follow-up clinic team based on the extent of the infant's developmental disability and the status of his enrollment in a community-based program. Clinics can adopt different time frames and protocols for follow-up evaluations. Care must be taken, however, to see the infant when significant milestones should be occurring at his particular age level. The initial follow-up clinic appointment should be given to the parents when the infant is discharged from the hospital. Also at that time, parents should be told of the function and importance of the clinic to ensure compliance in keeping their appointments.

The functions of the follow-up clinic should be:

1. To assess regularly the neurodevelopmental status of the high-risk infant to ensure that he is attaining milestones appropriate for his age level.

2. To provide parents and care givers with medical information updates in regard to the infant's current medical status, prognosis, and medical and therapeutic needs.
3. To make parents and care givers aware of and assist them in making application to the financial resources and community agencies available to them and their child.
4. To evaluate the child for equipment needs and the writing of necessary prescriptions.
5. To recommend the appropriate mode for treatment if therapeutic intervention is indicated as a result of the infant's neurodevelopmental examination.

The follow-up clinic team should consist of, but not be limited to, a physician with a strong neurodevelopmental background, a physical therapist, an occupational therapist, a registered nurse, and a social worker. A speech pathologist may or may not attend every clinic, but is usually available for consultation and treatment if necessary. A translator should be made available to the clinic if a portion of the population served is non-English speaking.

The follow-up clinic team should be aware of the community agencies in their area and of the services they offer. The most commonly referred to agencies available in most large cities are:

School-based programs
Cerebral palsy or developmental disability
   treatment centers
Home health agencies (physical therapy,
   occupational therapy, speech)
Mental health and mental retardation programs
Residential care facilities
Hospital-based or private practice physical
   therapy services
Psychological testing or services
Parent support groups

Discharge criteria vary for parents in a follow-up clinic setting. Some clinics follow children for their developmental needs until they are 16 years of age even if they are receiving services from a community agency. The reason for this is that many community agencies do not provide medical intervention for these children, and unless they acquire the services of a private physician, they have no method for obtaining prescriptions for equipment needs as they get older. Frequently, older children who regularly attend school-based programs visit the follow-up clinic every few years for a "tune up" that consists of an evaluation of their existing equipment, an update of their home program, and a projection of future needs. Some clinics follow children from birth to 3 years of age and then refer them to other facilities for the continuation of their medical care. There are no hard and fast guidelines for establishment of a follow-up clinic. Every facility should develop a follow-up clinic setting based on the resources available to them.

REFERENCES

1. Campbell SK (ed): Pediatric Neurologic Physical Therapy. p. 109. Churchill Livingstone, New York, 1984
2. Ensher GL, Clark DA: Newborns at Risk: Medical Care and Psychoeducational Intervention. p. 26. Aspen Publishers, Rockville, Maryland, 1980
3. Pritchard JA, MacDonald PC, Gant NF: Williams Obstetrics. Appleton-Century-Crofts, East Norwalk, CT, 1985

SUGGESTED READINGS

Allen ME, Jones MD: Medical complications of prematurity. Obstet Gynecol 67:427, 1986

Amiel-Tison C: Neurological evaluation of maturity of newborn infants. Arch Dis Child 43:89, 1968

Barnes M, Crutchfield C, Heriza C: The Neurophysiological Basis of Patient Treatment. Vol. 2. Reflexes in Motor Development. Stokesville Publishing, Atlanta, 1979

Behrman RE: Preventing low birth weight: a pediatric perspective. J Pediatr 107:842, 1985

Blackman JA (ed): Medical Aspects of Developmental Disabilities in Children Birth to Three. Aspen Systems, Rockville, Maryland, 1984

Brazelton TB: Neonatal behavioral assessment scales. Clinics in Developmental Medicine. No. 50. William Heinemann Medical Books, London, 1973

Campbell SK, Wilhelm IJ: Development from birth to 3 years of age of 15 children at high risk for central nervous system dysfunction: interim report. Phys Ther 65:463, 1985

Chamberlin RW: Developmental assessment and early intervention programs for young children: lessons learned from longitudinal research. Pediatr Rev 8:237, 1987

Chapman Y, James T: Handling of the premature, light for dates and "at risk" babies in the special care unit. Totline 11:16, 1985

Cohen SE, Parmelee AH, Beckwith L, Sigman M: Cognitive developmnent in preterm infants: birth to 8 years. J Dev Behav Pediatr 7:102, 1986

Dickson JM: A model for the physical therapist in the intensive care nursery. Phys Ther 61:45, 1981

Dunn DW, Epstein LG: Decision Making in Child Neurology. BC Decker, Toronto, 1987

England MA: Color Atlas of Life Before Birth: Normal Fetal Development. Year Book Medical Publishers, Chicago, 1983

Evans OB: Manual of Child Neurology. Churchill Livingstone, New York, 1987

Finnie NR: Handling the Young Cerebral Palsied Child at Home. EP Dutton, New York, 1974

Fiorentino MR: Reflex Testing Methods for Evaluating CNS Development. Charles C Thomas, Springfield, IL, 1973

Garland KR: Grief: the transitional process. Neonatal Network 5:7, 1986

Gardner SL, Merenstein GB: Perinatal grief and loss: an overview. Neonatal Network 5:7, 1986

Goldberg K: The high-risk infant. Phys Ther 55:1092, 1975

Goldberg S, DiVitto BA: Born Too Soon: Preterm Birth and Early Development. WH Freeman, San Francisco, 1983

Goodman M, Rothberg AD, Houston-McMillan JE, et al.: Effect of early neurodevelopmental therapy in normal and at-risk survivors of neonatal intensive care. Lancet 2:1327, 1985

Gottfried AW, Gaiter JL (eds): Infant Stress Under Intensive Care. University Park Press, Baltimore, 1985

Graham GG: Poverty, hunger, malnutrition, prematurity, and infant mortality in the United States. Pediatrics 75:117, 1985

Greene JG, Fox NA, Lewis M: The relationship between neonatal characteristics and three-month mother-infant interaction in high-risk infants. Child Dev 54:1286, 1983

Harel S, Anastasiow NJ (eds): The At-Risk Infant: Psycho/Socio/Medical Aspects. Paul H. Brooks Publishing, Baltimore, 1985

Harrison H, Kositsky A: The Premature Baby Book: A Parent's Guide to Coping and Caring in the First Years. St. Martin's Press, New York, 1983

Harrison L: Effects of early supplemental stimulation programs for premature infants: review of the literature. Maternal-Child Nursing J 14:69, 1985

Janowsky JS, Nass R: Early language development in infants with cortical and subcortical perinatal brain injury. Dev Behav Pediatr 8:3, 1987

Klaus MH, Fanaroff AA (eds): Care of the High-Risk Neonate. 3rd Ed. WB Saunders, Philadelphia, 1982

Knobloch H, Stevens F, Malone AF: Manual of Developmental Diagnosis. Harper & Row, Hagerstown, Maryland, 1980

Magyary D: Early social interactions: preterm infant-parent dyads. Issues Compr Pediatr Nursing 7:233, 1984

Mast J: A review of infant reflexes and the emergence of normal development. Totline 11:17, 1985

Mast J: Therapeutic management of the high-risk infant. Totline 11:14, 1985

Stern FM: Screening the high-risk infant in a follow-up clinic. Totline 13:24, 1987

Stern FM: Physical and occupational therapy on a newborn intensive care unit. Rehabilitation Nursing, p. 26, 1986

Sweeney J, Metcalf V: Early intervention for high risk infants: an outline of regional physical therapy services. Military Med 147:143, 1982

Sweeney J: Neonatal physical therapy: crisis intervention for military families. Totline 11:13, 1985

Sugar M: The Premature in Context. SP Medical and Scientific Books, New York, 1982

Towbin A: The depressed newborn: pathogenesis and neurologic sequels. Perinatol Neonatol 11:16, 1987

Ungerer JA, Sigman M: Developmental lags in preterm infants from one to three years of age. Child Dev 54:1217, 1983

Verzemnieks IL: Developmental stimulation for infants and toddlers. Am J Nursing, p. 749, 1984

Volpe JJ: Neurology of the Newborn. 2nd Ed. WB Saunders, Philadelphia, 1987

32 Cardiovascular Responses to Exercise in Children

Manuela J. Giannini

Knowledge of exercise performance in children is essential for the physical therapist involved in the care of children with any chronic illness or of the healthy child involved in recreational sports. The increased awareness of the role of regular exercise in health maintenance of adults has now, fortunately, been expanded to children. A current role of the pediatric physical therapist is the evaluation of exercise tolerance in the healthy child and the child with a chronic illness. This also includes the provision of an appropriate exercise prescription aimed at improving cardiovascular fitness and maintaining an active life-style, regardless of the chronic illness.

Maximal exercise performance has been well documented in healthy children. Of particular interest are the changes that occur as a result of growth. During childhood, the capacity for work increases with body size. Between the ages of 5 and 15 years, there is an approximate threefold increase in body weight, lung volume, heart volume, and maximal oxygen uptake. There is a parallel increase in the muscle mass of the child and an increase in working capacity.[1,2] In this chapter, the normal physiological changes related to growth affecting the child's performance during dynamic exercise are discussed. In addition, the possible effects of disease on exercise-related functions in the sick child are specified. Guidelines for making exercise and activity recommendations to sick children and their parents are given.

RESPONSE OF HEALTHY CHILDREN TO EXERCISE

The role of the cardiovascular system during exercise is to supply the exercising muscles with oxygen and remove carbon dioxide. The adaptations that occur to accomplish this task are illustrated by the Fick equation:

$$\dot{V}O_{2max} = \dot{Q}_{max} \times (CaO_2 - C\bar{v}O_2)_{max}$$

where maximal oxygen uptake ($\dot{V}O_{2max}$) is the product of maximal cardiac output ($\dot{Q}_{max}$) and the maximal arterial-mixed venous difference in O_2 content $(CaO_2 - C\bar{v}O_2)_{max}$. Increased oxygen requirements of the working muscles during exercise are met by increasing cardiac output and increasing oxygen extraction by the working muscles from the blood.[3,4]

Oxygen Cost of Work

The standard method of measuring exercise is in terms of the oxygen consumption needed to perform work. With an increase in work, there is a parallel increase in oxygen demand and carbon dioxide production. In many types of muscular exercise, the oxygen uptake increases roughly linearly with an increase in workload. The maximal oxygen uptake, or $\dot{V}O_{2max}$, is the highest oxygen uptake the individual can attain despite increasing workloads while breathing at sea level.[4]

During the first minutes of progressive exercise, there is a slow increase in oxygen uptake owing to the slow adjustment of the oxygen transporting systems to work. Oxygen uptake then levels off to a steady state. At steady state, the oxygen uptake equals the oxygen requirement of the tissues, and there is no lactic acid accumulation.[3,4]

Maximal oxygen uptake is related to age. The maximal oxygen uptake of a 5-year-old is about 1.0 L/min and rises to its peak of about 3.8 L/min in the early 20s. Beyond this age, there is a gradual decline so that at 60 years maximal oxygen uptake is about 70 percent of the maximum at the early 20s. To some extent this decline is due to hypoactivity that comes with aging and partially due to the decrease in maximal heart rate[1,4] (Fig. 32-1).

There is a wide distribution of $\dot{V}O_{2max}$ values for healthy children when expressed in relation to age (Fig. 32-2). When expressed as milliliters per minute per kilogram of body weight (ml/min/kg), there is less variation in younger subjects.[1,5,6] However, even when based on body weight, a wide variation remains.

VO_{2max} is also dependent on sex. Girls have a lower VO_{2max} than boys at any age. The reason for this sex differnce is not apparent, especially before the onset of puberty when both sexes are active physically to similar degrees. Although maximal oxygen uptake of boys keeps increasing until about 18 years of age, there is little increase in girls beyond age 14. However, when VO_{2max} is expressed relative to lean body mass or the muscle mass performing the activity, the sex difference is no longer apparent[5-7] (Fig. 32-3).

Cardiac Output

The intensity of the work performed dictates the oxygen requirements for the skeletal muscles performing the work. Thus, the cardiovascular system must be regulated so that cardiac output is sufficient and the metabolic demands of the working skeletal muscles are met. The increased oxygen requirements during exercise are met by increasing the amount of blood flowing through the muscle and extracting more of the available oxygen flowing through the muscle (widening the arteriovenous oxygen difference).[1,4] Cardiac output is the product of heart rate and stroke volume. Both increase with exercise. With progressively increasing work, the stroke volume reaches maximum at 10 percent of the resting value, and further increase in cardiac output is due to an increase in heart rate.[1,3,4]

Vasodilation of the large vascular bed within skeletal muscle requires compensatory vasoconstriction in other vasculatures so that the blood may be diverted from organs that are metabolically less active to the working skeletal muscles. During exercise, the percentage of cardiac output and

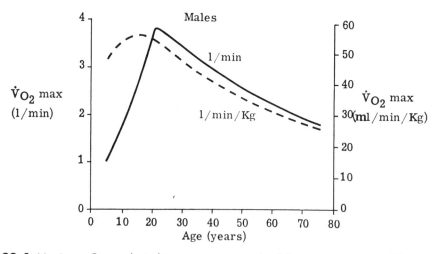

Fig. 32-1 Maximum O_2 uptake in liters per minute and milliliters per minute per kilogram of body weight in relation to age based on data collected from the literature. (From Godfrey S: Growth and development of cardiopulmonary responses to exercise. p. 271. In Davies JA, Dobbing J (eds): Scientific Foundations of Paediatrics, Heinemann Medical Books, London, 1974, with permission.)

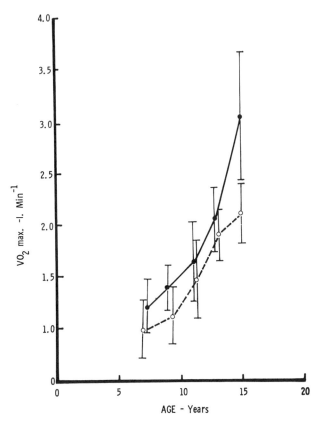

Fig. 32-2 Maximum O_2 uptake (VO_{2max}) in relation to age for boys (●) and girls (○). (Redrawn from Davies,[6] with permission.)

blood flow are decreased below resting levels in the visceral organs with the exception of the heart. The summation of local vasodilation in muscle together with vasoconstrictive diverting mechanisms in other organs increases blood flow to working muscles so that muscle oxygen consumption increases 50 to 75 times above the resting condition. This results in a cardiac output of 5 L/min at rest to a cardiac output of 15 L/Min with moderate exercise in adults.[3,4]

The maximal cardiac output of a child is limited by the size of his heart. Children have smaller stroke volumes than adults, and the maximal heart rate does not alter below the age of 25. Cardiac output increases with increasing stroke volume. As the child grows, there is an increase in maximal stroke volume with little change in maximal heart rate. Thus, increase in cardiac output during growth is due primarily to the increase in stroke volume.[1,5]

There is a nonlinear increase in cardiac output with an increase in oxygen uptake. Increases in cardiac output in response to increasing exercise in children are similar to the adult response in that an increase in cardiac output for a given increase in oxygen consumption is constant throughout life. Cardiac output response in children is about 1 to 1.5 L/min below and parallel to the adult values. The compensatory mechanism of

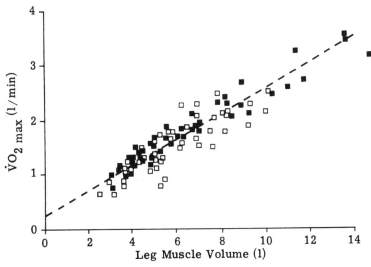

Fig. 32-3 Maximum O_2 uptake in boys (■) and girls (□) related to leg-muscle volume. (Redrawn from Davies,[6] with permission.)

the lower cardiac output is the higher arterial-mixed venous oxygen difference. Cardiac ouput in children during steady-state exercise is significantly related to VO_2 with no sex difference and a small size difference[1,5,8] (Fig. 32-4).

Stroke volume in children, unlike cardiac output, is affected by both size and sex. As the size of the child increases, stroke volume increases, and boys have larger stroke volumes than girls for any given size. Stroke volume reaches its maximal value at submaximal levels of exercise[1,5,8] (Fig. 32-5).

Lactic Acid

A criteria of maximal exercise is high levels of blood lactate. Maximal oxygen uptake measures the limit of aerobic exercise. As $\dot{V}O_{2max}$ is approached and passed, a point is reached at which lactate production exceeds its elimination from the blood. The level of blood lactate is used as a measure of the degree of anaerobic metabolism. The peak level of blood lactate is reached approximately 3 minutes after stopping maximal exercise and then there is a steady decline. Blood lactate is related to size at any given workload. Peak blood lactate level obtained in children increase from about 6 mmol/L in 5 year olds to about 11 mmol/L in 16 year olds.[1,9,10]

Heart Rate Response

Maximal heart rate is dependent on age and ranges between 195 and 215 beats/minute in children and adolescents (Fig. 32-6). Thereafter, it decreases with age, and the decline is independent of sex or level of fitness. At maximal exercise, the heart rate

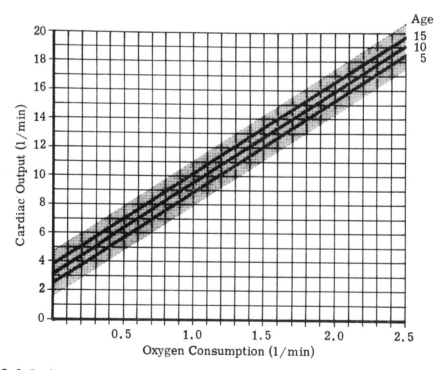

Fig. 32-4 Cardiac output in relation to oxygen consumption allowing for size (converted to age) in healthy children. The shaded band indicates the approximate 95 percent confidence limit for the 10-year-old line. (From Godfrey,[1] with permission.)

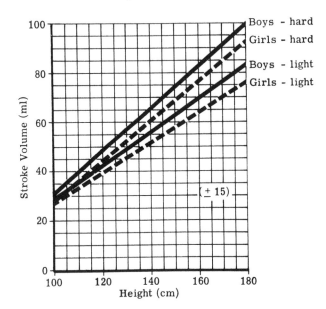

Fig. 32-5 Stroke volume in relation to size and sex during light or heavy work equivalent to approximately one-third and two-thirds W_{max}. (From Godfrey,[1] with permission.)

have higher heart rates at any work level than larger children, and their increases in heart rate per unit increase in work is also greater. At steady-state work, heart rate is also positively correlated with oxygen uptake.[1,5]

Working Capacity

Maximum working capacity (W_{max}) is defined as the highest rate of working that the child is able to achieve. Maximum power output increases linearly with age and size. There is also a modest correlation with sex. Boys will achieve a higher working capacity than girls at a given age or size. However, the sex difference becomes much

reaches a limiting value and then there is no further increase with harder work.[1,4]

At submaximal work levels, the heart rate depends on size, workload, and sex, girls having higher heart rates than boys. Smaller children

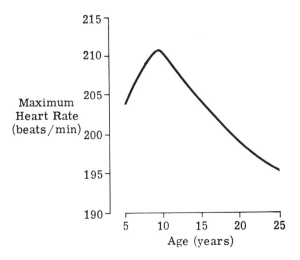

Fig. 32-6 Maximal heart rate during exercise in relation to age. (From Godfrey,[1] from data in Astrand PO: Experimental studies of physical working capacity in relation to sex and age. Munksgaard, Copenhagen, 1952)

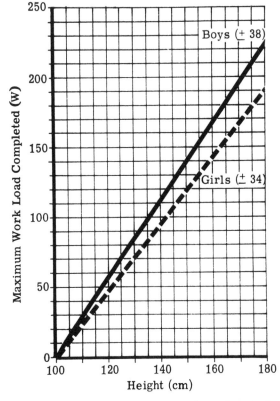

Fig. 32-7 Maximum power output achieved in simple progressive exercise related to height in boys and girls. The numbers in brackets in this and subsequent illustrations indicate the approximate 95 percent confidence limits. (Redrawn from Godfrey et al.,[5] with permission.)

greater by 14 years. The growth spurt seen in males between 13 and 14 years is paralleled by a sharp increase in working capacity. In contrast, the working capacity in girls actually demonstrates a small decrease at adolescence[1,11,12] (Fig. 32-7).

Blood Pressure

Systolic and diastolic blood pressure rise with age, although the rise in diastolic blood pressure in healthy individuals is small. Systolic blood pressure rises with increased intensity of exercise but often does not go much above 180 mmHg in normotensive individuals. Diastolic blood pressure becomes only slightly elevated, or may remain constant. The greatest increase in systolic blood pressure in children occurs in the first minute of exercise; thereafter the increase becomes more gradual until peak exercise is reached. There is a progressively higher rise in systolic pressure with size and age. Systolic blood pressures in boys are higher than in girls at peak exercise. Systolic and diastolic pressure at rest become significantly higher in blacks than in whites with increasing age. The difference

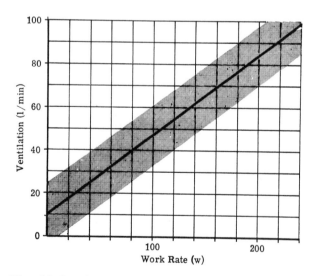

Fig. 32-8 Relationship between ventilation and power output during simple progressive exercise in children. The shaded area in this and subsequent illustrations indicates the approximate 95 percent confidence limit. (From Godfrey,[1] from data in Godfrey et al.,[5] with permission.)

is small, however, in healthy children and adolescents.[13,14]

Tidal Volume and Minute Ventilation

Total movement of gas by the lungs is usually expressed as the expired minute ventilation ($\dot{V}_E$), the product of tidal volume (V_T) and respiratory frequency (f). Tidal volume can be divided into that portion of gas that reaches the alveoli for respiratory exchange (alveolar ventilation or V_A) and that which occupies the anatomical dead space and nonperfused alveoli (dead space ventilation or V_D). Dead space ventilation does not participate in gas exchange with the circulation. Both dead space ventilation and perfusion remain a constant fraction of total ventilation as children grow.[1,5]

The physical dimensions of the heart and lungs increase throughout childhood. As size increases, maximum ventilation increases, tidal volume increases, and frequency falls. With increasing size, there is a fall in airway resistance and a rise in compliance. The resting frequency of a child is that which minimizes the work of breathing for the given mechanical condition. The smaller child must operate at a relatively higher heart rate and respiratory frequency.[1,5]

In children exercising at submaximal levels of work, tidal volume increase initially with increasing $\dot{V}O_2$, up to 60 percent of the child's vital capacity. It then remains relatively constant, and further increases in ventilation are due primarily to an increase in the frequency of breathing. The total minute ventilation increases with increasing $\dot{V}O_2$ in an almost linear fashion until $\dot{V}O_{2max}$ is approached. At this point, the increments in ventilation become larger owing to the added stimuli of anaerobic metabolism. At submaximal levels, ventilation is significantly related to workload and independent of sex (Fig. 32-8). There is only a small degree of variation between children of different sizes and sexes at any given $\dot{V}O_2$ (Fig. 32-9). Older children ventilate less than younger children, older girls ventilate more than boys, and the minute ventilation of children is a few liters per minute more than that of adults. Tidal volume is positively correlated to VO_2 and to size and is independent of sex[1,5,15].

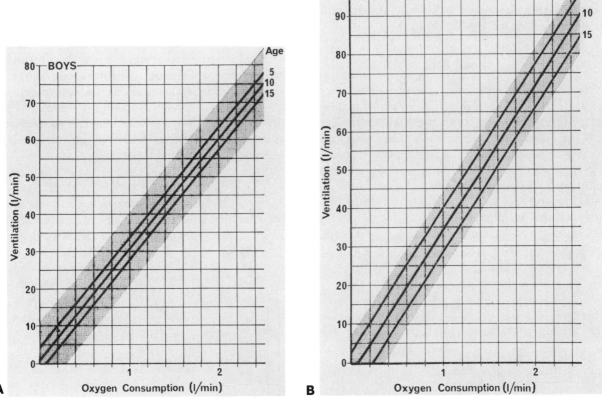

Fig. 32-9 (A) Relationship between steady-state ventilation and O_2 consumption in boys. The effective of age on the mean line is indicated. The shaded area indicates the approximate 95 percent confidence limits for the 10-year-old line. (From Godfrey,[1] with permission.) **(B)** Relationship between steady-state ventilation and O_2 consumption in girls with the same format as in part **A**. (From Godfrey,[1] with permission.)

EXERCISE RESPONSE IN SICK CHILDREN

Knowledge of exercise response in sick children is essential for the physical therapist involved in the care of any child with a chronic illness. It provides information of the impact of the chronic illness on the child's functional ability, and it allows the clinician to assess the efficacy of treatment interventions aimed at improving exercise performance. The physical therapist is then better equipped for prescribing appropriate exercise and rehabilitation programs and recommending recreational and vocational activities.[16]

The consequence of a chronic illness in a child is a reduced physical work capacity. This may be secondary to hypoactivity, which leads to detraining, and specific pathophysiological factors that limit one or more exercise-related functions. Disease can directly or indirectly affect aerobic capacity in the child by reducing cardiac output or the arteriovenous oxygen difference, both functions of the Fick equation. The following is a discussion of specific pathophysiological factors that limit exercise capacity in the sick child.

Stroke Volume

Outflow obstructions frequently found in children with congenital heart defects will prevent a sufficient rise in stroke volume during exercise. An insufficient rise in stroke volume may also occur as a result of low venous return secondary to severe hypohydration or a decrease in myocardial contractility caused by detraining.[7,16]

Heart Rate

The child with complete congenital heart block will be unable to reach an age-appropriate maximal heart rate, and subsequently there is a low maximal cardiac output. In other diseases, a low peak heart rate is a result, rather than the cause, of low maximal aerobic power. Compensation for the low cardiac output may be achieved at rest and submaximal exercise by a higher stroke volume or an increase in peripheral oxygen extraction. However, this may not be sufficient at exercise of higher intensity. Medications, for example, β-blockers, will also lower the heart rate in the child.[7,16,17]

Low Arterial Oxygen Content

Low arterial oxygen content occurs in children with severe respiratory disorders such as bronchial asthma, restrictive lung syndromes, or cystic fibrosis. In conditions such as severe scoliosis or extreme obesity, alveolar ventilation is low. Anemia of any origin will result in a reduced O_2-carrying capacity and thus a low maximal aerobic power and poor exercise tolerance.[7,16,18–20]

High Mixed Venous Oxygen Content

A high mixed venous oxygen content indicates poor oxygen utilization by the exercising muscles. This may occur when muscles are atrophied or

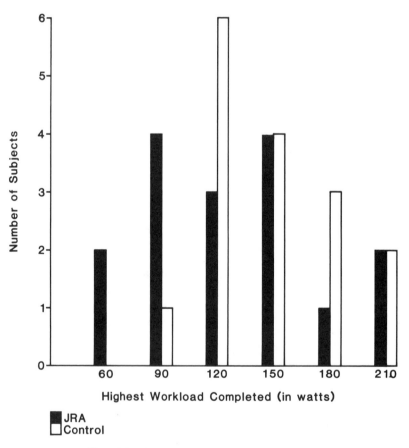

Fig. 32-10 Highest workload completed.

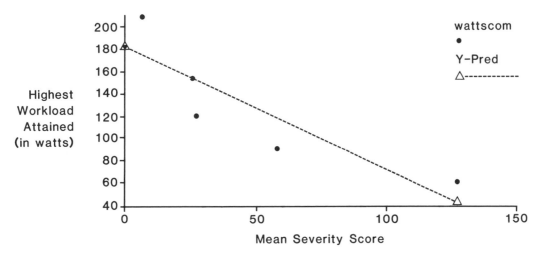

Fig. 32-11 Regression of the highest workload attained onto the mean severity score. There was an inverse correlation between the mean severity score and the highest workload completed ($R = -0.89$, $P = 0.02$).

dystrophied (e.g., juvenile rheumatoid arthritis or muscular dystrophy). A reduction in the oxidative capacity of muscle fiber occurs with detraining.[7,16]

Submaximal Oxygen Cost

Children with orthopaedic deformities or abnormal muscle tone as well as obese children have a high mechanical inefficiency. This results in a high metabolic cost of performing simple tasks such as activities of daily living. The work of breathing in the child with lung disease is also metabolically expensive.[7,16,21]

Exercise Performance in Children with Arthritis

Recent studies have shown that children with juvenile rheumatoid arthritis (JRA) have a reduced aerobic capacity compared with healthy children of similar age and size. Peak oxygen uptake in patients with JRA averaged 33 ml/kg/min compared with 47 ml/kg/min in matched controls during bicycle ergometer exercise. Maximum power output was also shown to be reduced (Fig. 32-10). In addition, disease severity is inversely proportional to both peak oxygen consumption and maximal power output[22–24] (Fig. 32-11).

Joint deformities and muscle atrophy occur sec-

ondary to the chronic arthritis. This results in a poor mechanical efficiency and a high metabolic cost of performing daily living activities. However, energy costs during specific activities have not been demonstrated in children with chronic arthritis.

EXERCISE AND ACTIVITY RECOMMENDATIONS FOR THE CHILD WITH A CHRONIC ILLNESS

Four factors to be considered when recommending exercise and activity for the child with a chronic illness include (1) the type of exercise to be recommended, (2) frequency of exercise sessions, (3) duration of exercise, and (4) intensity of exercise. All recommendations must be based on risk factors and symptomatology (contraindications to exercise and the child's present level of fitness and activity). In addition, the child must have the physical ability to perform the activity and the activity must be something the child enjoys.[25,26]

The child with a heart or lung disease should undergo a thorough cardiopulmonary examination by a physician, including a graded exercise test, before engaging in an exercise program. Normal exercise tolerance is present in some children with cardiac disease. Exercise testing helps determine whether a child has a lower than normal reserve to perform exercise. The exercise test can help prescribe a ssafe and effective exercise program based on the patient's measured functional capacity.[2,25]

Type of Exercise and Activity

Highly competitive sports in which there is a pressure for children to exercise beyond their limit should be avoided. It is important to instruct the child in the adverse effects of high-intensity anaerobic exercise such as sprints and heavy weight lifting. Low-impact, rhythmic activities that utilize large muscles groups are recommended, for example, walking, bicycling, and swimming. For the child with exercise-induced bronchoconstriction, swimming is believed to be the least asthmogenic. In addition, intermittent activities have been found to be better tolerated than continuous, prolonged activities.[27] Swimming is the activity of choice for the child with arthritis as it imposes less stress on arthritic joints. Elements of flexibility, endurance, and strength should be combined whatever the activity.

Intensity

The intensity of an activity is determined by either the metabolic demands (O_2 uptake) or the strain on the cardiovascular system (heart rate).[7] The intensity of the activity should be prescribed in relation to the current level of fitness of the child rather than in absolute terms.[7]

The linear relationship between heart rate and $\dot{V}O_2$ may be used to make exercise recommendations. The relationship is unique for each individual and will change as conditioning occurs so that at a given work rate, the heart rate will be lower. For cardiovascular benefits to occur, the intensity of exercise to be recommended for healthy individuals is that which brings about 60 to 90 percent of the individual's maximal heart rate. For the child with a chronic illness, 50 to 65 percent of maximal heart rate may be better tolerated, although specific data on the conditioning effect at this intensity are currently unavailable.

The child can be taught by the physical therapist to approximate the recommended level of aerobic exercise by "listening to his body" rather than counting his heart rate. By means of the "talk

test," children can regulate the intensity by starting out slowly and gradually increasing the intensity of exercise until their breathing has increased moderately but they can still carry on a conversation. This teaches children to recognize a safe level of exercise and the symptoms that may occur when the cardiovascular system is overstressed.[25]

Frequency

Optimum frequency to achieve cardiovascular benefits is three to four times a week.[26] Benefits have also been derived at a frequency of two times a week.

Duration

Children with severe disease who are deconditioned may begin with a duration as brief as 10 to 15 minutes. Intermittent exercise with frequent rest periods may be best tolerated. As conditioning improves, duration is increased to a duration of 30 to 40 minutes. It is essential to monitor the child for fatigue at all stages of the exercise program. In addition, the duration should be tailored to the attention span of the child.

Benefits

Benefits to both parents and children are derived from regular exercise. Physiological benefits include improved cardiovascular performance, flexibility, and strength. Possible psychological benefits are improved self-esteem, improved school attendance, and increased level of function and independence. By prescribing exercise to the sick child as a form of treatment, his abilities rather than his disabilities are emphasized. In addition, a characteristic of exercise is that the more it is done the easier it becomes and the greater the sense of accomplishment.[7,25]

Example of a Recommended Exercise Program

A walk or walk/jog program is appropriate for the child with heart or lung disease, obesity, diabetes mellitus, or chronic arthritis, especially if a pool is not available year-round. This type of program is easily performed, and no specific facilities or equipment are needed. Owing to the level of skill, it is not appropriate for children with advanced neurological or primary muscle disease (muscular dystrophy, spina bifida, etc).

The child can begin walking for 10-minute intervals 4 or 5 days a week. Walking to school or walking to a friend's house are options. The duration of walking can be increased by 5-minute intervals per week until 30 minutes of brisk walking is tolerated with the talk test. The child without chronic arthritis can modify this to a walk/jog program of walking for 2 minutes and jogging for 2 minutes and gradually increase the duration of jogging. For the child who is unable to jog or increase walking speed because of the increased biomechanical stress, hand-held weights may be used to increase exercise intensity. To avoid excess pressure on joints, weights that do not require a tight grasp and can be worn proximal to the metacarpophalangeal joints are preferred.[28]

A warm-up and cool-down session of 5 to 10 minutes should begin and end each session. This may include active range of motion exercise for upper and lower extremities and the trunk and static stretching.

REFERENCES

1. Godfrey S: Exercise Testing in Children. WB Saunders, Philadelphia, 1974
2. American Heart Association on Cardiovascular Disease in the Young. Ad Hoc Committee on Exercise Testing: Standards for exercise testing in the pediatric age group. Circulation 66:1377A, 1982
3. Bove AA, Lowenthal DT: Exercise Medicine. Physiological Principles and Clinical Applications. Academic Press, Orlando, FL, 1983
4. Astrand PO, Rodahl K: Textbook of Work Physiology. McGraw-Hill, New York, 1970
5. Godfrey S, Davies CTM, Wozniak E, Barnes CA: Cardiorespiratory response to exercise in normal children. Clin Sci 40:419, 1971
6. Davies CTM, Barnes C, Godfrey S: Body composition and maximal exercise performance in children. Hum Biol 44:195, 1972
7. Bar-Or O: Pediatric Sports Medicine for the Practitioner: From Physiologic Principles to Clinical Applications. Springer-Verlag, New York, 1983
8. Eriksson BO: Physical training, oxygen supply and muscle metabolism in 11–13 year old boys. Acta Physiol Scand (Suppl) 384:1, 1972
9. Wasserman K, Whipp BJ, Koyal SN, Beaver WL: Anaerobic threshold and respiratory gas exchange during exercise. J Appl Physiol 35:236, 1973
10. Wasserman K, McIlroy MB: Detecting the threshold of anaerobic metabolism in cardiac patients during exercise. Am J Cardiol 14:844, 1964
11. Adams FH, Linde LM, Miyake H: The physical working capacity of normal school children. Pediatrics 28:55, 1961
12. Bengtsson E: The working capacity in normal children, evaluated by submaximal exercise on the bicycle ergometer and compared with adults. Acta Med Scand 154:91, 1956
13. James FW, Kaplan S, Glueck CJ, et al.: Responses of normal children and young adults to controlled bicycle exercise. Circulation 61:902, 1980
14. Riopel DA, Taylor AB, Hohn AR: Blood pressure, heart rate, pressure-rate product and electrocardiographic changes in healthy children during treadmill exercise. Am J Cardiol 44:697, 1979
15. Hey EN, Lloyd BB, Cunningham DJC, Jukes MGM, Bolton DPG: Effects of various respiratory stimuli on the depth and frequency of breathing in man. Respir Physiol 1:193, 1966
16. Bar-Or O: Pathophysiological factors which limit the exercise capacity of the sick child. Med Sci Sports Exerc 18:276, 1986
17. Thoren C: Effects of β-adrenergic blockade on heart rate and blood lactate in children during maximal and submaximal exercise. Acta Paediatr Scand (Suppl) 177:123, 1967
18. Anderson SD: Exercise-induced asthma: current views. Patient Management 15:43, 1982
19. Cerny FJ, Pullano TP, Cropp GJA: Cardiorespiratory adaptations to exercise in cystic fibrosis. Am Rev Respir Dis 126:217, 1982
20. Whipp BJ, Davis JA: The ventilatory stress of exercise in obesity. Am Rev Respir Dis (Suppl) 129:590, 1984
21. Molbech S: Energy cost in level walking in subjects with an abnormal gait. p. 146. In Evang K, Andersen KL (eds): Physical Activity in Health and Disease. Universitets Forlaget, Oslo, 1966
22. Jasso MS, Protas EJ, Giannini EH: Assessment of physical work capacity in juvenile rheumatoid arthritis patients and healthy children. Arthritis Rheum 29:S75, 1986
23. Brewer EJ, Giannini EH, Person DA: Juvenile Rheumatoid Arthritis. WB Saunders, Philadelphia, 1982
24. Cassidy JT: Textbook of Pediatric Rheumatology. John Wiley & Sons, New York, 1982
25. Ruttenberg HD, Moller JH, Strong WB, et al.: Recommended guidelines for graded exercise testing and exercise prescription for children with heart disease. J Cardiac Rehabil 4:110, 1984
26. American Heart Association. The Committee on Exercise: Exercise Testing and Training of Apparently Healthy Individuals: A Handbook for Physicians. American Heart Association, 1975
27. Fitch KD: Comparative aspects of available exercise systems. Pediatrics 56:942, 1975
28. Zarandona JE, Nelson AG, Conlee RK, Fisher AG: Physiological responses to hand-carried weights. Physician Sports Med 4:113, 1986

33 Adapting Physical Therapy Intervention to the Elderly

Osa Littrup Jackson

"Movement is life—without movement life is unthinkable."
Moshe Feldenkrais (1904–1984)

What is unique about physical therapy for the elderly? Three things immediately come to mind: disease and disability, age-related changes in physiological and psychological systems, and changes in motivation for and goals of therapy. Let us look briefly at each one of these. One's first impression might be of disease and disability, yet one would be hard pressed to name any disease or disability that is reserved *exclusively* for those over 65 years of age. Certain conditions such as hip fracture and stroke are *more common* in the elderly, but they are not exclusively conditions of the senior years. Even Alzheimer's disease typically begins in persons in their 50s. Therefore, disease and disability in the elderly will not be further discussed in this chapter; these topics have been dealt with very adequately in the three major sections of this manual. The therapeutic techniques are the same for all alert adults; pacing and dosage may change with the elderly, and approaches to motivation may be somewhat different.

The second possible factor that might make physical therapy for the elderly unique is the area of age-related changes in physiological and psychological systems. Several years ago, gerontologists produced a long list of changes that they thought *might* result strictly from the aging process itself without any input from pathological conditions. As these changes are investigated more rigorously through research, the list grows smaller and smaller, yet there do appear to be some changes that fall into this category.

The final set of factors that may be unique to the elderly and that are important to physical therapists relates to concerns over motivation and goal setting for the elderly. Even if these factors are not, strictly speaking, unique to those over 65 years of age, their magnitude in this age group makes them very important.

NORMAL AGING

Fitness

The factors that enhance the likelihood of a long life as described by Gardner and Beatty[1] include the need for a strong self-concept, extended social contacts, belief in something beyond self, and mental and physical fitness. As a physical therapist, it is important to acknowledge the impact of the nonphysical parameters (self-esteem, social contacts, and belief in something beyond self) in defining the life satisfaction of every individual. The primary focus of physical therapy intervention is to evolve those functional (physical) abilities that are a part of defining the individual's self-concept. It is well known that physical fitness has a direct impact on a person's sense of well-being, and this phenomenon exists into old age. Fitness is a concept that involves choices in daily activities, habits, and related attitudes that maintain or enhance short term as well as long term the overall sense of well-being. The physical aspect of fitness involves a modification in the daily plan of care as the person ages from 30 years to 85 years or more. As the physical therapists work with the healthy elderly person, consultation and education involve the aspects of how to maintain desired levels of endurance, flexibility, coordination, and habitual postures. The one known fact of normal aging is that the older the individual, the more methodically he needs to train to gain functional improvements. It takes a little longer to obtain peak athletic levels of performance than it would for a younger person starting from the same initial level of fitness. Physical therapy for the elderly person should emphasize prevention of unnecessary deconditioning and support the development of lifelong habits of physical recreation.

The physical therapist may also interact with the older person in the role of a patient who is seeking physical therapy because a functional problem has developed related to acute or chronic causes. Before or during the initial assessment, a preventive emphasis is crucial in the form of education about the potential fun and physical benefits of enhanced levels of physical fitness of all uninvolved body parts. All fitness activities should be perceived by the participant as *pleasurable*, otherwise the physical benefits are minimized and compliance with the desired program is unlikely. The goal of all education is to plant the seed of knowledge with the patient that fitness at any age is a choice. The old saying "use it or lose it" holds true for the older person as well.

What are the normative abilities that can be expected of an 85-year-old person after a hip fracture?

This question can best be answered by using the PMI system developed by Edward de Bono.[2] The P stands for pluses and is an inventory of all the assets that the patient perceives he has (all the positive life experiences and learning that he has to draw from). The M stands for minuses and involves a survey of what the patient perceives are the liabilities in the current situation. The I stands for interesting, and this is anything that the patient is excited about or interested in doing. The interesting data are often the information that the clinician will focus on to enhance patient motivation. A person who was swimming 1 mile per day and was hiking 6 to 10 miles every Sunday and who had an active role in shaping the local swim club will likely have better endurance, flexibility, coordination, and habitual postures than an individual who is not making a conscious choice to

maintain a minimum level of physical fitness. The patient who develops an acute pathological condition while in a state of fitness is likely to recover more rapidly from that acute injury.

All the statements above point to the logic of all individuals developing and maintaining a fitness program so that their body maintenance is not neglected as they grow older. The reality of life is that human beings do not act on the basis of logic, but on the basis of feelings, to the degree that the individual feels good about self. Each individual makes choices that support and enhance overall personal well-being. The pivotal factor for compliance with a physical fitness program is self-concept or self-esteem (feelings about self). The degree that an individual is able to adapt effectively to the demands of life supports an internal sense of adequacy. Normal aging, taken apart from physical losses (acute or chronic) and emotional demands for adaptability, shows few major changes that directly affect the functional abilities needed to live a happy, meaningful existence.

BIOLOGICAL CHANGES WITH NORMAL AGING: ADAPTATIONS IN PHYSICAL THERAPY INTERVENTION

The normal biological changes that occur with advanced age increase the risk of the person developing problems adapting to certain types of situations or stimuli. The following discussion is based on the summary developed by Pickles[3] of normal age-related changes in those tissues of the body of particular significance to the physical therapist. The lower the level of physical fitness, the greater is the distortion in overall performance since it becomes a combination of deconditioning and normal age-related changes. Presuming a normative level of physical fitness, the normative levels and ability to perform physical activities at the age of 70 or 85 are directly affected by the body's altered mechanisms. The following principles apply.

Initial Physiological Response

To get an initial physiological response, the older person will usually need to have a slightly greater stimulus or else to have the stimulus applied for a longer period than a younger person with the same clinical problems.

Clinical Implications

The protocol for all modalities of heat, cold, and other stimuli must incorporate a method of monitoring for response to the stimuli that acknowledges the small but common need for slightly more stimulus than in the young patient to obtain the initial physiological response.

Environmental adaptation is needed to ensure that there is adequate (a little more) stimulation for visual, auditory, and kinesthetic input (for example, more light).

Response of the Older Patient

The response of an older patient to pathological conditions or therapeutic stimulus is not usually as large or as predictable as the response of a younger patient.

Clinical Implications

Primary care nursing is needed to ensure that the unique individual differences are well known to all care givers. The better the patient is known to each member of the rehabilitation team, and especially the aide, the more likely it is that small but significant changes will be noted and treated in a timely fashion.

The rehabilitation team interaction is important since diagnosis of pathological conditions in the elderly patient is often based on data contributed by many observers of the patient, so that unique patient responses can be interpreted in light of how the patient responded to similar events in the past. For example, one patient may have no fever with an infection, whereas another elderly person may manifest acute dementia, and another will develop episodes of falling or incoordination in response to infection.

The older patient needs to be educated to interpret body signs (e.g., changes in patterns of tiredness, heaviness of a body part, localized sense of pressure, unusual sense of irritability or need for drastic amounts of rest or changes in eating patterns) and to take responsibility for reporting changes early so that treatment can be initiated in a timely fashion. The team needs special training so that there is an attitude of receptivity as the

patient presents with vague but clear signs of bodily distress. The problem-oriented record as developed by Weed[4] and refined by Feitelberg[5] is an excellent tool for organizing the process of clinical decision making to organize the geriatric patient's plan of care.

Peak Level of Response

The elderly patient experiences the peak level of therapeutic response sooner than the younger patient does.

Clinical Implications

The total range of safe therapeutic interaction is smaller for the elderly than for the young. Clinically, the elderly patient requires a treatment protocol in which continued therapeutic progress is verified at shorter intervals to avoid overstimulating and potentially harming the elderly patient.

A safe therapeutic dose for a younger patient may prove to be too large a dose for the elderly patient. The individualization of geriatric physical therapy is the key to effective clinical outcomes.

Biorhythms

As an individual ages, the biorhythms (physiological functions that vary in a regular cyclic fashion) become less regular and greater variations occur between the high and low of a particular bodily variable.

Clinical Implications

When planning physical therapy and all major physical activities of daily living, it is important to ask for the patient's perception of his peak time of day and to utilize his peak performance time to the degree possible within the restraints of the treatment setting (e.g., a patient who feels best in the early morning should be treated as early in the morning as possible).

The patient's final plan of care should be based on more than one assessment.

It is important to prioritize the stabilization of biorhythms as a first step toward being able to evaluate the patient's true potential for functional improvement.

The elderly patient needs a predictable schedule of activity to perform at his highest level of ability, including regulation of such functions as waking and sleeping, eating, and activity and rest.

Connective Tissue

The tensile strength of connective tissue in the elderly individual is greater than that of the young. With inactivity, the oxygen concentration in the cellular matrix is moderately low and the secretion of collagen is encouraged.

Clinical Implications

If any type of immobilization is needed, it is crucial that all uninvolved body parts are maintained at a near normal activity level to prevent development of undue stiffness.

Regular physical exertion should be expected by asking the patient to use all activities and abilities that are uninvolved in the current disability and to perform as many normal activities of daily living as is possible (i.e., the patient does all activities of daily living that he is capable of and gets special recognition and emotional interaction for taking the responsibility to attempt to do for himself).

Elastin

With advanced age, elastin is no longer produced by the ribosomes.

Clinical Implications

The elastic properties of the skin are progressively reduced with advanced age, increasing the risk of developing pressure irritation (e.g., the patient will need more attention to proper fitting of a prosthesis and will need ideal skin care to avoid developing pressure sores).

The elastic properties of the bronchial tree are progressively reduced with advanced age. Therefore, preventive health care to maintain the normal resting tone of the intercostal muscles and diaphragm will allow full use of the existing functional capacity of the bronchial tree.

The arterial walls have progressively decreasing elasticity with advanced age. Thus, there is a need to consciously add warm-up and cool-down times to all aerobic and endurance work to allow a sense of natural ease and to support the urge to be physically active. It is recommended that severe explosive efforts be avoided, so, for example, to

avoid the Valsalva maneuver as an assist to bowel evacuation, a bowel management program is a key part of effective geriatric rehabilitation.

Glycoproteins

The production and liberation of glycoproteins by the connective tissue cells is considerably reduced with advanced age.

At a cellular level, it is more difficult for the tissues to retain their normal fluid content, and so progressive dehydration will occur with advancing age.

Clinical Implications

The patient will need ongoing monitoring to ensure normal intake of fluids.

The risk of skin breakdown is enhanced as cellular dehydration increases, so closer attention must be paid to basic skin care.

Hyaluronic Acid

With advanced age, the ability of the connective tissue cells to secrete hyaluronic acid is reduced and the viscosity of the connective tissues is altered.

Clinical Implications

At a cellular level, movement and the resulting friction between different cellular components will be increased by some amount. The open acceptance by the physical therapist of this concept will place greater importance on the therapist and patient finding motions and activities that are personally meaningful to the patient and that also progress in a manner that is enjoyable to the patient. In other words, the cognitive and emotional experience can in many cases completely counteract the functional implications of the normal age related changes that occur at a cellular level.

Contractile Proteins

As a person ages, the connective tissue cells have a reduced number of contractile proteins.

Clinical Implications

At a cellular level, the connective tissues will have a reduced motility (i.e., the ability to push out a pseudopodium to ingest a particle of tissue debris), a reduced ability of some cells to move bodily within tissue spaces, and a reduced capacity of the cells to force their way through the wall of a capillary or a lymphatic vessel. Since the normal age-related changes occur at the cellular level, the functional implications relate to the importance of using emotional and cognitive support to enhance the individual's urge to move. Also, disuse atrophy can bring about many of the same physical changes as normal aging. Therefore, in physical therapy intervention with the older patient population, the emphasis on creating ways to enhance and maintain a high level of physical fitness is a priority in treatment planning.

Cartilage

With advanced age, the cartilage experiences a reduced production of chrondroitin sulfate,[3] the osmotic attraction forces are lessened, and the ability of the cellular matrix to attract and retain fluid is impaired.

Clinical Implications

Overall, the functional health of hyaline cartilage (cartilage that covers the articular surfaces in synovial joints) is guaranteed by regular intermittent compression and release of force on these tissues. The normal age-related cellular changes in cartilage reinforce the importance of avoiding unnecessary periods of bed rest and of maintaining the urge to do for oneself. In all planning with the nursing staff, the patient's daily schedule should include meaningful activity that is spread across the day in a normal manner to encourage the patient to take responsibility for his own well-being.

Bone Density

With advanced age, there appears to be a normal developmental tendency toward a reduction in bone density.

Clinical Implications

Bone is a very active tissue and is therefore subject to a constant remodeling process. Reduction in bony density can be impacted greatly by various pathological conditions. The one focus for physical therapy intervention involves evaluating resting muscle tension and the overall activity level of the patient. Weight bearing and muscle action are two important factors in the maintenance of normal density of the bones.

First, in the evaluation of a patient with a history of one or more fractures, it is important to examine the habitual resting tone of the major muscle groups of the entire body. Muscle groups that manifest resting postures with a high level of tone are likely to be contributing to dysfunctional cellular nutrition to the bones and joints they surround. Clinical evaluation would specifically involve taking the patient through very slow passive range of motion and looking for holding or resistance on the part of the patient. Similarly, the ability of a patient to lie supine (propped with towels to create comfort, with a roller under the knees to place the iliopsoas on a slack) and the patient's ability to feel intermittent pressure applied through the foot upward toward the head would indicate potential points of excessive muscle fixation. Any muscle group that cannot easily allow passive motion to travel through the area has a resting muscle tone that is too high and that will contribute to distorted cellular nutrition for the bones and joints that the muscles surround. Therefore, if excessive resting muscle tone is found, physical therapy intervention should focus on normalizing muscle tone, on kinesthetic awareness, and on the ability to allow slow passive range of motion from all angles through the joints.

The second point for physical therapy evaluation is the overall activity level of a patient through the entire day and, specifically, the amount of natural weight bearing and weight shift that is occurring. All physical therapy and restorative intervention should support the natural urge to do for oneself (a sense of self-determination) and normalization of life style. A part of the physical therapy assessment will evaluate the patient's self-image since many people, including health practitioners, expect a major decrease in all physical activity and vigor with advanced age. The older person can remain active and vital, presuming that there is a willingness to first accept that this is a goal that is potentially attainable. Overall, avoiding unnecessary inactivity (e.g., if there is a hip fracture, all unaffected body parts need to function in performing meaningful activities of daily living and facilitating the urge to move and a sense of self-determination) is the key to avoiding secondary bony changes in the elderly.

Skeletal Muscles

Skeletal muscles, if they are used frequently, show remarkably few structural changes with advanced age.

Clinical Implications

Normal muscle function depends on an intense homeostasis involving adequate hydration and mineral balance. If there is a doubt that symptoms of tiredness or lethargy are related to dehydration, the blood chemistry should be checked before active physical therapy intervention. While the results of the blood chemistry tests are being processed, basic work using intervention to normalize the parasympathetic and sympathetic nervous systems can be used within the patient's sense of comfort. Preventive care, that is, a maintenance of fitness, is the key to effective muscle function with advanced age. It is again important to note that all fitness activities need not be related to sports, but can be regular activities of daily living (including normal sexual activities). The fitness activities should be perceived as pleasurable to avoid noncompliance and, more important, to avoid unnecessary overstimulation of the parasympathetic and sympathetic nervous systems, which will occur if a person dislikes or hates a repeated activity performed over a long period.

Nervous System

There is a gradual reduction in the level of nervous system function with advanced age based on biochemical changes that take place in the neurons.

Clinical Implications

The elderly are likely (to varying degrees) to experience some negative changes in fine motor coordination. A thorough evaluation should be made to determine the need for assistive devices to compensate for changes in fine motor coordination.

The older patient is more prone to depression and Parkinson's disease owing to normal biochemical changes with advanced age. A review of med-

ication to ensure the minimum side effects that would reinforce depression and Parkinson's disease is essential. Secondarily, a preventive fitness program that emphasizes pleasurable activities with an emphasis on easy, smooth, and controlled rotational motions (no matter how small) is a core preventive consideration for the elderly.

The older patient may need environmental modifications to enhance visual and auditory input to enhance his adaptive skills.

The older patient will take longer to successfully integrate new data and create a plan of action, act, and review the effectiveness of the outcome. Overall, the older person will need a more thorough and structured orientation to new concepts and places. The use of a "buddy system," in which a liason is available throughout the day, is a help for older patients attempting to adjust to a new setting.

Timed tasks or timed learning should be avoided. The older patient needs to be in control of the pace of learning to ensure a positive outcome.

Pain is a special problem for elderly patients, and they are likely to experience an altered threshold of pain. A systematic review of the pain problem should be first in all therapeutic intervention to avoid unnecessary secondary complications. With advanced age, the early signs and symptoms of disease as well as the final manifestations may be different from what is seen in the young. The ability to recognize the signs and symptoms of diseases common to the elderly begins with screening out the common parasympathetic and sympathetic reactions to overstimulation. It is only possible to evaluate the real medical problem for the older patient when he is (ideally) pain free, feeling at ease and in control.

NURTURING MOTIVATION

Smiling, laughing, winking, waving, shaking hands, hugging, kissing, caressing, and holding hands are among the ageless experiences that nurture the urge to move, to do, and to choose to live. Age alone is only a measure of time, and these timeless things do not, or need not, change. The unique individuality of a person's life experience, one's response to that experience, and the wisdom gained on the journey through life are the predictors of life satisfaction. Life satisfaction stimulates the motivation to pursue a meaningful life despite changes caused by aging or impairment and subsequent disability. Physical therapy intervention, properly approached, can promote and develop the capacity for the patient to create a unique definition of life and determine those activities that give satisfaction and meaning to life.

Adaptation as a Goal

Life is never static, so it requires the ongoing ability to adjust or adapt to change. The ability to adapt to life situations is as important to all daily activities as is movement. Elderly people (over 65) live in a unique set of life circumstances that require an unusually large amount of adapting that is enforced by factors beyond their control (e.g., changes in physical appearance, changes in personal, family, social and, work roles, changes in habitual daily activities, a decreased speed of assimilating new information, changes in expectations from others, decreased income, and death of family and friends). The ability to adapt effectively involves the ability to accept loss, to grieve, and to dare to set new goals and focus on the positive parts of life. There is at any moment in life a limit as to how many requirements for adapting a person can effectively meet in a defined period. Adapting is a process of learning, and it requires a certain amount of time to get used to the novelty of the new situation. In the process of physical therapy for the elderly person, an inventory should be taken *jointly* by the physical therapist and the patient of (1) the physical, emotional, cognitive, and environmental resources that the patient is aware of; (2) the physical, emotional, cognitive, and environmental resources that the patient *feels* comfortable using at this moment; (3) the abilities and resources that the patient is aware of that he is willing to work with and to become comfortable using; and (4) the abilities and resources that are truly missing that need to be developed jointly in the work between the physical therapist and the patient. For example:

1. Working with a physical therapist, an elderly person may develop a list of resources known

to be available to him, such as the physician, visiting nurse, pharmacist, etc. The physical therapist may notice that several community agencies of potential use to people similar to this patient are missing from the list, for example, senior citizen support groups, Meals-on-Wheels, etc., as well as the availability of several devices of potential use for activities of daily living.
2. The patient states that, at present, he is using only the physician and the physical therapist as resources in handling his problems.
3. During discussion it becomes clear that, although the patient is aware of the services of the visiting nurse, he doesn't feel comfortable using that service at the present time, *but is willing* to explore that possibility and become comfortable in seeking appropriate help from that agency.
4. Through discussion, demonstration, and experimentation, the patient becomes aware of several devices to assist activities of daily living, such as quad canes and adapted eating utensils, and agrees to work with some of them on a trial basis to see whether their use will increase his abilities to deal effectively with his environment.

Motivating an elderly person to deal effectively with change and to meet the many challenges of learning useful and meaningful adaptations in response to age-related physical, psychological, and socioenvironmental changes is frequently the first goal a physical therapist must achieve before the more kinesiological and therapeutic goals can be addressed successfully.

Nurturing Motivation

A person who is motivated to participate in working out his life is a person who is open to learning new things (this is not altered with age). At the moment when the average elderly person is in need of physical therapy intervention, it is likely that he has experienced a major loss or a change in his physical abilities. The personal history (all the events that combine to mold this unique individual) of each patient will be the determining factor that will influence motivation. Personal history is not only all the events that a person has experienced, but it is also a series of automatic coping mechanisms that can control how an individual will respond to a given situation. The first questions to be posed as a part of the evaluation and treatment program for an elderly person are: Does the person feel safe in the moment, and does he feel in control of his life?

The fundamental essence of the rehabilitation experience is that there is something positive to be gained from every negative experience. Automatic coping mechanisms can occasionally be helpful; however, the conscious checking of the suitability of responses to a specific situation enhances the likelihood of a positive outcome. A basic part of the desired rehabilitation attitude is a sense of safety in the moment. As a sense of physical and emotional safety is experienced by a person, the natural abilities to solve problems and to integrate various pieces of new information are greatly enhanced.

Self-talk (the internal dialogue that is constantly going on in a person's head) is the essential foundation for all goal setting.[6] It is important to help the older patient to perform an inventory on his self-talk. The physical therapist often needs to help elderly clients examine their internal dialogue to see precisely what it is saying to the patient about the reality of change, abilities to adapt, need to adapt, etc. This material needs to be brought out into the open to enable the patient to develop more precise and more positive self-talk and to set into action more meaningful personal goals. For a patient with very high level of life stress and very poor motivation, the focus may be to develop self-talk to support goals for achieving self-determination in the basic activities of daily living. As a patient experiences an enhanced self-esteem (the ability to feel good about himself), the development of precise self-talk is the foundation for the normalization of his life. Normalization of a person's life involves developing a daily schedule of events and activities that support habits that lead to a high degree of life satisfaction and not to an emphasis on illness or loss.

Enhancing the potential for patient motivation (Fig. 33-1) involves very specific actions to be taken

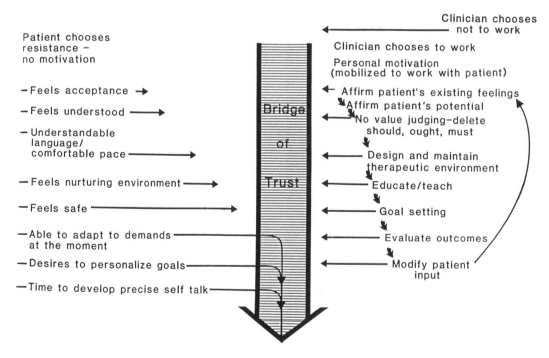

Fig. 33-1 Enhancing the potential for patient motivation.

by the health care team members (including the physical therapist) in response to the unique reactions and emotional state of the patient at any given moment. Physical therapy intervention that is guaranteed to enhance the potential for patient motivation is like a dance, and it is the patient who is leading. The physical therapist's actions are based on the ongoing inventory that is being done by the therapist to ensure that the patient experiences the following:

1. A sense of acceptance.
2. A feeling of being understood.
3. The ability to understand the language and follow the pace of interaction.
4. A feeling that the surroundings and people are nurturing and supportive.
5. A feeling of safety in the moment.
6. A feeling of adequacy to meet the demands of the moment and recognize the early signs of overload, that is, loss of the urge to move, to speak, to do for oneself, and other specific body symptoms of chronic hyperactivity of the autonomic nervous system.[7]
7. A desire to develop personal goals.
8. A feeling of comfort about taking the time to develop precise self-talk and affirmations.
   It is important to note that it is the patient's *feelings* that need to be openly accepted, acknowledged, and supported to get to the rehabilitation attitude—an urge to do for yourself (an urge is a feeling).

Peterson and Orgren[8] describe rehabilitation as a *process* of relearning tasks and movements and the associated attitudes. To enhance patient motivation, it is often necessary to involve the older patient in the process of habilitation—the learning of entirely new and unfamiliar tasks and movements and the associated attitudes. In the summary of the specific instructional strategies that facilitate learning for persons in the later years, Peterson and Orgren note that positive reinforcement is a key factor. A physical therapist working with the older patient population should avoid the use of value-judging comments as a teaching tool. The desired approach is to avoid value-judging words such as "should," "ought," and "must" and to incorporate active listening and nurturing psycholinguistics (i.e., using words such as "need," "want,"

and "consider"). A key motivational factor for the older patient is that the learning will occur most rapidly for the average person if the individual is given the physical therapist's undivided attention for short periods (avoid all interruptions such as phone calls, talking to other professionals, etc.)

The psycholinguistics of learning enable the patient to become an expert about how his body works best. The primary intent is to urge the patient to focus on or become aware of how his body responds. The foundation of the process is the question of stimulus and response.

1. How does your body feel at this moment? (Describe the sensory experience starting at the feet and proceeding up to the head in the amount of detail that is needed to ensure developing a complete picture of all the sensations for the patient and the physical therapist. Patients will have the urge to tell historical data, such as "This hurts sometimes." Attempt to use and explore all historical details but conclude with a refocusing: How does this part feel now?)
2. Provide a stimulus (a therapeutic activity as deemed appropriate).
3. Repeat step 1. The goal is to determine, by repeating the body scan, what is the difference, if any, in the body after the stimulus was applied. What are you aware of in your body that was not present previously? For example, contact with the floor may feel more complete, or the foot may feel heavier. A comparison of sensory experiences and any noted changes can enhance the patient's awareness of how his body responds and begin to make the patient feel safe enough to initiate movement.

Please note that not all elderly patients will need to work on enhancing their total body awareness. However, if there is any postural distortion into *flexion at the trunk* and associated changes in the rest of the body, for example, it is likely that sensory awareness will be below the level desired for ease of motion in the upright position.

The therapeutic experiment involves (1) noting the current status, (2) providing a stimulus, and (3) noting the overall response. The therapeutic experiment is a process in which the patient is in charge of the therapy. The patient is in control since the physical therapist is at all times working to enhance the patient's awareness of how he is responding (physically and emotionally) to the treatment activities. The physical therapist working with the older patient will consciously choose to listen so the patient can clarify his current status. As the physical therapist attempts to develop a plan of intervention from a realistic perception of the patient's current emotional and physical abilities, the likelihood of supporting motivation for self-directed behavior is enhanced. The attitude that supports a positive rehabilitation outcome is an acceptance and nurturing of the innate value and dignity of each human being and a focus on what the assets, resources, and abilities are for the patient at this moment as well as looking for the untapped potential.

Adaptability

The therapeutic stage has been set by taking the time to ensure that the patient feels safe in the moment and feels a sense of control over his life in this interaction. The basic foundation for motivation has been created since self-determination, at whatever level is possible within the patient's abilities, forms the core of motivation. The next question to ask is to what degree it is necessary for the physical therapist as well as the entire rehabilitation team to make special adaptations to meet the emotional needs of the frail elderly patient. A frail elderly person may quickly move into a state in which there is no urge to do for himself. The patient may be seen sitting with toes resting off the floor and perhaps with arms and hands not resting in a natural position (a natural position would be with the hands and arms supported on a body part or resting on a chair or table). The patient may be uncommunicative or withdrawn. One possible cause for this syndrome is transportation shock, that is, the shock of being moved from familiar surroundings to a new environment. The symptoms of transplantation shock can include all the changes that occur with acute activation of the sympathetic and parasympathetic nervous systems. The critical question to ask is the following: within the last 2 weeks to 3 months, was this person functioning independently living in

the community? Transplantation shock and the apparent collapse of all urge for self-directed behavior is the extreme result when a person is faced with too many requirements for adaptation over a short period. The majority of elderly patients who come to physical therapy are not in a severe state of transplantation shock, but there may be early warning signs of overstimulation. Such a person may be in need of a modified pace and a special restorative nursing plan of care in collaboration with other rehabilitation strategies. The common changes that signal potential problems can include the following:

1. The person wants to go home and that appears to be all he talks about.
2. The person does not accept small changes in scheduling or in the routine of daily activities.
3. The person expresses an unwillingness to try new things or a fear of trying new activities.
4. The person states that he is overwhelmed and may refuse to get out of bed, refuse to go to therapy, etc.
5. The person may abdicate all responsibility and indicate that the physical therapist is the expert and that he wants the therapist to decide for him.

These examples of maladaptive behavior are signals that a patient may be experiencing a state of overstimulation with too many things to adjust to over a short period.

Before any initiation of treatment, the physical therapist should evaluate the degree to which the emotional strain has affected the patient's physical abilities (e.g., overactivation of the sympathetic and parasympathetic nervous systems contributing to a forward flexed posture, poor concentration, need for frequent urination, etc.). One test of a patient's level of adaptability is to evaluate his ability to allow passive range of motion of various body parts. The process would involve the following steps.

Ask the patient to lie down in his favorite position (supine, lying on the right or left side, or prone). (With elderly persons, the prone position is only used for therapy if it is chosen by the patient as a favorite position.)

Add layers of towels (a measurable height) as

props under any and all body parts so that the body is well supported and comfortable. For example, a wrist that is arched up off the table and is held in that position by chronic habitual hyperactivation of the forearm musculature by the central nervous system should be supported. In such a case, if you wish to work on refining patterns of motion that involve the upper extremity, it becomes necessary to support the wrist and hand in a position of comfort so that the forearm musculature can rest or relax. A muscle group that is resting at ease in a normal amount of elongation with normalized joint alignment is likely to produce a more precise and coordinated motion when it is activated.

Verbally request that the patient note what you are doing and indicate that your intent is to move the body part for him and that "he gets a free ride."

Quiet yourself and begin the actual process by noting the ease and regularity of your own breathing and noting whether you are at ease and physically comfortable. The patient will sense if you are tense and respond with tension. If for any reason you are not at ease physically or your mind is wandering and not focused, then stop. It is crucial to make necessary adjustments and then start from a position of personal ease, both physically and emotionally.

Note the patient's breathing pattern (depth and rate) before touching him.

Now simply make contact and allow the patient the time to get used to the novelty of the situation. Note the breathing response in the patient and wait to continue until the quality of breathing appears to be reasonably at ease.

Work now to attempt to simply lift those body parts that are least involved in the patient's primary complaint (it is presumed that the ability to release control and allow passive range of motion in a small excursion would be easiest for those muscle groups).

Evaluate the degree to which passive range of motion done *very* slowly, and initially just involving lifting a body part and returning it to the resting position, is successfully completed. Guided by the patient's tolerance, proceed to evaluate this ability throughout the body, gradually moving to the more involved body parts.

To the degree that the attempt to slowly lift a body part and perform passive range of motion meets with resistance (conscious or unconscious), standardized neurological facilitation techniques (light touch, stroking, light tapping, slow rotational motion, holding body part in muscles' shortened position, reinforcement of activity by using breathing or actual breathing facilitation) can be used. Heat and vibration in the form of whirlpool baths can also be utilized. If with neurological cuing the patient is able to allow passive range of motion to the major body parts involved in the primary complaint within a 30- to 60-minute session of physical therapy, the patient has functional adaptive abilities. The special neurological cues that were used to enhance the patient's adaptability should be taught to the patient and meaningful others (primary persons who the patient identifies as source of emotional support) and also incorporated into the restorative nursing plan of care. It is here that cost-effective rehabilitation programs begin. The restorative nursing plan of care is responsible for maintaining the patient at the current functional status. The physical therapy, occupational therapy, and other special interventions proceed in collaboration with restorative nursing and the patient to develop new, needed functional abilities. The patient who can adapt to slow, gentle passive range of motion is likely to be able to feel at ease with actively concentrating to learn new skills and abilities.

If the patient is resistant when you attempt passive range of motion combined with basic neurological rehabilitation techniques, then it is necessary to use basic techniques to quiet the autonomic nervous system and the limbic system before initiating active exercises. Among the common tools available to the physical therapist for this purpose are therapeutic massage, light touch facilitation, breathing facilitation, and Feldenkrais techniques. The patient can function as a receiver of input that feels easy and safe to integrate. A clinician working in geriatrics needs to have a heightened proficiency in one of these techniques, especially if major functional gains are to be noted in a long-term care setting. It is hoped that by decreasing excessive chronic activation of the sympathetic and parasympathetic nervous systems, many symptoms that were presumed to be related to the primary complaint may prove to be secondary adaptive changes that can be eliminated.

Of course, not all elderly patients will need to start that far back in the basics. But it is only when the autonomic nervous system is at a normalized state that the true functional losses can be measured. Using Figures 33-2 and 33-3 as a checklist, if any symptoms are present that can be attributed to chronic activation of the sympathetic and parasympathetic nervous systems, active exercise is *not* the desirable therapeutic intervention.

SUMMARY

The goal of rehabilitation intervention with an older patient is to enhance the urge to do for oneself and to facilitate abilities that allow the patient a meaningful quality of life. The older patient, owing to his life experiences, is more likely than the young person to manifest symptoms of overstimulation of the parasympathetic and sympathetic nervous systems. A patient who has the common and normal age-related changes and whose parasympathetic-sympathetic nervous systems are in a hyperactive state will need special therapeutic intervention before traditional physical therapy intervention is initiated. The physical therapist working with older patients should begin treatment by evaluating the patient's normal age-related changes and the patient's current abilities to adapt to the degree of overload present. Specific treatment should start to normalize the state of the parasympathetic and sympathetic nervous systems. The majority of physical disabilities and functional losses seen in the elderly population are not unique to that age group. The process of evaluation and treatment of an older individual should consider the patient's overall readiness to adapt and learn new concepts and skills. The older individual has the ability to learn if the pace and input are adapted to meet his special needs so that there is a personal sense of safety and control. Overall, the success of a rehabilitation program with an older patient is built on enhancing the patient's sense of self-determination and self-esteem (how you feel about yourself) and understanding and working with the normal age-related changes.

REFERENCES

1. Gardner DC, Beatty GJ: Stop Stress and Aging Now. American Training and Research Association, Inc., Concord, New Hampshire, 1985
2. deBono E: New Think. Avon, New York, 1971
3. Pickles B: Biological aspects of aging. In Jackson O (ed): Physical Therapy of the Geriatric Patient. Churchill Livingstone, New York, 1983
4. Weed LL: Medical Records, Medical Evaluation and Patient Care. Case Western Reserve University Press, Cleveland, 1971
5. Feitelberg SB: The Problem Oriented Record System in Physical Therapy. University of Vermont, Graphic Printing, Burlington, 1975
6. Helmstetter S: What to Say When You Talk to Yourself. Grindle Press, Scottsdale, AZ, 1986
7. Murray RB, Huelskoetter MMW: Psychiatric Mental Health Nursing—Giving Emotional Care. Prentice-Hall, Englewood Cliffs, NJ, 1983
8. Peterson DA, Orgren RA: Older adult learning. In Jackson O (ed): Physical Therapy of the Geriatric Patient. Churchill Livingstone, New York, 1983

Index

Page numbers followed by an f refer to figures; those followed by a t designate tables.